W0036634

Essentials of Pediatric Endoscopic Surgery

Amulya K. Saxena · Michael E. Höllwarth (Eds.)

Essentials of Pediatric Endoscopic Surgery

With 701 Figures

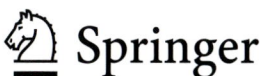
Springer

Amulya K. Saxena, MD
Associate Professor
Department of Pediatric
and Adolescent Surgery
Medical University of Graz
Auenbruggerplatz 34
A-8036 Graz
Austria

Michael E. Höllwarth, MD
Professor and Chair
Department of Pediatric
and Adolescent Surgery
Medical University of Graz
Auenbruggerplatz 34
A-8036 Graz
Austria

ISBN 978-3-540-78386-2   e-ISBN 978-3-540-78387-9

DOI 10.1007/978-3-540-78387-9

Library of Congress Control Number: 2008924191

© Springer-Verlag Berlin Heidelberg 2009

This work is subject to copyright. All rights are reserved, wether the whole or part of the material is concerned, specifically the rights of translation, reprinting, reuse of illustrations, recitation, broadcasting, reproduction on microfilm or any other way, and storage in data banks. Duplication of this publication or parts thereof is permitted only under the provisions of the German Copyright Law of September 9, 1965, in it current version, and permission for use must always be obtained from Springer. Violations are liable to prosecution under the German Copyright Law.

The use of general descriptive names, registered names, trademarks, etc. in this publication does not imply, even in the absence of a specific statement, that such names are exempt from the relevant protective laws and regulations and therefore free for general use.

Product liability: the publishers cannot guarantee the accuracy of any information about dosage and application contained in this book. In every individual case the user must check such information by consulting the relevant literature.

Cover illustration: Frido Steinen-Broo, eStudio Calamar, Spain

Printed on acid-free paper

9 8 7 6 5 4 3 2 1

springer.com

Preface

General pediatric surgery has undergone a revolutionary change in the last decade, with the widespread acceptance and adoption of endoscopic surgery in the neonatal, pediatric and adolescent age groups. The establishment of pediatric endoscopic surgery was due to the combined efforts of dedicated pediatric surgeons who devoted precious time in implementing, evaluating, innovating and adapting procedures for the pediatric age group, manufactures who invested into research and development of pediatric instruments and equipments despite being aware of the relatively small market share in pediatric surgery and the establishment of an international forum to exchange and compare experiences as well as support advances and promote research.

Pediatric endoscopic surgery requires the knowledge of and familiarity of existing equipment with the ability to constantly adapt to ongoing innovations. The perception of the three-dimensional operation field in two-dimension requires good hand-eye coordination and hours of practice to familiarize with the basic procedures while acquiring skills for advanced procedures. The spectrum of patients treated using pediatric endoscopic surgical procedures ranges from premature infants to adolescents, which adds another dimension to the technical complexity in terms of extreme variations in size encountered by pediatric surgeons. Techniques in endoscopic surgery might be new initially and may require additional training to accomplish, however the surgical goal remains the same as in open procedures. As these techniques become standard practice, the ease to perform endoscopic procedures will increase.

The Editors have selected a distinguished team of contributors from around the world to provide practical guidance and their expertise on various issues dealing with pediatric endoscopic surgery. Topics dealt with include theoretical concepts pertaining to endoscopic surgery, video-assisted thoracoscopic surgery, laparoscopic surgery and retroperitoneal endoscopic procedures. Technological strides in pediatric endoscopic surgery have also been explained with emphasis laid on instrument refinement, evolving role of ergonomics in the development of operation room design, and the progress in the field of robotics. Constant training and evaluation of coordinated skills which can be estimated using virtual reality simulators and the capabilities of these systems have been elaborated.

Since a picture speaks more than thousand words, this monograph is designed to acquaint both the novice and the experienced surgeon with pediatric endoscopic procedures using surgical images and diagrams. The text is concise and emphasis has been placed on the practical and technical aspects of performing procedures. Variations in procedures have also been mentioned to offer procedural options to the reader. Complications in endoscopic surgery arising due to limited knowledge of the instrument or equipment have been addressed, along with recommendations to overcome them and advice on their proper usage.

We wish to thank all the authors for their outstanding contributions and for offering their valuable experience in pediatric endoscopic surgery towards this compilation. We express our gratitude to Reiner Klostermann (Product Manager, Richard Wolf GmbH, Germany) for his continued assistance throughout the project. We also appreciate the assistance from our industry partners who have contributed generously toward this work. Finally, we wish to thank the editorial staff of Springer, Stephanie Benko and Gabriele Schroeder, for the excellent assistance during the entire publication process.

We hope that this work contributes to the better understanding of pediatric endoscopic surgery and benefits children throughout the world.

Amulya K. Saxena, MD
Michael E. Höllwarth, MD

Contents

List of Contributors

Stephanie P. Acierno, MD, MPH
Clinical Research Fellow and Acting Instructor
Department of Surgery
Children's Hospital and Regional Medical Center
W-7729
4800 Sand Point Way, NE
Seattle, WA 98105
USA

Craig T. Albanese, MD
Professor of Surgery, Pediatrics,
Obstetrics and Gynecology
Stanford University Medical Center
Chief, Division of Pediatric Surgery
John A. and Cynthia Fry Gunn Director of Surgical
Services
Lucile Packard Children's Hospital
780 Welch Road, Suite 206
Stanford, CA 94305
USA

Richard G. Azizkhan, MD, PhD (hon)
Professor of Surgery and Pediatrics
Lester W. Martin Chair of Pediatric Surgery
Surgeon-in-Chief
Department of Pediatric General and Thoracic
Surgery
Cincinnati Childrens Hospital
3333 Burnet Avenue
Cincinnati, OH 45229
USA

Klaas N.M.A. Bax, MD, PhD, FRCS (Ed)
Professor of Pediatric Surgery
Head of the Department of Pediatric Surgery
Sophia Children's Hospital
Erasmus Medical Center
PO Box 2060
3000 CB Rotterdam
The Netherlands

François Becmeur, MD, PhD
Professeur des Universités
Service de Chirurgie Infantile
Hôpital de Hautepierre
Hôpitaux Universitaires de Strasbourg
67098 Strasbourg
France

Francisco J Berchi, MD
Professor and Chief
Department of Pediatric Surgery ONG
"Infancia sin Fronteras"
Margarita 69
Soto de la Moraleja
28109 Alcobendas
Madrid
Spain

Marcos Bettolli, MD
Clinical Research Fellow Pediatric General Surgery
Children's Hospital of Eastern Ontario
401 Smyth Rd
Ottawa, Ontario, K1H 8L1
Canada

Luigi Bonavina, MD, FACS
Professor of Surgery
Department of Medical and Surgical Sciences
Section of General Surgery
University of Milano
Ospedale Maggiore Policlinico
IRCCS
Via Francesco Sforza, 35
20122 Milan
Italy

Venita Chandra, MD
Surgery Fellow Lucile Packard Children's Hospital
Stanford University Medical Center
780 Welch Road
Stanford, CA 94305
USA

Roshni Dasgupta, MD
Assistant Professor
Department of Pediatric General and Thoracic
Surgery
Cincinnati Childrens Hospital
3333 Burnet Avenue
Cincinnati, OH 45229
USA

Ivan R. Diamond, MD
Surgery Resident
Division of General Surgery
The Hospital for Sick Children
555 University Avenue
Toronto, M5G 1X8
Ontario
Canada

Sanjeev Dutta, MD, MA, FRCSC, FACS
Assistant Professor of Surgery and Pediatrics
Lucile Packard Children's Hospital
Stanford University Medical Center
780 Welch Road
Stanford, CA 94305
USA

Hans G Eder, MD
Professor
Department of Neurosurgery
Medical University of Graz
Auenbruggerplatz 34
8036 Graz
Austria

Ciro Esposito, MD, PhD
Associate Professor of Pediatric Surgery
Department of Clinical and Experimental
Medicine
Chair of Pediatric Surgery
Magna Graecia University of Catanzaro
School of Medicine
Campus delle Bioscienze
Viale Europa, Germaneto
88100 Catanzaro
Italy

Chiara Grimaldi, MD
Chef de Clinique
Chirurgie Pédiatrique
Hôpital Robert Debré
48, Boulevard Sérurier
Paris, 75019
France

Anton Gutmann, MD
Attending Physician
Department of Pediatric Anesthesiology
Medical University of Graz
Auenbruggerplatz 34
8036 Graz
Austria

Munther J Haddad, FRCS, FRCPCH
Consultant Pediatric Surgeon
Chelsea and Westminster Hospital
369 Fulham Road
London SW14 7DQ
UK

George W. Holcomb III, MD, MBA
The Katharine B. Richardson Endowed Chair
in Pediatric Surgery
University of Missouri - Kansas City
Surgeon-in-Chief and Director
Center for Minimally Invasive Surgery
The Children's Mercy Hospital
2401 Gillham Road
Kansas City, MO 64108
USA

Celeste Hollands, MD
Associate Professor of Surgery
Director, Division of Pediatric Surgery
University of South Alabama Children's
and Women's Hospital
CWEB 1, 251 Cox St, Room 1157
Mobile, AL 36604
USA

Michael E. Höllwarth, MD
Professor and Chair
Department of Pediatric and Adolescent Surgery
Medical University of Graz
Auenbruggerplatz 34
8036 Graz
Austria

Ramin Jamshidi, MD
Adjunct Professor of Physics
University of San Francisco
Pediatric Surgery Research Fellow
University of California San Francisco
513 Parnassus Ave, S-321
San Francisco, CA 94143-0470
USA

Troels M. Jorgensen, MD, FEBU, FEAPU, DMSci
Professor
Department of Urology
Section of Pediatric Urology
Aarhus University Hospital – Skejby
Institute of Clinical Medicine
University of Aarhus
Brendstrupgaardsvej 100
8200 Aarhus N.
Denmark

Timothy D. Kane, MD
Assistant Professor of Surgery
Clinical Director
Division of Pediatric General & Thoracic Surgery
Children's Hospital of Pittsburgh
University of Pittsburgh Medical Center
3705 Fifth Avenue
Pittsburgh, PA 15213-2583
USA

Francis X. Keeley Jr, MD, FRCS (Urol)
Consultant Urologist
Bristol Urological Institute
North Bristol NHS Trust
Southmead Hospital
Westbury-on-Trym
Bristol, BS10 5NB
UK

Sergey Keidar, MD
Dana Children's Hospital
Tel Aviv Sourasky Medical Center
Sackler Faculty of Medicine
6 Weitzman St
Tel Aviv
Israel

Jerry Kieffer, MD
Pediatric Orthopedic Surgeon
Department of Pediatric Surgery
Kannerklinik / Clinique Pédiatrique de
Luxembourg
4, rue Barblé
1210 Luxembourg
Luxembourg

Jacob C. Langer, MD
Division Chief and Robert M. Filler Chair
Division of General Surgery
The Hospital for Sick Children
555 University Avenue, Rm1526
Toronto, M5G 1X8
Ontario
Canada

Hanmin Lee, MD
Associate Professor
Department of Surgery
University of California San Francisco
513 Parnassus Ave, HSW-1601
San Francisco, CA 94143-0570
USA

Michael K. Li, MB BS, FRCS
Chief of Service
Department of Surgery
Pamela Youde Nethersole Eastern Hospital
3 Lok Man Road
Chai Wan
Hong Kong SAR
China

Mario Lima, MD, PhD
Professor and Chair
Department of Pediatric Surgery
University of Bologna
Via Massarenti, 11
40138 Bologna
Italy

Marcelo H Martinez-Ferro, MD
Professor of Surgery and Pediatrics
Chief of Surgery Department
"Fundacion Hospitalaria" Private Children´s
Hospital
Cramer 4601
Buenos Aires, C1429AKK
Argentina

Martin L Metzelder, MD
Attending Surgeon
Department of Pediatric Surgery
Hannover Medical School
Carl-Neuberg-Straße 1
30625 Hannover
Germany

Philippe Montupet, MD
Associated Member of National Academy
of Surgery
Senior Consultant
Department of Pediatric Surgery
CHU Bicêtre
74 rue du Général Leclerc
94275 Le Kremlin-Bicêtre (F)
France

Oliver J. Muensterer, MD, PhD
Assistant Professor of Surgery
University of Alabama at Birmingham
Department of Pediatric Surgery
Children's Hospital of Alabama
1600 7th Avenue South ACC 300
Birmingham, AL 35233
USA

Kiyokazu Nakajima, MD
Assistant Professor
Department of Surgery
Osaka University Graduate School of Medicine
2-2, E-1, Yamadaoka
Suita
Osaka 565-0871
Japan

Toshirou Nishida, MD, FACS
Associate Professor
Department of Surgery
Osaka University Graduate School of Medicine
2-2, E-1, Yamadaoka
Suita
Osaka 565-0871
Japan

Tadaharu Okazaki, MD, PhD
Assistant Professor
Department of Pediatric General and Urogenital
Surgery
Juntendo University School of Medicine
2-1-1, Hongo, Bunkyo-ku
Tokyo, 113-8421
Japan

Lars H. Olsen, MD, FEBU, FEAPU
Associate Professor
Department of Urology
Section of Pediatric Urology
Aarhus University Hospital – Skejby
Institute of Clinical Medicine
University of Aarhus
Brendstrupgaardsvej 100
8200 Aarhus N.
Denmark

Chinnusamy Palanivelu, MCh, FRCS(Ed), FACS
Director
Department of Gastroenterology and Minimal
Access Surgery
GEM Hospital & Postgraduate Institute
45-A, Pankaja Mills Road
Ramanathapuram
Coimbatore-641045
India

Gloria Pelizzo, MD
Attending Surgeon
Children's Hospital
IRCCS Burlo Garofolo Trieste
Via dell`Istria 65/1
34124 Trieste
Italy

Thomas Petnehazy, MD
Pediatric Surgery Resident
Department of Pediatric and Adolescent Surgery
Medical University of Graz
Auenbruggerplatz 34
8036 Graz
Austria

Paul Philippe, MD
Chirurgie Pédiatrique
Clinique Pédiatrique
Centre Hospitalier de Luxembourg
4, rue Barblé
1210 Luxembourg
Luxembourg

J. Duncan Phillips, MD
Associate Professor of Surgery
Division of Pediatric Surgery
Department of Surgery
School of Medicine
University of North Carolina
3010 Old Clinic Bldg.
Chapel Hill, NC 27599
USA

Prem Puri, MS, FRCS, FRCS (Ed), FACS
Newman Clinical Research Professor
University College Dublin
Consultant Paediatric Surgeon & Director
of Research
Children's Research Centre
Our Lady's Hospital for Sick Children
Crumlin
Dublin 12
Ireland

Muthukumaran Rangarajan, MS, DipMIS (Fr), FACS
Professor of Surgery
Department of Gastroenterology and Minimal
Access Surgery
GEM Hospital & Postgraduate Institute
45-A, Pankaja Mills Road
Ramanathapuram
Coimbatore-641045
India

Steven S. Rothenberg, MD
Chief of Pediatric Surgery
The Rocky Mountain Hospital for Children
1601 E th Ave. Suite 5500
Denver, CO 80218
USA

Steven Z. Rubin, MD
Professor of Surgery
Chief Pediatric General Surgery
Children's Hospital of Eastern Ontario
401 Smyth Rd
Ottawa, Ontario, K1H 8L1
Canada

Amulya K. Saxena, MD
Associate Professor
Department of Pediatric and Adolescent Surgery
Medical University of Graz
Auenbruggerplatz 34
8036 Graz
Austria

Johannes Schalamon, MD
Associate Professor
Department of Pediatric and Adolescent Surgery
Medical University of Graz
Auenbruggerplatz 34
8036 Graz
Austria

Jürgen Schleef, MD
Director of the Department of Surgery
Children's Hospital
IRCCS Burlo Garofolo Trieste
Via dell`Istria 65/1
34124 Trieste
Italy

Julia Seidl
Research Assistant
Department of Pediatric and Adolescent Surgery
Medical University of Graz
Auenbruggerplatz 34
8036 Graz
Austria

Felix Schier, MD, PhD
Professor and Chair
Department of Pediatric Surgery
University Medical Center Mainz
Langenbeckstr. 1
55101 Mainz
Germany

Hideki Soh, MD
Assistant Professor
Department of Pediatric Surgery
Osaka University Graduate School of Medicine
2-2, E-1, Yamadaoka
Suita
Osaka 565-0871
Japan

Shawn D. St. Peter, MD
Director
Center for Prospective Clinical Trials
The Children's Mercy Hospital
2401 Gillham Road
Kansas City, MO 64108
USA

Lutz Stroedter, MD
Attending Surgeon
Department of Pediatric and Adolescent Surgery
Medical University of Graz
Auenbruggerplatz 34
8036 Graz
Austria

Chung N. Tang, MB BS, FRCS
Consultant Surgeon
Department of Surgery
Pamela Youde Nethersole Eastern Hospital
3 Lok Man Road
Chai Wan
Hong Kong SAR
China

Holger Till, MD, PhD
Professor and Chair
Department of Pediatric Surgery
Children's University Hospital of Leipzig
Oststraße 21–25
04317 Leipzig
Germany

Stefano Tursini, MD
Department of Pediatric Surgery
University of Bologna
Via Massarenti, 11
40138 Bologna
Italy

Benno M Ure, MD
Professor and Chair
Department of Pediatric Surgery
Hannover Medical School
Carl-Neuberg-Straße 1
30625 Hannover
Germany

Jean-Stéphane Valla, MD
Professor of Pediatric Surgery
Head of Department of Pediatric Surgery
Fondation Lenval
Hôpital pour Enfants
57, Avenue de la Californie
06200 Nice
France

Cornelia van Tuil, MD
Pediatric Surgery Fellow
Department of Pediatric Surgery
Ruprecht- Karls University Heidelberg
Im Neuenheimer Feld 110
69120 Heidelberg
Germany

David C. van der Zee, MD, PhD
Department of Pediatric Surgery
Wilhelmina Children's Hospital
University Medical Center Utrecht
P.O.Box 85090
3508 AB Utrecht
The Netherlands

Kari Vanamo, MD, PhD
Department of Pediatric Surgery
Kuopio University Hospital
70211 Kuopio
Finland

Itzhak Vinograd, MD
Dana Children's Hospital
Tel Aviv Sourasky Medical Center
Sackler Faculty of Medicine
6 Weitzman St
Tel Aviv
Israel

John H.T Waldhausen, MD
Professor of Surgery
Department of Surgery
Children's Hospital and Regional Medical Center
W-7729
4800 Sand Point Way, NE
Seattle, WA 98105
USA

Mark L. Wulkan, MD
Associate Professor of Pediatrics and Surgery
Surgical Director, Pediatric Intensive Care Unit
Director, Minimal Invasive Surgery Center
Division of Pediatric Surgery
Emory Children's Center
2015 Uppergate Dr., NE
Atlanta, GA 30322
USA

Atsuyuki Yamataka, MD, PhD
Professor of Pediatric Surgery
Department of Pediatric General and Urogenital
Surgery
Juntendo University School of Medicine
2-1-1, Hongo, Bunkyo-ku,
Tokyo, 113-8421
Japan

Sani Yamout, MD
Pediatric Surgery Research Fellow
University at Buffalo
Women and Children's Hospital of Buffalo
219 Bryant Street
Buffalo, NY 14222
USA

James G. Young, MA, PhD, FRCS (Urol)
Consultant Urologist
Bristol Urological Institute
North Bristol NHS Trust
Southmead Hospital
Westbury-om-Trym
Bristol, BS10 5NB
UK

Section 1
Concepts in Endoscopic Surgery

1 History of Endoscopic Surgery

Amulya K. Saxena

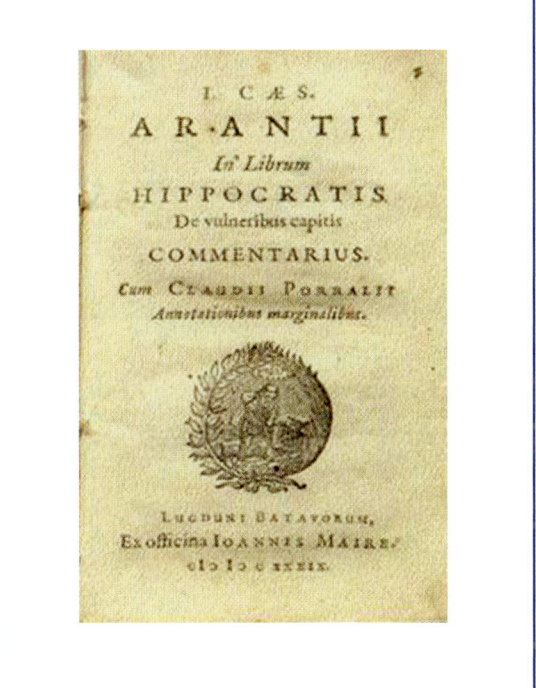

1.1 Giulio Cesare Aranzi

In 1585, Giulio Cesare Aranzi (1530–1589), from Bologna, was the first to use a light source to visualize a cavity in the human body. To achieve this, Aranzi focused sunlight through a flask of water and projected it to visualize the nasal cavity. *From Aranzi GC: Hippocratis librum de vulneribus capitis commentarius cum Claudii Porralii annotationibus marginalibus MDC XXXIX.* (Courtesy Austrian Literature Online, Graz University Library, Graz, Austria)

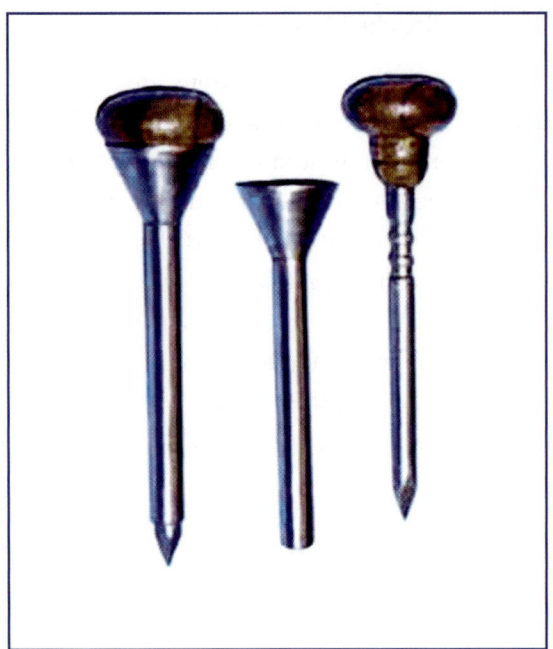

1.2   Origin of Trocar

The term *trocar* was first used by the British in 1706. However, it is believed to be derived from French "*trois-quarts,*" a three-faceted instrument consisting of a cutter in a metal sleeve that was used for withdrawing fluids from a body cavity. (Courtesy of G. Gedney Godwin, Valley Forge, PA, USA)

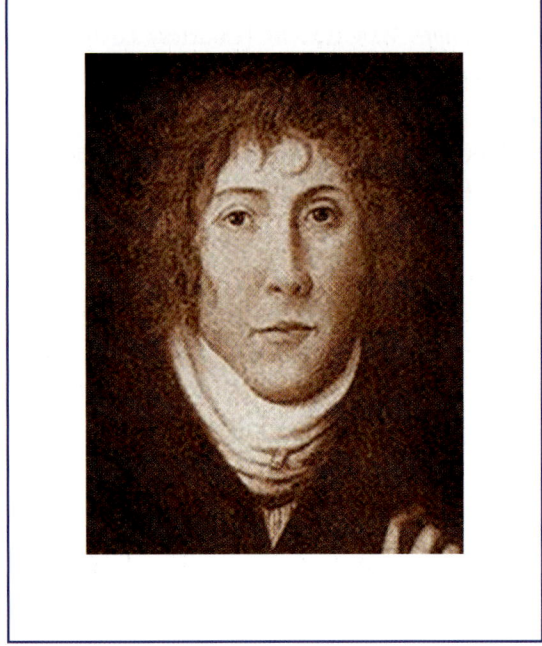

1.3   Philip Bozzini

Philip Bozzini (1773–1809) from Frankfurt was the first to design and build a self-contained instrument with light source and mechanics to illuminate the interior cavities and spaces of the living body. He called this device the "*Lichtleiter,*" or "light conductor." Bozzini first presented his idea to the public in 1804 and officially on February 7, 1805. In July of 1806 the instrument was demonstrated at a scientific session in Frankfurt. (Courtesy of William P. Didusch Center for Urologic History, American Urological Association, Linthicum, MD, USA)

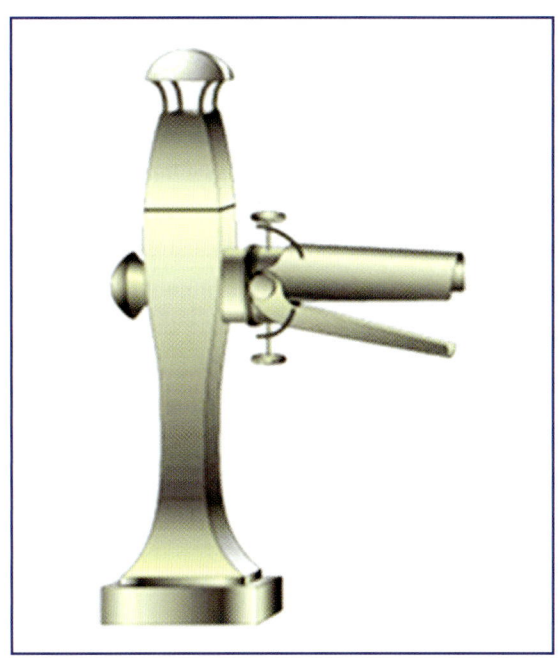

1.3.1   Bozzini's *"Lichtleiter"*

The *"Lichtleiter"* was made from an aluminum tube. The tube was illuminated by a wax candle and had mirrors fitted to it in order to reflect the images. Bozzini published his invention in 1806 in the Hufeland's Journal of Practical Medicine, Volume 24, under the title "Light Conductor, An Invention for the Viewing of Internal Parts and Diseases with Illustration." Incidentally, Bozzini was censured for "undue curiosity" by the Medical Faculty of Vienna for this invention. (Courtesy of Olympus Austria, Vienna, Austria)

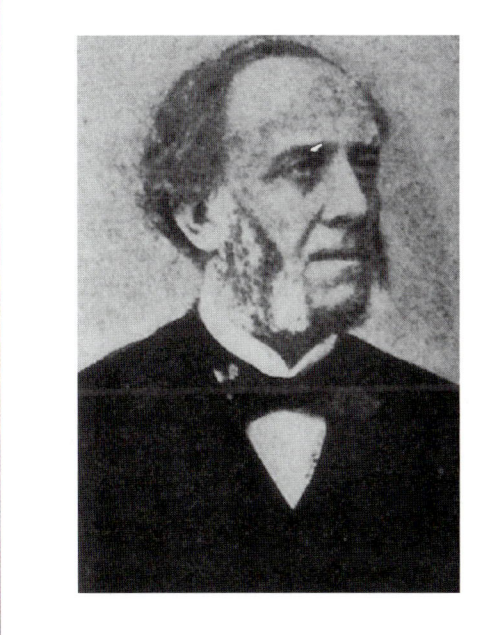

1.4   Antoine Jean Desormeaux

Antoine Jean Desormeaux (1815–1894), a French Surgeon, was the first to introduce the Bozzini's *"Lichtleiter"* into a patient. In 1853, he further developed the *Lichtleiter* and termed his device the *"Endoscope."* It was the first time this term was used in history. Desormeaux presented the *endoscope* in 1865 to the Academy in Paris. He even used his endoscope to examine the stomach; but due to an insufficient light source he was not quite successful. (Copyright Verger-Kuhnke AB. The life of Philipp Bozzini (1773-1809), an idealist of endoscopy. Actas Urol Esp. 2007;31:437-444)

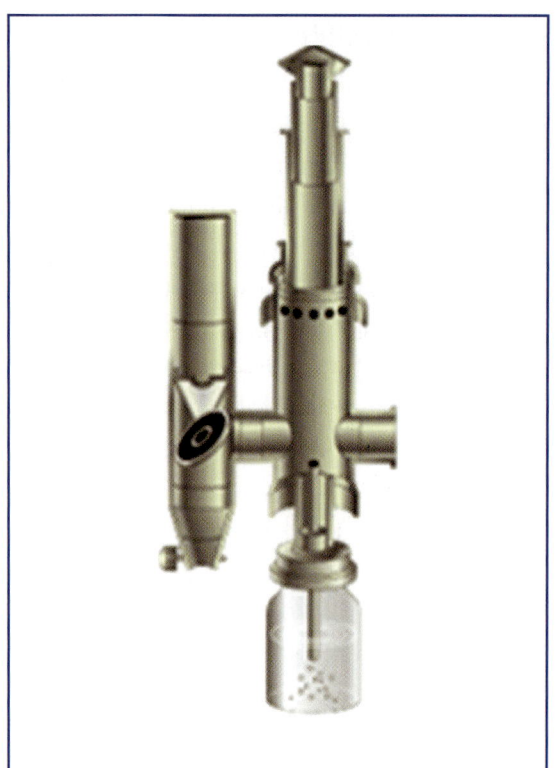

1.4.1   Desormeaux's *"Endoscope"*

Desormeaux's *endoscope* used as a light source a kerosene lamp burning alcohol and turpentine, with a chimney to enhance the flame and a lens to condense the beam to a narrower area to achieve a brighter spot. He used this instrument to examine the urethra and bladder. As might have been expected, burns were the major complication of these procedures. Interestingly, he thought of using electricity but felt it unsafe. (Courtesy of Olympus Austria, Vienna, Austria)

1.5   Adolf Kussmaul

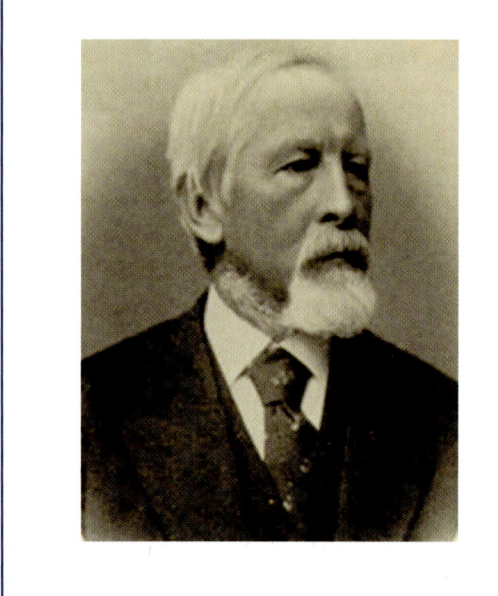

In Freiburg, Adolph Kussmaul (1822–1902), a German physician, succeeded in looking inside the stomach of a human body. The direct esophagoscopy had been undertaken using a tube-shaped speculum to which he had attached Desormeaux's *endoscope* for illumination. His device, two 47-cm-long metal tubes, one round with a diameter of 13 mm and the other elliptical, was gulped down and tested on a sword-swallower.

1.6　Maximillian Carl-Friedrich Nitze

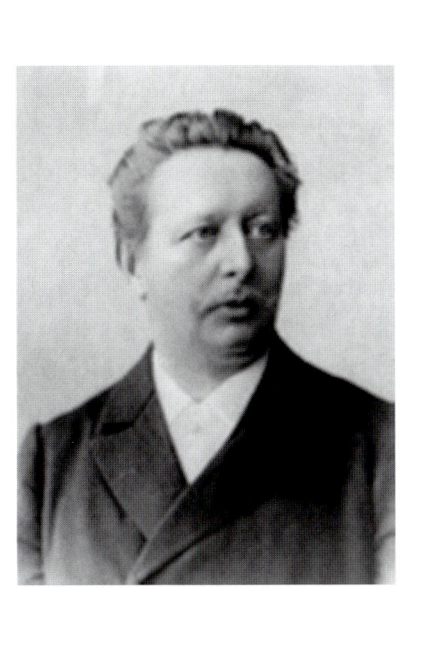

In 1877, Maximillian Carl-Friedrich Nitze (1848–1906), a German urologist from Dresden, with the help of two opticians – Wilhelm Deicke and Louis Beneche – constructed a "*zystoscope*" to view corpse bladders. Attempts to further improve the "*zystoscope*" were hampered in Dresden and Nitze left for Vienna. With the aid of a Viennese electro-optician, Joseph Leiter, Nitze is credited with the invention of the modern cystoscope. The *Nitze-Leiter cystoscope* used a prism and a glowing platinum wire, the end of which was cooled by water, to illuminate a 7-mm scope. In 1879, while still in Vienna, Nitze demonstrated this device in a living patient. Nitze is also credited with producing the first endoscopic photographs. (Copyright: Reuter M. Maximillian Nitze: (1848–1906) Geburtshelfer der Urologe. Urologe 2006; 45:1076-1083 Springer Verlag)

1.7　Thomas Alva Edison

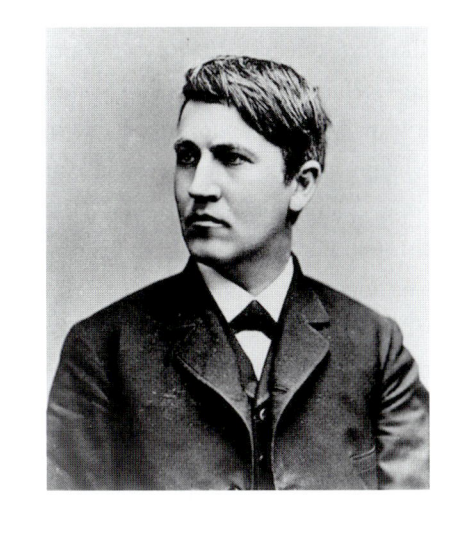

Thomas Alva Edison (1804–1896) invented the incandescent light bulb in Menlo Park, NJ, USA. After many experiments with platinum and other metal filaments, Edison returned to a carbon filament. His incandescent lamp, which had a filament of carbonized sewing thread, burned for 13.5 h on October 22, 1879. Edison patented an electric distribution system in 1880, which was essential to capitalize on the invention of the electric lamp. Thomas Edison's invention of the incandescent light bulb in 1879 laid the foundation for major strides in the field of endoscopic illumination.

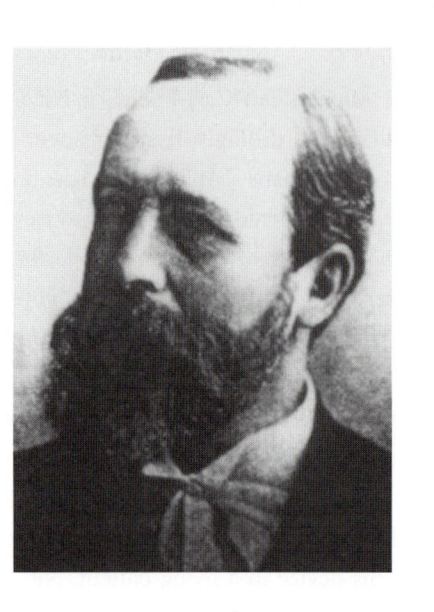

1.8   Johannes Freiherr von Mikulicz-Radecki

Johannes Freiherr von Mikulicz-Radecki (1850–1905), a surgeon of Polish-Lithuanian descent born in Bukowina, Romania, constructed the first rigid endoscope in 1880 and was the first to use Edison's light bulb for his gastroscope in practice. He modified the instrument so that it could be angled by 30° near to its lower third to achieve better visualization. He added a separate channel for air insufflation. In one of the first interventional endoscopic procedures, he pushed a large swallowed bone from the esophagus into the stomach, thus avoiding surgery. (Copyright: Morgenthal CB. The role of the surgeon in the evolution of flexible endoscopy. Surg Endosc 2007: 21; 838-853 Springer Verlag)

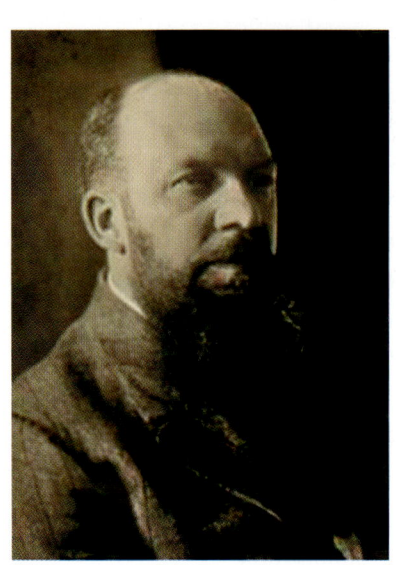

1.9   Georg Kelling

Georg Kelling (1866–1945), a German physician from Dresden, was introduced to endoscopy and gastrointestinal surgery when he worked with Professor Mikulicz-Radecki at the Royal Surgical Clinic in Breslau, Germany. In Hamburg on September 23, 1901, he visualized the abdominal cavity of a dog with the help of Nitze's *cystoscope*, and coined this laparoscopic examination "*celioscopy.*" He used air filtered through sterile cotton to create pneumoperitoneum in dogs. For insufflation he used a trocar developed by Alfred Fiedler, an internist from Dresden. (Copyright: Hatzinger M: Georg Kelling (1866–1945) Der Erfinder der modernen Laparoskopie. Urologe A 2006; 45 (7):868-71 Springer Verlag)

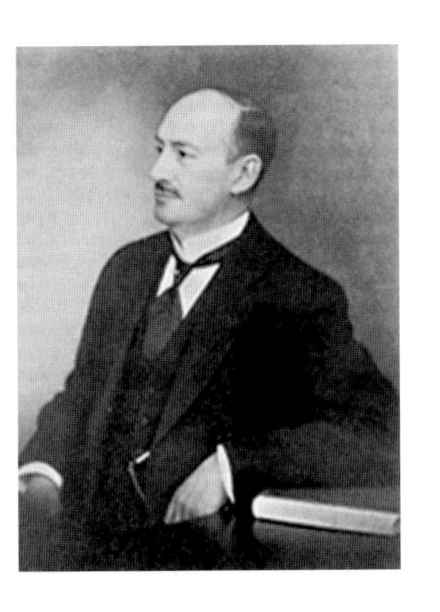

1.10 Hans Christian Jacobaeus

In 1910, Hans Christian Jacobaeus (1879–1937), a Swedish internist, used the term *"laparothoracoscopy"* for the procedure he used to visualize the thorax and the abdomen. Unlike Kelling, he did not employ pneumoperitoneum. The Stockholm internist evacuated ascites using a trocar with a trapvalve. In a 1912 monograph, Jacobaeus gave an exact description of the patients' conditions and the 97 laparoscopies performed between 1910 and 1912 in Stockholm's community hospital. (Copyright: Hatzinger M.: Hans-Christian Jacobaeus (1879-1937): The inventor of human laparoscopy and thoracoscopy. Urologe A 2006; 45:1184-6. Springer Verlag)

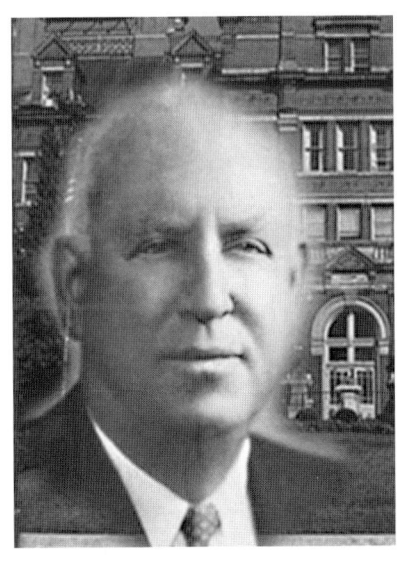

1.11 Bertram Moses Bernheim

Bertram Moses Bernheim (1880–1958) graduated from the Johns Hopkins School of Medicine in 1905 and thereafter undertook clinical research, a prerequisite for all surgeon-scientists, in the Hunterian Laboratory of experimental surgery which had been established in 1904 by Harvey Cushing. In 1911 he introduced laparoscopy in the USA and named the procedure *"organoscopy-cystoscopy of the abdominal cavity."* Bernheim commented on the limited angle of vision of 90° using a cystoscope as a laparoscope. (Adapted with permission to reprint: Archives of Surgery, 2004, 139:1110–1126, Copyright 2004, American Medical Association. All rights reserved)

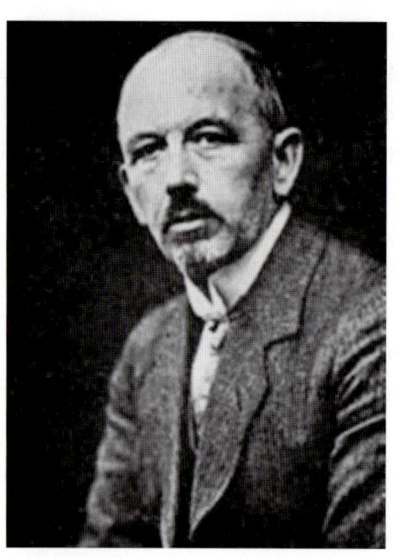

1.12   Severin Nordentoft

Severin Nordentoft (1866–1922), a Danish radiologist and surgeon from Aarhus reported on the successful endoscopic visualization of the knee in 1912 at the 41st Annual Meeting of the German Society of Surgery in Berlin. Along with the help of his brother, Jacob Nordentoft, he designed the "*trocar endoscope*," which consisted of a 5-mm trocar, a fluid valve, and an optic tube. This trocar went into production at the Louis and Lowenstein Company in Berlin. Nordentoft used the device for the diagnosis of early meniscal lesions of the knee using saline or boric acid solution. He termed the procedure "*arthroscopy*." (Copyright: Kieser C. Severin Nordentoft und die Priorität für die Arthroskopie. Arthroskopie 2000; 13: 197-199. Springer Verlag)

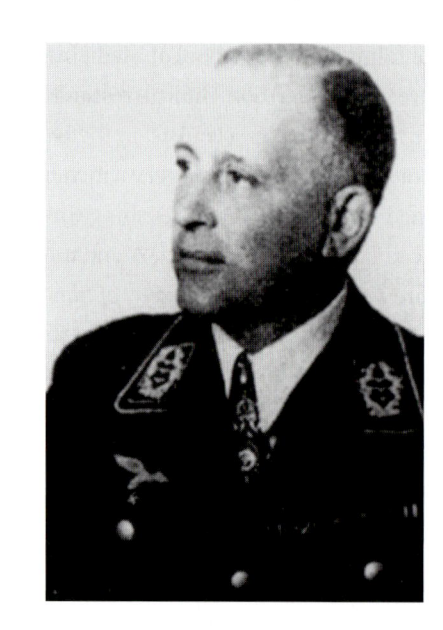

1.13   Heinz Kalk

Heinz Kalk (1895–1973), from Frankfurt am Main, was drafted into the German army while a medical student. After the war, he completed his medical studies and was later appointed as a physician at the Charité Hospital in Berlin. In 1928, he asked the Heynemann Company to construct a scope with a 135° optical system for laparoscopy. He advocated the use of a separate puncture site for pneumoperitoneum and published his findings in 1929. By 1942, he had carried out 750 laparoscopies, and in 1943 reported on 123 laparoscopic-assisted liver biopsy procedures. His "dual-puncture techniques" opened the door for operative laparoscopy. (Reprinted from JSLS, Journal of the Society of Laparoendoscopic Surgeons, 1997, 1:185–188)

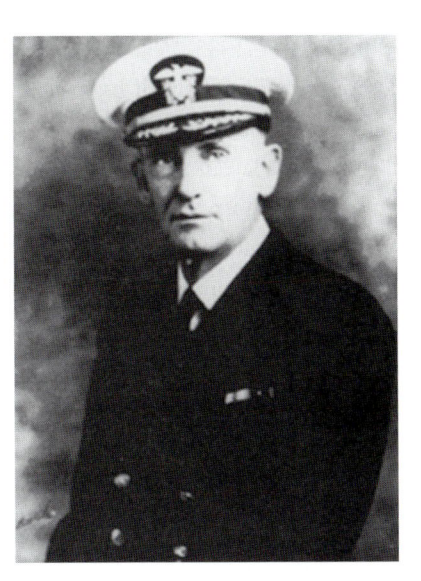

1.14 John Carroll Ruddock

Ruddock (1891–1964), an American internist, left the United States Naval Hospital San Diego after the war to enter private practice in Los Angeles. Ruddock was interested in laparoscopy and initially used a McCarthy cystoscope for his patients. Later, in 1934, he developed and presented his "*peritoneoscope*." Ruddock used his peritoneoscope with built-in monopolar forceps for electrocoagulation during procedures. However, he expressed great concerns at "*audible explosions*" and "*flashlights*" in the abdomen due to electric current in the presence of oxygen. (Reprinted from JSLS, Journal of the Society of Laparoendoscopic Surgeons, 1997, 1:185–188)

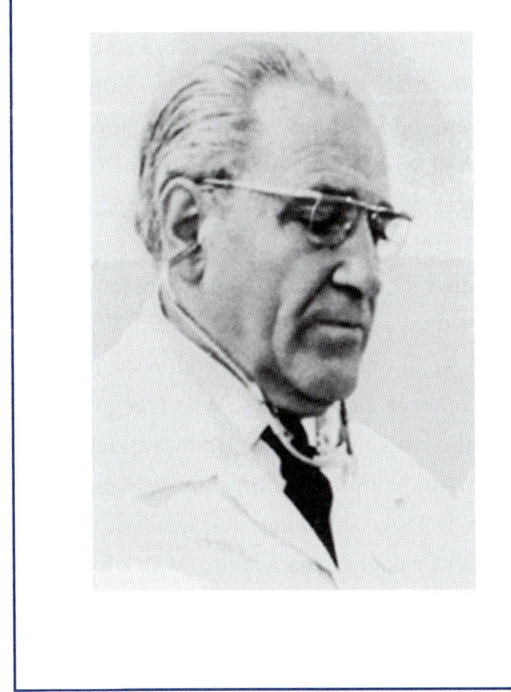

1.15 János Veres

János Veres (1903–1979) was born in Kismajtény, Hungary, where his father was a stationmaster at the Royal Hungarian Railways. He completed his medical education in Debrecen and was later appointed as the Head of Internal Medicine in Kapuvar. Since 1932, in Kapuvar, he had to deal with tuberculosis patients and used a spring-loaded needle to create an artificial pneumothorax in these patients. After 960 successful interventions he reported his experiences in Hungarian in 1936. However, he became known to the international medical world after his publication in German in 1938. His report from 1938 additionally indicated that he also used his needle for pneumoperitonuem. Veres wrote his name both with single and double "s". However, his birth certificate showed the name Veres. (Copyright: Sandor J. A needle puncture that helped to change the world of surgery. Surg Endosc 2000; 14: 201-202 Springer Verlag)

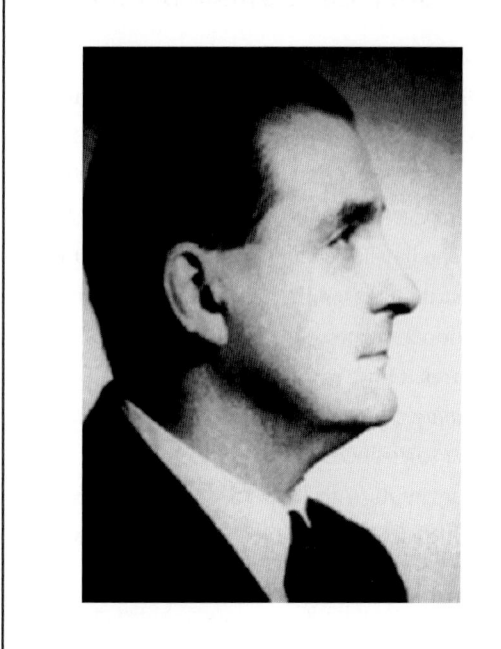

1.16   Raoul Palmer

Raoul Palmer (1904–1985) began his first attempts in laparoscopy with the help of his wife, Elisabeth Palmer, amidst the hardships of the German invasion of Paris in 1943. Palmer had to make most of the instruments, as most of the manufacturers were out of business or were prisoners of war. After the war, in 1947, Palmer published his experience on 250 gynecological celioscopies performed by placing the patients in the Trendelenburg position. He stressed the importance of continuous monitoring of intra-abdominal pressure during laparoscopy. (Reprinted from JSLS, Journal of the Society of Laparoendoscopic Surgeons, 1997, 1:289–292)

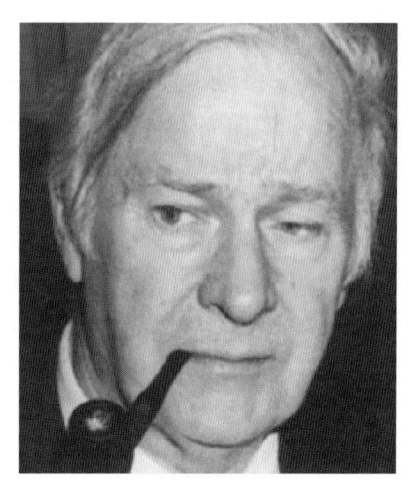

1.17   Harold Horace Hopkins

Hopkins (1918–1994) obtained a degree in physics and mathematics at Leicester University in 1939. After the war, in 1947, Hopkins became a research fellow at Imperial College, London, UK. Hopkins invented the rigid rod-lens system for scopes, which allows double light transmission, requires short and thin spacer tubes, and gives a larger and clearer aperture. He filed a patent for the rod-lens system in 1959. However, the English and American companies to whom he offered the system displayed little interest. The situation changed however in 1965 when Professor George Berci, who recognized the potential of this invention, introduced Hopkins to Karl Storz to manufacture the scopes. (Courtesy of William P. Didusch Center for Urologic History, American Urological Association, MD, USA)

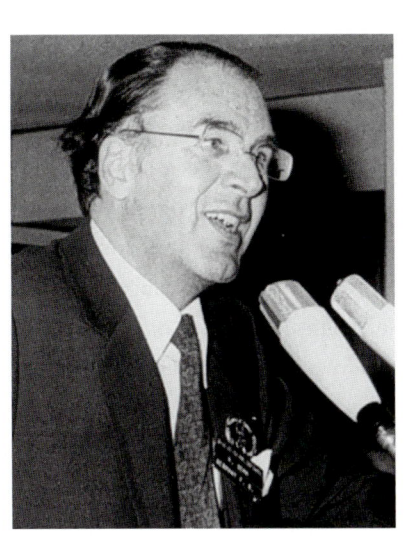

1.18   Kurt Karl Stephan Semm

Kurt Karl Stephan Semm (1927–2003) was born in Munich, Germany, where he also studied medicine at the Ludwigs-Maximillian University. In 1958, he wrote his medical thesis under the guidance of Nobel laureate Adolf Butenandt. Semm began his career in gynecology under Professor Fikentscher in Munich. In 1970s, as the Head of Gynecology in Kiel, he: (1) introduced an automatic insufflation device capable of monitoring intra-abdominal pressures, (2) introduced endoscopic loop sutures, (3) introduced extra- and intracorporeal suturing techniques, and (4) created the pelvitrainer. He performed the first laparoscopic appendectomy in 1982. (Courtesy of Monika Bals-Pratsch MD, Zentrum für Gynäkologie, Universität Regensburg, Germany)

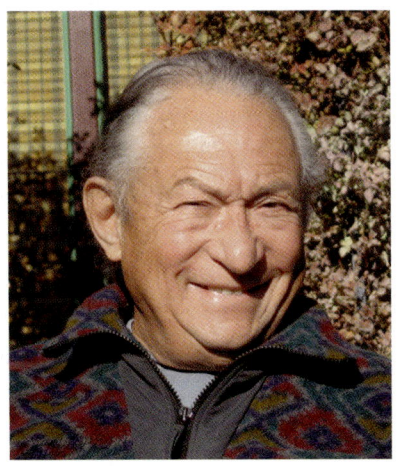

1.19   Harrith Hasson

In 1978, Harrith M. Hasson, a gynecologist in Chicago, IL, USA, introduced an alternative method of port placement. He proposed a blunt minilaparotomy that permitted direct visualization of the port entrance in the cavity. The Hasson trocar system was initially developed for laparoscopy in patients who have had a previous laparotomy. Hasson served as Assistant Professor at Northwestern University, Associate Professor at Rush University, Director of the Gynecologic Endoscopy Center and Chairman of the Division of Obstetrics & Gynecology at Weiss Memorial Hospital in Chicago, and Clinical Professor at University of Chicago. He retired from clinical practice in 2003. (Courtesy of RealSim Systems LLC, Albuquerque, NM, USA)

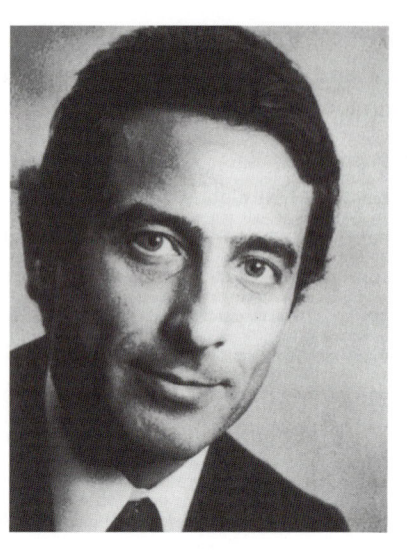

1.20   Erich Mühe

Erich Mühe (1938–2005) completed his medical education in 1966 and training in surgery in 1973 under Professor Gerd Hegemann at the University of Erlangen, Germany. He was later appointed as the Head of Surgery in Böblingen County Hospital in 1982. In 1985, Mühe performed the first laparoscopic cholecystectomy. He used a modified rectoscope and employed carbon dioxide insufflation for this procedure. As surgical instruments, he used a pistol grip applier with hemoclips to ligate, and pistol grip scissors to cut between the clipped cystic duct and artery. (Reprinted from JSLS, Journal of the Society of Laparoendoscopic Surgeons, 1998, 2:341–346)

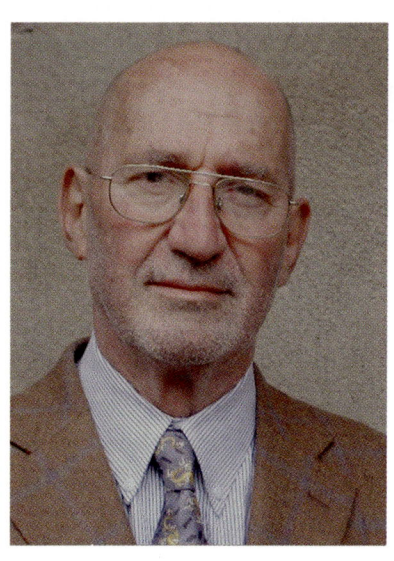

1.21   Philippe Mouret

Philippe Mouret, a French general surgeon, rotated on a gynecology service in the 1960s, during which he had his first contact with laparoscopy. Mouret further developed interest in laparoscopy as he also shared his surgical practice with a gynecologist and had access to laparoscopic instruments and, importantly, to patients requiring laparoscopy. In 1987, Mouret performed the first videolaparoscopic cholecystectomy in Lyons, France. Cholecystectomy is the first laparoscopic procedure that "revolutionized" general surgery and was the stimulus in the development of operative laparoscopic surgery. (Courtesy of the Honda Foundation, Tokyo, Japan)

1.22   Michael Harrison

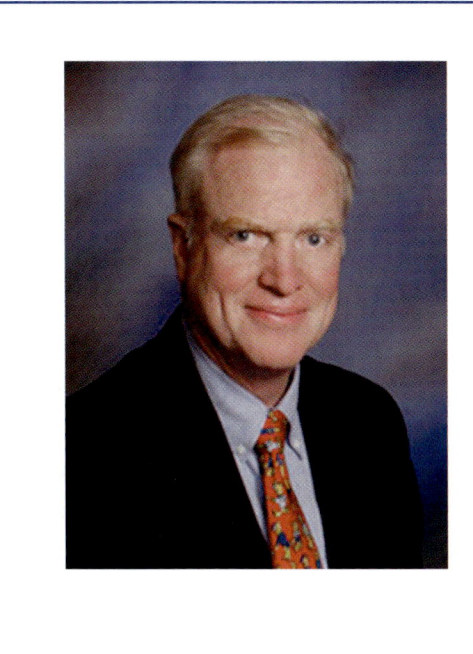

Since the 1980s, Michael R. Harrison, a pediatric surgeon in San Francisco, California, USA, has been involved in fetal medicine. He performed the first open fetal surgical procedure in 1981. In 1997, Harrison performed the first successful clipping of the trachea using minimal access "fetoscopic techniques" by placing the Fetendo clip into a human fetus with a congenital diaphragmatic hernia. Michael Harrison is the Director of the Fetal Treatment Center, University of California, San Francisco. Over the past two decades he has developed various techniques for minimal-access treatment of fetuses. (Courtesy of Michael Harrison, UCSF, San Francisco, CA, USA)

Recommended Literature

1. Modlin IM, Kidd M, Lye KD (2004) From the lumen to the laparoscope. Arch Surg 139:1110–1126
2. Spaner SJ, Warnock GL (1997) A brief history of endoscopy, laparoscopy, and laparoscopic surgery. J Laparoendosc Adv Surg Tech A 7:369–373
3. Vecchio R, MacFayden BV, Falazzo F (2000) History of laparoscopic surgery. Panminerva Med 42:87–90

2 Instrumentation and Equipment

Amulya K. Saxena

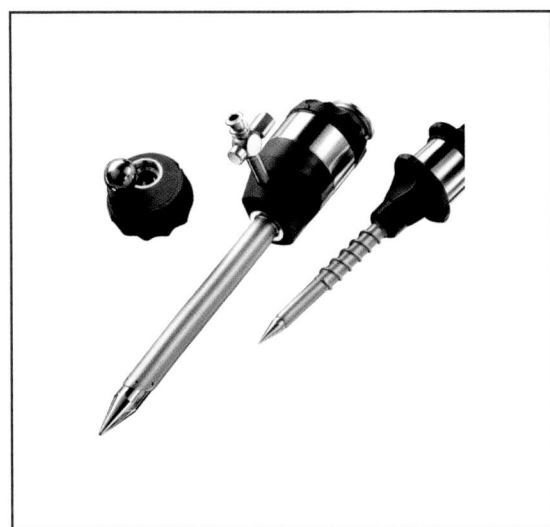

2.1   Port and Trocar

A port is a tubular sleeve-like device through which operative access is obtained in endoscopic surgery. A trocar is a spike-like device (conical- or pyramidal-tipped) that is placed inside the port sleeve with its tip exposed toward the end of the port. The port and trocar are inserted as a set through the abdominal or chest wall, and the trocar is removed after the port is in place. The port has a valve mechanism to allow instruments to be passed through it without the loss of insufflated gases. (Courtesy of Richard Wolf, Knittlingen, Germany)

2.2 Veress Needle

A Veress needle is used for creating the initial pneumoperitoneum so that the subsequent trocars and ports can enter safely. It consists of an inner cannula that is spring-loaded and retracts within the sharp outer needle while passing through the anterior wall, and then springs forward when it is in the open cavity. The inner cannula is sealed at the distal end, but has a hole on the side of the tip *(inset)* for the gas to flow through. The Veress needle should be checked for its patency and spring action prior to use. (Courtesy of Richard Wolf, Knittlingen, Germany)

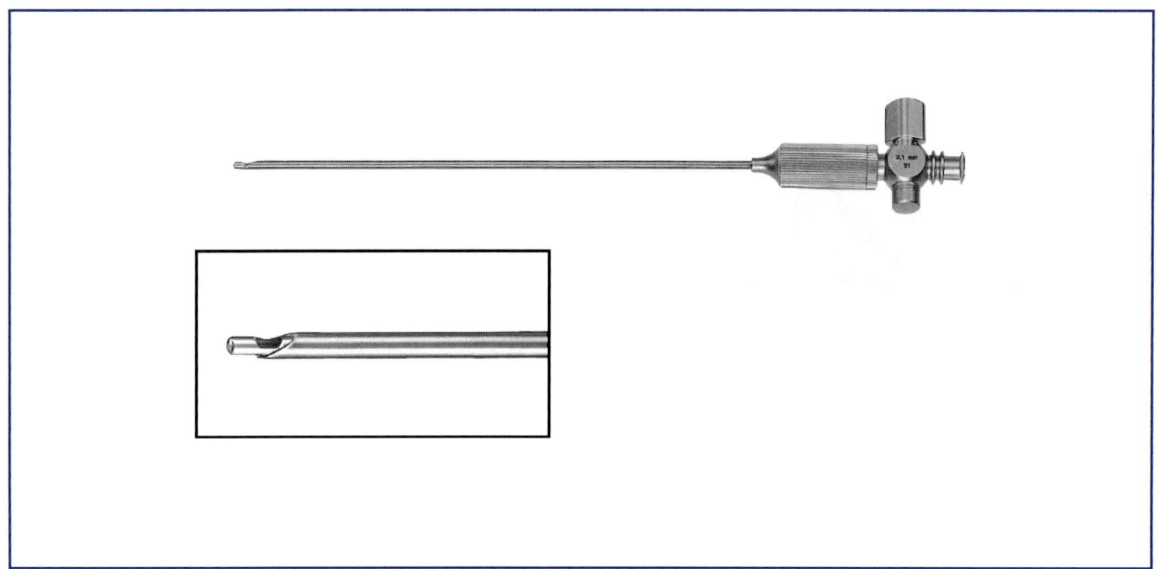

2.3 Blunt Grasping Forceps

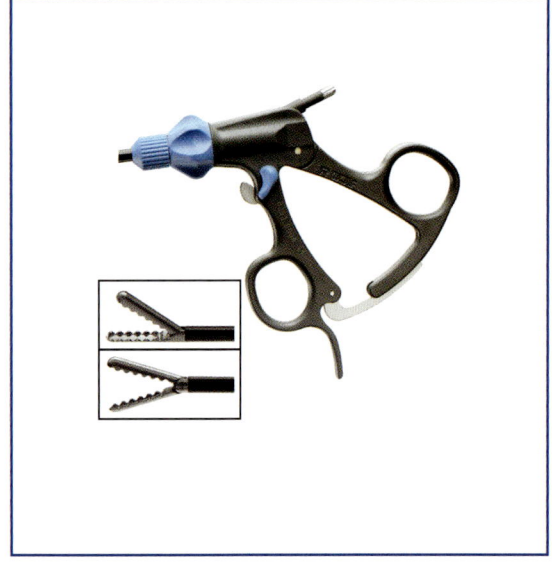

Blunt graspers are the principle means of manipulating tissue and providing exposure to the operation site. It is compulsory that each endoscopic surgery set has at least two pairs of graspers. Blunt graspers have opposing jaws with fine, parallel grooves. They may have a single-action *(inset above)* or double-action *(inset below)* jaw mechanism. The handle may be a scissor grip, spring loaded or ratcheted (see Figure). The handles and bodies of the graspers should be insulated, but should have the possibility for use with electrosurgery. (Courtesy of Richard Wolf, Knittlingen, Germany)

2.4   Dissectors and Tissue Extractors

Various types of endoscopic scissors are available for sharp dissection. However, the hook scissor *(inset)* is a special scissor used in endoscopic surgery in that its unique blade shape helps to withdraw the tissue into the grasp prior to completing the cut. This is advantageous when a relatively large amount of tissue has to be cut. (Courtesy of Richard Wolf, Knittlingen, Germany)

Tissue extractors are single-action jaw forceps with ratchet teeth that permit a greater force to be applied to extract tissues.

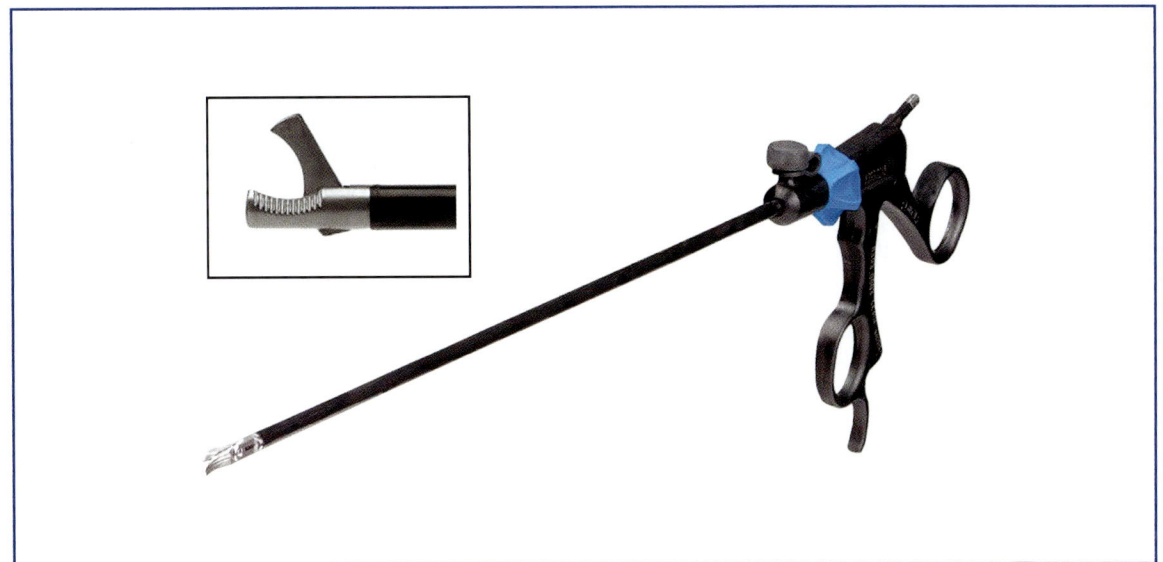

2.5   Biopsy Forceps

Biopsy forceps facilitate the removal of small tissue specimens for pathological studies. Spoon forceps have been specially developed for this purpose as they provide an alternative to dissecting a portion of the tissue and retrieving it with ordinary graspers, which may crush the tissue in the process of retrieving. On the other hand, spike biopsy forceps have special pins that prevent accidental drop of tissue inside the abdominal cavity. (Courtesy of Richard Wolf, Knittlingen, Germany)

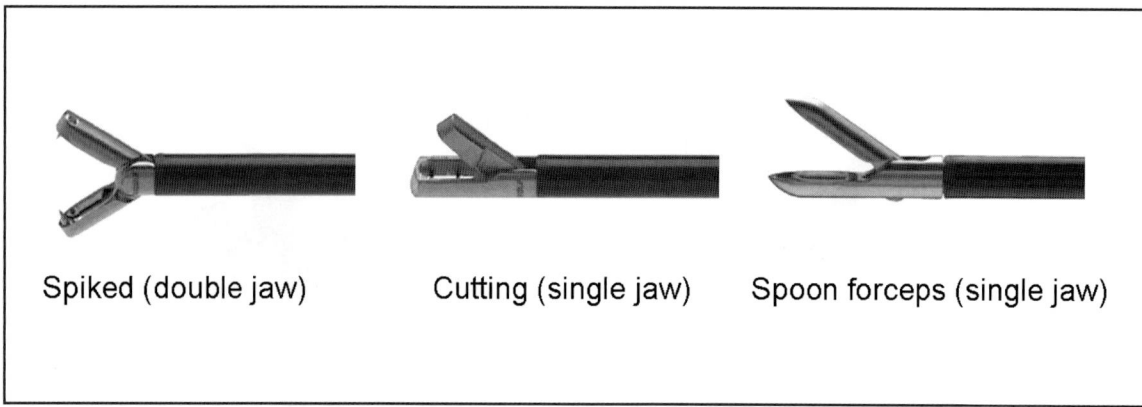

Spiked (double jaw)   Cutting (single jaw)   Spoon forceps (single jaw)

2.6   Endoscopic Retractor Instruments

Endoscopic retractors are used for manually maneuvering tissue that would otherwise obstruct the view of the operative site. They may be straight or curved. The retractor instrument is sized for insertion through the endoscopic ports and comprises a pair of arms that are opened with a scissors motion *(inset)*. Care must be taken to ensure that tissue out of sight is not injured when endoscopic retractors are used. (Courtesy of Richard Wolf, Knittlingen, Germany)

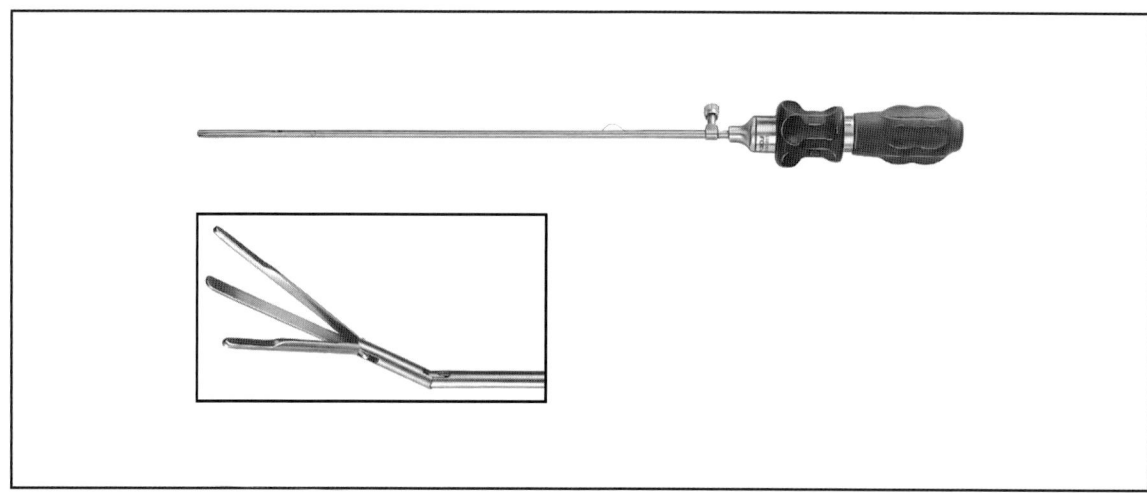

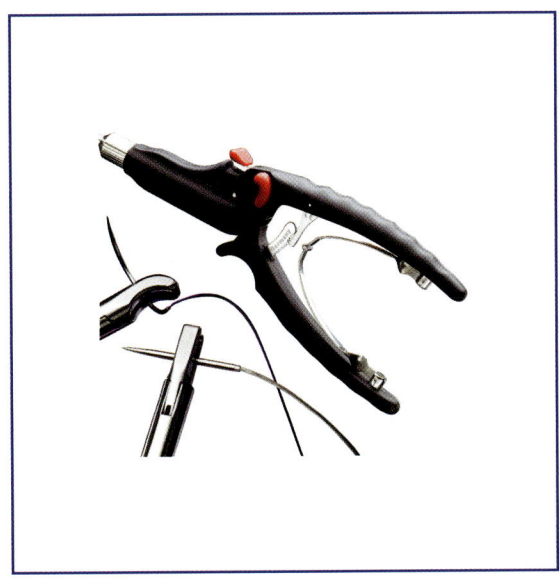

2.7   Needle Holders

Various types of handle grips are offered to maximize the ergonomics of suturing and knot tying. However, most surgeons prefer the axial handle as this ergonomic design reduces hand fatigue and provides optimal as well as efficient needle control. A variety of tip styles (straight to curved) have been developed over the years, leading to an improvement in the design of needle holders. However, the curved tip is used at most centers to tie knots. (Courtesy of Richard Wolf, Knittlingen, Germany)

2.8   Knot Pushers

A surgical knot-pusher device allows a prepared knot to be pushed down through the length of the suture. The device includes a handle and an elongated body extending from it *(above)*. The elongated body has a curved tip that is tapered and has a groove along the length of the tip *(inset)*. Modular knot pushers *(below)* have grooves in both the prongs and function on the same principle as the rod type. (Courtesy of Richard Wolf, Knittlingen, Germany)

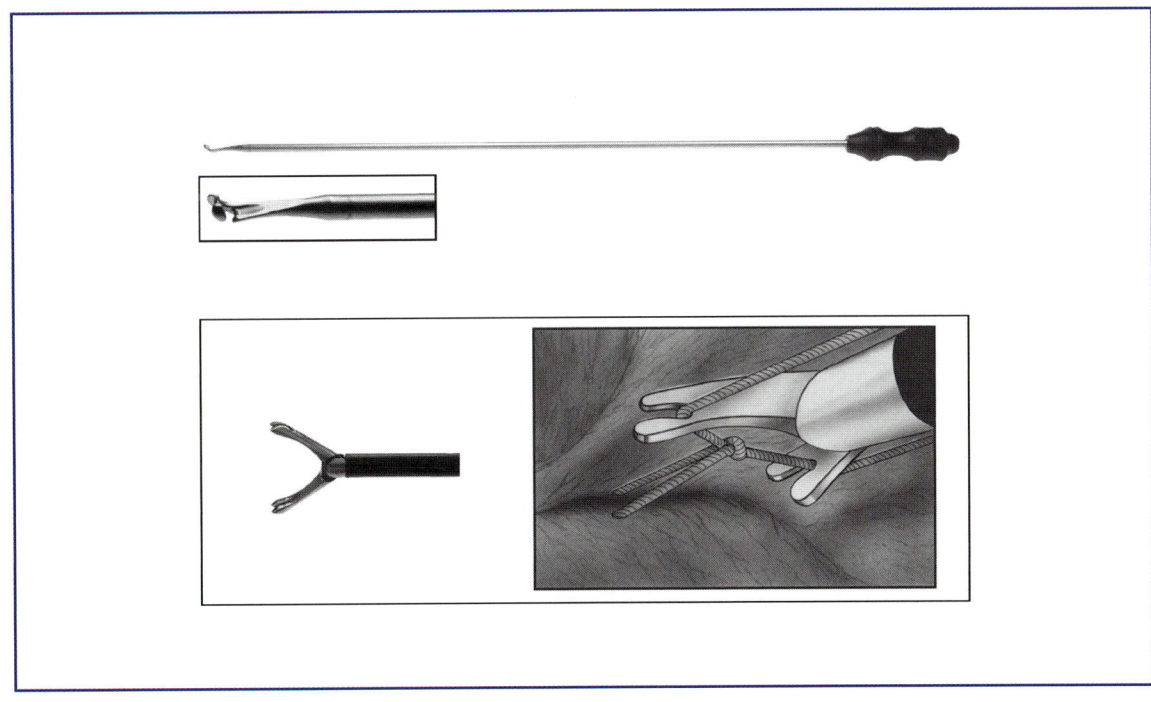

2.9   Probes

Probes are blunt instruments that are utilized to manipulate tissues. Depending on the type of manipulation required, the following types can be used: (1) graduated, (2) hook, and (3) palpation. Hooked probes are generally used for lifting structures that also need to be palpated. (Courtesy of Richard Wolf, Knittlingen, Germany)

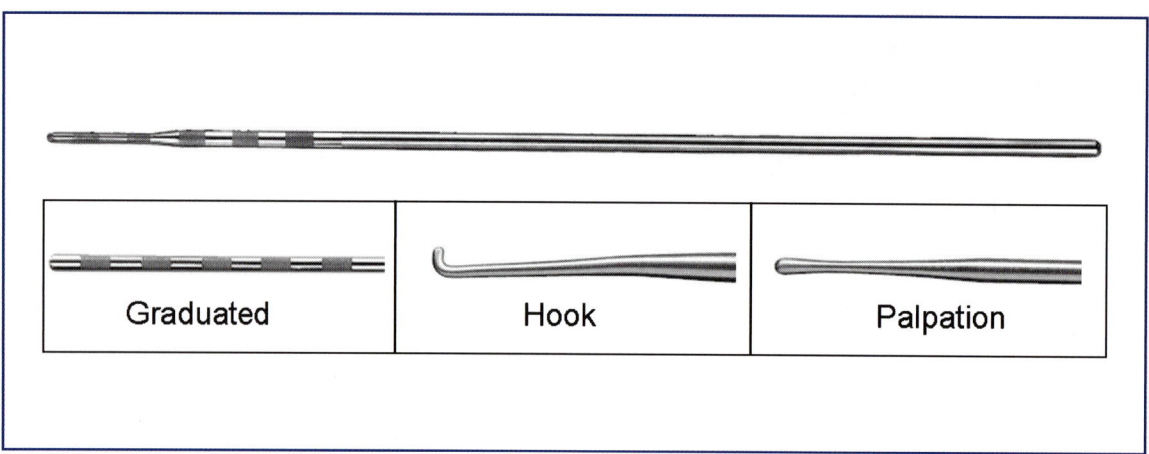

2.10   Goldfinger® Dissector

The Goldfinger® dissector (Johnson & Johnson Medical Products, Ethicon Endo-Surgery, Cincinnati, OH, USA) is a tool developed for bariatric surgery that aids in the placement of the gastric band. The tip of the Goldfinger dissector can flex 90° in the vertical axis, which is similar to the movement obtained by flexing a finger. The tool is passed behind the esophagus and is pushed back up through the opening made in the gastrophrenic ligament, where the thread loop of the gastric band is secured to it. (Courtesy of Johnson & Johnson Medical Products, Ethicon Endo-Surgery, Vienna, Austria)

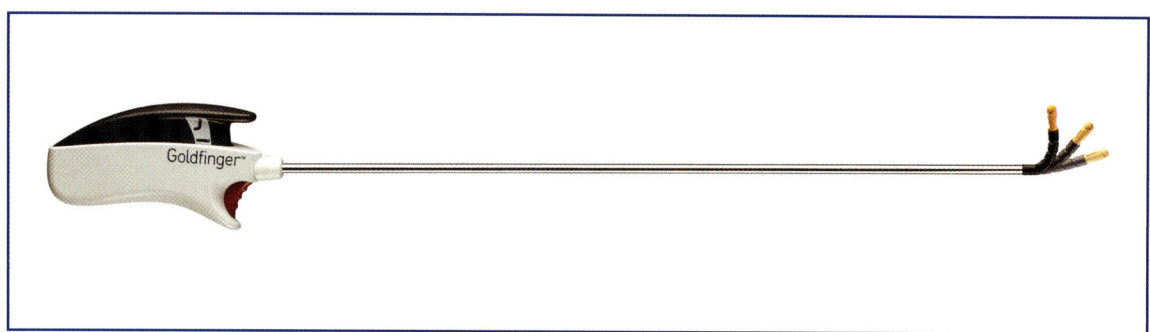

2.11   Endoscopic Clip Applicators

Titanium is the most widely used metal in minimal-access surgery for tissue approximation. An endoscopic clip applicator is a device that allows application of clips within body cavities. Titanium clips are held in position by a dumbbell formation of the tissue they are applied on. If the clips are applied very close to each other, the dumbbell formation will be nullified and the clips will fall loose. (Courtesy of Richard Wolf, Knittlingen, Germany)

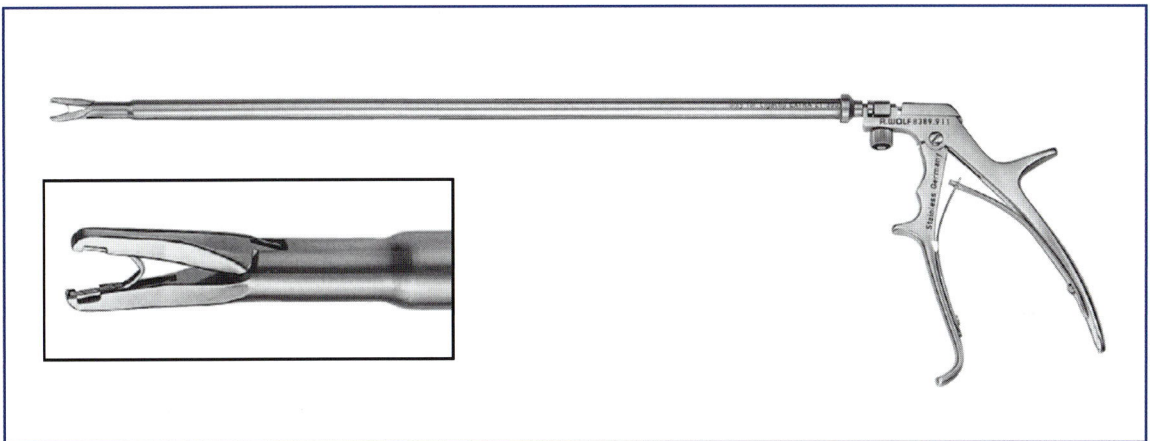

2.12   Endoscopic Linear Stapler

An endoscopic linear stapler device is able to eliminate most of the need for suturing within the surgical cavity. It comprises a single-use loading unit with titanium staples for resection, transection and anastomosis. Care should be taken in port selection, as endoscopic staplers are only available in the 10-mm size. (Courtesy of Johnson & Johnson Medical Products, Ethicon Endo-Surgery, Vienna, Austria)

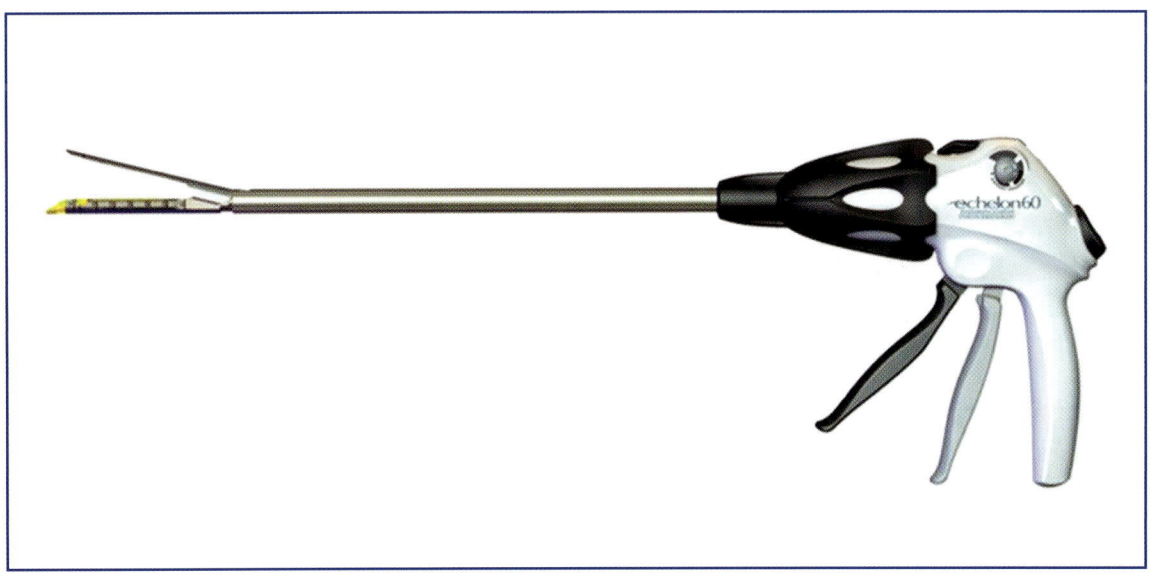

2.13   Circular Intraluminal Anastomosis Stapler

The end-to-end anastomosis stapler enables a circular intraluminal anastomosis of the bowel by placing a double-staggered row of titanium staples.

The instrument is activated by squeezing the handles firmly. Immediately after staple formation, a knife blade in the instrument resects the excess tissue. (Courtesy of Johnson & Johnson Medical Products, Ethicon Endo-Surgery, Vienna, Austria)

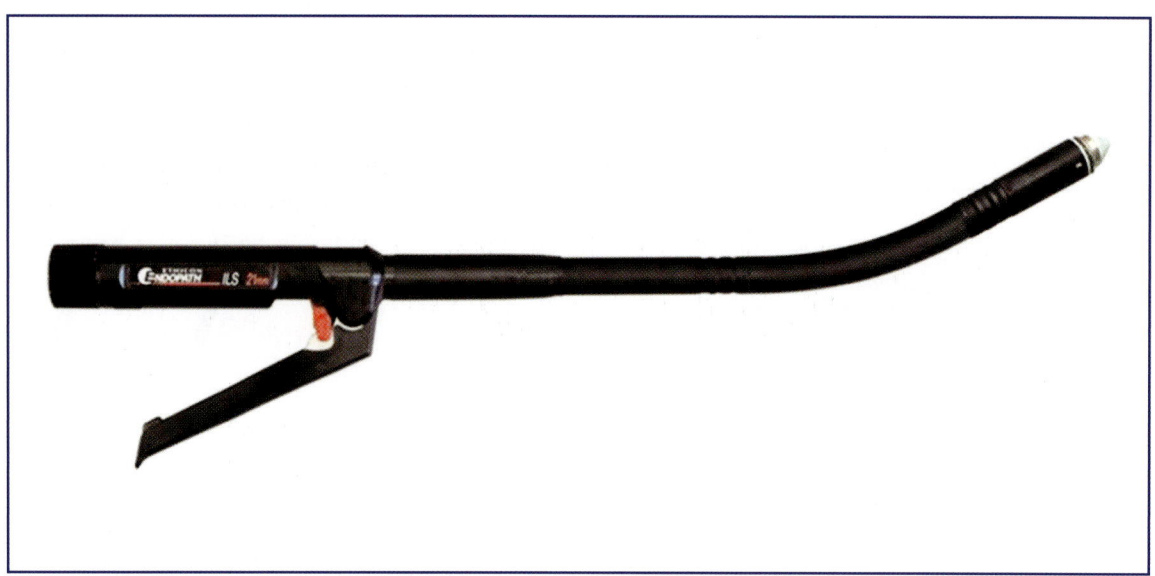

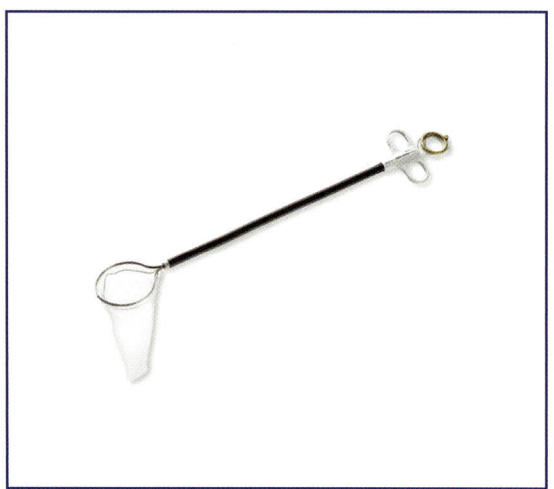

2.14   Specimen Retrieval Bags

Specimen retrieval bags are designed to enable the safe retrieval and extraction of tissues from the body without spillage or contamination. The bags are made of polyurethane to eliminate porosity and provide the necessary strength. Two support arms help to facilitate bag opening and tissue capture. The bag and support arms are attached to a shaft and introducer to facilitate their use in laparoscopic procedures. Each bag is a sterile, single-patient-use, disposable product. (Courtesy of Covidien Austria, Brunn am Gebirge, Austria)

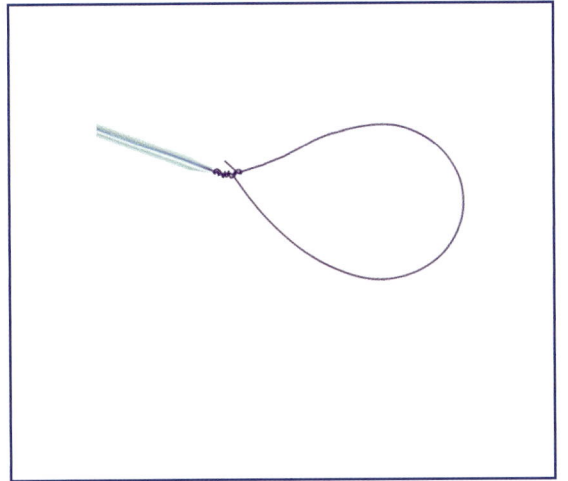

2.15   Endoscopic Loop Suture

Endoscopic sutures are available as pretied loops. In order to apply the suture, the loop and its applicator are placed through an appropriate cannula and inserted into the cavity. The tissue to be ligated is grasped through the loop and then pulled to allow the loop to slide over it. The external end of the applicator is then broken free and pulled to tighten the loop. The pretied Roeder knot slips forward along the suture and will stay relatively in the area where it is applied. (Courtesy of Johnson & Johnson Medical Products, Ethicon Endo-Surgery, Vienna, Austria)

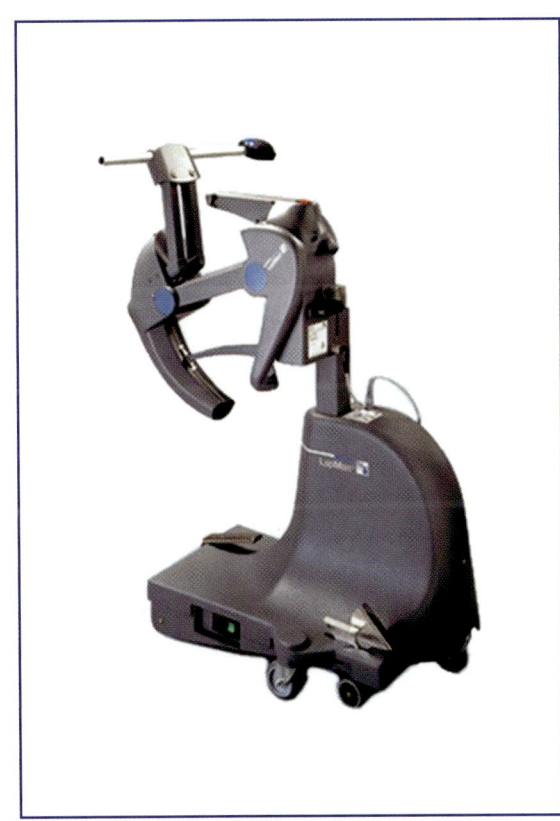

2.16   Automated Laparoscope Assistance

Automatic laparoscope manipulators are systems that render an additional hand for movement or positioning of the scopes during a procedure. Such systems help in autonomous coordination of the hand and eye, directly by the surgeon. The systems are generally composed of a base unit, a mobile and mechanically adjustable arm, and a shaft holder. Recently developed units (Lapman™, Richard Wolf, Knittlingen, Germany) are delivered with an autoclavable "hand control remote" that can be held in position in the palm of the surgeon's hand under the sterile gloves. (Courtesy of Richard Wolf, Knittlingen, Germany)

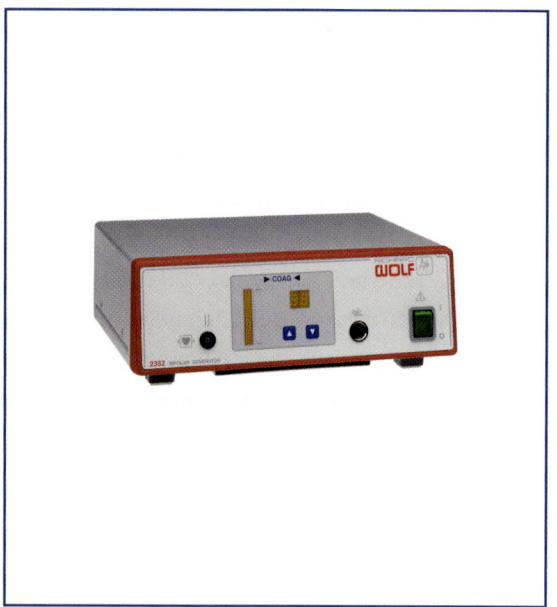

2.17   Electrosurgery Devices

2.17.1   Coagulation and Dissection

Coagulation by desiccation is performed when the instrument comes into contact with the tissue, to slowly heat and evaporate water from the tissue. This process continues until the tissue becomes desiccated to the point that it no longer conducts electric currents and an eschar is produced.

Electrosurgery equipments have controls for setting waveforms. The waveforms represented are *cut* and *coagulate*. The electrosurgery solid-state generators start with 50 cycles of current and transform them to frequencies of more than 50,000 cycles, which is above the level of neuromuscular stimulation, to achieve the desired result in the tissue. (Courtesy of Richard Wolf, Knittlingen, Germany)

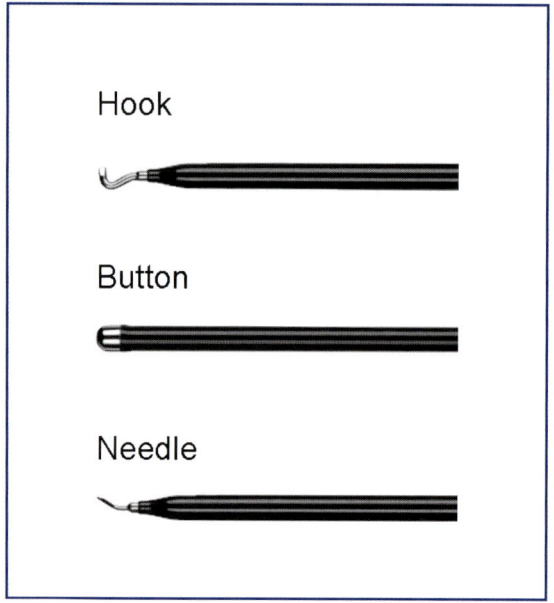

Hook

Button

Needle

2.17.2   Monopolar Coagulation

In monopolar electrosurgery, current passes through the body from the active electrode (instrument) to the grounding electrode pad, which is attached to the patient's body. Monopolar electrosurgery is widely used and enables the surgeon to both, *cut* and *coagulate*. Along with the power level used, the efficacy of coagulation or cutting is also determined by the shape of the electrode. The hooked-shaped electrode is one of the most useful devices, since cutting may be achieved either by pulling or alternatively using the heel of the hook. (Courtesy of Richard Wolf, Knittlingen, Germany)

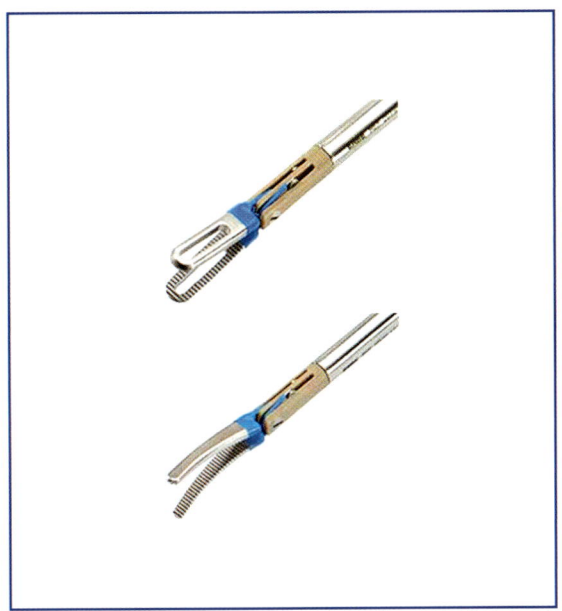

2.17.3   Bipolar Coagulation

In bipolar electrosurgery, the functions of both the active electrode and return electrode are performed at the site of surgery. Only the tissue grasped is included in the electrical circuit. Because the return function is performed by one tine of the forceps, no patient return electrode is needed. This eliminates most of the safety concerns associated with monopolar electrosurgery. Bipolar electrosurgery is generally employed for captive hemostasis; however, sharp hemostatic dissection is possible with the newer configurations available. (Courtesy of Erbe Elektromedizin, Tübingen, Germany)

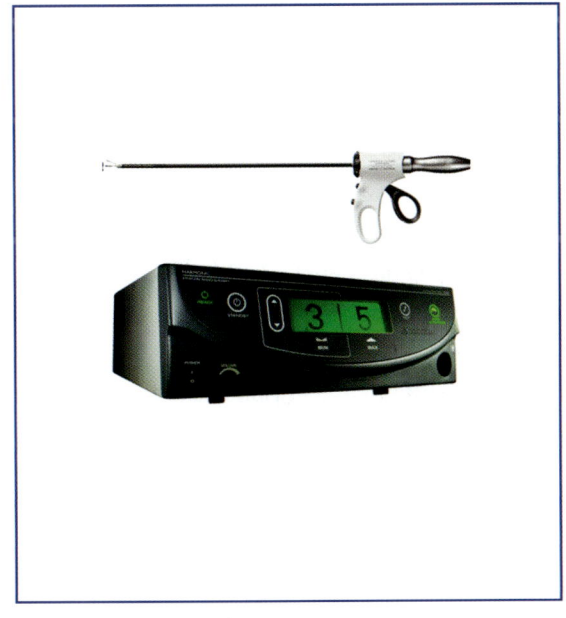

2.17.4   Harmonic Technology/Instruments

The Ultracision® harmonic scalpel (Johnson & Johnson Medical Products, Ethicon Endo-Surgery, Cincinnati, OH, USA) uses ultrasound technology for precise cutting and controlled coagulation. The main benefits of this instrument are:

1. Greater precision near vital structures.
2. Fewer instrument exchanges.
3. Minimum charring and desiccation.
4. Reduced need for ligatures.
5. Coagulation/cutting at lower temperatures.
6. Less lateral thermal damage.
7. Heat development in the tissue rather than the instrument.
8. No electrical circuit through the patient.

(Courtesy of Johnson & Johnson Medical Products, Ethicon Endo-Surgery, Vienna, Austria)

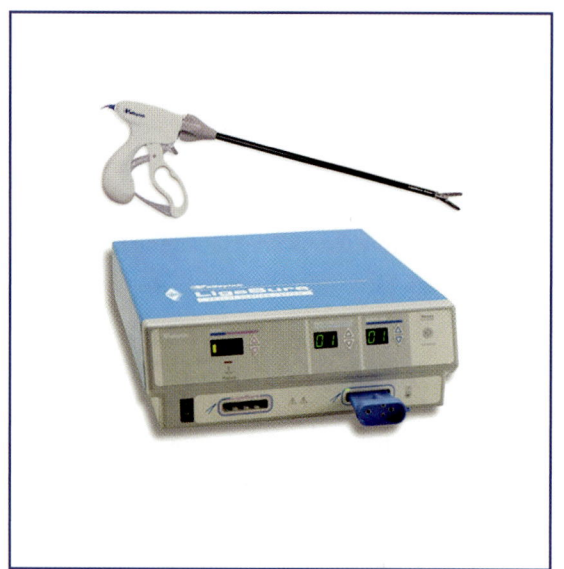

2.17.5 LigaSure™ Sealing Device

The LigaSure™ (Valleylab, Boulder, CO, USA) sealing device uses an optimized combination of pressure and energy to create seals by melting the collagen and elastin in the vessel walls and reforming it into a permanent, plastic-like seal. It fuses vessels up to and including 7 mm in diameter and tissue bundles without dissection or isolation. Furthermore, when the instrument determines that the seal is complete, a tone sounds and output to the handpiece is automatically discontinued. Lateral thermal spread is minimal (1–2 mm) and the unique energy output results in no sticking or charring. (Courtesy of Covidien Austria, Brunn am Gebirge, Austria)

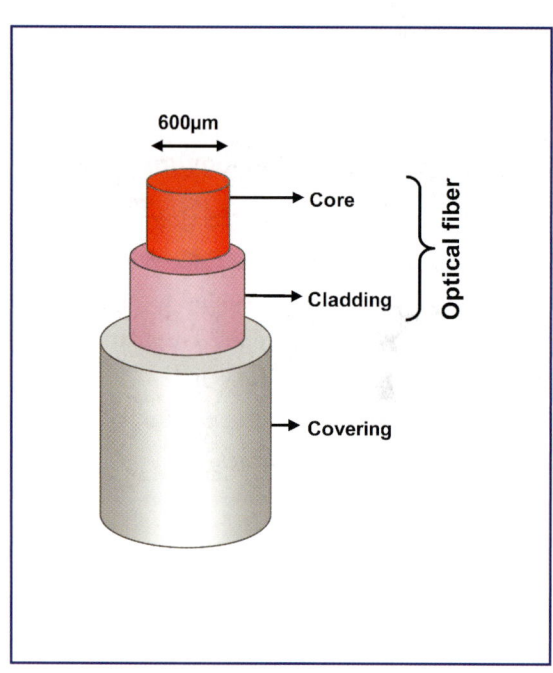

2.18 Laser Fiber Optics

The most frequently used lasers in operative procedures are argon, potassium-titanyl-phosphate (KTP) and neodymium-doped yttrium-aluminum-garnet (Nd:YAG). Laser energy is delivered to the tissues through optical fibers – fiber optics. The optical fiber consists of a 600-μm pure silica core surrounded by a low-refractive-index silica cladding. In order to prevent breakage, a covering of silicone rubber and nylon is applied. The 600-μm fiber optics offer the best combination of coagulation and cutting, which is combined with the appropriate amount of stiffness and flexibility. For laser application in endoscopic surgery, various laser fiber-optic delivery device options (operating scopes/reducing valve ports) are available.

2.18.1   Scopes and Video Camera Systems

2.18.1.1 Anatomy of a Rigid Scope

Central to the instrumentation is the scope. Its backbone is the rod lens system designed by Hopkins. The shaft of scopes houses both light fibers and viewing optics. The viewing optics consist of three distinct parts: the objective lens, rod lenses, and ocular lens.

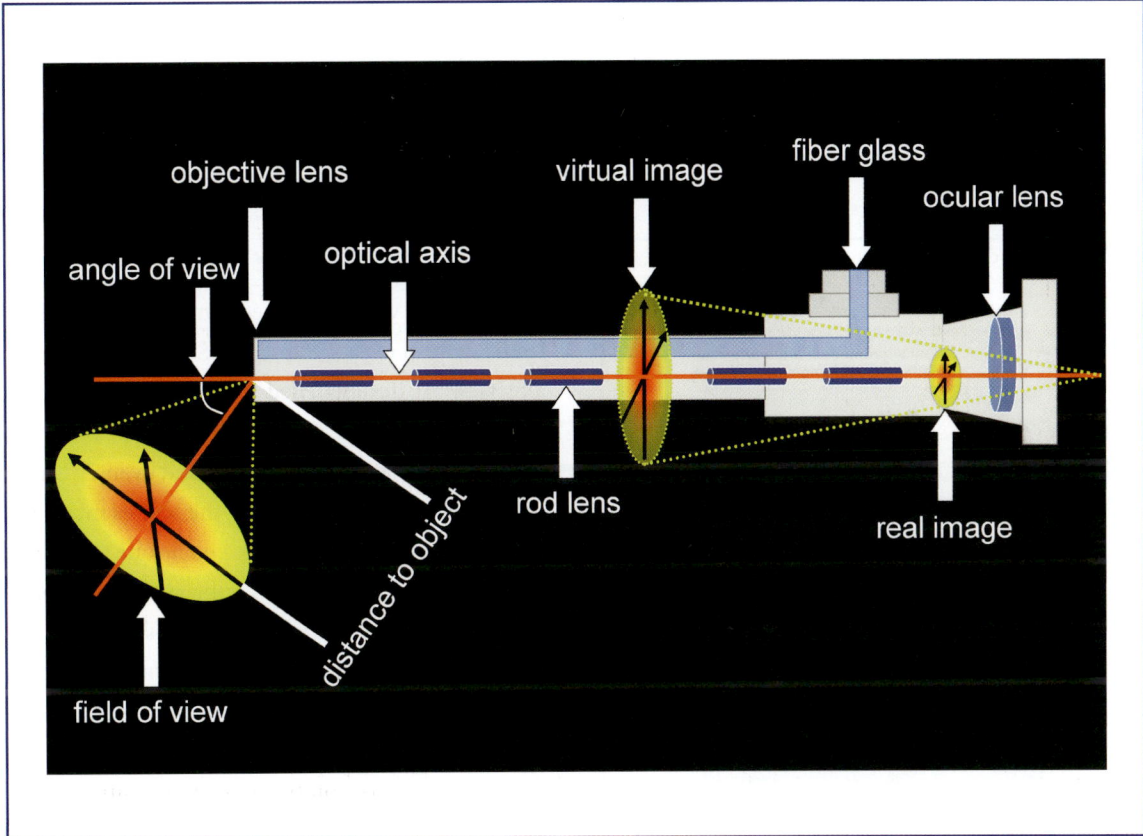

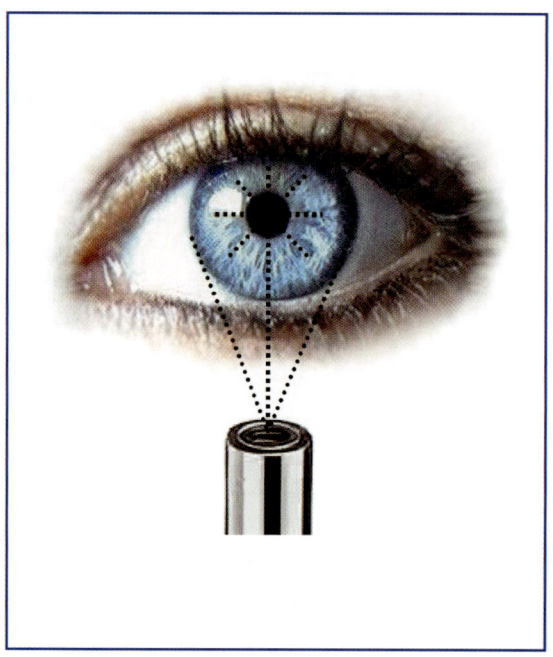

2.18.1.2 Field of View

The field of view (also field of vision) is the angular extent of the observable area that is seen at any given moment. The field of view in scopes for endoscopic surgery can vary from 60° to 82° depending up on the type of instrument. Wider angles of view provide a greater depth of field in the image with better utilization of illumination. A smaller field of view allows the scope to be farther from the tissue, for the same to be observed.

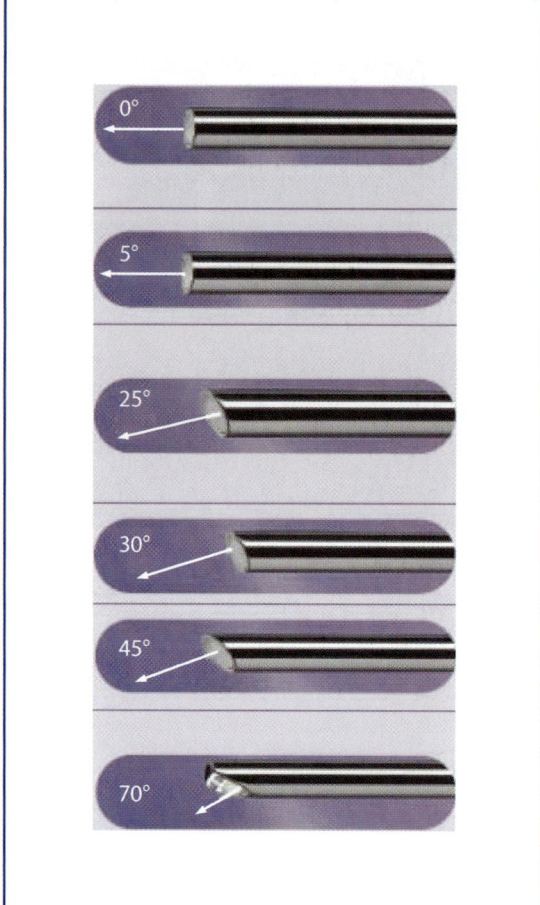

2.18.1.3 Angle of View

The angle of view in scopes can vary with respect to the central axis of the scope. Scopes that offer an axis view are designated as 0° and provide a straight view of the structure in question. Scopes are also available with a 5°, 25°, 30°, 45°, and even 70° angle of view, allowing utilization of the scopes much as a periscope. The off-axis scopes enable one to observe down into the gutters and up the anterior abdominal wall as well as sideways. Off-axis scopes are difficult to work with; however, they provide an excellent means of obtaining close inspection of tissues at difficult angles and positions.

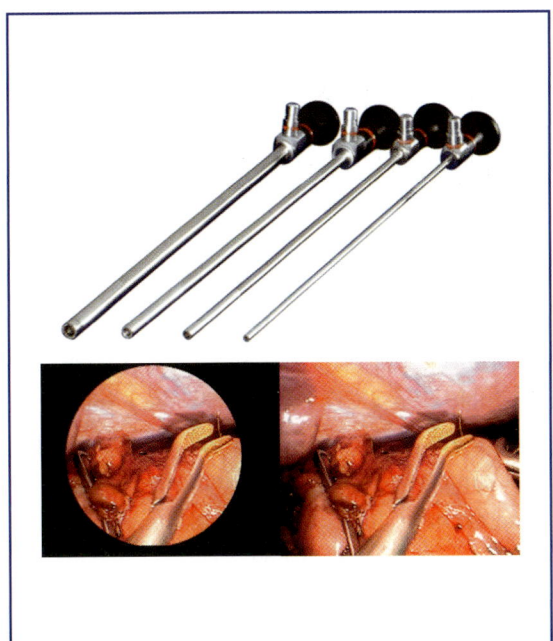

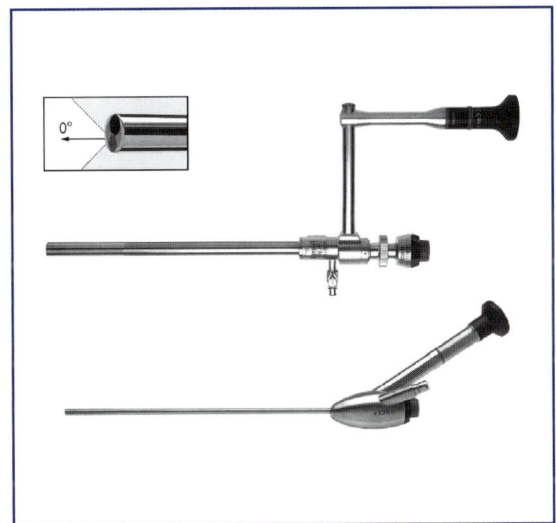

2.18.1.4   Scope Size and Screen Image

The decrease in the size of scopes was an important factor in the advancement of minimally invasive surgery in the pediatric age group. Although scopes are available in sizes from 1.9 mm to 12 mm in diameter, the majority of the procedures are performed using 5- or 10-mm scopes.

When compared to the reduced view obtained in the previous generation of scopes *(left)*, modern 5-mm, full-screen scopes provide a bright, distortion-free, full-screen image *(right)*. In addition, the image size in modern 5-mm scope is equivalent to that obtained by the previous-generation 10-mm scope. (Courtesy of Richard Wolf, Knittlingen, Germany)

2.18.1.5   Operating Scopes

Beside the optical component and the lens system, operating scopes posses an additional work channel that allows the introduction of instruments (between 3.5–5.0 mm in diameter and 220 mm in length) through the scope. These scopes have a 0° angle of view and 85° field of view. Operating scopes have been used frequently in gynecology for tubal ligations; however their use in pediatric surgery has risen with the increasing trend in single-port laparoscopic applications. (Courtesy of Richard Wolf, Knittlingen, Germany)

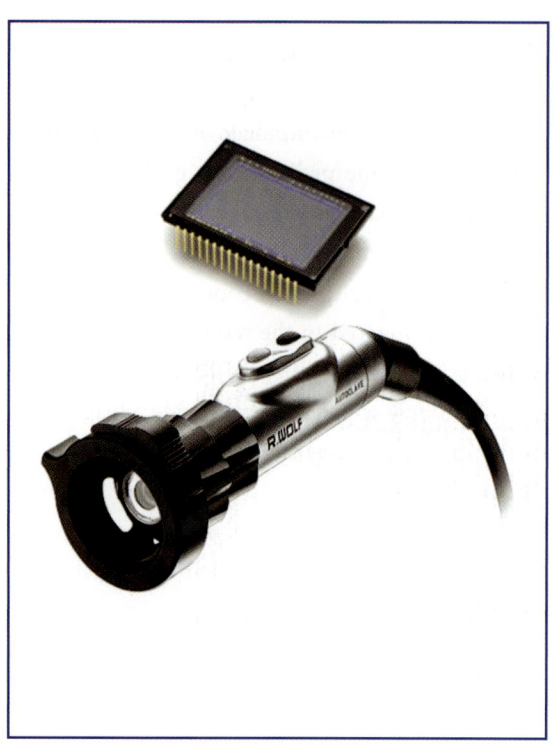

2.18.1.6 Charge Coupled Device (CCD) Video Cameras

Scope cameras are available in either single-chip or three-chip versions (one chip offers 300,000 pixels/cm²). In single-chip CCD cameras, all the three primary colors (red, blue and green) are sensed by a single chip. In three-chip CCD cameras, there are three chips for separate capture and processing of the primary colors.

Single-chip CCD cameras produce images of 450 lines/inch resolution and are ideal for outpatient surgery. On the other hand, three-chip CCD cameras have high fidelity with unprecedented color reproduction to produce images of 750 lines/inch resolution that can be viewed optimally on flat-panel screens and are best suited for endoscopic surgery. (Courtesy of Richard Wolf, Knittlingen, Germany)

2.19   Light Sources

2.19.1   Light-Source Generators and Transmission Pathways

There are two commonly utilized light sources: halogen and xenon. A schematic overview of light transmission is outlined in the diagram (*next page*).

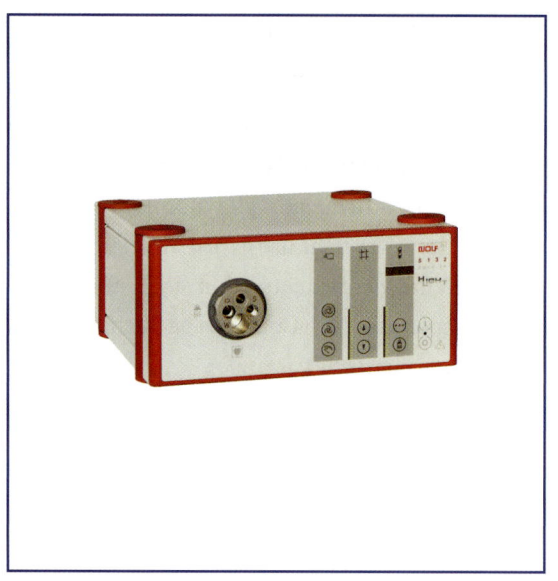

Halogen bulbs (250 W) provide a highly efficient white light source with excellent color rendering. Electrodes in halogen gas lamps are made of tungsten and reach color temperatures up to 5000–5600 K.

Xenon bulbs (300 W) consist of a spherical or ellipsoidal envelope made of quartz glass. The color temperature of a xenon lamp is 6000–6400 K. Xenon bulbs last longer than halogen, but are significantly more expensive. (Courtesy of Richard Wolf, Knittlingen, Germany)

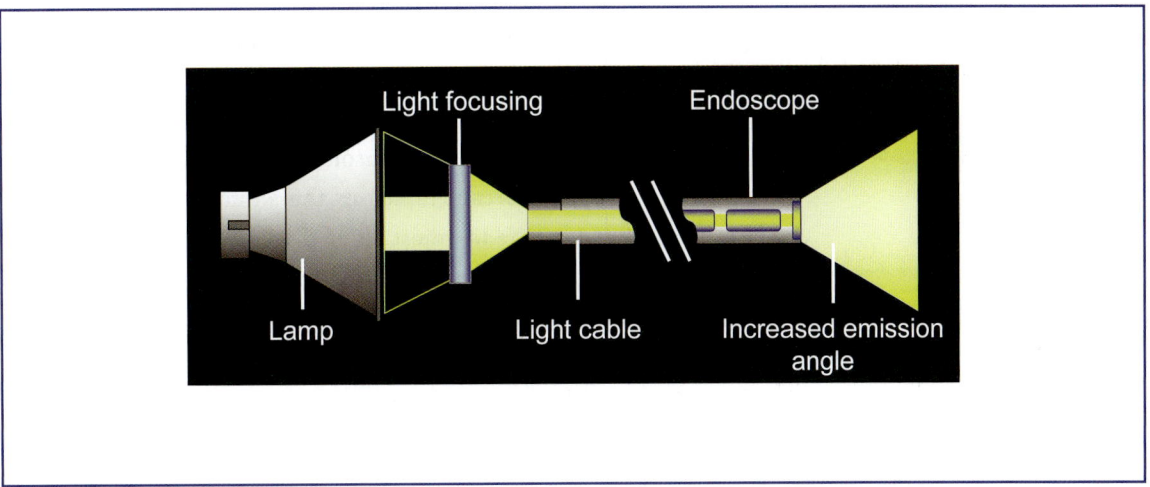

2.19.2 Fiber-Optic Cables for Light Transmission

A fiber-optic cable is used to transmit light from the light source to the scope. Fiber-optic bundles are very flexible and are made of small, 5-μm-diameter fibers. Since individual fibers are subject to breakage, fractured optical cable fibers reduce the capacity to transmit light. To prevent cable breakage, the cable should be handled with care, and inserted and removed from its socket without angling at the flexible as well as the rigid junction. Cables should never be bent at acute angles. Fiber-optic cables should be discarded when less than 75% of the fibers transmit light. (Courtesy of Richard Wolf, Knittlingen, Germany)

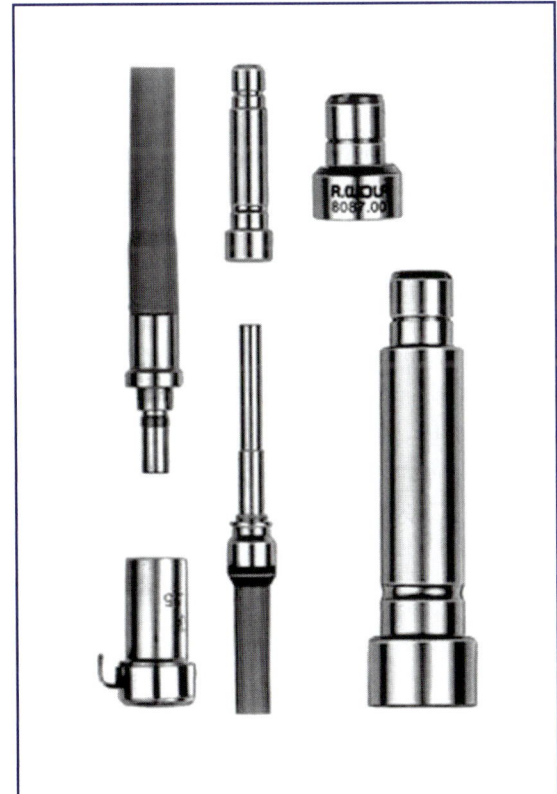

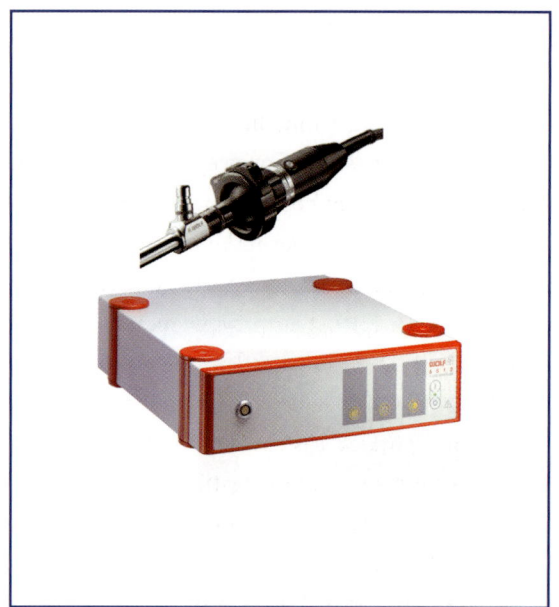

2.19.3   The Concept of White Balancing

White balancing should be performed before inserting the camera inside the abdominal cavity. This is necessary before commencing surgery to diminish the added impurities of color that may be introduced due to a variety of reasons such as: (1) voltage difference, (2) staining of the tip by cleaners, and (3) scratches and wear of the eyepiece.

White balancing is achieved by keeping a white object in front of the scope and activating the appropriate button on the video system or camera. The camera senses the white object as its reference to adjust all of the primary colors (red, blue and green). (Courtesy of Richard Wolf, Knittlingen, Germany)

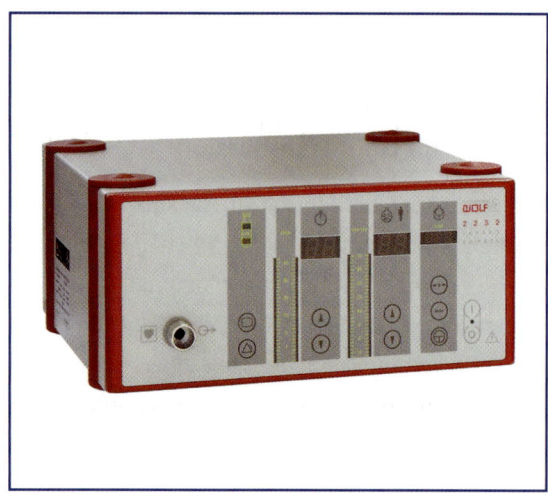

2.20   Insufflation, Irrigation and Aspiration Devices

2.20.1   Insufflation Devices

Modern insufflators automatically monitor and regulate the internal pressure of the abdominal cavity. Insufflators have four clearly visible gauges: (1) a carbon dioxide (CO_2) flow rate indicator (maximum 10 l/min), (2) a CO_2 cylindrical pressure indicator, (3) a total volume of gas delivered indicator, and (4) an intra-abdominal pressure indicator. A filter is placed between the insufflators and sterile tubing attached to ports. The required values for pressure and flow can be set precisely using digital displays. (Courtesy of Richard Wolf, Knittlingen, Germany)

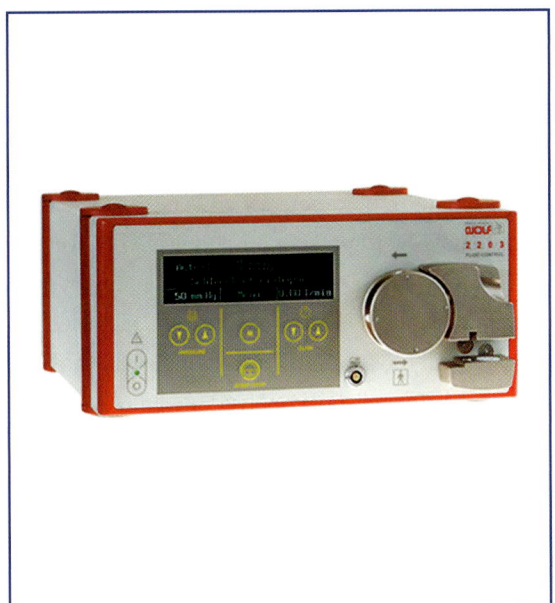

2.20.2 Concepts in Irrigation and Aspiration

Vision is one of the limitations of endoscopic surgery. Blood has the darkest color inside the abdominal cavity and excess of blood therein absorbs most of the light. So, whenever there is bleeding during endoscopic procedures, blood should first be aspirated before irrigating to prevent reduction of vision. Aspiration of fluids and washing of tissues to enable better visualization is accomplished with an irrigation/aspiration system. The instrument that is used to gently spray the irrigation solution is also employed to aspirate the irrigant. Suction/irrigation instruments can also be used for blunt dissection. (Courtesy of Richard Wolf, Knittlingen, Germany)

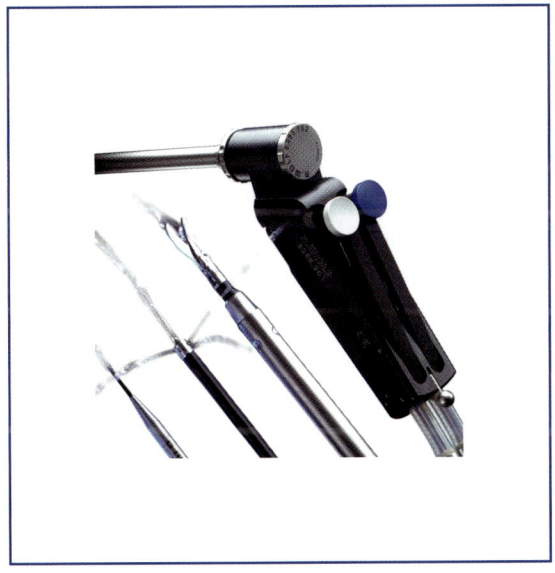

2.20.3 Instruments for Irrigation and Aspiration

Irrigation/aspiration instruments for endoscopic procedures are available in a variety of handle- and tip-form combinations. Furthermore, some hand instruments, especially those designed for electrosurgical dissection, have channels within for aspiration of smoke from the surgical site.

At the time of using suction, it is important to visualize the tip of the irrigation/suction instrument and ensure that it is dipped inside blood or other fluid to be evacuated. If not completely immersed, a loss of insufflated gas will occur. (Courtesy of Richard Wolf, Knittlingen, Germany)

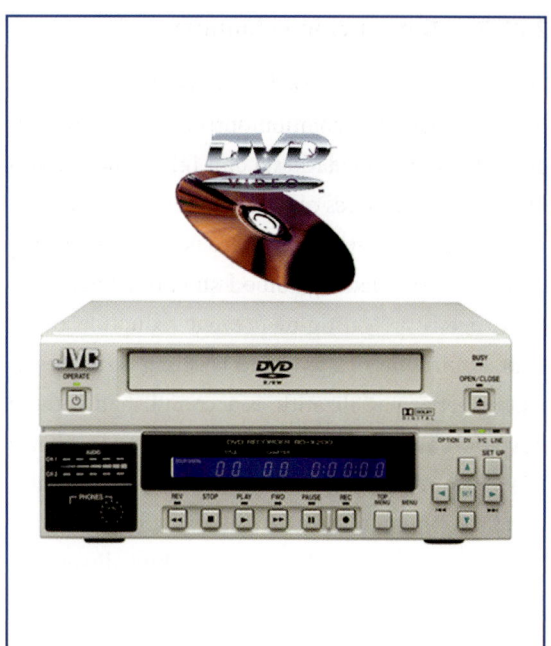

2.21 Video and Data Storage Equipment

2.21.1 Digital Video Recorders

Modern endoscopic surgery towers are generally equipped with digital video disc (DVD) recorders (DVRs), which enable recording of a procedure in digital quality. The procedures are recorded on commercially available DVDs, which can later be viewed on normal DVD players or edited on personal computers.

DVRs have evolved into devices that are feature rich and provide services that exceed the simple recording of video images that was previously achieved using video cassette recorders (VCRs). DVR systems provide a multitude of advanced functions, including video searches by event and time.

2.21.2 Digital Video Printers

A variety of printers from small print format to large A5 print format are available. These printers offer high-resolution prints, quick, 20-s print time, and high-quality, curl-free prints at 400 dpi resolution. Most modern printers come with a four-frame memory. The new compact design of printers allows for easy integration with other video equipment. Small, compact printers are ideal for the office setting, but large-print format printers are preferable in the operating room.

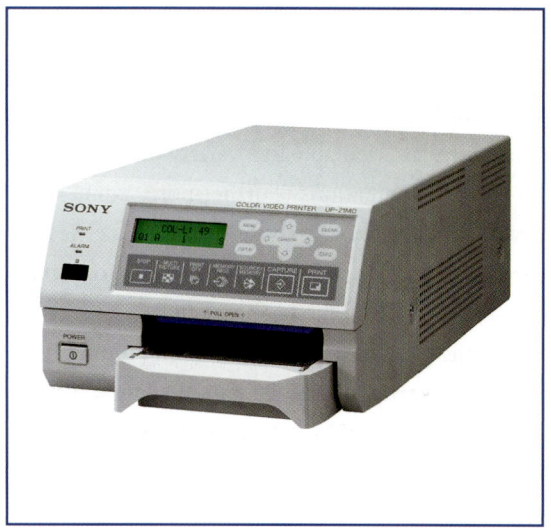

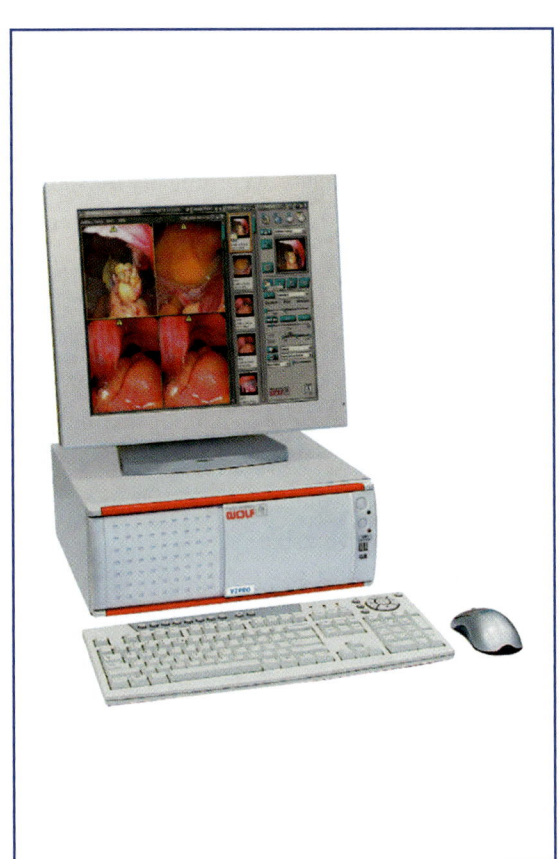

2.21.3   Digital Video Managers

These are computer-based systems that display intuitive patient information screens that allow for quick and easy input of vital data. The data is stored on hard drives and can be viewed as images or videos, and may be stored or deleted. The editing screen enables viewing and editing procedures.

Current systems allow storage of up to 50 patient archives for multiple procedures. These systems are compatible with personal computers and hospital network software. (Courtesy of Richard Wolf, Knittlingen, Germany)

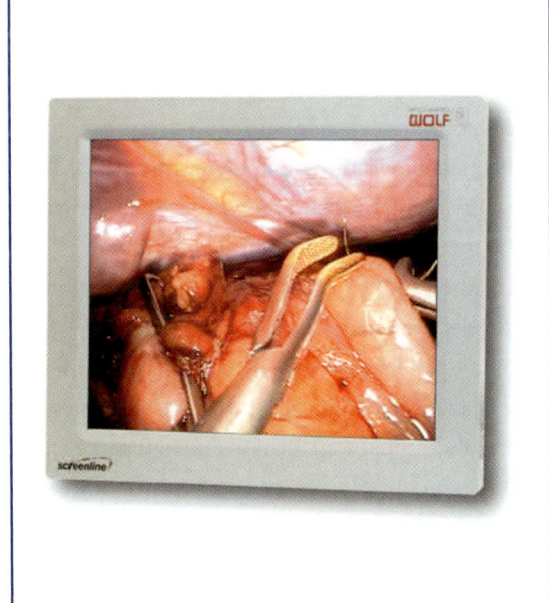

2.21.4   Flat-Panel Screens

The industry offers a variety of high-quality LCD monitors with ultrasharp detail and perfect color rendition. The 14-inch medical and non-medical-grade monitors including stand-alone and built-in audio speaker are ideal for office endoscopy; however, 19-, 21-, and 23-inch medical-grade monitors are presently an integral component of video carts and are ideal for endoscopic surgery visualizations. Due to their light weight, flat-panel monitors can be held by swivel arms on video carts. (Courtesy of Richard Wolf, Knittlingen, Germany)

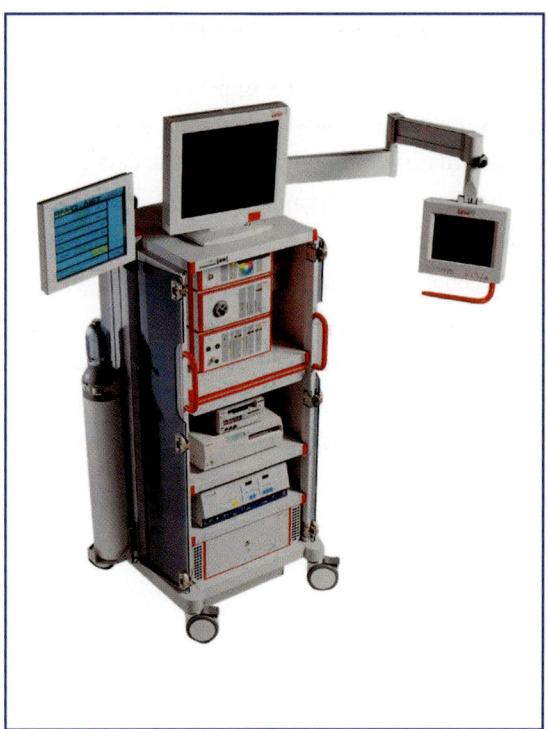

2.21.5 Endoscopic Surgery Towers

Endoscopic surgery towers are mobile carts that house the equipment. Their mobility enables the placement of equipment according to the procedure and position of the team. Standard towers consist of:

1. Monitors.
2. Video processing equipment.
3. Light-source generator.
4. Gas (CO_2) insufflator.
5. Aspiration/suction device.
6. Documentation equipment.
7. Stand for CO_2 cylinder.

(Courtesy of Richard Wolf, Knittlingen, Germany)

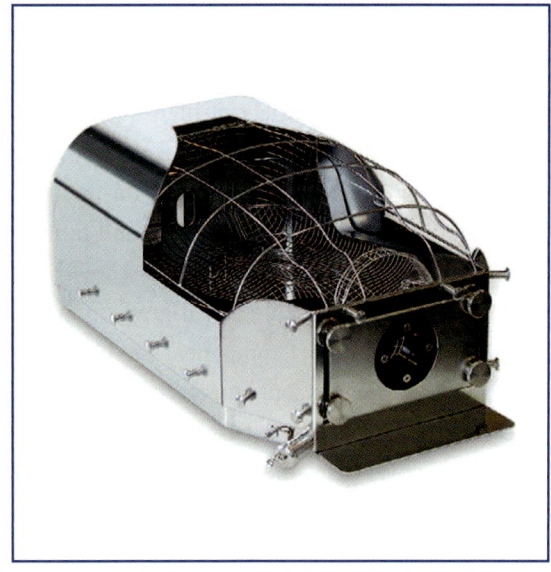

2.22 Trainers for Endoscopic Surgery

2.22.1 Pelvitrainers

A realistic surgical training requires an anatomical model that allows the easy integration of animal organs. The regular repetition of procedures demands quick preparation of the training setup with optimal fixation of the organs within the pelvitrainers.

Modern trainers such as the Tübingen MIC Trainer™ (Richard Wolf, Knittlingen, Germany) have realistic anatomical shape that simulates the frontal abdominal wall of an insufflated patient, and covers that deliver a reality effect for the introduction of the trocars and ports. (Courtesy of Richard Wolf, Knittlingen, Germany)

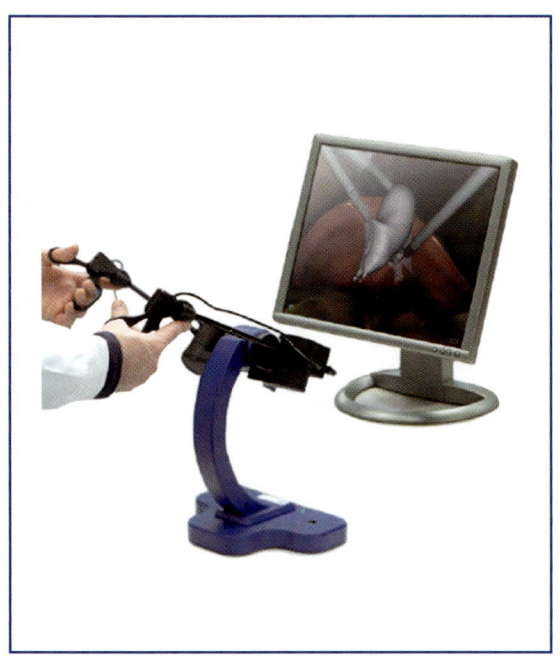

2.22.2   Virtual Reality Simulators

The LapSim® System (Surgical Science Sweden, Göteburg, Sweden) is a digital training aid that replaces the vulnerable patient with expendable pixels. By recreating digitally the procedures and environment of endoscopic surgery, LapSim® provides an effective training tool for endoscopic surgeons. Augmenting surgical training with simulation offers great promise because maneuvers can be practiced over and over until they are mastered. (Courtesy of Surgical Science Sweden, Göteborg, Sweden)

NOTE

Tyco Healthcare is now Covidien (Covidien, Mansfield, MA, USA) with endoscopic surgery product brands- Autosuture (division of United States Surgical -USS), Valleylab and Syneture.

Recommended Literature

1. Chmarra MK, Grimbergen CA, Dankelman J (2007) Systems for tracking minimally invasive surgical instruments. Minim Invasive Ther Allied Technol 17:1–13
2. Mercy CM, Cooke DT, Chandra V, Shafi BM, Tavak-kolizadeh A, Varghese TK (2007) The road to innovation: emerging technologies in surgery. Bull Am Coll Surg 92:19–33
3. Eriksen JR, Grantcharov T (2005) Objective assessment of laparoscopic skills using a virtual reality stimulator. Surg Endosc 19:1216–1219

3 Ergonomics of Endoscopic Surgery

STEVEN Z. RUBIN AND MARCOS BETTOLLI

3.1 Introduction

3.1.1 Indications for Endoscopic Surgery

There must be a demonstrable advantage to the patient (i.e., rapid return to normal function; cosmetic advantage; decreased complications).

3.1.2 Requirement for Procedures

Endoscopic surgery requires advanced surgical and nursing training in the purchase and use of the equipment and instrumentation.

3.1.3 Complications

Most are related to equipment misuse/failure and improper surgical access.

3.2 Definition and Aim

Ergonomics is the application of scientific information to the design of objects, systems, and the environment for human use (International Ergonomic Association). The aim of ergonomics in endoscopic surgery is to improve human performance, decrease surgical fatigue, and minimize the dangers and disadvantages. Thus, operating room design requires input from an ergonomic expert, and surgeons and nurses trained in endoscopic surgery.

3.3 Operating Room Requirements

1. Adequate room size.
2. Room/endoscopic surgery light sources.
3. Multiple adjustable and mobile monitors.
4. Carbon dioxide insufflation.
5. Endoscopic suction and irrigation.
6. Electrosurgery, laser, harmonic scalpel.
7. Radiological imaging.
8. Anesthetic equipment.
9. Specialized operating table.

3.4 Manpower Requirements

1. Surgeon trained in endoscopic surgery.
2. Surgical assistant experienced in use of the camera.
3. Second surgical assistant.
4. Nurses trained in endoscopic surgery.
5. Anesthetist trained in endoscopic surgery.

3.5   Technical Requirements

1. Functional instruments compatible with the size of the patient and the surgeon.
2. A monitor directly facing the surgeon in a line so that the level of vision is neutral or with a slight inclination of cervical spine (Fig. 1).
3. Surgeon, assistant, and nurse on same side of the patient.
4. Triangulation of the ports with the camera centrally placed.
5. Mechanized assistance for camera and retraction.
6. Needle driver port in the same axis (0°) as the suture line.

Figure 3.1

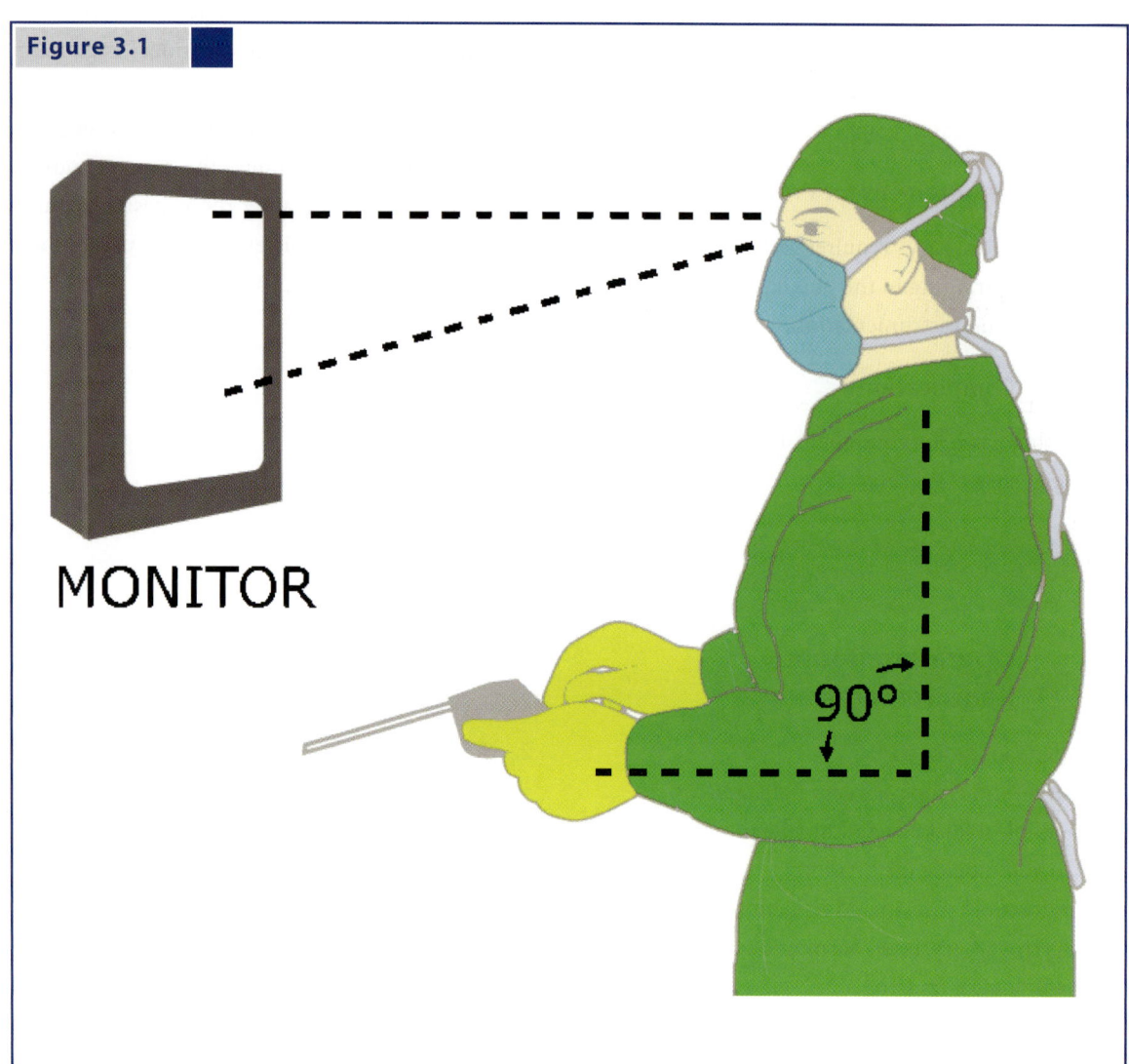

MONITOR

90°

Line of vision

3.6   Robotics

The advantages of robotic systems are many since they overcome many of the obstacles of endoscopic surgery. They increase dexterity, restore proper hand-eye coordination and an ergonomic position, and improve visualization. In addition, these systems make possible surgeries that were previously technically difficult. However, at present there is no evidence-based ergonomic advantage for robotics in pediatric endoscopic surgery.

3.7   Improvement of Team Performance

1. Using training courses and human reliability analysis.
2. Using a surgical team; this is better than one bimanual surgeon.
3. The surgeon is preferably seated.
4. Using ultrasound, computed tomography, and magnetic resonance imaging to display vessels, nerves and tumors.
5. Team review of advanced procedures both pre- and postoperatively.
6. Improve procedure visualization using overhead illumination, gravity, and optimizing camera position.

3.8   The Future

1. Improved ergonomic operating room and equipment design with integrated systems under the control of the operating surgeon.
2. The development of an endoscopic pointer using ultrasound, computed tomography, and magnetic resonance imaging to identify vessels and anatomical relationships.
3. Instruments that intraoperatively adjust to the surgeon's hand size and the size of the patient.

3.9 Operating Staff Positions and Ergonomics

3.9.1 Single-Monitor Option

If a single monitor or flat screen panel is used, it should be positioned suitably to allow sufficient vision to the operating team (Fig. 2). This option is practical when the entire operating team stands on one side.

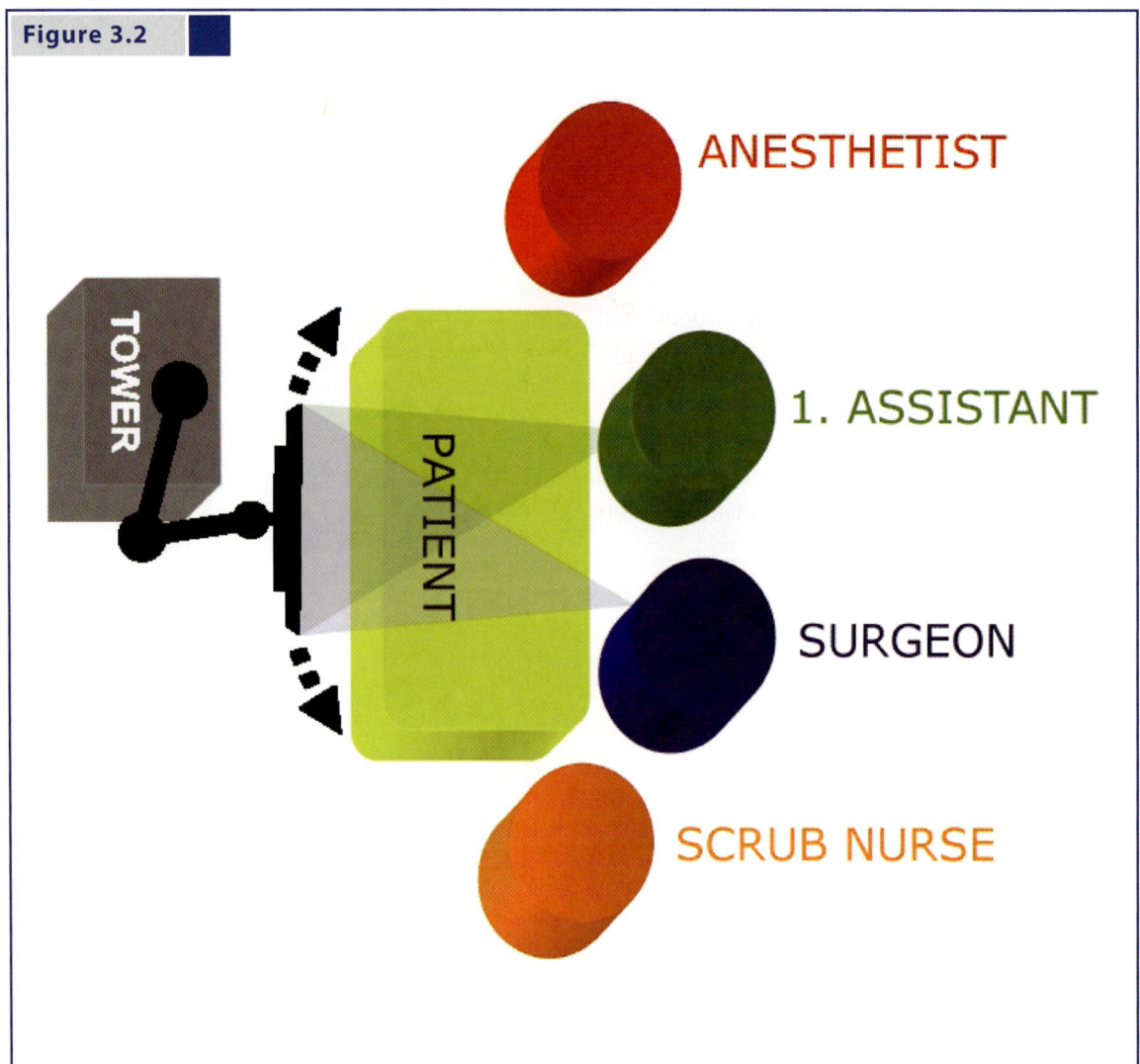

Figure 3.2

Single-monitor option

3.9.2   Dual-Monitor Option

If the operating team is dispersed around the operating table it is advisable to have two monitors so that the entire team has visible access irrespective of their position (Fig. 3).

Figure 3.3

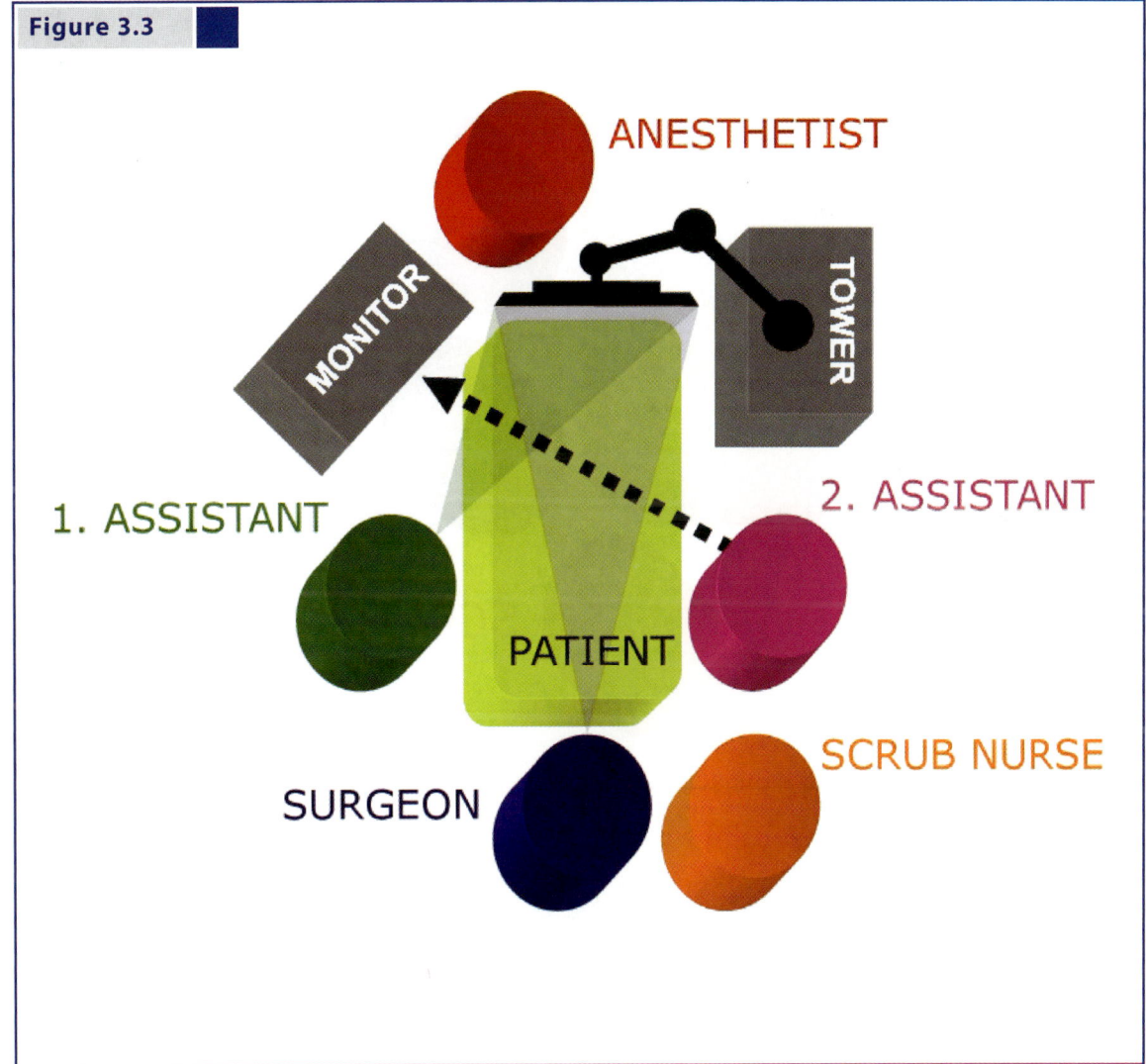

Dual-monitor option

3.9.3   Ventilator vs. Monitor Placement

It is often difficult to position the tower toward the head of the patient since this place is occupied by the anesthetist and the ventilation equipment. A swivel flat screen is helpful to overcome this problem (Fig. 4).

Figure 3.4

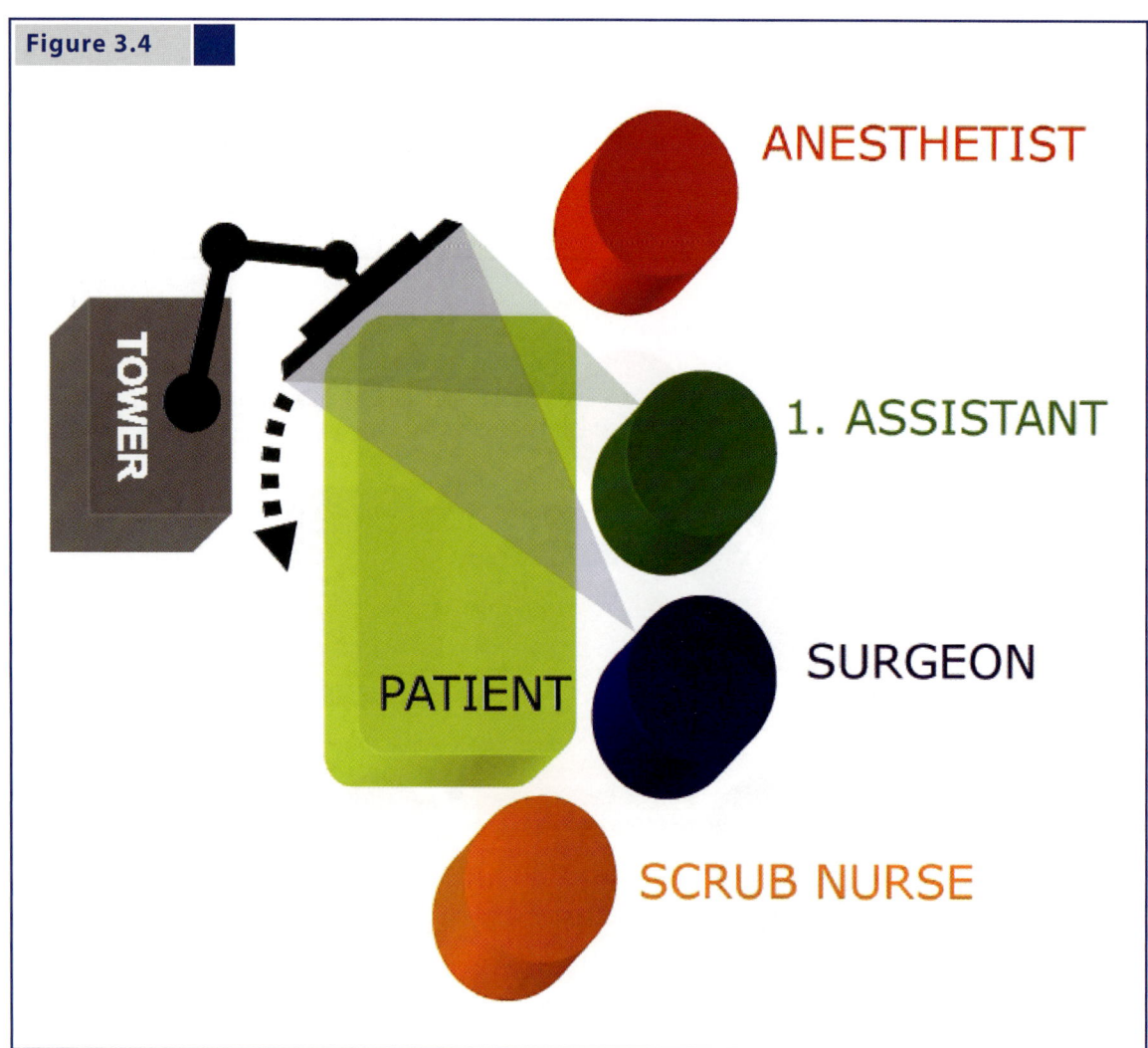

Ventilator vs. monitor placement

Recommended Literature

1. Catchpole K, Mishra A, Handa A, McCulloch P (2008) Teamwork and error in the operation room: analysis of skills and roles. Ann Surg 247:699–706
2. Hanna GB (1999) Ergonomics of task performance in endoscopic surgery. In: Bax NMA, Georgeson KE, Najmaldin A, Valla J-S (eds) Endoscopic Surgery in Children. Springer-Verlag, Berlin, pp 37–47
3. Zehetner J, Kaltenbacher A, Wayand W, Shamiyeh A (2006) Screen height as an ergonomic factor in laparoscopic surgery. Surg Endosc 20:139–141

4 Instrument Ergonomics

Amulya K. Saxena

4.1 Endoscopic Surgery and Surgeons

Although endoscopic surgery has proven beneficial for patients because it entails less trauma and a shorter hospital stay, the procedure is quite strenuous for the surgeon. Often, limited knowledge of port placement and its dynamics accentuates this problem and adds to technical challenges faced during surgery. Surgeons often experience muscle fatigue and injuries in their hands and upper extremity because of awkward grasping and arm positioning over long periods of time.

4.2 Ergonomics and Instruments

The present working conditions for endoscopic surgeons are not satisfactory and there is a clear need for more awareness regarding instrument ergonomics. Both manufacturers and surgeons focus almost entirely on the functionality of the instrument tip, leaving the hand–handle interface unattended. Surgeons are commonly too concentrated on performing the task to notice the inconveniences of the instrument during surgery.

4.2.1 Paradoxical Port Movement

The working ports inserted into the abdominal cavity have a tendency to move in different directions since the area securing the port lies approximately in the mid point. In addition, the weight of the port is not evenly distributed, which further accentuates the various degrees of movement.

Although ports are fixed at the point of entry into the abdomen, paradoxical movements of the port are encountered every time the instruments are changed. Coordination of the surgical assistant or the scrub nurse is important to secure the ports (if required) during introduction of the instruments.

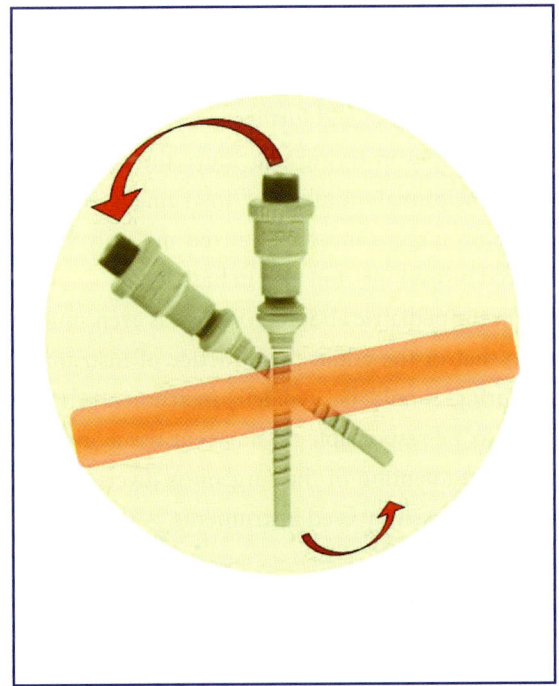

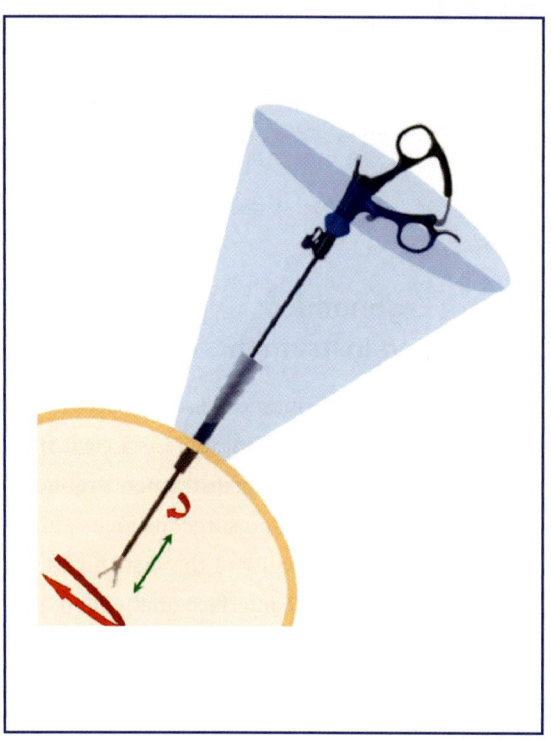

4.2.2   Working Field Perimeters

Working ports have a cone-shaped field inside and outside the abdomen. The degree of movements of both of the fields should be borne in mind when introducing the ports through the body cavities. The limitations of work fields require good understanding so as to enable the easy manipulation of tissue. Narrow work field parameters can lead to extreme technical difficulties when suturing and knot tying. An optimal work field must be worked out before any endoscopic surgery procedure is carried out.

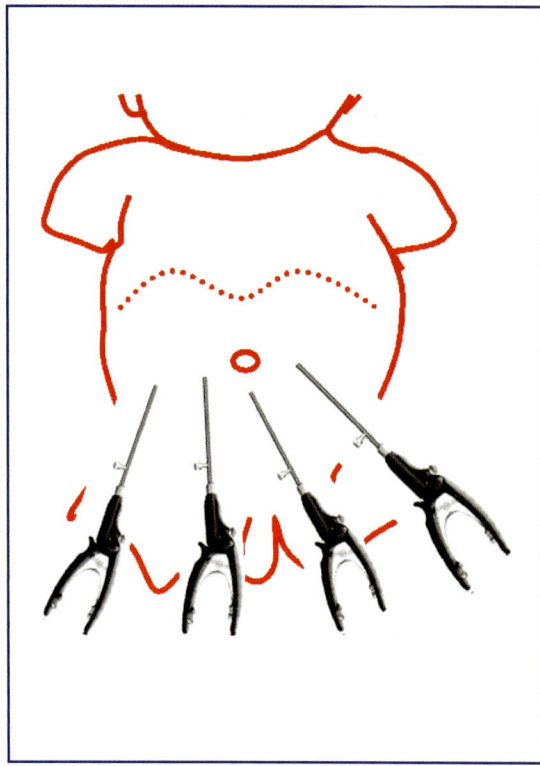

4.2.3   Instrument Cluttering

Crowding of instruments in the abdominal cavity does not provide better access. It only leads to increased confusion and further increases the technical difficulties in trying to achieve the desired objective. Optimal number of instruments for endoscopic surgery must be utilized not only in advanced procedures, but also in basic ones.

In the pediatric abdomen, which is even smaller than that of the adult, this practice of instrument cluttering should be avoided. Instrument cluttering may be responsible for adjacent tissue injuries, since the attention of the surgeon is diverted away from the passively used instruments.

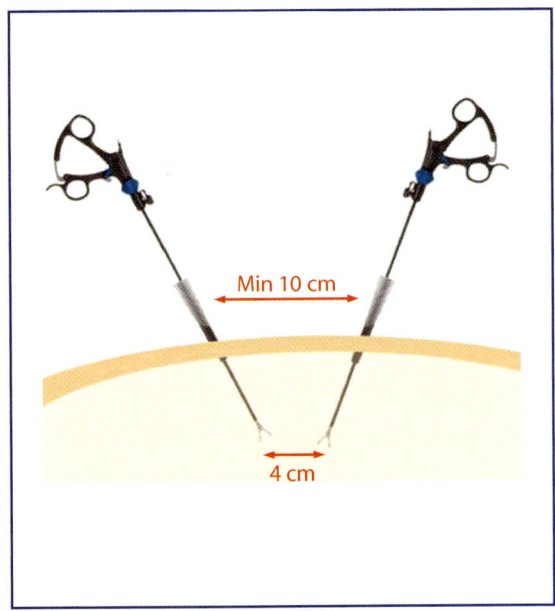

4.2.4 Working Angles

Optimum working angles are necessary for desired tissue manipulation. However, it is of paramount importance to have the best working angles in endoscopic procedures that require suturing and knotting.

A distance of 10 cm between the working ports outside the body cavity, if possible, provides a relatively good suturing field. However, inside the body cavity, a working distance of 4 cm is desired at the point where the tips of the needle holders meet to enable comfortable suturing and knotting.

4.2.5 Handle Design

The handle is the instrument's interface, where the surgeon can interact with the instrument. A good indication of a functional instrument is when the surgeon can forget about the tool and just concentrate on the job. The hand–handle interface should be "invisible" so that the tool can function merely as an extension of the arm.

4.2.6 Power Grip and Precision

The classic categorization of grips distinguishes power grips from precision grips. A power grip requires great force but little precision and vice versa. Both power-, precision, and combination grips function optimally when the hand is in its neutral position. This characteristic of grips stresses the importance of keeping the wrist in a neutral position.

4.2.7 Hand and Wrist Movements

The most important positioning of the hand is called the neutral position, or the position of rest. This occurs typically when the hand is resting in a palm-medial position with fingers slightly flexed. It is the most comfortable hand position and it is also the situation in which the hand can perform optimally with both force and precision.

4.2.8 Adaptation for Various Hand Sizes

The instrument handle should provide usability for all surgeons or be adjustable to all its users' various hand sizes, as individual fitting is often not possible with today's mass-production. For endoscopic instruments, hand size is an important determinant of difficulty of use. Individuals with small hands experience problems more commonly than those with large hand sizes.

4.2.8.1 Handle Grip Diameter

The handle should be of such a size that it permits slight overlap of the thumb and fingers of a surgeon with small hands. A handle diameter of 40–50 mm can provide sufficient support as well as allow strength to be applied for most surgeons. If the handle is too small it will not allow proper force exertion, but at the same time, strength deteriorates with a handle size above 50 mm.

4.2.8.2 Handle Length and Cross-Section

Handle lengths should be at least 115 mm and allow clearance for extra large hands. If gloves are to be used, extra length must be added depending on glove type and thickness. Handles of circular cross-section (and appropriate diameter, e.g., 30–50 mm) are the most comfortable to grip.

4.2.9 Buttons and Springs

In endoscopic surgery the result of the procedure is determined by the surgeon's ability to keep the instrument steady during manipulation. Awkwardly positioned buttons and springs that require great force to be operated can result in jeopardizing the movements of the instrument tip. It should be possible for the user to operate buttons and springs without major repositioning of the fingers.

4.2.10 Multifunctionality of Handles

Putting too many functions in one handle can render its use more difficult to learn, harder to remember, or simply confusing for surgeons. It is especially important to keep the functionality of the handle simple when the task itself is complicated, as in endoscopic surgery.

When it comes to endoscopic surgical instruments, less is really a lot more.

Recommended Literature

1. Berguer R, Hreljac A (2004) The relationship between hand size and difficulty using surgical instruments: A survey of 726 laparoscopic surgeons. Surg Endosc 18:508–512
2. van Veelan MA, Meijer DW, Goossens RHM, Snijders CJ, Jakimowicz JJ (2001) Improved usability of a new handle design for laparoscopic dissection forceps. Surg Endosc 16:201—207
3. Vereczkel A, Bubb H, Feussner H (2003) Laparoscopic surgery and ergonomics – it's time to think of ourselves as well. Surg Endosc 17:1680–1682

5 Suturing Techniques

Lutz Stroedter

5.1 Endoscopic Suturing

The endoscopic knots presently practiced are basically a modification of knots used by seamen, fishermen, weavers, or hangmen.

There are three stages of knot tying:

1. configuration (tying),
2. shaping (drawing), and
3. securing (locking or snuggling).

For a knot to be perfect, all the stages of knot tying should be accurate.

5.2 Parameters Influencing Intracorporeal Suturing

1. Angle of the instruments at the suture area.
2. Space around the suture site.
3. Length of the suture.
4. Constant and stable view and quality of the screen picture.
5. Angle of the needle in the needle holder.
6. Angle of the needle to be passed through the tissue.
7. Conflicts of the needle holder with other instruments.
8. Natural bias of the suture.
9. Tension of the tissue to be approximated.
10. Personal skill and technique.

5.3 Endoscopic Needle Shapes

Half-circle needles are too large to pass through the ports. Flattened needle forms are preferred to overcome the shape and size disparity of half-circle needles. Ski-shaped needles are the most reliable ones for endoscopic suturing and combine the advantages of the curved and flattened designs.

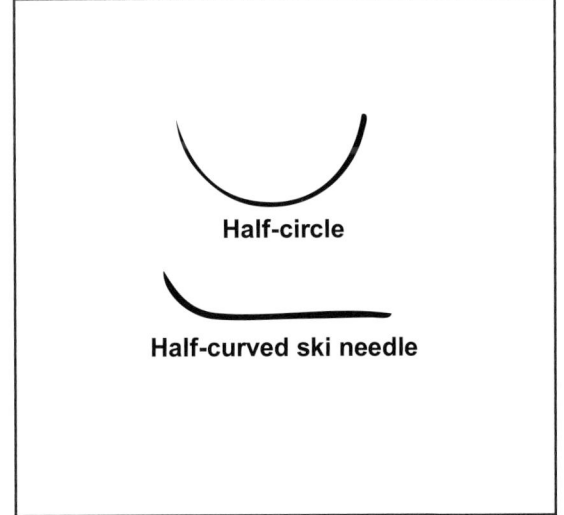

Half-circle

Half-curved ski needle

5.4 Endoscopic Suture Materials

Sterile, packed, absorbable and nonabsorbable suture materials are available for endoscopic procedures:

1. Polydiaxone (PDS™ ‡) is a monofilament, absorbable, long-lasting, and strong suture material.
2. Polyglactin (Vicryl™ ‡) is a plaited, absorbable, medium-lasting, and strong suture material.
3. Polyester (Ethibond™ ‡) and silk. Polyester is a plaited, nonabsorbable, strong suture material for permanent organ fixation.
4. Polypropylene (Prolene™ ‡) is a monofilament, nonabsorbable suture that can also be used for permanent fixation.

    (‡ Ethicon, Somerville, NJ, USA)

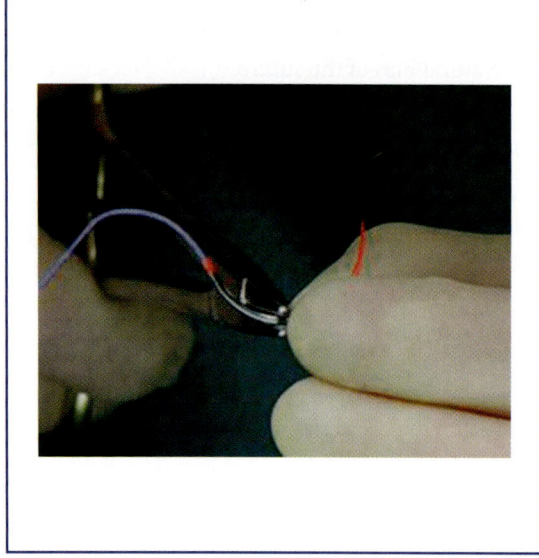

5.4.1 Ski Needle

Ski needles are available in different sizes and armed with different suture material. The surgeon can bend the proximal two-thirds of a normal circled needle and convert it into a ski needle.

5.4.2   Extracorporeal Knot Tying

Extracorporeal knot tying is a method of avoiding the difficult and time-consuming skill of intracorporeal knot tying, and is equally effective. The knot is tied outside the body and then slipped inside using a knot-pusher device. The suture has to be long enough (45–90 cm) to pass from outside the port to the target tissue and back out through the port. The only disadvantage is the wastage of suture material.

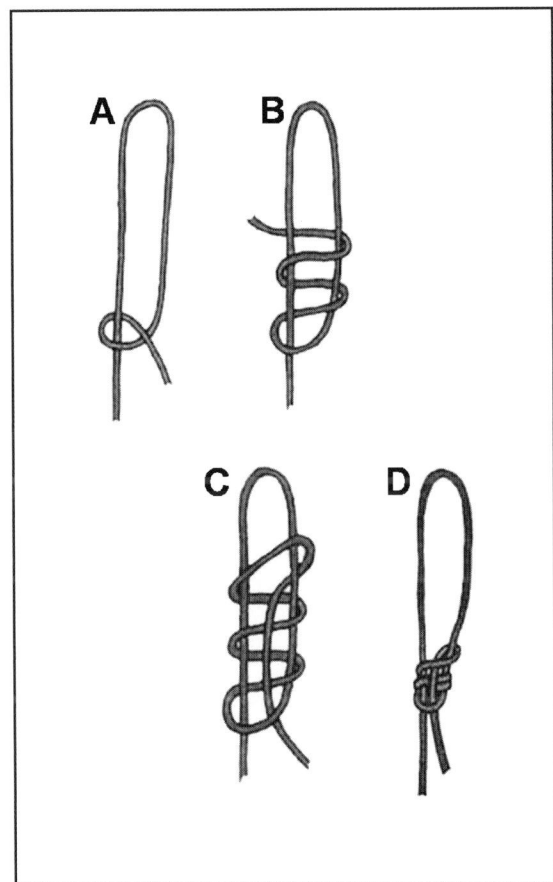

5.4.2.1   Types of Extracorporeal Knots

Extracorporeal knots are normal single- or double-hitch knots followed by one or two single-hitch knots, all of which are slid down separately, like in open surgery. However, extracoporeal tied slip knots can also be employed. The most commonly used extracorporeal tied slip knots are the Roeder knot (see figure for technique), Meltzer slip knot, and the Tayside knot.

5.4.2.2 Extracorporeal Knot-Tying Technique

Please see Figs. 1–6.

Figure 5.1

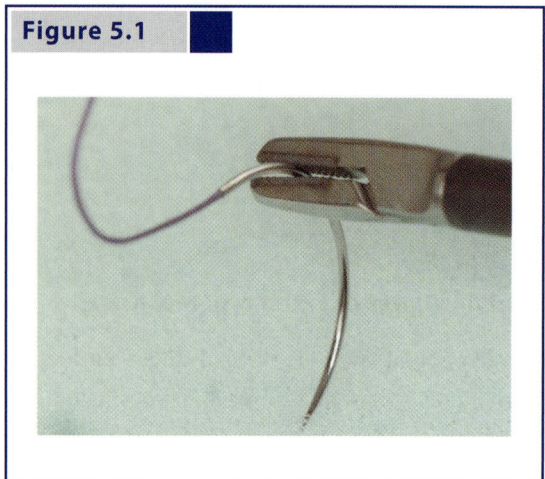

The full-length suture is introduced and the tissue is approximated with the suture

Figure 5.2

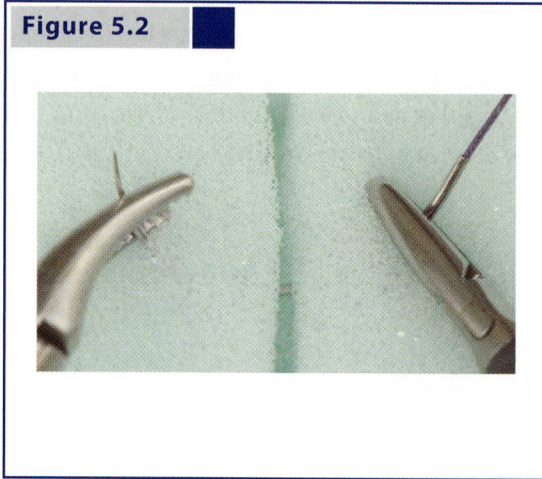

The suture is retrieved from the same port where it was introduced. The suture site should be observed on the monitor to avoid excessive tension and tears of the tissue

Figure 5.3

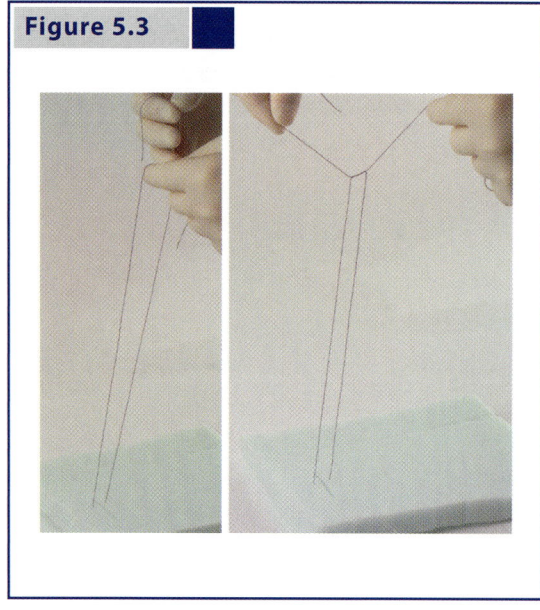

The suture ends are tied extracorporeally

Figure 5.4

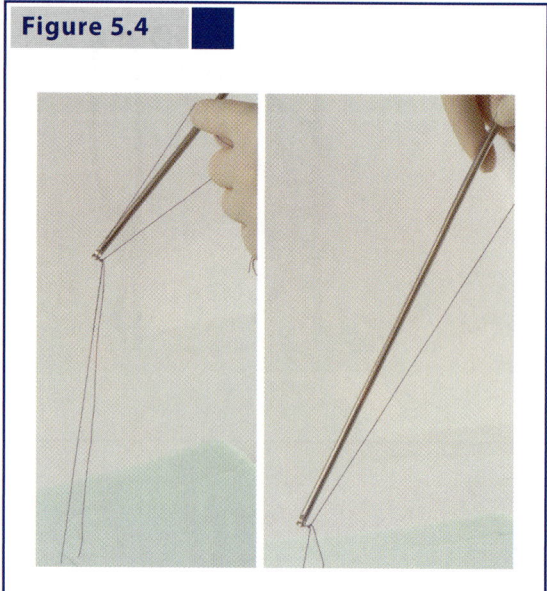

Holding both the sutures in one hand, the knot is then pushed using a knot-pusher

Figure 5.5

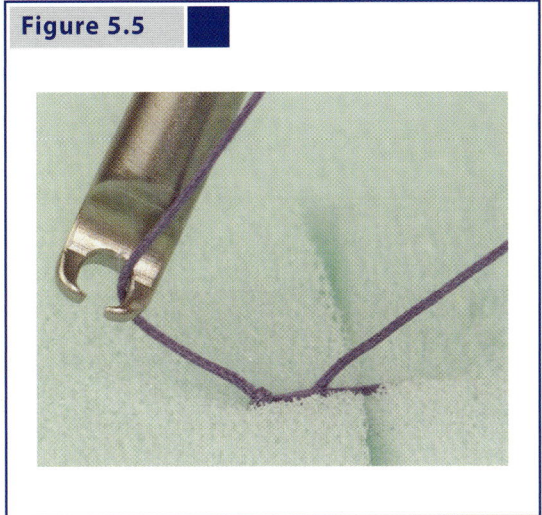

Figure 5.6

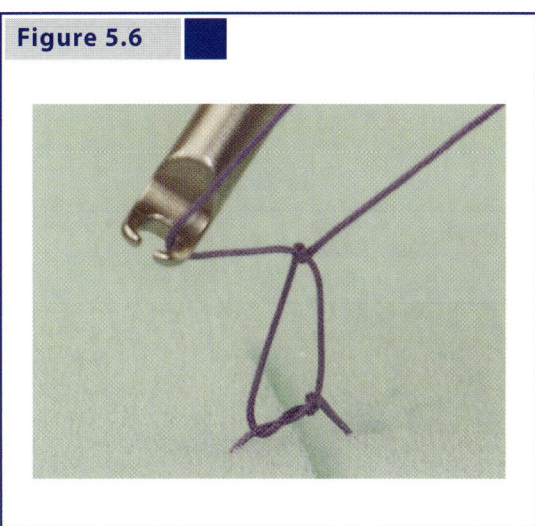

Care should be taken to direct the knot-pusher away from the wound edge

The second knot is tied and pushed holding one suture end under slight tension

5.4.3 Intracorporeal Knot Tying

Intracorporeal knots are tied with the help of a needle holder within the body cavity. The suture should have a minimum length of approx 10 cm and should not exceed 20 cm for comfortable tying.

There are five types of intracorporeal knots:

- square knot
- surgeon's knot
- tumble square knot
- Dundee jamming knot
- Aberdeen termination knot

5.4.3.1 Tips for Intracorporeal Knot Tying

1. If the tissue is under tension and a double wrap is insufficient to hold the tension, two single wraps can be made to create a slip knot.
2. Never pull the needle in the needle holder when not sighted on the monitor. This can lead to tissue damage.
3. Do not pull the needle to tighten the suture. This can cause the suture to detach from the needle.
4. Tying intracorporeal knots is easiest when the instruments meet at an angle of 45–80° at the target tissue.

5.4.3.2   Intracorporeal Suturing with a Half-Circle Needle

Please see Figs. 7 and 8.

Figure 5.7

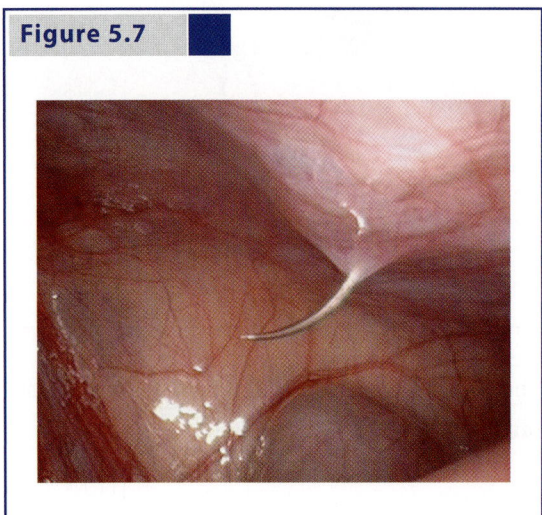

Figure 5.8

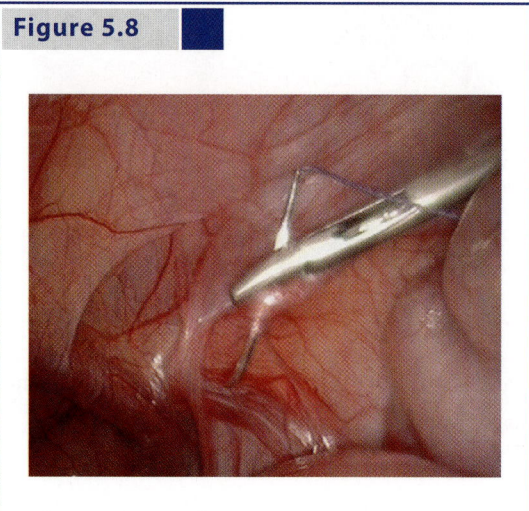

Half-circle needles are too large to pass through the ports and can be introduced directly through the abdominal wall

The needle is grasped and the suture is tied intra-corporeally. After this, the needle can be removed either (a) back through the abdominal wall or (b) through the port site along with the port as a single unit (with loss of insufflation in this case)

5.4.3.3 Intracorporeal Knot-Tying Technique

Please see Figs. 9–14.

Figure 5.9

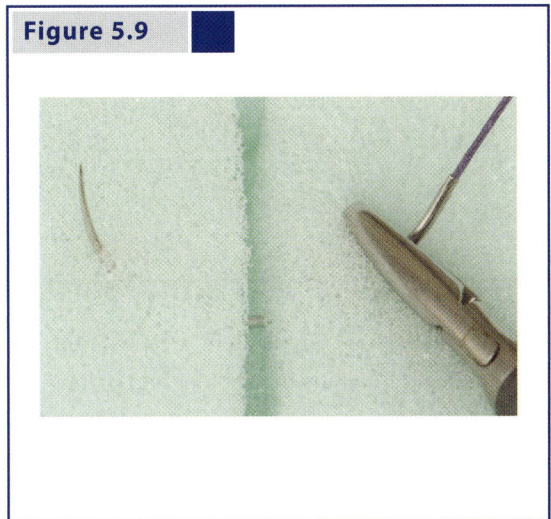

The needle is approximated. The suture is passed through the tissue with the needle held by the dominant needle holder

Figure 5.10

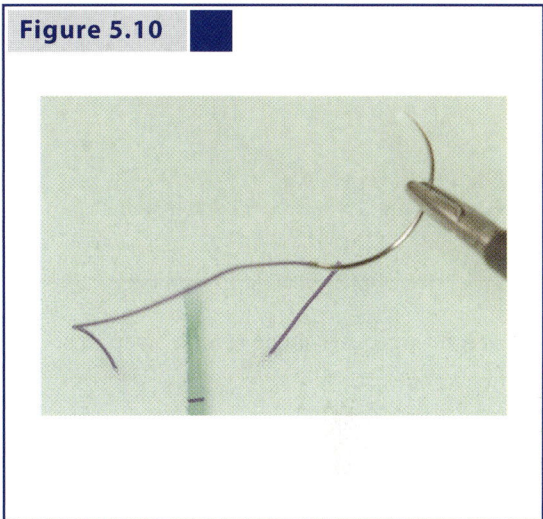

The needle is received by the nondominant needle holder and pulled so that it can be grasped by the dominant needle holder. The suture is pulled and laid in the form of a tension-free C-loop

Figure 5.11

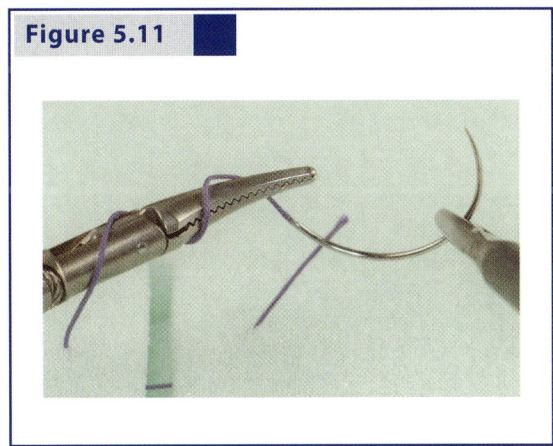

With the needle held in the dominant needle holder, the suture is then wrapped twice over the nondominant needle holder

Figure 5.12

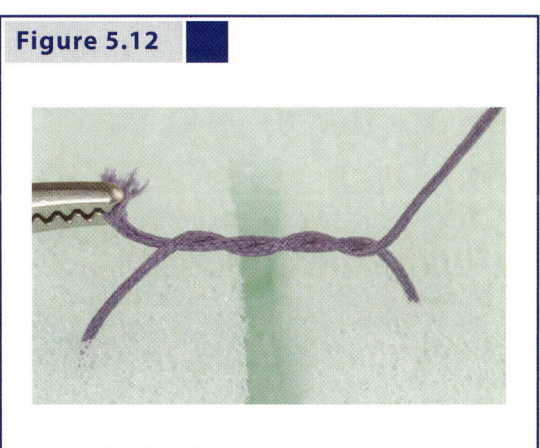

The nondominant needle holder is used to grasp the tail of the suture and pull to cinch down the knot

Figure 5.13

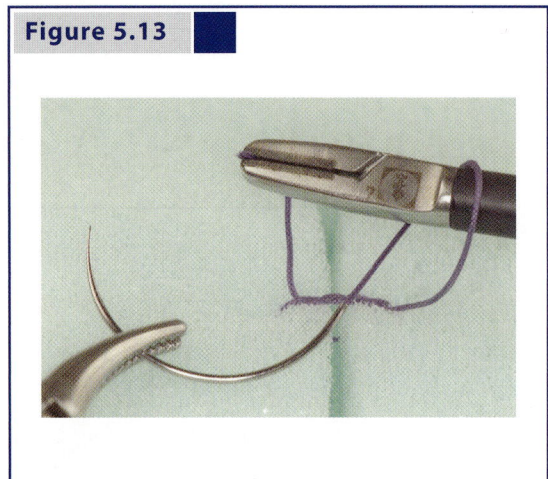

Figure 5.14

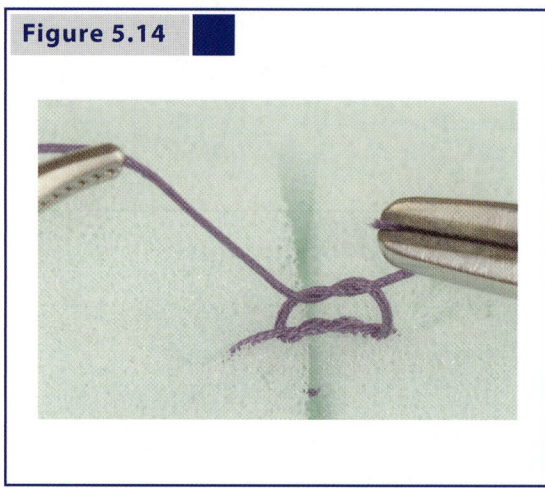

The second wrap is a single reverse wrap to secure the first knot

The second wrap is completed by wrapping the suture on the dominant needle holder and pulling the free end to tie the first knot. The third single wrap is made to place a second knot on the first one

Recommended Literature

1. Brown SI, White G, Witpat K, Frank TG, Cuschieri A (2004) Improving the retention of suturing needles in surgical graspers. Surg Endosc 18:1605–1607
2. Croce E, Olmi S (2000) Intracorporeal knot-tying and suturing techniques in laparoscopic surgery: technical details. JSLS 4:17–22
3. Joice P, Hanna GB, Cuschieri A (1998) Ergonomic evaluation of laparoscopic bowel suturing. Am J Surg 176:373–378

6 Effects of Insufflation

Amulya K. Saxena

6.1 Insufflating Gas Properties

The ideal properties of insufflation gas are:
1. Minimal peritoneal absorption.
2. Minimal physiological effects.
3. Rapid excretion.
4. Noncombustible.
5. Minimal effect after vascular embolization.
6. High solubility in blood.

No gas at present fulfils all of these criteria; however, carbon dioxide (CO_2) could be considered as the closest for endoscopic surgery.

This chapter deals on the effects of insufflated gases in laparoscopic surgery (for thoracoscopic surgery see Chap. 10).

6.2 Gas Delivery Systems

Gas delivery systems are composed of a containment cylinder, insufflator, tubing, filter, and abdominal entry device or port. The cylinders contain the gas as a liquid under pressure of 57 atm (5775.5 kPa). Over time, the cylinders build up inorganic and organic contamination, thus requiring filtration of the gas prior to insufflation of a patient's thorax or abdomen.

6.3 The Jewel-Thompson Effect

The pressure change from the containment cylinder to the insufflator and into the patient's abdomen/thorax causes cooling according to the Jewel-Thompson effect. The temperature of CO_2 gas is about 20.1°C as it enters the abdomen. Gas flow contributes to hypothermia by convection effects. The net effect is a loss of 0.3°C per 60 l of gas insufflated.

6.4 Insufflation Flow Values

Flow should be started at an initial rate of 0.5 l/min to rule out any obstruction. Once the pneumoperitoneum/pneumothorax has been established the insufflation rate can be changed to a higher setting of approximately 0.5–2 l/min to speed up the process. When the limit is reached, the rate of flow can be decreased to 0.1–0.2 l/min.

6.5   Water Content of Gases

The gases used for pneumoperitoneum have low water content. The water content of CO_2 is less than 200 ppm. Dry insufflation gases cause drying of the peritoneum and result in intact mesothelial cells being lost or desiccated from the peritoneum surface. Continuous or intermittent moistening should be performed in order to preserve peritoneal surface integrity and to decrease the tendency toward adhesion formation.

6.6   Insufflation Pressures

The surgeon decides upon the desired pressures required for the pneumoperitoneum. Although no absolute values can be recommended, pressures in the following ranges are considered to be safe:
1. 6–8 mmHg for infants.
2. 8–12 mmHg for small children.
3. 12–15 mmHg for older children/adolescents.

For thoracoscopic procedures lower pressures between 4–8 mmHg are recommended.

6.7   Dynamic Condition

The inactive and invisible pneumoperitoneum is not a static condition and must not be ignored in endoscopic surgery. The pneumoperitoneum is a dynamic space that affects the patient's condition and specific physiologic cellular processes.

The insufflation gas needs to be:
1. filtered to reduce contamination,
2. heated to reduce hypothermia, and
3. hydrated to preserve cellular integrity and reduce adhesion formation.

6.8   Stress/Immunologic Responses

Changes in systemic inflammatory and anti-inflammatory parameters (mainly cytokines) as well as in stress response parameters are less pronounced after laparoscopic surgery than after conventional surgery. Whether this leads to clinically relevant effects (e.g., less pain, fatigue, and complications) remains to be proven. There is no compelling clinical evidence that specific modifications of the pneumoperitoneum alter the immunological response.

6.9   Physiological Changes From CO_2

Physiological changes during laparoscopic surgery are related mainly to the increased intra-abdominal pressure (IAP) associated with CO_2 insufflation of the abdomen, the patient's postural modifications (head-up or head-down), and CO_2 absorption. During pneumoperitoneum, younger children absorb proportionately more CO_2 than older individuals.

6.10   Cardiopulmonary Effects

Increases in IAP affect both ventilation and circulation. Increased IAP induces a mechanical compression of the diaphragm that reduces pulmonary compliance, vital capacity, functional residual capacity, basilar alveolar collapse, and total lung volume. Pneumoperitoneum in children has a major impact on cardiac volumes and function, mainly through the effect on ventricular load conditions.

6.11 Combustion Under Low Oxygen Content

1. Combustion processes that occur in low-oxygen environments cause elevated carbon monoxide emissions.
2. Peritoneal absorption of carbon monoxide causes carboxyhemoglobin formation.
3. The affinity of carbon monoxide for hemoglobin is 200–240 times greater than that of oxygen.
4. Carbon monoxide can cause cardiac arrhythmias and exacerbate complications.
5. Hence, smoke within the pneumoperitoneum should be intermittently evacuated.

6.12 Venous Blood Return

1. During laparoscopy, both the head-up position and elevated IAP independently reduce venous blood return from the lower extremities.
2. Intraoperative sequential intermittent pneumatic compression of the lower extremities effectively reduces venous stasis during pneumoperitoneum and is recommended for prolonged laparoscopic procedures.
3. The true incidence of thromboembolic complications after pneumoperitoneum is not known.

6.13 Methemoglobinemia

1. Methemoglobinemia may occur during tissue combustion.
2. Methemoglobin is the oxidative product of hemoglobin causing the reduced ferrous to be converted to the ferric form.
3. The difference between methemoglobin and oxyhemoglobin in the ferric state is that methemoglobin is formed from unoxygenated hemoglobin and is not capable of carrying either oxygen or CO_2.
4. This property shifts the oxyhemoglobin dissociation curve to the left, inhibiting oxygen delivery to tissues.

6.14 Intra-abdominal Organ Perfusion

Although in healthy subjects changes in kidney or liver perfusion and also splanchnic perfusion due to an IAP of 12–14 mmHg have no clinically relevant effects on organ function, this may not be the case in patients with already impaired perfusion. In particular, in patients with impaired hepatic or renal function or atherosclerosis, the IAP should be as low as possible to reduce microcirculatory disturbances.

6.15   CO$_2$ Elimination After the Procedure

The short-lived increase in CO$_2$ elimination post-desufflation may be related to an increase in venous return from the lower limbs after release of the abdominal pressure. CO$_2$ absorbed by the peritoneal surfaces can cause hypercapnia, respiratory acidosis, and pooling of blood in vessels resulting in decreased cardiac output. This effect is controlled by the anesthesiologist by increasing minute ventilation to maintain normocapnia.

Recommended Literature

1. Balick-Weber CC, Nicholas P, Hedreville-Montout M, Blanchet P, Stephan F (2007) Respiratory and haemodynamic effects of volume-controlled vs pressure-controlled ventilation during laparoscopy: a cross-over study with echocardiographic assessment. Br J Anaesth 99:429–435
2. De Waal EE, Kalkman CJ (2003) Haemodynamic changes during low-pressure carbon dioxide pneumoperitoneum in young children. Paediatr Anaesth 13:18–25
3. Tobias JD (2002) Anaesthesia for minimally invasive surgery in children. Best Pract Res Clin Anaesthesiol 16:115–130

6.16   Shoulder Pain after CO$_2$ Insufflation

Several causes of shoulder pain following laparoscopic surgery have been suggested:
1. The effect of CO$_2$ gas.
2. Peritoneal stretching.
3. Diaphragmatic irritation.
4. Diaphragmatic injury.
5. Shoulder abduction during surgery.

The pain after laparoscopic procedures is usually transient and disappears in a day or two.

7 Anesthesia Considerations

Anton Gutmann

7.1 Preoperative Evaluation

1. Thorough preoperative history.
2. Complete physical examination.
3. Identifying underlying medical conditions.
4. Length of procedure.
5. Severity of disease.
6. Routine versus additional blood investigation.
7. Blood loss assessment with surgeon.
8. Chest films (if required).
9. Electrocardiogram (if required).

7.2 Premedication

1. Topical anesthetic (EMLA) cream is applied to the skin to relieve the pain of peripheral venous access.
2. Cessation of oral intake prior to the procedure depending on hospital protocol.
3. Oral administration of midazolam (0.5–1.0 mg/kg body weight; maximum dose of 15 mg) 30 min prior to the procedure.

7.3 Induction of Anesthesia

1. Induction of anesthesia can be done by inhalation or the intravenous route.
2. Peripheral intravenous access must permit rapid fluid and blood administration in major procedures.
3. Venous access above the diaphragm is preferred to bypass the elevated intra-abdominal pressure compression of the inferior vena cava.

7.4 Muscle Relaxants and Analgesics

1. Good muscle paralysis provides optimal surgical conditions and a more secure airway. This also facilitates controlled ventilation in the case of elevated intra-abdominal pressure.
2. Rocuronium and cis-atracuronium are the muscle relaxants of choice.
3. Ventilation must be appropriate to maintain end-tidal carbon dioxide within the physiological range of 35–45 mmHg.
4. Do not use nitrous oxide as it supports combustion and crosses swiftly to any gas-filled space.

7.5   Decompression

1. After induction of anesthesia a nasogastric tube is inserted to deflate the stomach. This tube is left in place for intermittent suction and gravity drainage.
2. Decompression of the stomach improves visualization and reduces the risk of accidental stomach perforation.
3. Placement of a urethral catheter allows urinary bladder decompression and monitoring of intraoperative urine production.

7.6   Intraoperative Monitoring

1. Continuous electrocardiography.
2. Blood pressure monitoring.
3. Pulse oximetry.
4. Temperature.
5. Capnography.
6. Invasive monitoring (in high risk patients):
   a. Arterial blood pressure.
   b. Central venous pressure.

7.7   Intraoperative Cardiovascular Complications

7.7.1   Venous Gas Embolus

A venous gas embolus can occur due to inadvertent placement of a Veress needle into a vessel. When large volumes of gas reach the right ventricle, an airlock is created in the pulmonary outflow tract. This leads to a sudden drop in pulmonary venous flow and left ventricular output and evident drop in end-tidal CO_2.

7.7.2   Hypotension

Factors involved in hypotension are:
1. Decreased venous return and cardiac output due to high intra-abdominal pressure.
2. Drop in the volume of circulating blood.
3. Bradycardia resulting from vagal stimulation.
4. Hypoxia.
5. Venous gas embolism.
6. Pneumothorax.
7. Anesthetic overdose.

7.7.1.1   Management of a Venous Gas Embolus

1. Cessation of abdominal insufflation.
2. Immediate deflation of intra-abdominal gas.
3. Place the patient in the head-down, left lateral decubitus position to minimize the right ventricular outflow tract obstruction.
4. Increase the fraction of inspired oxygen to 1.0.
5. If possible, the central venous pressure catheter should be advanced to aspirate the gases from the right side of the heart.

7.7.2.1   Management of Hypotension

1. Immediate deflation of intra-abdominal gas.
2. Rapid intravenous fluid administration.
3. Place the patient in the head-down position.
4. Atropine may be administered.
5. Vasopressors may be necessary.
6. Chest tube placement in case of pneumothorax.
7. Reduction of anesthetic concentration.

7.7.3 Hypertension

Hypercarbia may stimulate the sympathetic nervous system, resulting in tachycardia and hypertension. Other contributors to hypertension are inadequate depth of anesthesia, hypoxia, and increase in superior vena cava return. Treatment involves removal of the causative factor and administration of vasodilatory agents.

7.7.4 Dysrhythmias

Dysrythmias can occur:
1. During abdominal insufflation
2. Stretching of intra-abdominal structures
3. Inadequate anesthesia levels
4. Hypoxia
5. Myocardial sensitization to halothane (if used).

Treatment includes removal of the causative factor, immediate deflation, and administration of lidocaine.

7.8 Intraoperative Pulmonary Complications

7.8.1 Hypoxia

The major causes of hypoxia are ventilation–perfusion mismatch and increased pressure on the diaphragm due to increased intra-abdominal pressure. Hypoxia can also occur due to displacement of the endotracheal tube. Treatment involves removal of the causative factor.

7.8.2 Hypercarbia

Hypercarbia occurs secondary to absorption of insufflated CO_2 into the vascular system and ventilation–perfusion mismatching during surgery. Hypercarbia can be managed by increasing minute ventilation and reducing the insufflation pressure.

7.9 Postoperative Management

7.9.1 Patient Care

Monitoring must continue because excessive CO_2 must be cleared from the body. Patients with respiratory disease may have problems removing CO_2. Postoperative chest films must be obtained in certain procedures after laparoscopy and all procedures after video-assisted thoracoscopic surgery for careful evaluation of pneumothorax or pneumomediastinum.

7.9.2 Pain Management

- Local anesthetic infiltration (0.25% bupivacaine) at the port sites can help reduce pain in the incisions.
- Nonsteroidal anti-inflammatory drugs and opioids are used in general postoperative pain management.
- Regional blocks via epidural or intrapleural catheters can be beneficial after thoracic procedures.

Recommended Literature

1. Bickel A, Yahalom M, Roguin N, Frankel R, Breslava J, Ivry S, Eitan A (2002) Power spectral analysis of heart rate variability during positive pressure pneumoperitoneum: the significance of increased cardiac sympathetic expression. Surg Endosc 16:1341–1344

2. Fuentes JM, Hanly EJ, Aurora AR, De Maio A, Talamini MA (2005) Anesthesia-specific protection from endotoxic shock is not mediated through the vagus nerve. Surgery 138:766–771

3. Noga J, Fredman B, Olsfanger D, Jedeikin R (1997) Role of the anesthesiologist in the early diagnosis of life-threatening complications during laparoscopic surgery. Surg Laparosc Endosc 7:63–65

8 Preoperative Considerations

Amulya K. Saxena

8.1 Explanation of Procedures

Patients and their families should be informed about the procedure. Patients and parents may be more apprehensive because of the unique nature of such procedures and evolving technology. Information should be provided on:

1. The approximate number of incisions that will be required.
2. The possibility of conversion.
3. The benefits of minimal-access procedures.
4. Postoperative management.
5. Length of hospital stay.

8.2 Surgical Team Coordination

The procedure to be performed must be understood by all teams members. Briefing before a new procedure is recommended to reduce confusion during the procedure as well as to reduce operating time. Considerations regarding team coordination include:

1. Determination of staff for the procedure.
2. Instrument availability.
3. Assign a scrub nurse who is familiar with the equipment.
4. Ask the circulating nurse to position the equipment as desired for the procedure.

8.3 Operating Room Set Up

The procedure determines the operating room set up. The optimal set up is necessary for the operator, first assistant, and the cameraman (if not the first assistant). Considerations for the operating room are:

1. Complete the set up before the patient arrives.
2. Pay careful attention to the sterile field.
3. Avoid abundant instruments around the table.
4. Avoid contamination when connecting the cables.
5. Comfortable positioning for long procedures.

8.4 Instrumentation and Equipment

Perform a last-minute check even if critical components are functioning properly. The checklist includes:

1. Electrical/ digital instrument check.
2. Sufficient gas volume for the procedure.
3. Proper functioning of the video equipment.
4. Irrigation/aspirations devices within reach.
5. Desired values on electrosurgery device.
6. Decide scope required for the procedure.

8.5   Patient Preparation

The patient position for endoscopic procedures is quite similar to that for open procedures. Position preferences may differ between surgeons within the same group. Considerations for patient preparation are:

1. Constant urinary drainage with catheters.
2. Nasogastric tube (procedure dependent).
3. Drape patient for eventual conversion.
4. Place electrode pad on clean, dry skin.
5. Instruments for open procedure accessible.

8.6   Patient Safety Concerns

Electrosurgery is largely responsible for the complications that may arise during procedures. Factors regarding patient safety during electrosurgery are:

1. Safer when used with tissue contact.
2. Grounding pads must be secured.
3. Follow the hot point of the instrument on monitors.
4. Check for breaches in instrument insulation.
5. Avoid wet towels around the operative site.
6. Use certified standard instrumentation.

8.7   Video and Documentation Systems

The entire minimally invasive surgical procedure is dependant on the correct functioning of the video system. Considerations regarding the video systems are:

1. Monitors should be adjusted as desired.
2. Perform a video-imaging test run.
3. On-call service should be reachable in case of equipment malfunction.
4. Decide upon the recording medium: DVD or pictures.
5. Remember to switch "On" recording.
6. Check the light cables regularly.

8.8   Fogging of Endoscopes

A common problem in endoscopic surgery is fogging of the distal lens after the cavity is entered. A solution to this technical problem during procedures must be addressed in the team prior to the procedure and a method to combat it must be in place. Options to combat fogging are:

1. Apply an antifogging agent to the endoscope tip.
2. Use a hot water bath with chemical defogger.
3. Apply special lens attachments.

8.9   Endoscopes

The scrub nurse must be familiar with the various parts of the endoscopic equipment. It is recommended not to add on and mix instruments from multiple manufacturers, since this can lead to confusion during set up. The specific manufacturer's instructions, guidelines, and precautions should be followed in the maintenance of the endoscopes. With good maintenance, endoscopes will have a longer life.

8.10   Compatibility of Accessories

Before commencement of a procedure, ensure that all items of equipment and instruments are compatible, that all of the instruments will fit through the chosen ports, and that the various cables will connect with one another. In addition, the length of the connecting cables must be checked before the procedure to avoid restrictions of movement during procedures. It is frustrating to discover mismatches during the procedure and it is often too late to find immediate replacements.

8.11   Lasers in Endoscopic Surgery

Application of laser technology in endoscopic surgery has gained acceptance in a wide variety of procedures. Protective personnel precautions should be employed if the laser is used in endoscopic surgery, although the risk of retinal damage is much lower than in open surgical procedures. Signs should be posted outside the operating room door indicating the use of a laser. In addition, a suitable suction device should be present to properly evacuate the laser plume during procedures.

8.12   Preparation and Draping

Before placing the patient on the surgical table, the anesthetist may prefer that a warming blanket be applied below the table sheet, especially in infants and small children. For endoscopic procedures, the patient is prepped and draped in the same routine fashion as for open procedures, but all draping must be performed in a commonsense manner, taking into account the specific procedure being performed.

Recommended Literature

1. Chan SW, Hensman C, Waxman BP, Blamey S, Cox J, Farrell K, Fox J, Gribbin J, Layani L (2002) Technical developments and a team approach leads to an improved outcome: lessons learnt implementing laparoscopic splenectomy. ANZ J Surg 72:523–527
2. Hsiao KC, Machaidze Z, Pattaras JG (2004) Time management in the operating room: an analysis of the dedicated minimally invasive surgery suite. JSLS 8:300–303
3. Ohdaira T, Nagai H, S. Kayano S, Kazuhito H (2007) Antifogging effects of a socket-type device with the superhydrophilic, titanium dioxide-coated glass for the laparoscope. Surg Endosc 21:333–338

9 Closed- and Open-Access Techniques

Johannes Schalamon

9.1 Assortment and Definition of Ports

1. Insufflation port: used for carbon dioxide (CO_2) insufflation. This is the first port placed during a procedure and could be either a Veress needle or a combined port.
2. Optical port: this is used for camera introduction.
3. Work port: this is used for introduction of the instruments.
4. Combined port: port with a valve for CO_2 insufflation that can simultaneously be used for the camera, instruments, or both.

9.2 Main Access Techniques

1. Closed access: the closed technique is performed by the insertion of a Veress needle through the immediate subumbilical area in a previously unoperated abdomen.
2. Open access: access is gained into the cavities using open surgical methods with placements of ports under complete vision.

9.3 Umbilical Access Sites

Abdominal access through the umbilicus can be achieved through either (a) superior or inferior umbilical crease incision, (b) lateral umbilical fold incision or (c) directly transumbilical.

The advantages of umbilical access are:
1. Thinnest part of abdominal wall.
2. Center point of the abdomen for the best overview.
3. No major blood vessels present.
4. Good cosmetic results of scar concealment.

9.4 Trocar and Veress Needle Injuries

Open establishment of a pneumoperitoneum is safer compared to the closed (Veress-needle) technique. Injuries to the small bowel, bladder or vessels may occur in closed techniques due to forceful insertion of the trocars. In pediatric laparoscopic surgery the open-access technique is preferred and accepted at most centers worldwide.

9.5   Veress Needle Insertion

1. A stab incision is made in the umbilical fold.
2. The abdominal wall is elevated.
3. The Veress needle is held like a dart between the fingers and inserted at an angle of 45° to the abdominal wall.
4. The "hanging-drop" test is performed to confirm the free location of the Veress needle tip.
5. Gas is insufflated through the Veress needle to create a cushion over the bowel for insertion of the primary trocar.

9.6   Removal of the Ports

1. Removal of ports under vision is recommended to avoid omental incarceration.
2. Closure of large access wounds in layers to prevent port-hernia.
3. Absorbable sutures are preferred for closure of port sites.
4. Remove infected tissue using specimen retrieval bags to prevent contamination of the port sites.

9.7   Closed Abdominal Access Using a Veress Needle

Please see Figs. 1–4.

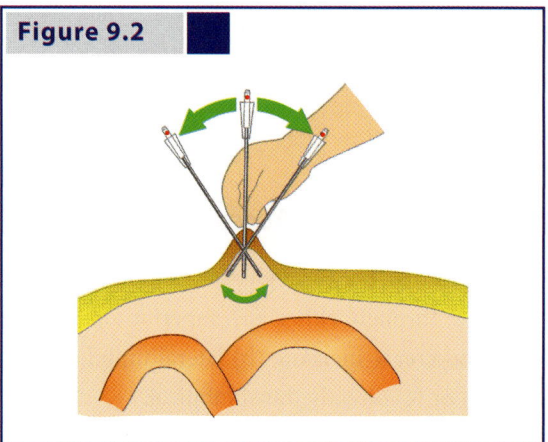

Figure 9.1

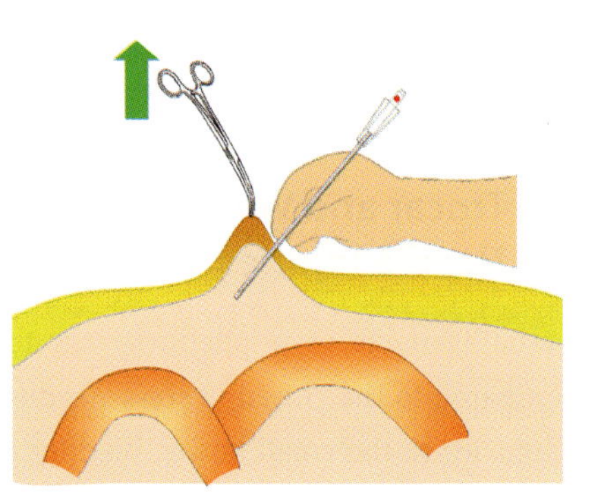

The abdomen is grasped and raised with clamp(s) to produce counter traction against the needle and allow the intestines to fall away from the site of needle insertion. The needle is held like a dart in the middle and inserted at angle of 45° towards the caudal part of the abdomen

Figure 9.2

A definitive "click" is felt in the hand as the needle enters the abdominal cavity. The needle is then moved side to side and its freedom is assessed to ensure that the inserted tip is free inside the peritoneal cavity

Figure 9.3

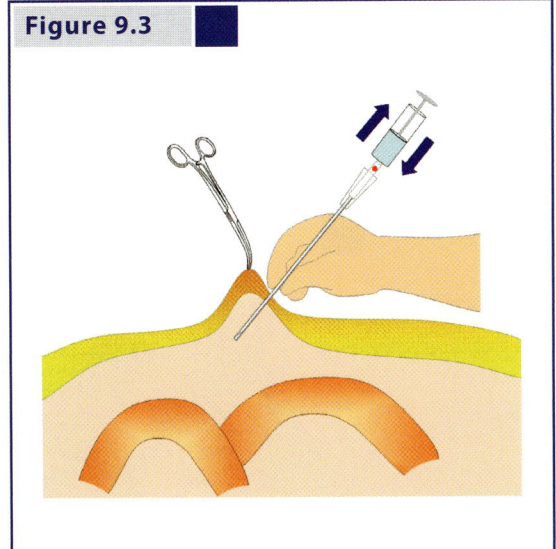

Figure 9.4

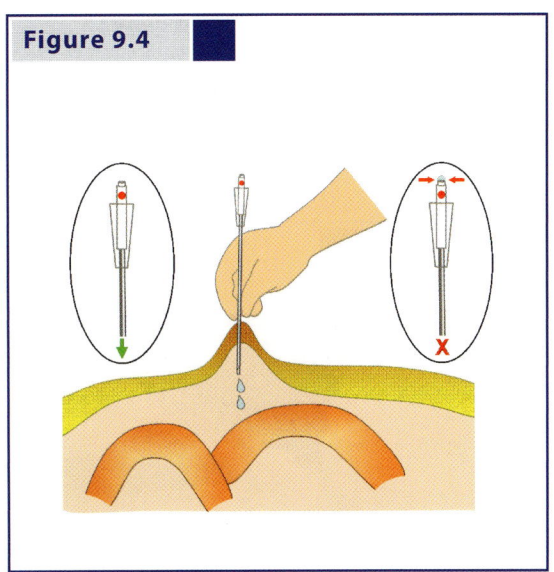

A 5 ml or 10 ml syringe filled with saline is used to flush the needle. The syringe is first used to aspirate (it should not aspirate blood or fluids) before it is flushed. If the needle tip is in the abdominal cavity, no resistance to flow of saline is experienced

Once the syringe is detached from the hub, the saline in the hub should disappear rapidly into the abdominal cavity. A saline drop "hanging" in the hub *(inset right)* should raise suspicion of tip obstruction. Otherwise correct placement of the needle can be confirmed *(inset left)*

9.8   Open Abdominal Access

Please see Figs. 5–10.

Figure 9.5

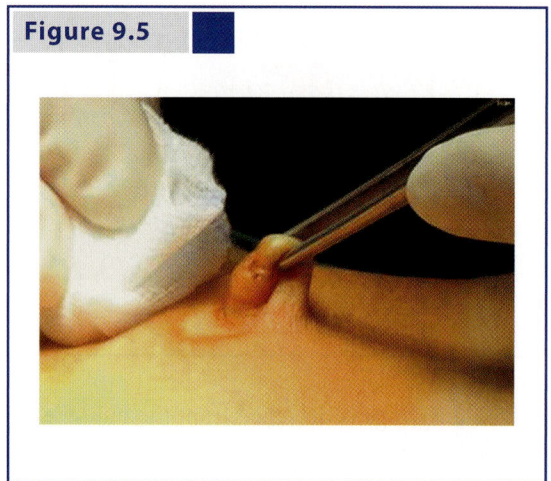

The umbilicus is meticulously cleansed/prepared with Betadine or alcohol

Figure 9.6

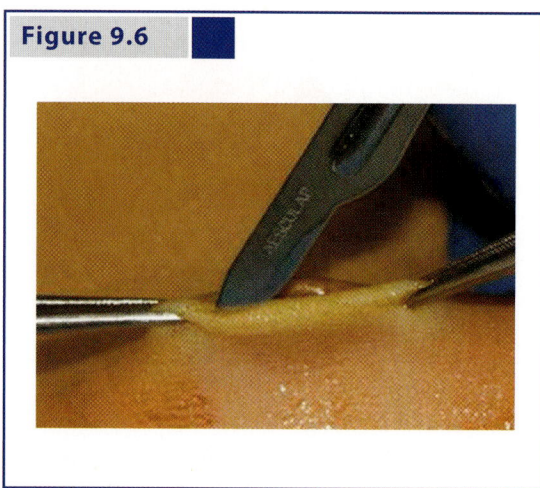

Holding the umbilical fold with forceps under tension the umbilical crease is incised

Figure 9.7

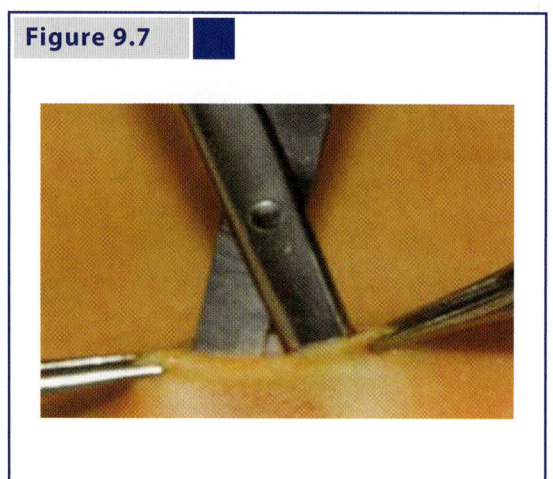

Blunt preparation through the subcutaneous tissue is done to expose the fascia

Figure 9.8

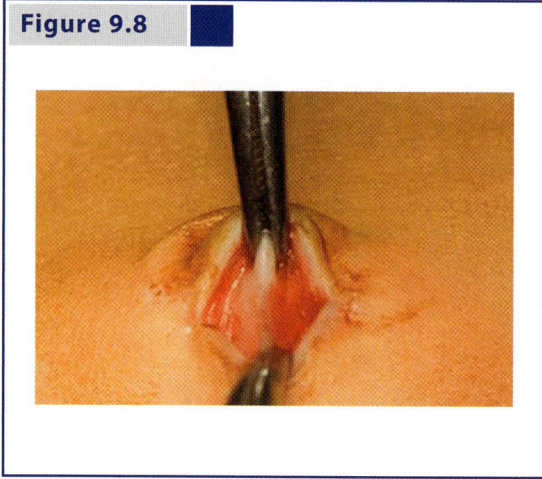

The fascia is incised and the peritoneum is identified and opened

Figure 9.9

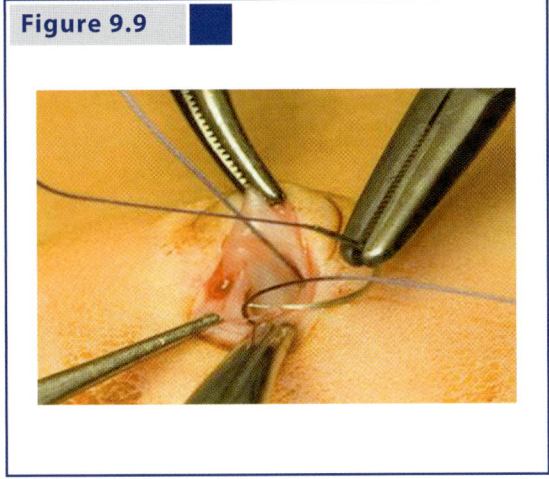

Figure 9.10

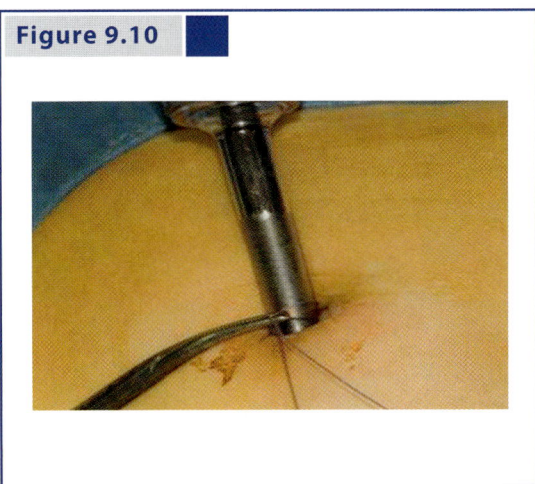

A purse-string suture is placed to secure the edges of the peritoneum and fascia

The purse-string suture is further used to secure the port and to minimize gas leaks. The suture can be tied to close the fascia after completion of the procedure

Literature Recommended

1. Ballem RV, Rudomanski J (1993) Techniques of pneumoperitoneum. Surg Laparosc Endosc 3:42–43
2. Schaefer M, Lauper M, Kraehenbuehl L (2001) Trocar and Veress needle injuries during laparoscopy. Surg Endosc 15:275–280
3. Zaraca F, Catarci M, Gossetti F, Mulieri G, Carboni M (1999) Routine use of open laparoscopy: 1006 consecutive cases. J Laparoendosc Adv Surg Tech A 9:75–80

10 Concepts in Video-Assisted Thoracic Surgery (VATS)

Stephanie P. Acierno and John H.T. Waldhausen

10.1 Introduction to Video-Assisted Thoracic Surgery

Video-assisted thoracic surgery (VATS) in the pediatric population has progressed rapidly since its development in the mid 1970. The indications for VATS in children have become diverse and continue to advance as instrumentation and skills improve. VATS procedures offer reduced patient discomfort, improved cosmetic outcome, prevention of functional disorders of the chest and shoulder as a result of thoracotomy incisions, and may shorten hospital stays when compared to traditional thoracotomy.

In this chapter, we will discuss important concepts in all VATS procedures, but leave the technical discussion of each specific procedure to other chapters.

10.2   Indications for VATS

Basic Techniques	
Intrathoracic	Mediastinum
Diagnostic evaluation of the pleura	Pericardial drainage
Empyemectomy	Pericardial window
Evacuation of hemothorax	Mediastinal tumor biopsy
Mechanical or chemical pleurodesis	Mediastinal lymph node biopsy
Bleb resection	
Lung biopsy	
Sympathectomy	
Transdiaphragmatic liver biopsy	

Advanced Techniques	
Intrathoracic	Mediastinum
Evaluation of trauma (diaphragm)	Vagotomy
Decortication	Thoracic duct ligation
Lobectomy	Patent ductus arteriosus ligation
Resection of sequestration	Esophageal dissection
Diaphragmatic plication	Esophageal myotomy
Congenital diaphragmatic hernia repair	Esophageal atresia repair
Anterior spine procedures	Tracheoesophageal fistula ligation
	Bronchogenic cyst surgery
	Neurogenic tumor resection
	Benign esophageal tumor resection
	Aortopexy
	Thymectomy
	Automatic implantable cardioverter defibrillators (AICD) implantation

10.3   Contraindications

10.3.1   Absolute Contraindications

The only absolute contraindications are conditions that prevent adequate visualization of the thoracic space such as:

1. Pleural symphysis.
2. Inability to tolerate single lung ventilation.
3. Contralateral pneumonectomy.
4. High positive-pressure ventilation.

10.3.2   Relative Contraindications

These do not eliminate VATS as an option, but must be carefully considered in operative planning:

1. Prior tube thoracostomy.
2. Previous thoracoscopy or thoracotomy.
3. Coagulopathy (if uncorrectable, is absolute contraindication).

10.4   Anesthesia Considerations

10.4.1   Preoperative Considerations

1. Thorough preoperative evaluation.
2. Assess need for blood availability.
3. Adequate intravenous access (if central access needed, place patient on operative side).
4. Standard monitoring as indicated by patient condition and specific procedure.
5. Recommended to be performed under general anesthetic to ensure adequate pain and airway control.

10.4.2   Double-Lung Ventilation Option

If the double-lung ventilation option is chosen, the following may allow adequate visibility:

1. Introduction of pneumothorax with spontaneous ventilation.
2. Insufflation of carbon dioxide (CO_2) into the thoracic cavity (low pressures 4–8 mmHg).
3. Use of retractors (will require an additional 3-, 5-, or 10-mm access site).
4. Fan (5 or 10 mm) or snake (3 mm) retractors can be placed into the chest without a port.

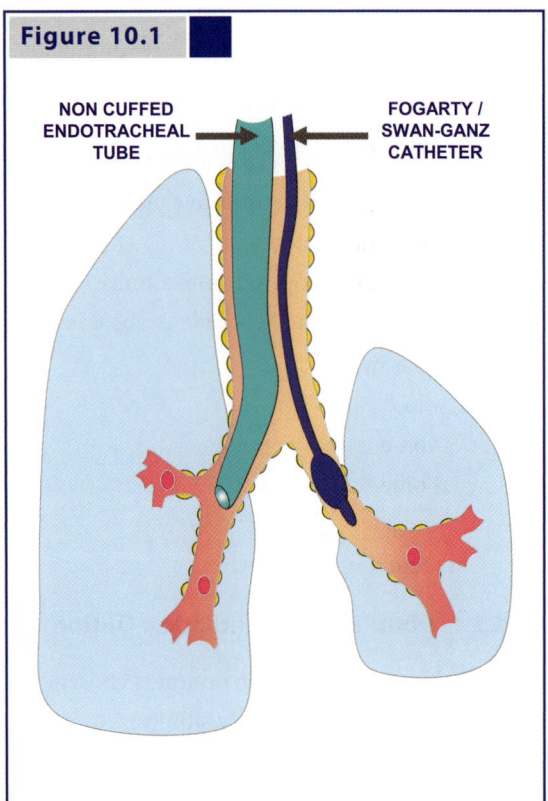

Figure 10.1

NON CUFFED
ENDOTRACHEAL
TUBE

FOGARTY /
SWAN-GANZ
CATHETER

Bronchial blocker method of single-lung ventilation

10.4.3 Single-Lung Ventilation Option – I

Dual-lumen endotracheal tubes:
1. Only widely available for patients older than 8 years of age (size 26 Fr).
2. Offers easy conversion from single- to double-lung ventilation if the need arises.

10.4.4 Single-Lung Ventilation Option – II

Bronchial blockers (Fig. 1):
1. Under bronchoscopic guidance, pass a Fogarty catheter or Swan-Ganz catheter into the involved side.
2. Inflate the balloon to occlude the desired side (Swan-Ganz allows oxygen delivery to the involved side to facilitate oxygenation if needed).
3. The noncuffed endotracheal tube can remain in the trachea or be advanced into the contralateral lung.
4. The Fogarty catheter may become dislodged during the procedure and obstruct the endotracheal tube, and so requires continuous monitoring of breath sounds and compliance.

10.4.5 Single-Lung Ventilation Option – III

Selective endobronchial intubation can be performed blindly for right-sided intubation, but may require bronchoscopy or fluoroscopy for left-sided placement
1. Use a cuffed endotracheal tube 0.5–1 size smaller than usual.
2. The balloon is inflated to prevent ventilation of the opposite lung.
3. May become dislodged with positioning or balloon inflation.

10.5   Technical Considerations for VATS

Figure 10.2

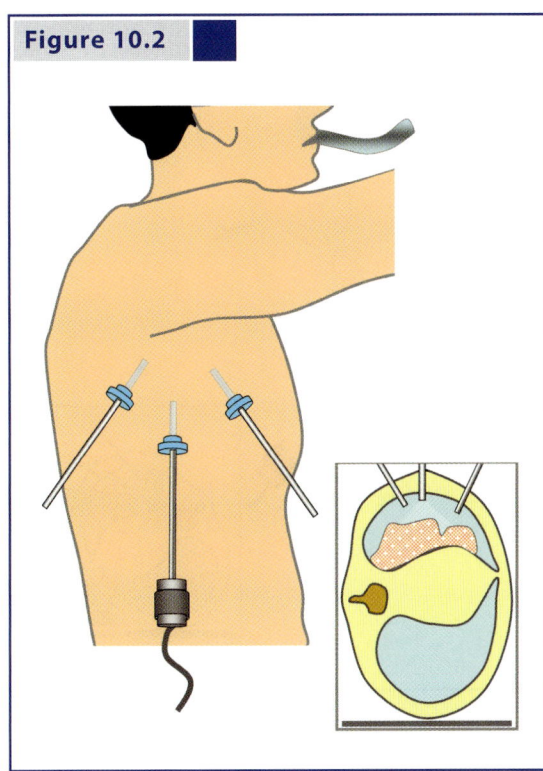

Patient positioning for lung biopsy for diffuse process. Full lateral decubitus position with operative side up. Lesions on the surface of the lung can be seen directly and the procedures can be performed accordingly (**inset**)

10.5.1   Preoperative Imaging

1. Thorough preoperative imaging will help with planning patient positioning and access sites in order to provide the best access to the lesion.
2. A chest-computed tomography (CT) is most helpful for masses and infiltrates.
3. Ultrasound can be used to find the largest fluid collection in cases of empyema.
4. For spontaneous pneumothoracies, anterior-posterior/lateral X-ray is usually adequate, although chest-CT may help identify blebs.

10.5.2   Positioning of the Patient

Proper positioning will assist with the retraction of uninvolved structures. Using the kidney rest in larger children or a rolled up blanket or foam pad placed under the flank on the dependent side will help mobilize the hip out of the way and open the intercostal spaces.

The positioning of the patient described herein are general guidelines only; they may need to be adjusted based on the specific lesion, patient size, or surgeon preference.

Patient positioning for the procedures of lung biopsy for diffuse process, anterior lesions (anterior, right middle lobe, or lingual), and posterior lesions are shown in Figs. 2–4.

Figure 10.3

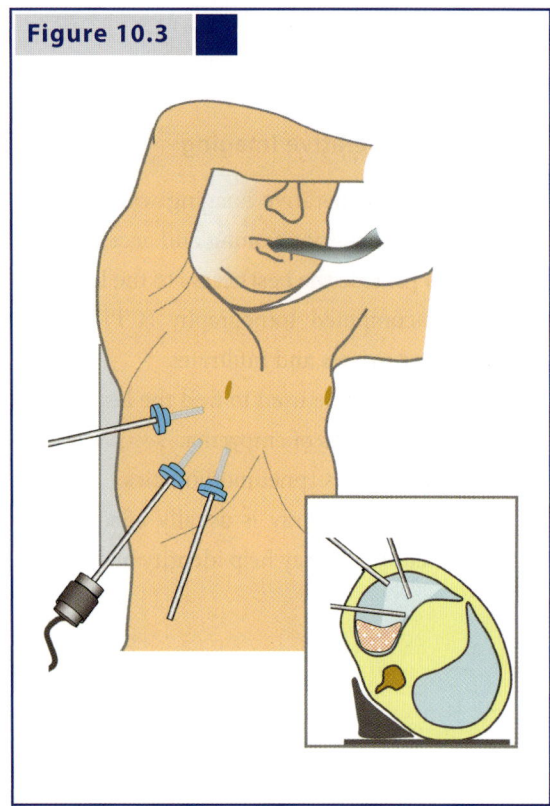

Figure 10.4

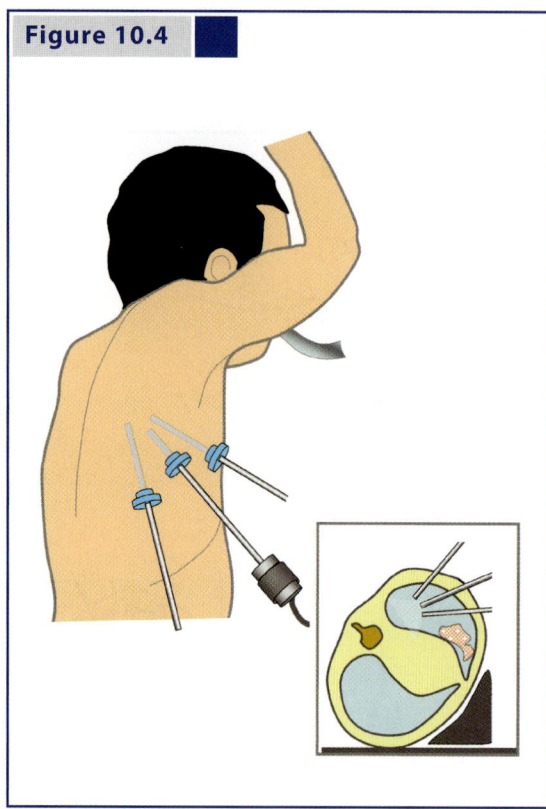

Patient positioning for anterior lesions. Lateral de-cubitus position, operative side up, tilted 30° pos-teriorly. This will allow gravity to retract the lung posteriorly, providing better visibility. The Tren-delenburg or reverse Trendelenburg position will provide improved access to the base or apex, re-spectively (***inset***)

Patient position for posterior lesions. Lateral decu-bitus position, operative side up, tilted 30° anteri-orly. This will allow gravity to retract the lung an-teriorly, providing better visibility. The Trendelen-burg or reverse Trendelenburg position will provide improved access to the base or apex, respectively (***inset***)

10.5.3   Access to Mediastinal Lesions

1. Select the side that provides the easiest access to the lesion.
2. Position as previously described to allow the lung to fall away from the lesion with gravity (usually tilted 30° posteriorly for an anterior mass and 30° anteriorly for a posterior mass, as positioned for intrathoracic lesions).
3. Approach these lesions transpleurally. Extra-pleural techniques have not yet been fully devel-oped.

10.5.4   Access to the Diaphragm

1. Lateral decubitus, operative side up. Anterior tilt for posterior lesions, posterior tilt for ante-rior lesions.
2. For plications, the patient should be in the full decubitus position.
3. Morgagni hernias are best approached via the abdomen.

10.6   Basic Instrumentation

1. High-intensity light source.
2. CO_2 insufflator.
3. High-resolution video monitors.
4. 2.7- or 5-mm telescope. The 5-mm scope is most commonly used as it provides greater flexibility in the costal interspace to allow a wide rage of camera movement. The 2.7-mm telescope is used in neonates and infants.
5. In larger children (> 8 years old) a 10-mm camera can be used, but is rarely necessary.
6. Generally 0° or 30° scopes are most commonly used, but 45–70° scopes may be helpful to improve visibility.
7. Camera.
8. Basic endoscopic instrument set (3 or 5 mm, shorter shafts will provide better intrathoracic tissue handling).
   a. Biopsy forceps.
   b. Irrigator/aspirator/cautery device.
   c. Grasper.
   d. Dissectors.
   e. Needle holder.
   f. Scissors.
9. Clip applier (5 mm size)

Other instruments that may be used:
1. Specimen retrieval bag.
2. Harmonic scalpel.
3. LigaSure™ (Valleylab, Boulder, CO, USA).
4. Endoscopic ultrasound.
5. Argon beam coagulator.
6. Automated tissue morcellator.
7. Endoscopic stapler: will need 12 mm access and at least 5 cm within the chest to allow the anvil to open. Therefore, the port must be placed low in the chest and often can not be used in children <5 years old. The endoscopic stapler is often passed directly into the chest without a port. Use 2.5- or 3.5-mm staple loads depending on patient size.
8. Cannulas or ports (3, 5, 10, 12 mm). Most often one will be utilized for the camera and two for operating. Thoracoports or laparoscopic ports can be used. The initial port (often the camera port) is placed using a direct cut down.
9. The positioning of the camera port will depend on the location of the target lesion and the child's body habitus; the camera must be placed far enough from the lesion to allow visualization of the lesion and the working instruments.

As a general guide, camera ports will usually be placed:
1. In the 4th or 5th intercostal space at the anterior axillary line for apex or pleural dome lesions.
2. In the 4th or 5th intercostal space, but more laterally for anterior pulmonary or superior mediastinal lesions.
3. In the 5th or 6th intercostal space at the midaxillary line for pericardial lesions.
4. In the 5th or 6th intercostal space slightly posterior to the midaxillary line for anterior mediastinal or hilar lesions.
5. In the 5th or 6th intercostal space slightly anterior to the midaxillary line for posterior mediastinal lesions.

The remaining cannulas should be placed under direct vision with the position determined after direct examination of the lesion and the chest cavity.

A configuration of cannulas that will give optimal visibility and maneuverability is the baseball diamond or clock configuration (Fig. 5). Placing the lesion at second base (12 noon), the camera port is placed at home plate (6 o'clock), and the two operating (work) ports are placed at first and third base (3 and 9 o'clock, respectively).

Ports or cannulas are not always required. Most instruments can be passed directly into the chest through an incision, even if insufflation is being used via a single port to help with lung retraction.

With selective intubation, the diaphragm may rise to the 3rd or 4th intercostal space, so care must be taken to avoid injury to the diaphragm or subdiaphragmatic organs. Avoid the area 1–2 cm from the sternal margin where the internal mammary arteries run.

Port sizes should be chosen based on the size of the instruments that are required. A 10- or 12-mm port should only be used if dictated by equipment size. Careful planning and positioning may allow one to use smaller ports.

Figure 10.5

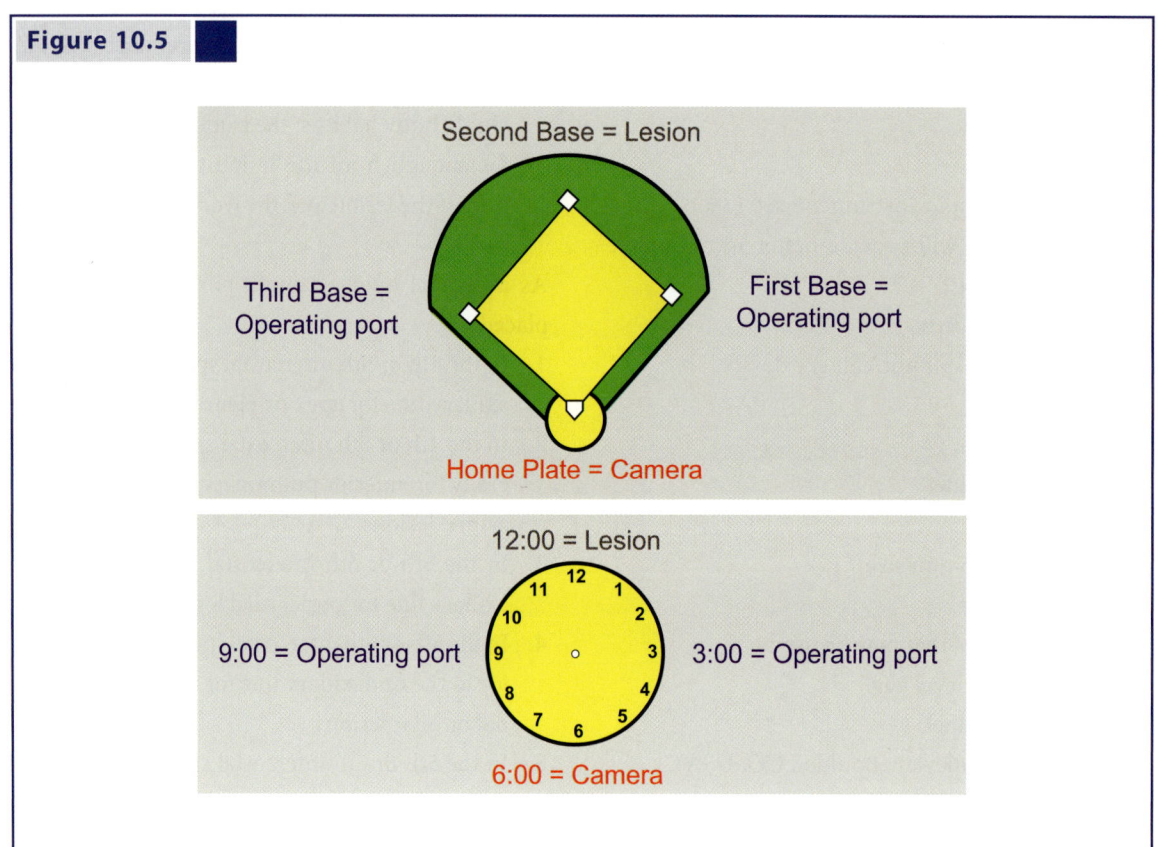

Baseball diamond or clock-face positioning of the camera and working ports to allow ergonomically appropriate positioning

10.7 Use of a Chest Tube Postoperatively

1. Chest tube can be placed under direct vision via one of the port sites, if necessary.
2. If a mediastinal mass or pleural lesion has been biopsied, a red rubber catheter can be used to evacuate any residual pneumothorax after wound closure, and then immediately removed.
3. Some surgeons may omit the chest tube if a surgical stapler is used in the parenchymal resection as long as prolonged mechanical ventilation is not necessary and no air leak is seen at the staple line on inflation.
4. If a chest tube is placed, it can be removed once the pneumothorax resolves and there is no air leak (can be as soon as 6–12 h postoperatively).

10.8 Complications of VATS

The majority of VATS complications reported in the literature are mild, but include:

1. Recurrent pneumothorax.
2. Tension pneumothorax during insufflation or initial air introduction.
3. Hemorrhage from a vessel or lung injury (an open thoracotomy is rarely required).
4. Air or CO_2 embolism.
5. Injury to the diaphragm or subdiaphragmatic organs.
6. Cardiac fibrillation due to the use of cautery too close to heart, vagus nerve, or pericardium.
7. Elevation of serum CO_2 levels.
8. Subcutaneous crepitus.
9. Organ injury from port or instrument insertion.

Recommended Literature

1. Lobe TE, Schropp KP (eds) (1994) Pediatric Laparoscopy and Thoracoscopy. Chapters 6, 9, 10, Saunders, Philadelphia
2. Rodgers BM (2003) The role of thoracoscopy in pediatric surgical practice. Semin Pediatr Surg 12:62–70
3. Rothenberg SS (2005) Thoracoscopy in infants and children: the state of the art. J Pediatr Surg 40:303–306

11 Robot-Assisted Pediatric Surgery

VENITA CHANDRA, SANJEEV DUTTA
AND CRAIG T. ALBANESE

11.1 Introduction

Since their introduction into clinical practice in the late 1990s, the use of computer-enhanced robotic surgical systems has grown rapidly. Originally conceived as a military tool for remote battlefield surgery, these systems are now used to enable complex endoscopic surgical procedures in a wide variety of pediatric surgical disciplines.

11.2 The Surgical Robotic System

The da Vinci® Surgical System (Intuitive Surgical, Sunnyvale, CA, USA), currently the primary system used in pediatric surgery is comprised of (Fig. 1):

1. The surgeon console, which includes a user interface panel, control handles that direct the robotic arms, and a stereoscopic visual display.
2. Patient side cart, which includes a two- to three-armed robot that controls the operative instruments, and a video endoscope.

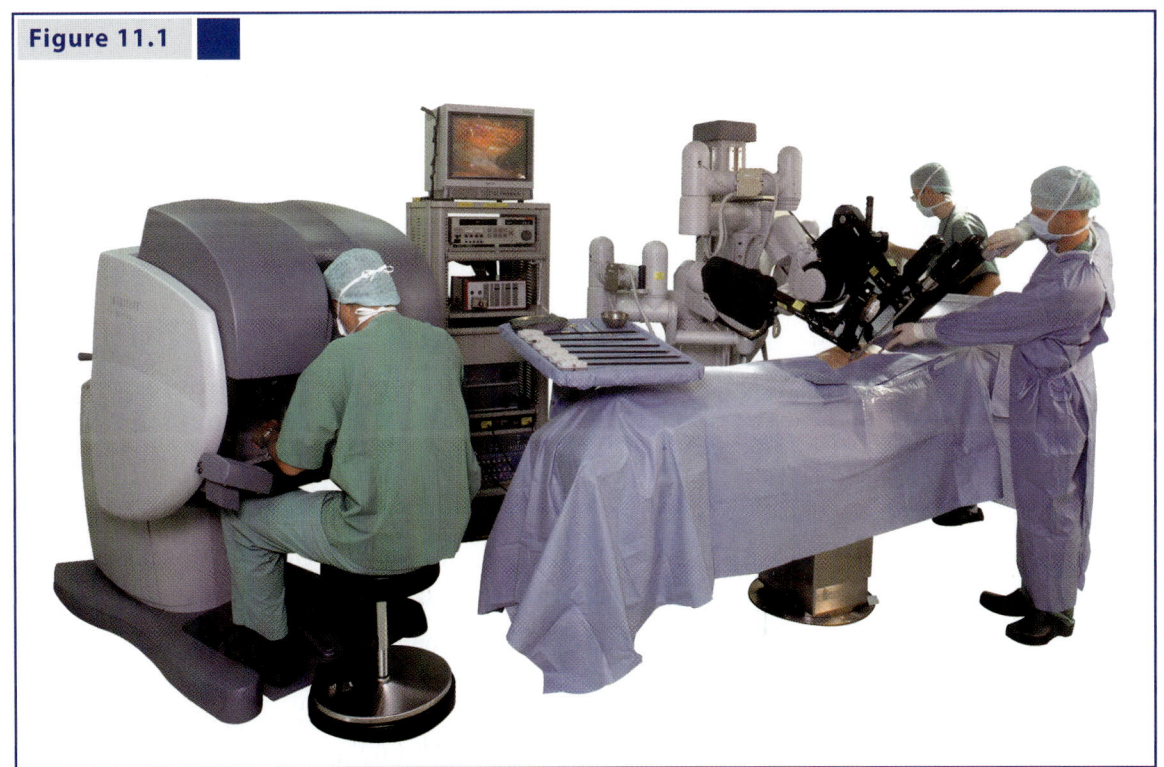

Figure 11.1

The da Vinci® robotic surgical system comprising of a surgeon's console and a patient side cart. (Courtesy of Intuitive Surgical, Sunnyvale, CA, USA)

Figure 11.2

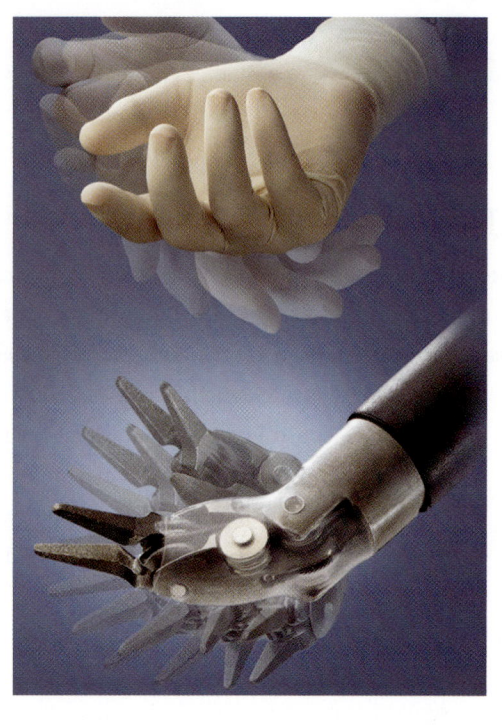

Demonstration of the seven degrees of freedom with a "wristed instrument" compared to the surgeon's hand. (EndoWrist®; Intuitive Surgical) (Courtesy of Intuitive Surgical, Sunnyvale, CA, USA)

11.3 Advantages of Robotics in Children

Robotic systems have the ability to overcome some of the limitations of conventional laparoscopy, including difficulties with dexterity and challenges of two-dimensional optics. Advantages include:

1. Improved hand-eye coordination.
2. Wristed instruments enabling seven degrees of freedom (Fig. 2).
3. Elimination of the fulcrum effect.
4. Tremor filtration.
5. Stereoscopic three-dimensional visualization.
6. Motion scaling.
7. Ergonomic positioning.

11.4 Disadvantages of Robotics in Children

1. Loss of force feedback (haptics). Surgeon must rely on visual cues such as tissue compression and blanching to compensate.
2. Complex and time-consuming set up, requiring specially trained operating staff.
3. High initial expense and maintenance costs.
4. Limited size and variety of available instrumentation.
5. Large size discrepancy between the typical patient and the overall size of the robotic system.

11.5 Anesthetic Considerations

1. Open communication between the anesthesiologist and surgeon is essential.
2. Pressure points must be carefully padded, and potential sites of instrument back-end collision identified.
3. Extension tubing may be required for intravenous and arterial lines.
4. The operating team must practice the crisis scenario of undocking the robotic equipment and gaining access to the patient rapidly, should the need arise.

11.6   Preoperative Considerations

1. The robot is usually placed at the head of the bed for upper gastrointestinal and hepatobiliary cases.
2. Elevate the child off the bed on foam and blankets to prevent instrument backend collisions with the bed.
3. Ports must be as widely spaced as possible to achieve proper orientation.

11.7   Current Applications in Pediatric Subspecialties

While the majority of clinical experience in robotic surgery is in the field of pediatric general surgery, robot-assisted techniques are being applied to a growing number of surgical subspecialties.

Cardiothoracic applications include ligation of the patent ductus arteriosus and division of vascular rings.

In pediatric urology, robotic assistance is described for nephrectomy, pyeloplasty, and appendicovesicostomy.

11.8   Clinical Utility in Pediatric Surgery

1. Robotics is an enabling technology for surgeons not proficient in laparoscopy, allowing them to perform advanced minimal-access procedures they would otherwise do as open procedures.
2. For advanced laparoscopists, robotics does not improve basic dissection; however, it enables the performance of complex tasks (e.g., suturing a portoenterostomy) that require precision in a limited operative field or at awkward angles.
3. Clinical utility in pediatric patients is currently limited by the lack of small instrumentation, high cost, and cumbersome setup.

11.9   Future of Robotic Surgery

The future of robotic surgery lies in its ability to transcend human capability. Emerging developments include high-fidelity force sensors to improve tactile sensation, overlying of imaging data onto the operative field (augmented reality), and device miniaturization, which will allow surgeons to access remote anatomy without extensive dissection and further apply robotics to neonates and fetuses.

11.10 Current Applications in Pediatric General Surgery

Robot-assisted endoscopic procedures have been described for cholecystectomy, splenectomy, fundoplication, the Kasai procedure, choledochal cyst excision, Heller myotomy, posterior mediastinal cyst excision, and subcutaneous giant lipoma excision. In addition, successful formation of an esophago-esophagostomy and treatment of diaphragmatic hernias have been reported in animal studies.

11.11 Conclusion

Robot-assisted surgery holds promise in the pediatric population; however, further technical advances must be made and cost must come down for robotics to be adopted widely.

Literature Recommended

1. Camarillo DB, Krummel TM, Salisbury JK Jr (2004) Robotic technology in surgery: past, present, and future. Am J Surg 188:2S–15S
2. Chandra V, Dutta S, Albanese CT (2006) Surgical robotics and image guided therapy in pediatric surgery: emerging and converging minimal access technologies. Semin Pediatr Surg 15:267–275
3. Woo R, Le D, Krummel TM, Albanese C (2004) Robot-assisted pediatric surgery. Am J Surg 188:27S–37S

Section 2

Video-Assisted Thoracoscopic Surgery (VATS)

12 Lobectomy

STEVEN S. ROTHENBERG

12.1 Operation Room Setup

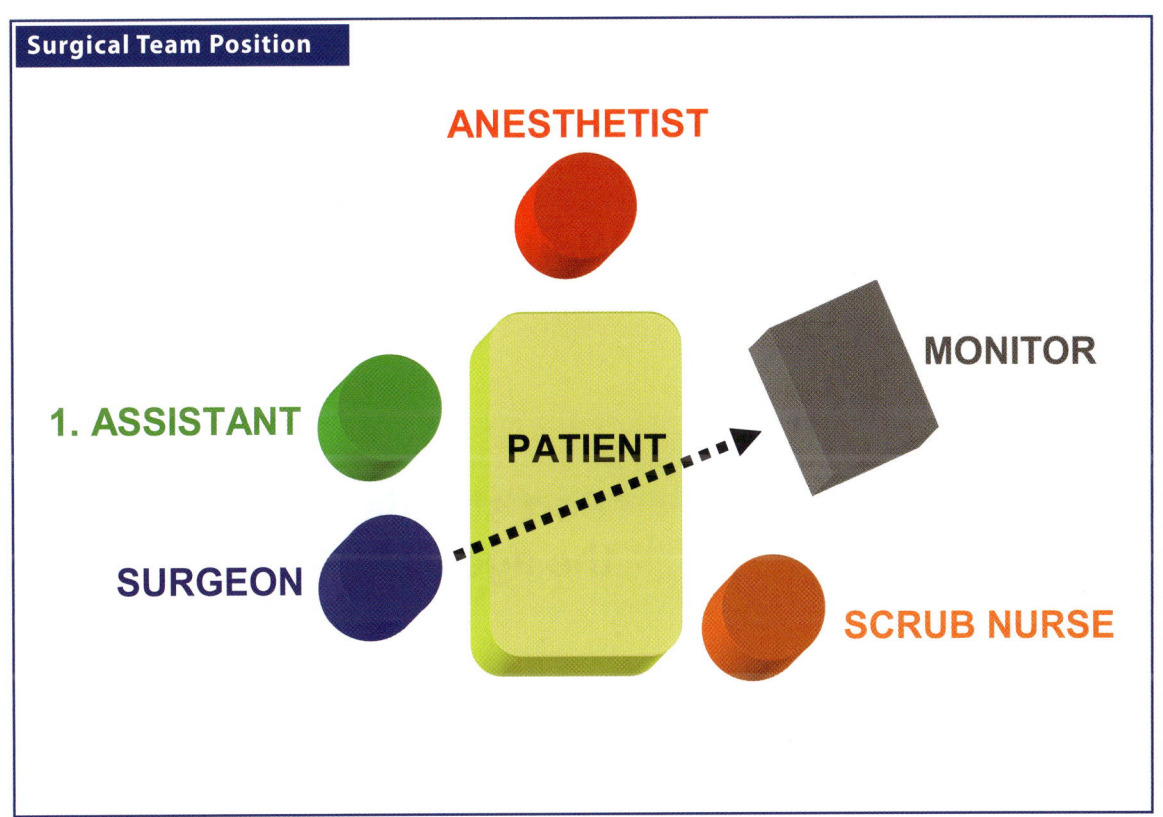

12.2   Patient Positioning

The patient is placed in a formal lateral decubitus position. The surgeon and assistant are at the front of the patient.

12.3   Special Instruments

- LigaSure™ (Valleylab, Boulder, CO, USA)
- Endoscopic clip applicator
- Endo GIA™ stapler (Auto Suture, Norwalk, CT, USA)

12.4   Location of Access Points

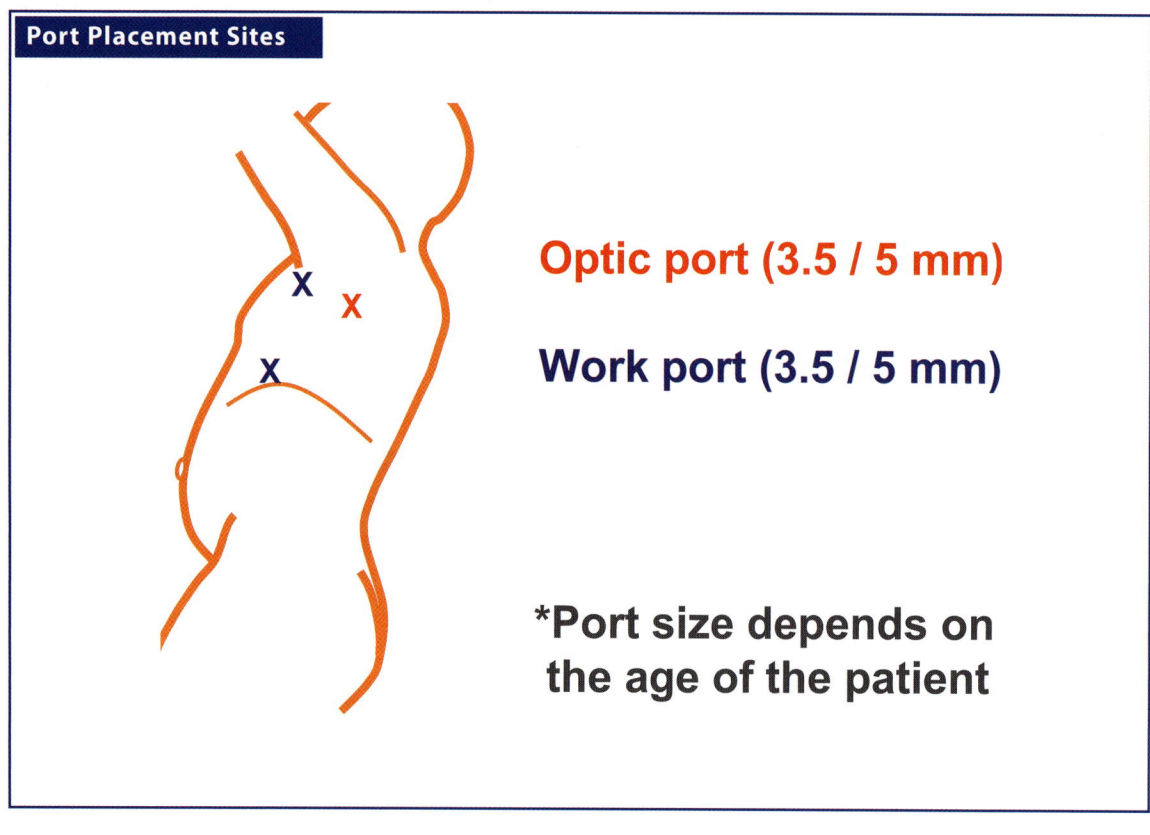

Port Placement Sites

Optic port (3.5 / 5 mm)

Work port (3.5 / 5 mm)

*Port size depends on the age of the patient

12.5 Indications

1. Congenital adenomatoid malformation.
2. Pulmonary sequestration.
3. Congenital lobar emphysema.
4. Severe bronchiectasis.
5. Right middle lobe syndrome.
6. Cystic fibrosis.

12.6 Contraindications

1. Severe respiratory distress associated with any of the above.
2. Necrotizing pneumonia and sepsis.
3. Malignancy.

12.7 Preoperative Considerations

1. Patient's respiratory status: the best chance for success is if the anesthetist can obtain single-lung ventilation of the contralateral side. Patients with significant mass effect or respiratory compromise may not tolerate this.
2. Patient size will determine the vessel and bronchus ligation technique. The appropriate equipment should be available prior to embarking on the procedure.
3. Appropriate antibiotics should be given preoperatively.
4. If there is a question of abnormal bronchial anatomy, a bronchoscopy should be performed at the beginning of the procedure.

12.8 Technical Notes

1. Valved ports and carbon dioxide insufflation should be used during the case to aide in lung collapse.
2. If there are large air- or fluid-filled cysts, they should be involuted or drained and decompressed to create more intrathoracic space and improve visualization.
3. An anatomic resection should be performed in all cases. Mass blind ligations are unsafe.
4. In general, the dissection should be performed from anterior to posterior. It is difficult to flip the lung thoracoscopically and doing so wastes time and results in increased parenchymal bleeding.

12.9 Procedure Variations

1. Most variation is due to the size of the patient and the lobe being resected. The upper lobe is the most difficult as the main pulmonary artery trunk must be preserved as it courses behind the upper lobe.
2. A hybrid approach instituting a combination of ports and a mini thoracotomy can be used, but this is rarely necessary if the surgeon is familiar with the anatomy and has the appropriate instrumentation.

12.10 Thoracoscopic Lobectomy Procedure

Please see Figs.1–6.

Figure 12.1

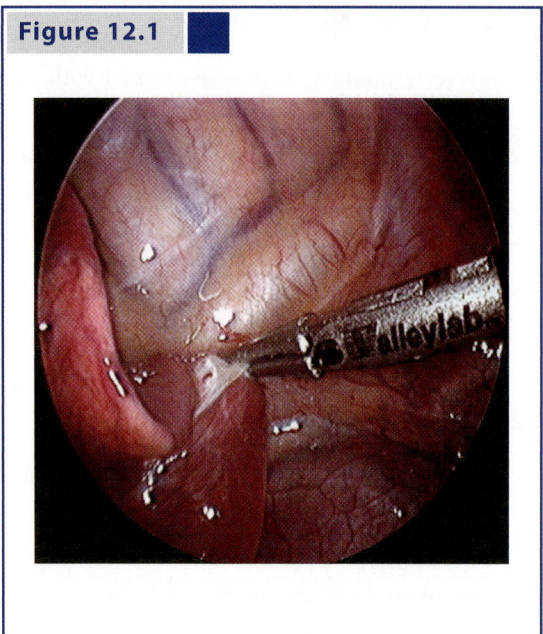

The inferior pulmonary ligament is divided exposing the inferior pulmonary vein

Figure 12.2

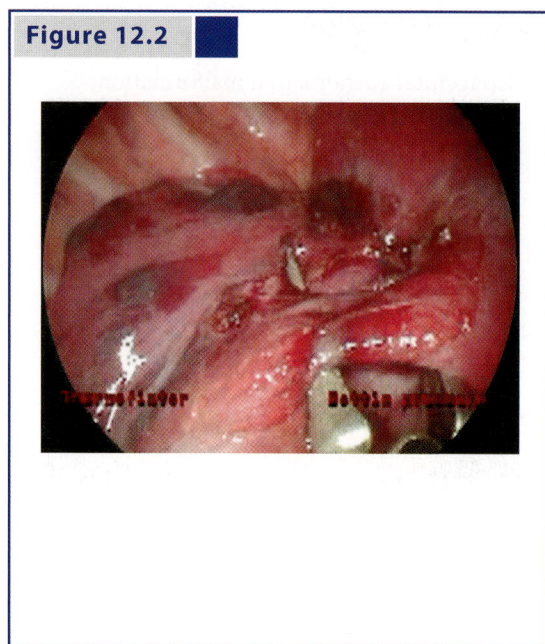

The major fissure is completely divided to expose the pulmonary artery to the lower lobe. This can be done in smaller patients with the LigaSure™ or in larger patients with the EndoGIA™ stapler

Figure 12.3

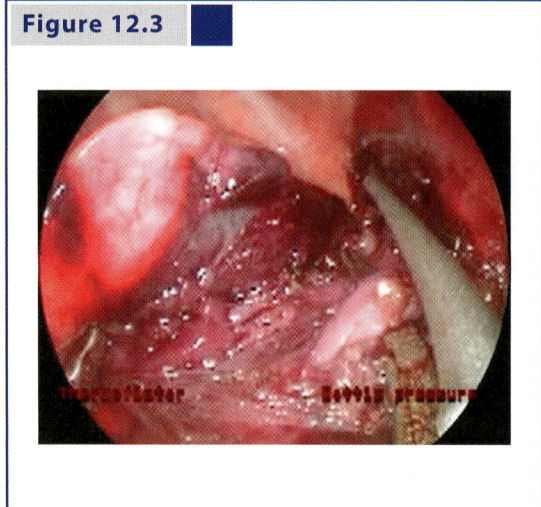

The pulmonary artery to the lower lobe is mobilized, ligated, and divided

Figure 12.4

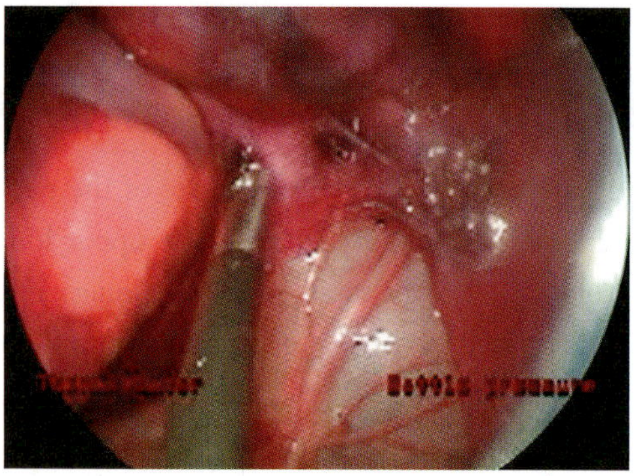

The inferior pulmonary vein is sealed and divided

Figure 12.5

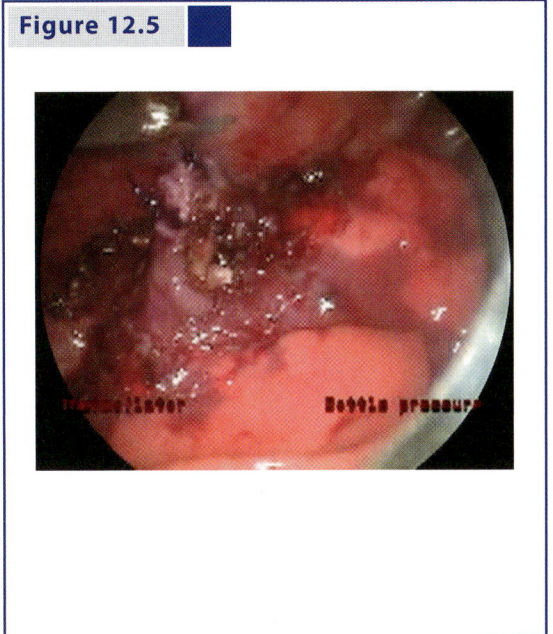

Figure 12.6

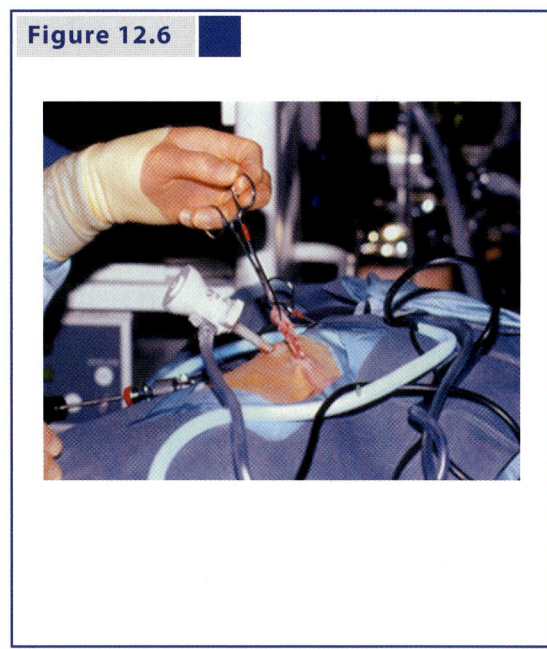

The bronchus is divided and sealed using sutures, clips, or a stapler

The specimen is brought out through the lower port site, which is slightly enlarged

Recommended Literature

1. Albanese CT, Rothenberg SS (2007) Experience with 144 consecutive pediatric thoracoscopic lobectomies. J Laparoendosc Adv Surg Tech 17:339–341
2. Rothenberg SS (2003) Experience with thoracoscopic lobectomy in infants and children. J Pediatr Surg 38:102–104
3. Truitt AK, Carr SR, Cassese J, Kurkchubasche A, Tracy TF Jr, Luks F (2006) Perinatal management of congenital cystic lung lesions in the age of minimally invasive surgery. J Pediatr Surg 41:893–896

13 Bronchogenic Cyst Resection

Roshni Dasgupta and Richard G. Azizkhan

13.1 Operation Room Setup

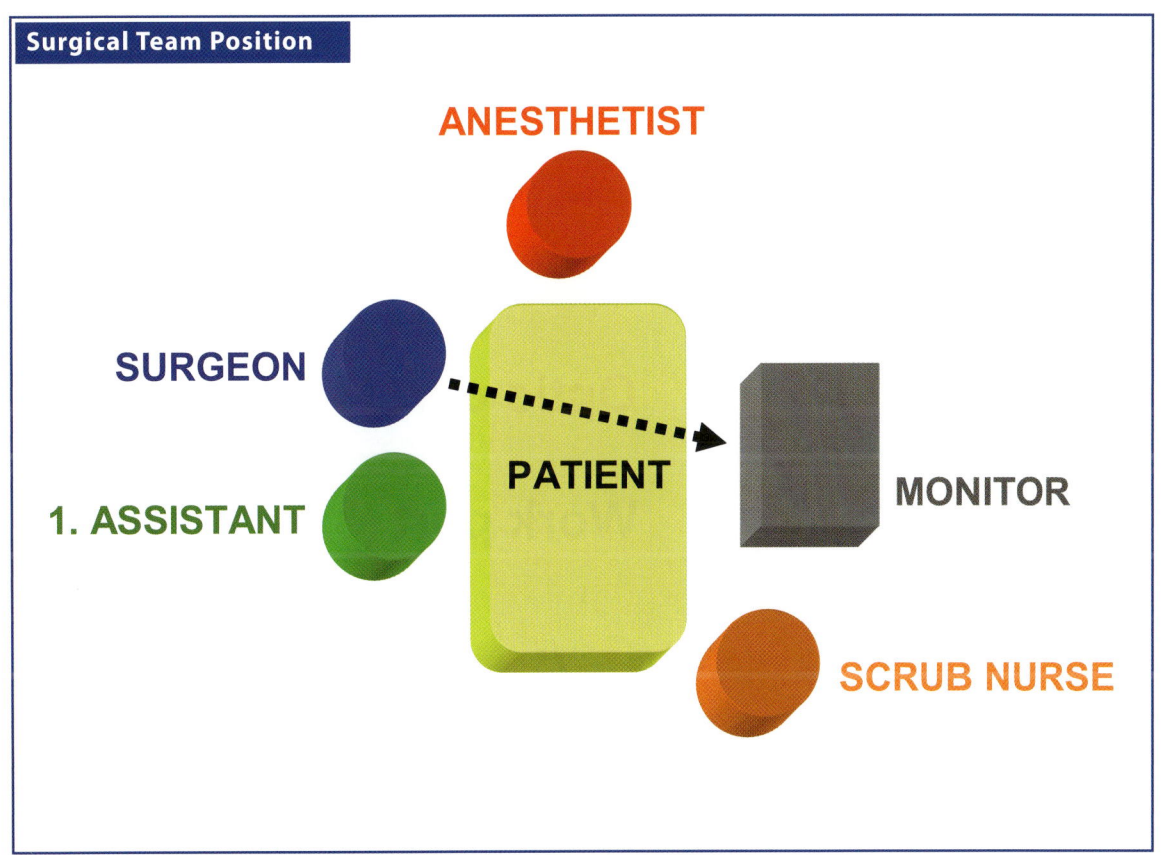

13.2   Patient Positioning

Ensure the patient is in a semiprone (45°)/lateral decubitus position, with the opposite arm elevated and supported well.

13.3   Special Instruments

1. Ultracision® harmonic scalpel (Johnson & Johnson Medical Products Ethicon Endo-Surgery, Cincinnati, OH, USA).
2. LigaSure™(Valleylab, Boulder, CO, USA)

13.4   Location of Access Points

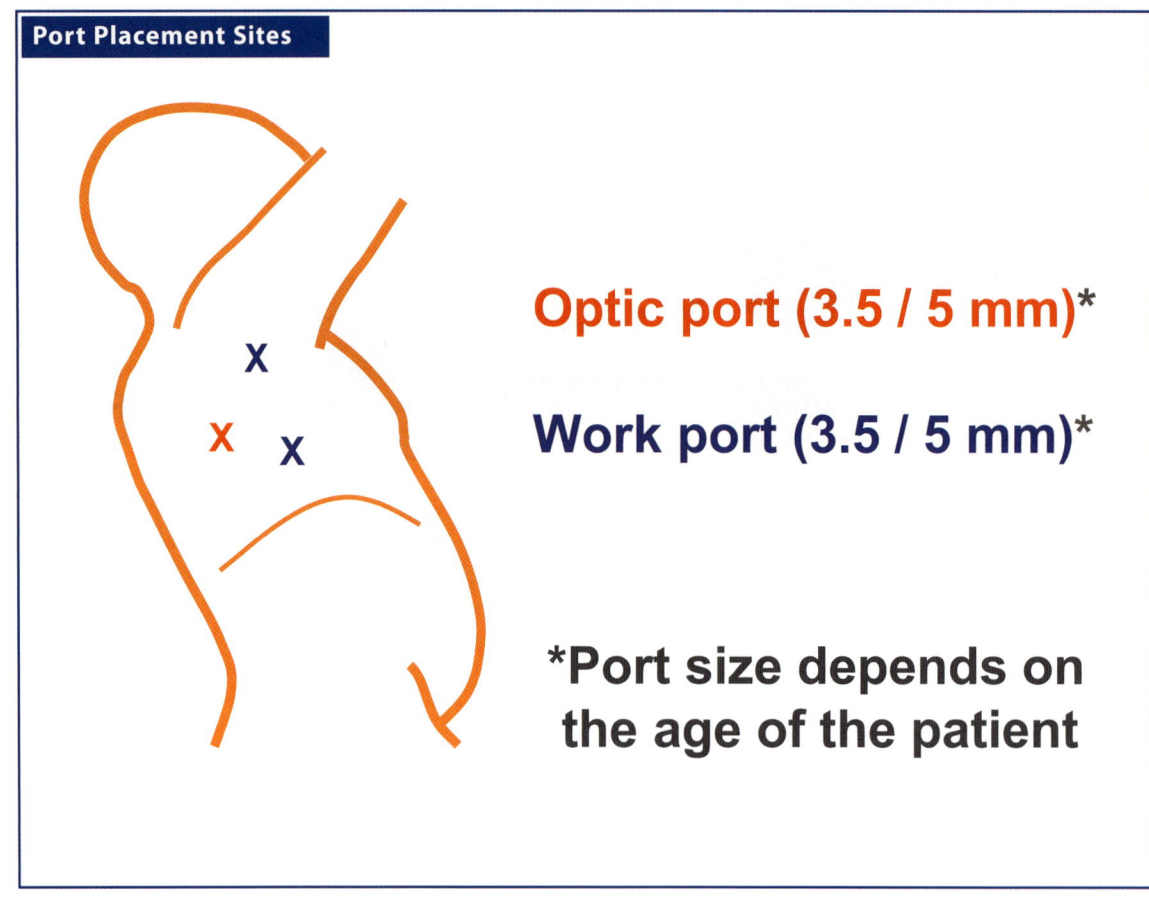

Port Placement Sites

Optic port (3.5 / 5 mm)*

Work port (3.5 / 5 mm)*

*Port size depends on the age of the patient

13.5   Indications

1. Bronchogenic cyst/lesion.
2. Resection performed to avoid complications of a lesion, including infection, hemorrhage, and expansion of cyst.

13.6   Preoperative Considerations

1. Obtain good imaging studies – computed tomography or magnetic resonance imaging scan of the chest to delineate the location of the bronchogenic cyst commonly found in the paratracheal, perihilar, paraesophageal, and intraparenchymal regions.
2. Avoid operation while there is an ongoing infection and ensure that the patient is adequately treated prior to attempting resection.
3. Preoperative antibiotics are generally administered

13.7   Technical Notes

1. Single-lung ventilation is preferred (tube position is checked using bronchoscopy).
2. Alternatively, insufflate with low pressure at 5–7 mmHg at a low flow rate (1 l/min) to allow for further collapse of the lung. Insufflation should be done slowly to prevent reflex bradycardia.
3. If it appears that vital structures may be compromised with resection, then it is essential to perform a mucosectomy or fulgurate the mucosa with a laparoscopic cautery, or argon beam coagulator to prevent recurrence.
4. Insert a chest tube to evacuate any residual pneumothorax, especially for central mediastinal cysts. This can usually be removed within 24 h.

13.8   Procedure Variations

1. Cyst resection can be performed with the hook cautery, harmonic scalpel, or LigaSure™.
2. Patient positioning and port sites can be varied according to the location of lesion.
3. In paraesophageal lesions perform a swallow study prior to feeding to ensure no leakage of the contrast medium.
4. Most small cysts can be removed from the 5-mm port sites; occasionally an incision may need to be enlarged, or a specimen retrieval bag can be used with a larger port.

13.9   Thoracoscopic Resection of Bronchogenic Cysts

Please see Figs. 1–4.

Figure 13.1

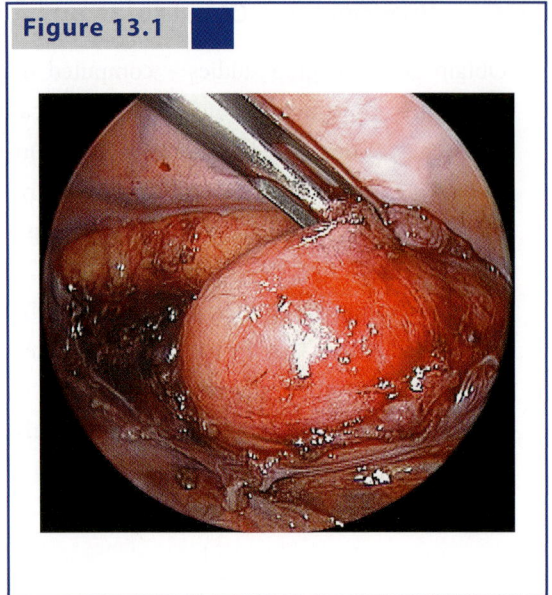

Thoracoscopic view of hilar bronchogenic cyst and initial dissection

Figure 13.2

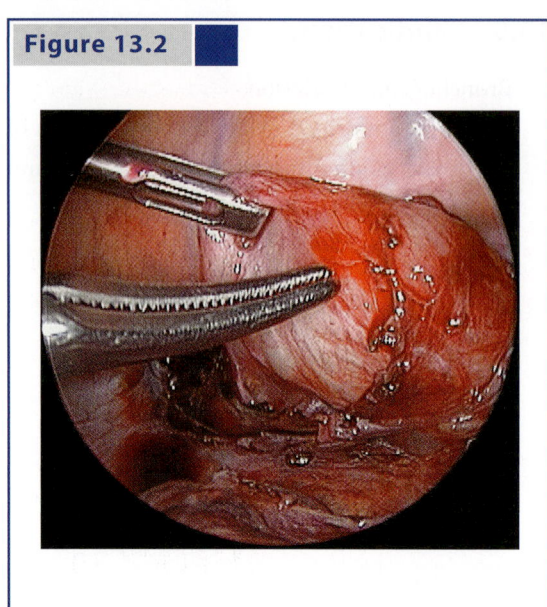

Dissection of the cyst from the mediastinal attachments

Figure 13.3

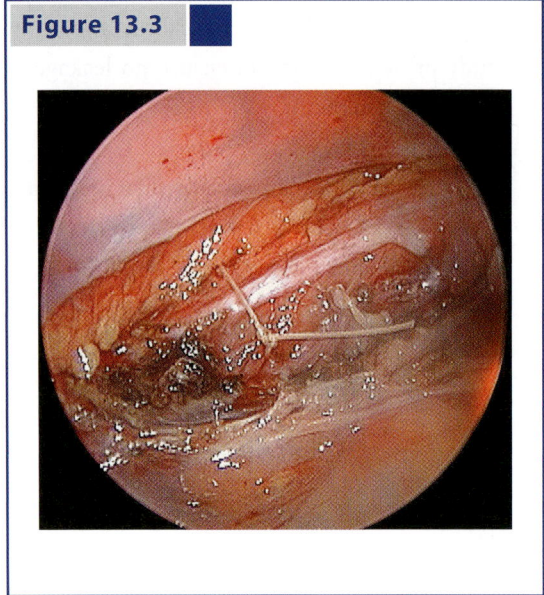

The thoracoscopic view of the mediastinum following removal of the bronchogenic cyst

Figure 13.4

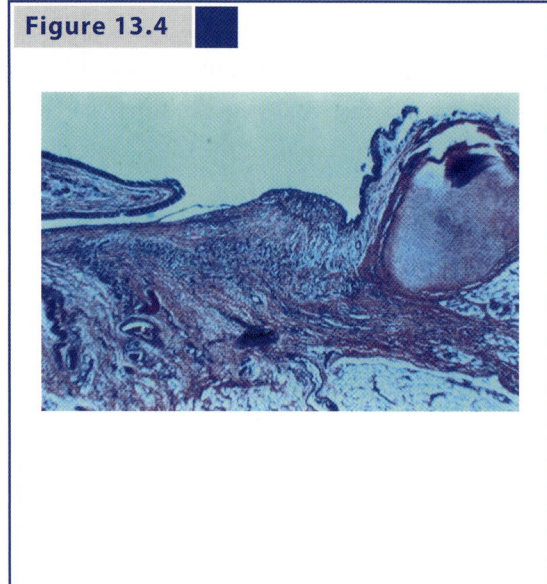

Histology of the bronchogenic cyst demonstrating a cartilage remnant and ciliated epithelium

Recommended Literature

1. Engum S (2007) Minimal access thoracic surgery in the pediatric population. Semin Pediatr Surg.15:14–16
2. Mercy C, Spurbeck W, Lobe TE (1999) Resection of foregut derived duplications by minimal access surgery. Pediatr Surg Int 15:224–226
3. Ure BM, Schmidt AI, Jesch NK (2005) Thoracoscopic surgery in infants and children. Eur J Pediatr Surg 15:314–318

14 Resection of Pulmonary Sequestrations

Lutz Stroedter

14.1 Operation Room Setup

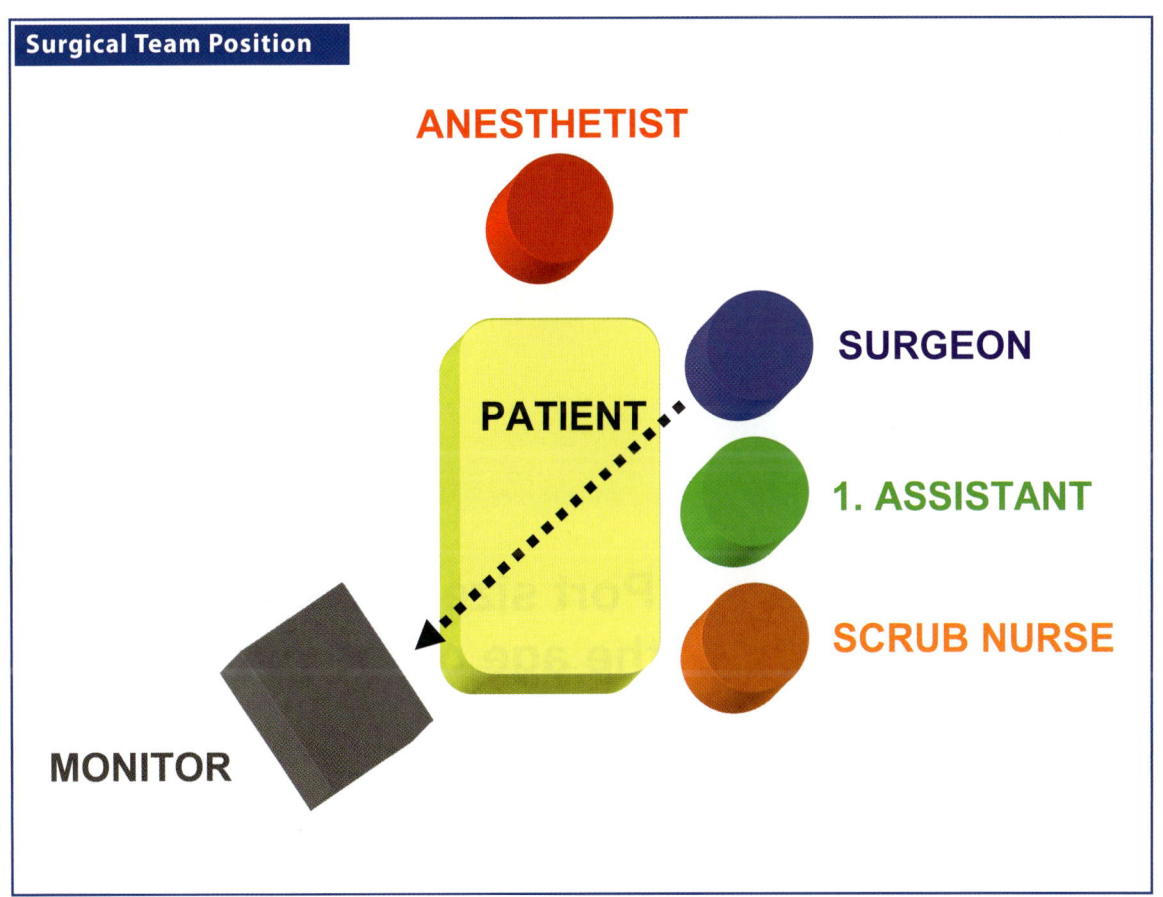

14.2   Patient Positioning

The patient is placed in a formal lateral decubitus position. The arm is elevated to move the scapula upward.

14.3   Special Instruments

- Endoscopic clips
- Endoscopic stapler
- Specimen retrieval bag (10 mm port)

14.4   Location of Access Points

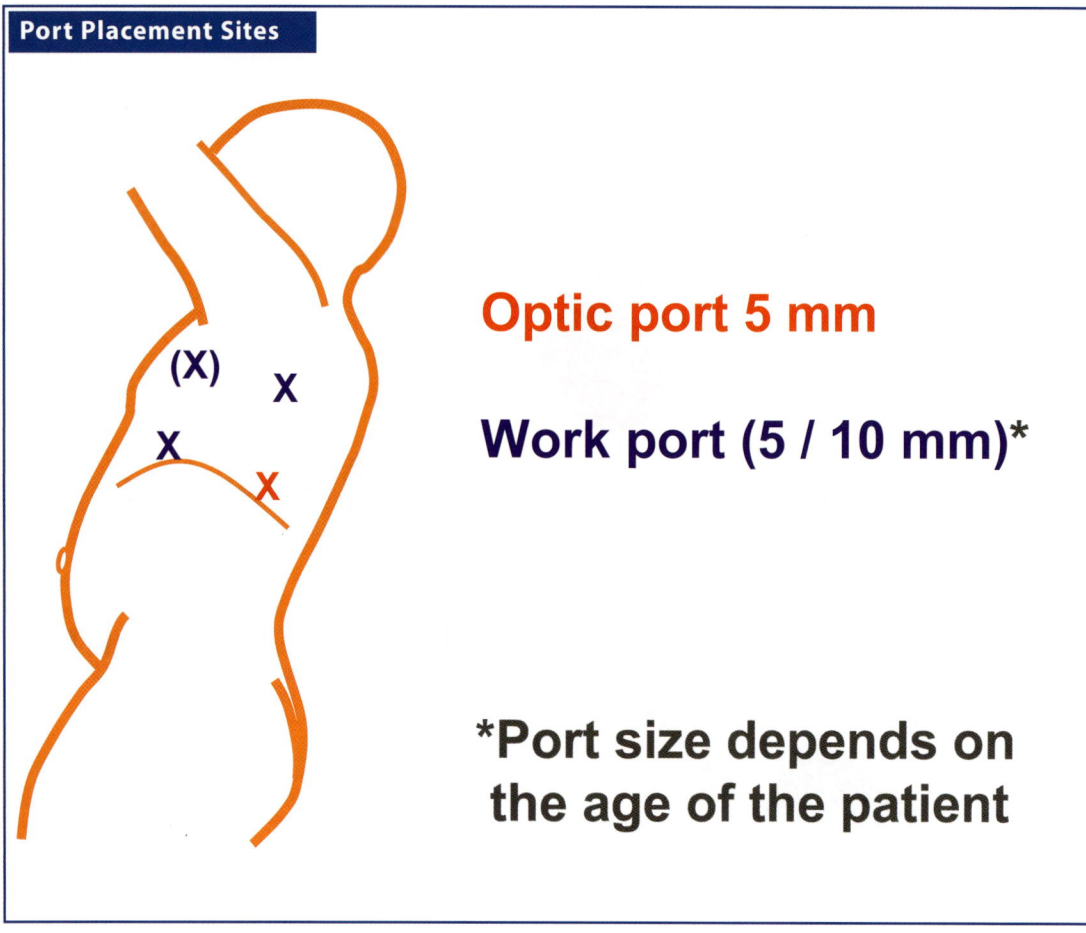

Port Placement Sites

Optic port 5 mm

Work port (5 / 10 mm)*

*Port size depends on the age of the patient

14.5   Indications

1. The resection of pulmonary sequestrations should be performed within the first year of life (when detected) because of the complications due to risk of infection.
2. Intralobar sequestrations (ILS) have a 9-fold higher risk of infection than extralobar sequestrations (ELS).
3. Most of the ELS lesions are diagnosed coincidentally during imaging investigations for surgery or for associated congenital anomalies.

14.6   Contraindications

1. General contraindications to Video-Assisted Thoracoscopic Surgery (VATS)
2. Since ELS patients have associated anomalies more frequently than ILS patients; the severity of these anomalies may be relative contraindications to VATS in ELS patients.

14.7   Preoperative Considerations

1. It is difficult to distinguish an ILS from ELS using plain films. However, ILS lesions tend to be heterogeneous and are not well defined. ELS masses are usually observed as solid, well defined, and retrocardiac.
2. Computed tomography (CT) with contrast or magnetic resonance angiography (MRA) provide valuable information. The arterial supply and venous drainage both should be outlined because of the unpredictability of vascular connections.
3. Upper gastrointestinal contrast examination may be useful if communication with the gastrointestinal tract is in question.

14.8   Technical Notes

1. ELS account for 25% of cases and have their own pleural covering. No tissue separation from lung is required.
2. ILS are surrounded by normal lung tissue and require endoscopic staplers utilization for surgical resection.
3. Both ELS and ILS receive their blood supply from anomalous systemic arteries, usually arising from the descending aorta.
4. Venous drainage is usually by the pulmonary veins for ILS and by the systemic venous system for ELS.
5. Multiple supply arteries are found in 15% of sequestrations; 73% originating from the abdominal aorta and 18% from the thoracic aorta.

14.9   Procedure Variations

1. The systemic artery can be ligated using three absorbable sutures and intracorporeal suturing.
2. Use of LigaSure™ (Valleylab, Boulder, CO, USA) for abberant vessels up to 7mm in diameter.
3. In ILS, lobectomy or wedge resection can be performed using bipolar cautery or harmonic scalpel.

14.10   Thoracoscopic Resection of Intralobar Sequestrations

Please see Figs. 1–6.

Figure 14.1

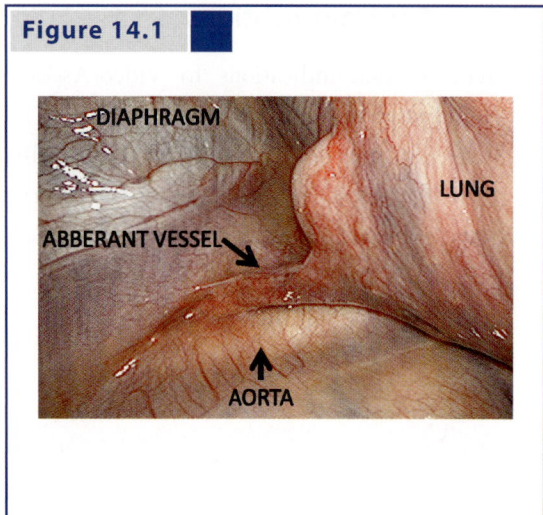

View of the left thoracic cavity showing the aberrant vessel as it enters the thorax through the diaphragm to provide vascular supply to the sequestration

Figure 14.2

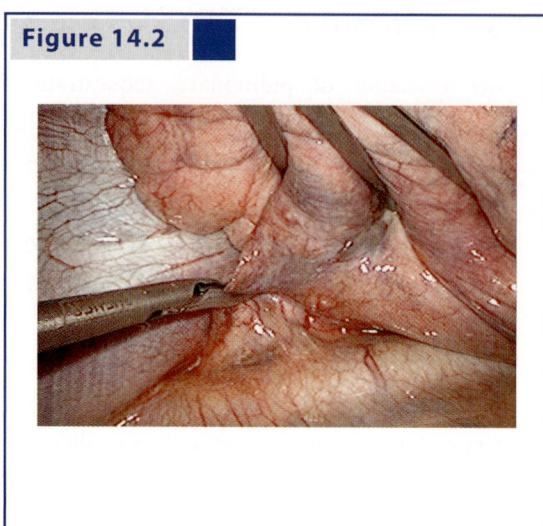

The lung is retracted using a retractor and the vessel feeding the ILS is carefully clamped using blunt forceps to confirm blanching of the sequestration

Figure 14.3

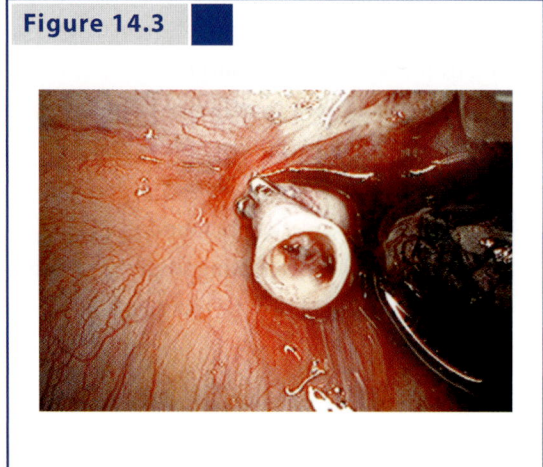

The feeding vessel is clipped twice centrally and once peripherally using endoscopic titanium clips and dissected. The disruption of vascular supply leads to visible demarcation of the ILS from the normal lung tissue

Figure 14.4

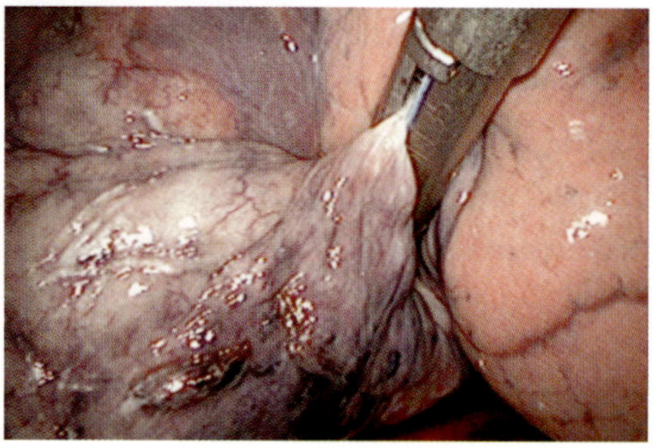

The endoscopic stapler is used to resect the sequestration from the normal lung tissue at the plane of demarcation. Multiple staplers may be required depending on the size of the sequester

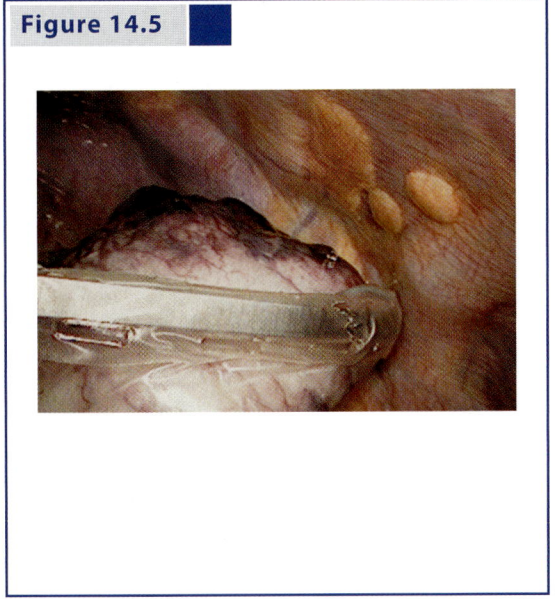

Figure 14.5

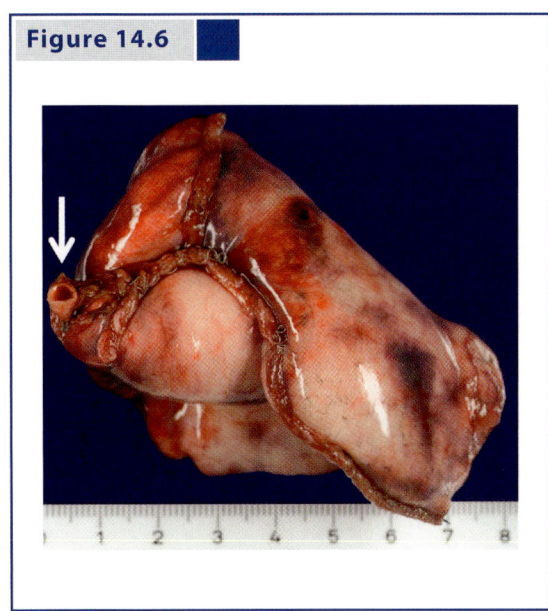

Figure 14.6

A specimen retrieval bag is used to retrieve the sequestration. The port incision is enlarged to extract the specimen out of the thoracic cavity

View of the ILS specimen resected using endoscopic staplers, along with the clipped supplying vessel (*arrow*)

Recommended Literature

1. Albanese CT, Sydorak AM, Tsao K, Lee H (2003) Thoracoscopic lobectomy for prenatally diagnosed lung lesions. J Pediatr Surg 38:553–555
2. de Lagausie P, Bonnard A, Berrebi D, Petit P, Dorgeret S, Guys JM (2005) Video-assisted thoracoscopic surgery for pulmonary sequestration in children. Ann Thorac Surg 80:1266–1269
3. Rothenberg SS (2008) First decade's experience with thoracoscopic lobectomy in infants and children. J Pediatr Surg 43:40–44

15 Treatment of Pulmonary Blebs and Bullae

Amulya K. Saxena

15.1 Operation Room Setup

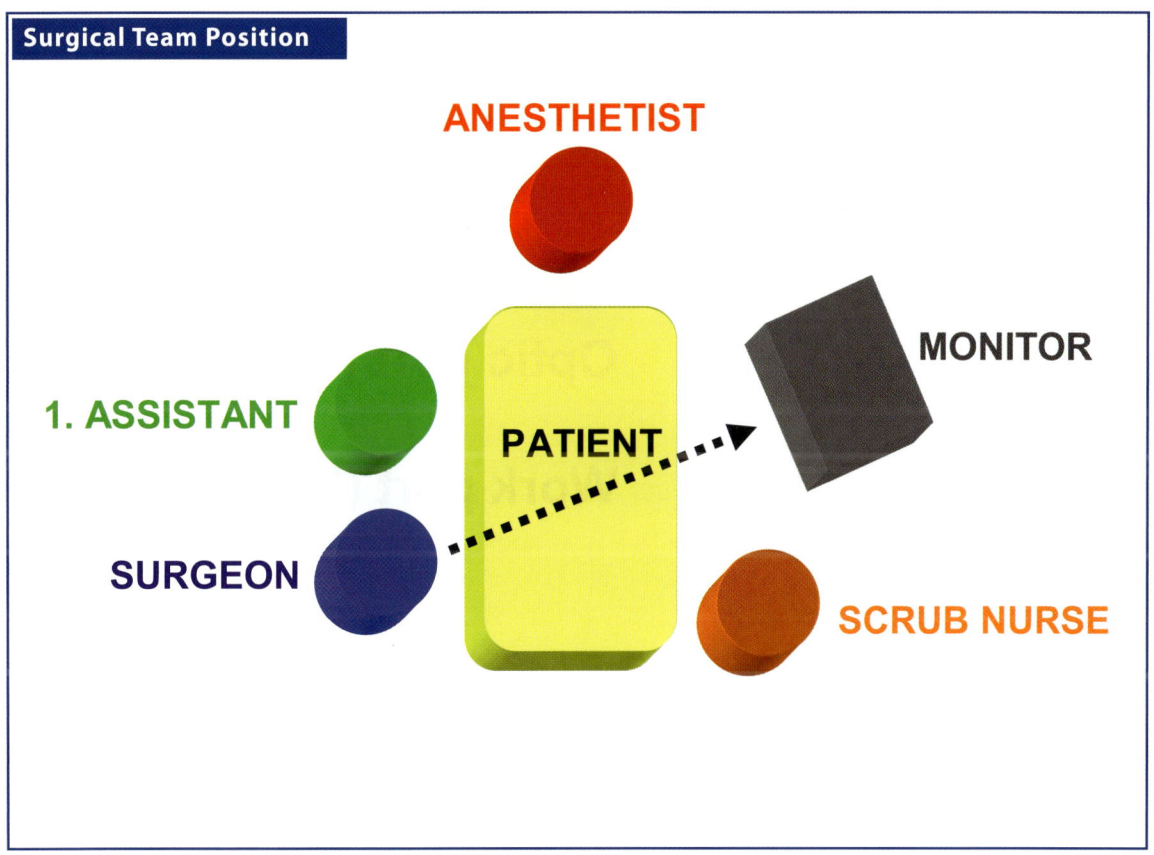

15.2   Patient Positioning

The patient is placed in a formal lateral decubitus position. The surgeon and assistant are at the back of the patient.

15.3   Special Instruments

- LigaSure™ (Valleylab, Boulder, CO, USA)
- Endo GIA™ stapler (Auto Suture, Norwalk, CT, USA)
- Laser
- PleuraSeal™ lung sealant (Covidien, Hazelwood, MO, USA)
- Fibrin glue

15.4   Location of Access Points

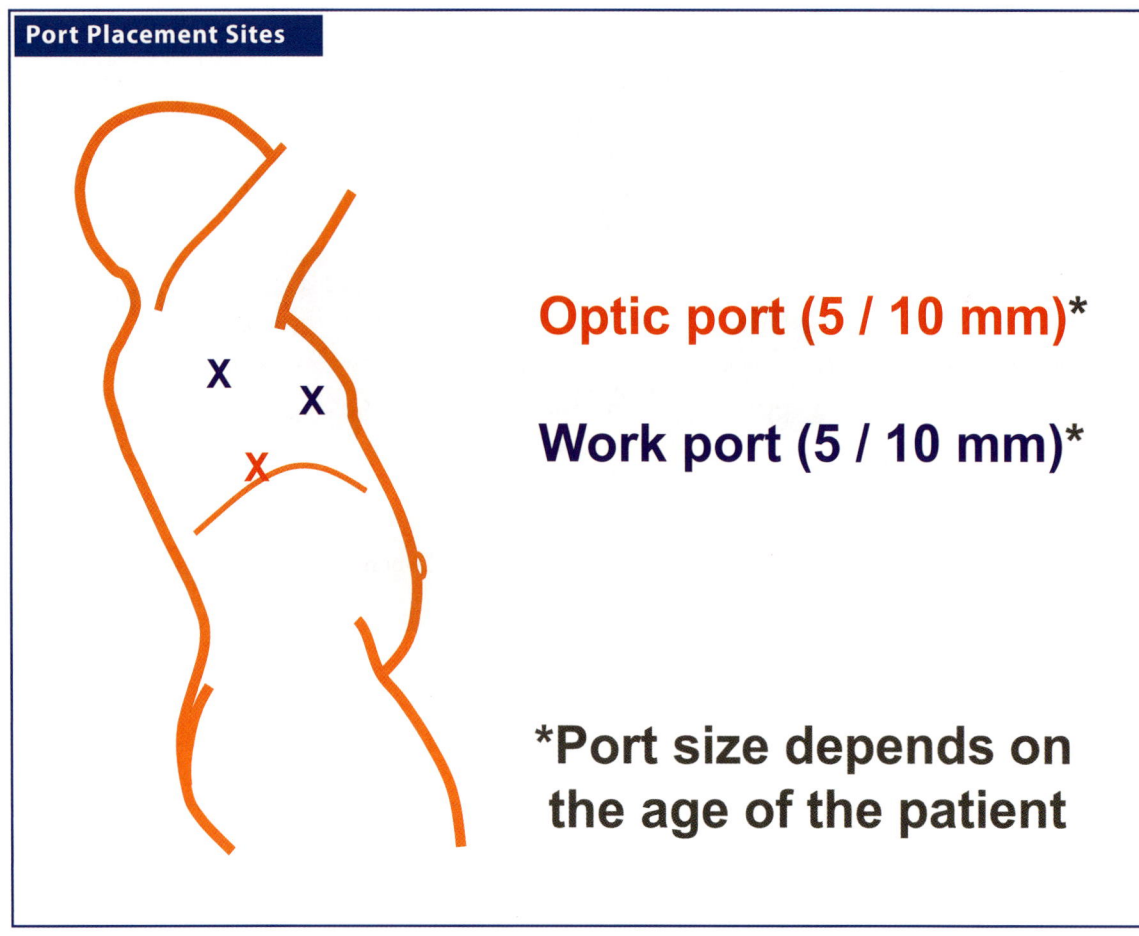

Port Placement Sites

Optic port (5 / 10 mm)*

Work port (5 / 10 mm)*

*Port size depends on the age of the patient

15.5   Indications

1. Blebs are small 1- to 2-cm subpleural air spaces that a frequently present on the apices of normal lungs.
2. Bullae are relatively large air-filled spaces that arise in the apices of the upper lobes and the superior segment of the lower lobes.
3. Indications for thoracoscopic treatment are limited to recurrent disease or episodes that last for 5 days or longer.

15.6   Contraindications

General contraindications to Video-Assisted Thoracoscopic Surgery (VATS)

15.7   Preoperative Considerations

1. Preoperative assessment with computed tomography scan should be performed to determine the size and location of the blebs.
2. The type of technique employed determines the number and size of ports used.
3. If endostapler devices are to be employed, ports of 10- or 12-mm should be used.
4. The surgeon must coordinate with the anesthetist and make sure that the concentration of oxygen being delivered to the lungs is less than 50%, since higher concentrations involve a danger of combustion with serious pulmonary burns.

15.8   Technical Notes

1. The entire lung should be inspected for air leaks.
2. Stapling must be performed with caution to prevent bleeding or removal of excess tissue.
3. On completion of the procedure ensure that there are no air leaks by irrigating the thorax and observing bubbles within the fluid.
4. PleuraSeal™ can be applied uniformly as a spray using the endoscopic spray applicator (MicroMyst™; Covidien, Hazelwood, MO, USA). The lung sealant hydrolyzes over a period of 4 to 8 weeks which gives sufficient time to allow for normal wound healing.

15.9   Procedure Variations

1. Lung tissue division and sealing using endoscopic linear stapler.
2. Lung tissue resection using LigaSure™.
3. Thoracoscopic ablation using Nd:YAG laser.
4. Tissue ligation using standard endoscopic loop suture.
5. Lesion sealing with fibrin glue.
6. Chemical pleurodesis by mechanical abrasion.

15.10   Thoracoscopic Options for Pulmonary Blebs and Bullae

Please see Figs. 1–5.

Figure 15.1

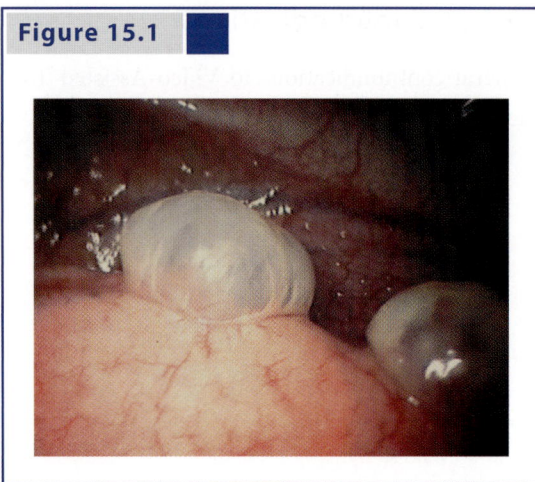

The entire lung surface is inspected so that the lesions are not missed. Pulmonary blebs (as seen in figure) generally present with a translucent or transparent surface

Figure 15.2

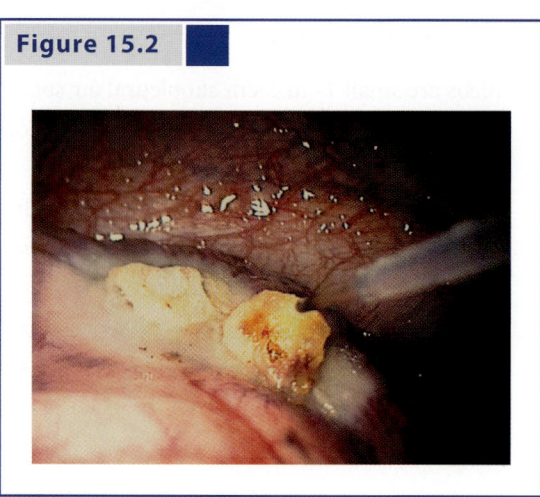

The blebs are ablated using Nd:YAG laser. Topical fibrin glue may be applied to strengthen the closure site

Figure 15.3

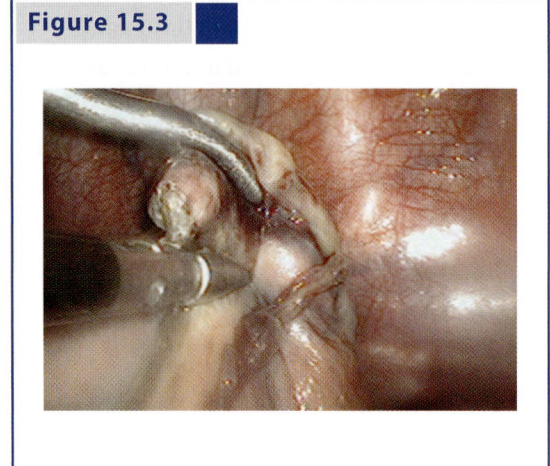

Alternatively, the blebs can be resected. If multiple blebs are present, each bleb must be resected separately and care must be taken to seal any communicating bronchii. The bleb is punctured and the tissue is held using graspers for resection using endoscopic staplers

Figure 15.4

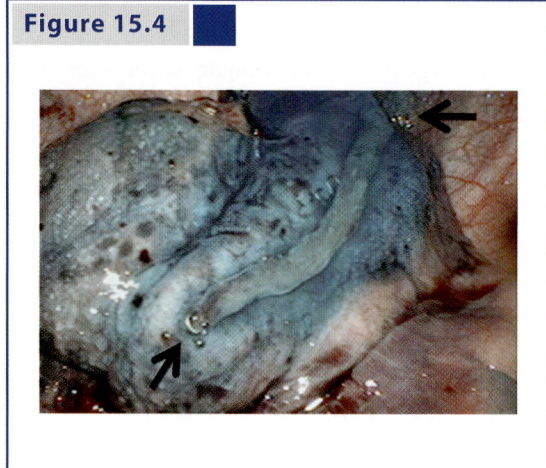

PleuraSeal™ is sprayed over the resected lung tissue (stapler line between *arrows* in figure) and forms an airtight and elastic sealant film. The blue color of PleuraSeal™ allows visual identification of the sealant on the area applied. PleuraSeal™ lung sealant is a 100% synthetic absorbable hydrogel

Figure 15.5

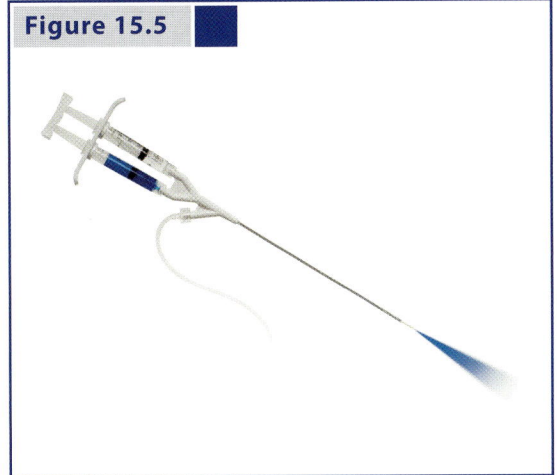

PleuraSeal™ is a two component lung sealant consisting of polyethylene glycol (PEG) ester and tri-lysine amine. When mixed together, the precursors link to form a surgical sealant. The mixing is accomplished as the materials exit the tip of the Mi-croMyst™ applicator. (Courtesy of Covidien Austria, Brunn am Gebirge, Austria)

Recommended Literature

1. Chang YC, Chen CW, Huang SH, Chen JS (2006) Modified needlescopic video-assisted thoracic surgery for primary spontaneous pneumothorax: the long-term effects of apical pleurectomy versus pleural abrasion. Surg Endosc 20:757–762

2. Cheng YJ, Kao EL (2004) Prospective comparison between endosuturing and endostapling in treating primary spontaneous pneumothorax. J Laparoendosc Adv Surg Tech A 14:274–277

3. Cho DG, Do Cho K, Kang CU, Seop Jo M (2008) Thoracoscopic apico-posterior transmediastinal approach for bilateral spontaneous pneumothorax. Interact Cardiovasc Thorac Surg 7:352–354

16 Thoracic Neuroblastoma Resection

Michael E. Höllwarth

16.1 Operation Room Setup

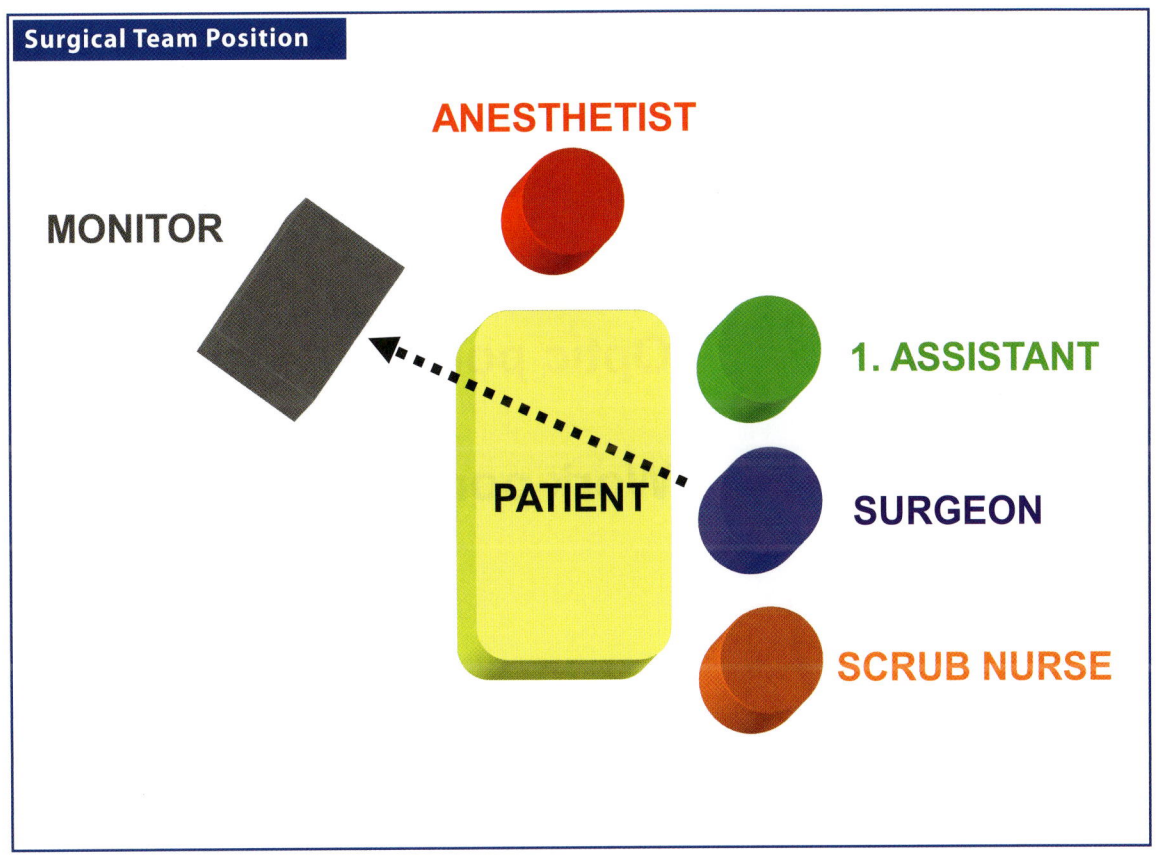

Surgical Team Position

ANESTHETIST

MONITOR

1. ASSISTANT

PATIENT

SURGEON

SCRUB NURSE

16.2   Patient Positioning

The patient is placed in a formal lateral decubitus or modified prone position. The surgeon and the assistant stand in front of the patient.

16.3   Special Instruments

- Specimen retrieval bag
- Bipolar electrocautery devices
- LigaSure™ (Valleylab, Boulder, CO, USA)

16.4   Location of Access Points

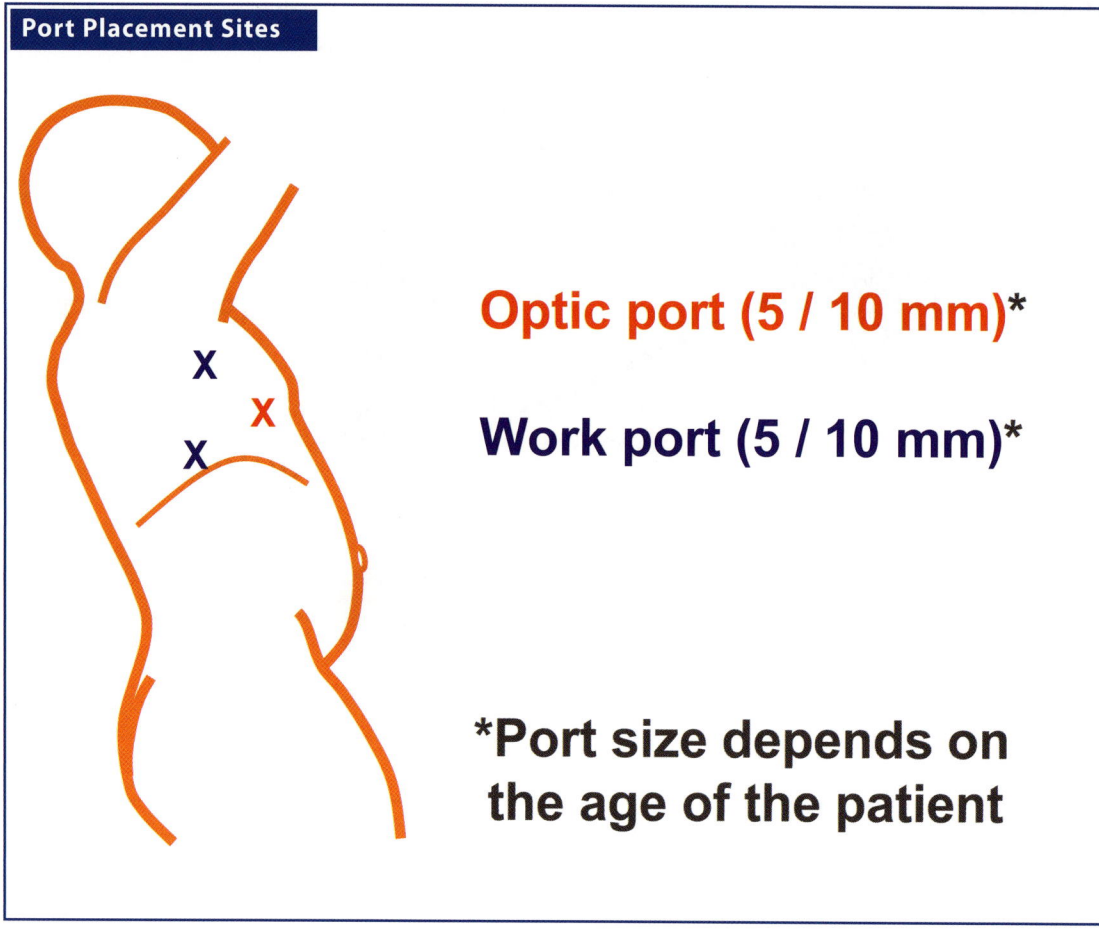

Port Placement Sites

Optic port (5 / 10 mm)*

Work port (5 / 10 mm)*

*Port size depends on the age of the patient

16.5   Indications

1. Localized neuroblastoma in Stage 1 according to the International Neuroblastoma Staging System (INSS) with sizes < 10 cm.
2. The primary goals of surgery are to:
   a) Determine an accurate diagnosis.
   b) Remove all of the primary tumor.
   c) To provide accurate surgical staging.
   d) Offer adjuvant therapy for delayed primary surgery.

16.6   Contraindications

1. Diffuse neuroblastoma Stage 3, Stage 4 and Stage 4S (INSS).
2. Tumor mass with involvement of vital structures.
3. Large neuroblastomas > 10 cm.

16.7   Preoperative Considerations

1. Preoperative assessment with computed tomography should be performed to determine the size and the location of the neuroblastoma in the thorax.
2. Specific investigations to stage neuroblastoma include (1) bone marrow aspirates and biopsy samples, (2) body CT scan (excluding head, if not clinically indicated), (3) bone scan, and (4) meta-iodobenzylguanidine (MIBG) scintigraphy.
3. Conventional mechanical ventilation with traction of the lung or single-lung ventilation options should be coordinated with the anesthetist.

16.8   Technical Notes

1. Apical tumors must be submitted to traction to allow proper dissected; this could result in temporary sympathetic lesions such as Horner's syndrome.
2. Precaution should be taken with electrocautery, since electrocoagulation associated lateral spread of current or heat could also induce temporary Horner's syndrome.
3. Roots of neurogenic tumors are easy to individualize and excessive traction should be avoided to prevent stretching of the medullar roots. The medullar roots can be divided at the neural foramen using harmonic scalpel.

16.9   Procedure Variations

1. Tumor resection using harmonic scalpel. This has the advantage of reduced thermal spread which decreases complications that are associated with electrosurgery.
2. Port number (3-, 4- or 5- ports) may vary depending on the age of the patient, size of the tumor, type of ventilation and location of the tumor.

16.10   Thoracoscopic Resection of Neuroblastoma

Please see Figs. 1–6.

Figure 16.1

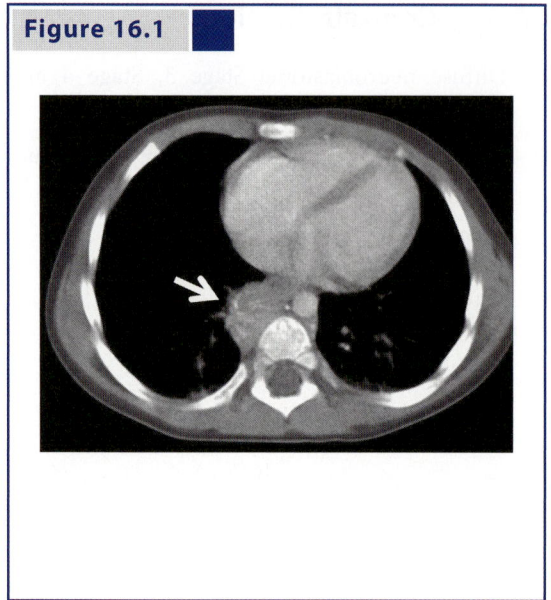

Nonenhanced axial CT scan of the chest in a patient with a thoracic neuroblastoma showing a right posterior mediastinal mass (***arrow***)

Figure 16.2

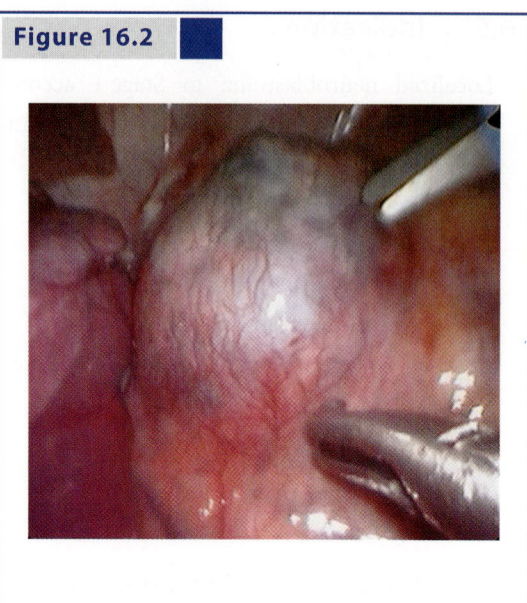

Endoscopic view of the thoracic neuroblastoma covered by the parietal pluera

Figure 16.3

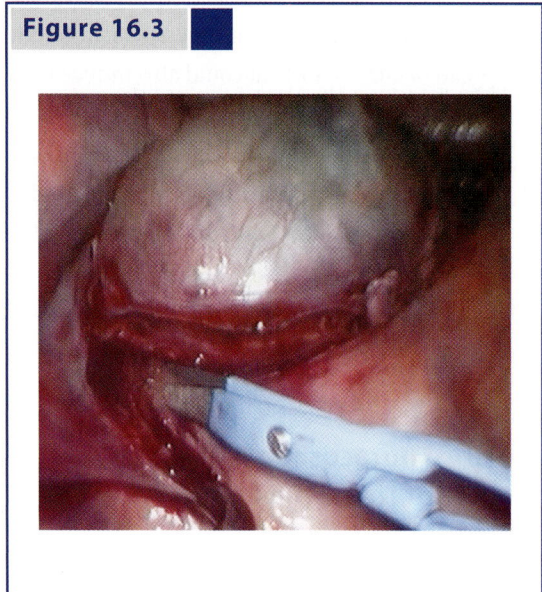

Using bipolar electrocautery scissors the parietal pleura covering the neuroblastoma is incised

Figure 16.4

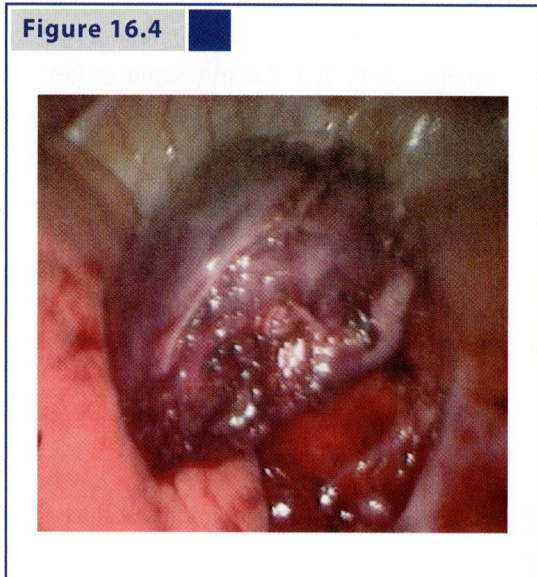

Further preparation of the neuroblastoma is carried out using a combination of bipolar electrocautery scissors and blunt dissection. The short intercostal vessels supplying the tumor have to be carefully cauterized

Figure 16.5

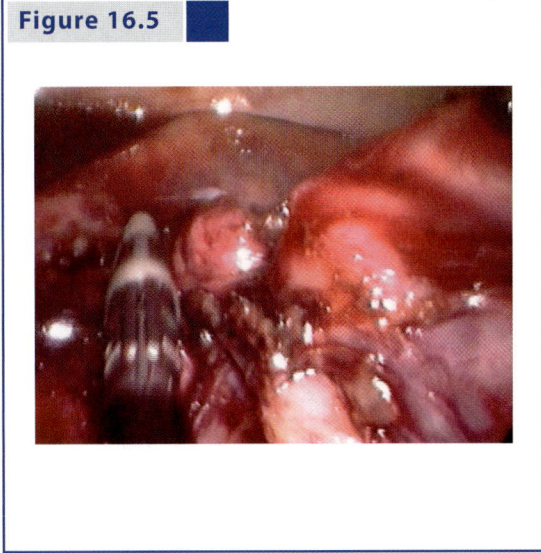

Figure 16.6

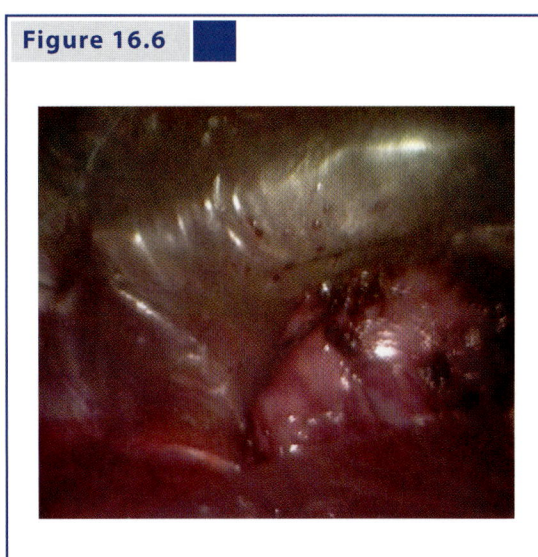

The medullar roots of the neuroblastoma are divided at the level of the neural foramen using Liga-Sure™

The neuroblastoma is placed in a specimen retrieval bag and the port incision is increased to an appropriate size to remove the tumor from the thoracic cavity

Recommended Literature

1. Lacreuse I, Valla J, de Lagausie P, Varlet F, Héloury Y, Temporal G, Bastier R, F . Becmeur F (2007) Thoracoscopic resection of neurogenic tumors in children. J Pediatr Surg 42:1725–1728
2. Nio M, Nakamura M, Yoshida S, Ishii T, Amae S, Hayashi Y(2005) Thoracoscopic removal of neurogenic mediastinal tumors in children. J Laparoendosc Adv Surg Tech A 15:80–83
3. Petty J, Bensard D, Partrick D, Hendrickson R, Albano E, Karrer F (2006) Resection of Neurogenic Tumors in Children: Is Thoracoscopy Superior to Thoracotomy? J Am Coll Surg 203: 699–703

17 Esophageal Atresia Repair

Klaas N.M.A. Bax and David C. van der Zee

17.1 Operation Room Setup

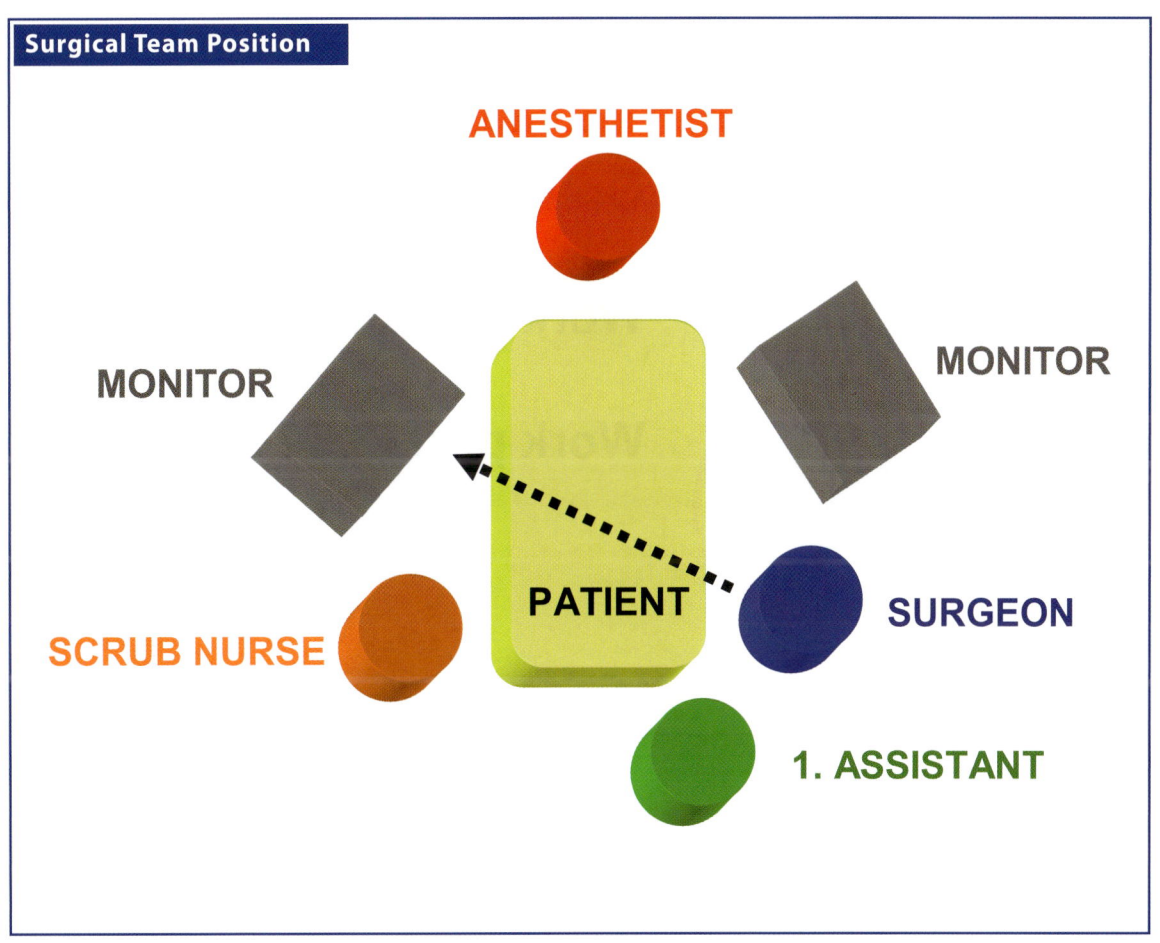

Surgical Team Position

ANESTHETIST

MONITOR

MONITOR

PATIENT

SCRUB NURSE

SURGEON

1. ASSISTANT

17.2   Patient Positioning

Left lateral decubitus at the left edge of the table, small pad below the chest, pelvis fixed to the table, right arm fixed over the head. A shortened operating table is preferred with a reversed Trendelenburg and a patient tilt to the left.

17.3   Special Instruments

See section on instrumentation.

17.4   Location of Access Points

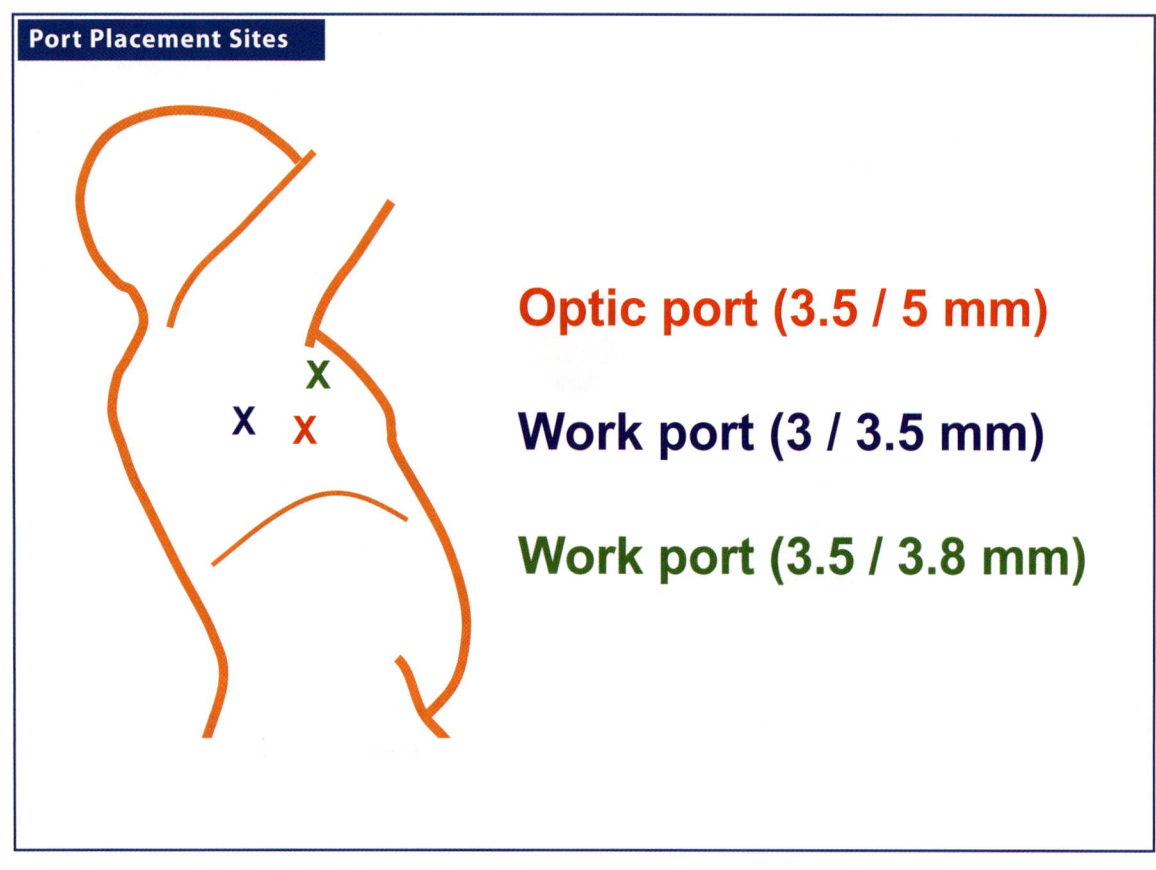

Port Placement Sites

Optic port (3.5 / 5 mm)

Work port (3 / 3.5 mm)

Work port (3.5 / 3.8 mm)

17.5   Indications

1. Esophageal atresia with distal fistula.
2. H-type fistula without atresia.
3. Esophageal atresia without fistula.

17.6   Contraindications

- There are no absolute contraindications.
- In esophageal atresia without fistula, one can opt for replacement instead for delayed primary repair. Even then, thoracoscopy may be useful for confirming the diagnosis of a long gap.

17.7   Preoperative Considerations

1. If the aorta descends on the right, the child is placed in a right lateral decubitus position and the esophagus is approached from the left.
2. A 10-Fr Replogle tube is placed in the upper esophageal pouch for identification.
3. The tip of the endotracheal tube should not be at the level of the carina in order to avoid accidental advancement into the right main bronchus or into the fistula if it originates from the carina.
4. Carbon dioxide is insufflated at a pressure of 5 mmHg and a flow of 0.1 l/min.

17.8   Technical Notes

1. Initial desaturation is the rule. Decreasing ventilatory pressure and increasing the frequency of respiration is desired. The anesthetist should be comfortable with the ventilatory parameters.
2. Transection of the azygos vein is only required when the fistula enters the trachea distally.
3. Commence the opening of the posterior mediastinal pleura above the azygos vein.

17.9   Instrumentation

1. In premature infants, a short, 3.3-mm, 30° telescope is used; otherwise a classic but short 5-mm 30° telescope is used.
2. Instruments utilized should have a 3-mm diameter and 24-cm length.
3. The working ports have a 3.5 or 3.8 mm diameter. Such ports allow introduction of 5-0 Vicryl™ sutures on a V-18 needle (Ethicon, Somerville, NJ, USA) with a 3-mm needle holder.

17.10   Thoracoscopic Esophageal Atresia Repair

Please see Figs. 1–6.

Figure 17.1

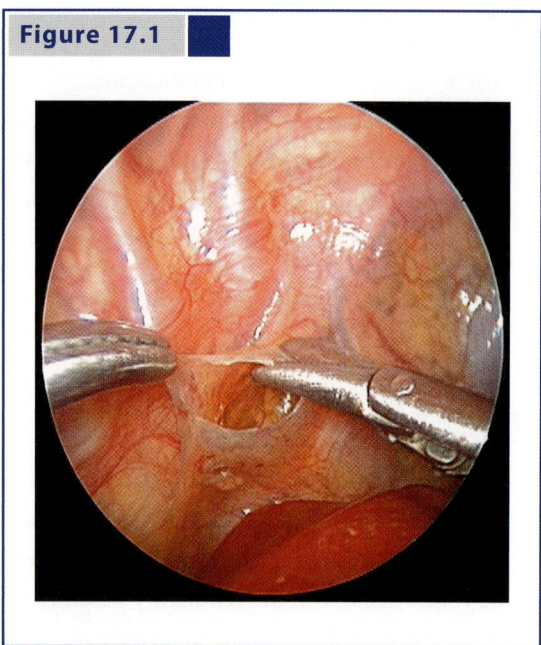

The mediastinal pleura is opened just anterior to the vertebral column

Figure 17.2

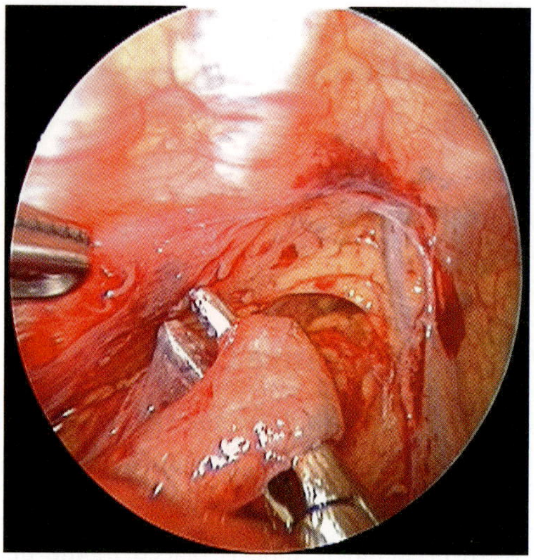

The distal fistula is freed close to the trachea and is suture ligated at this point. It is transected distally and its end is spatulated

Figure 17.3

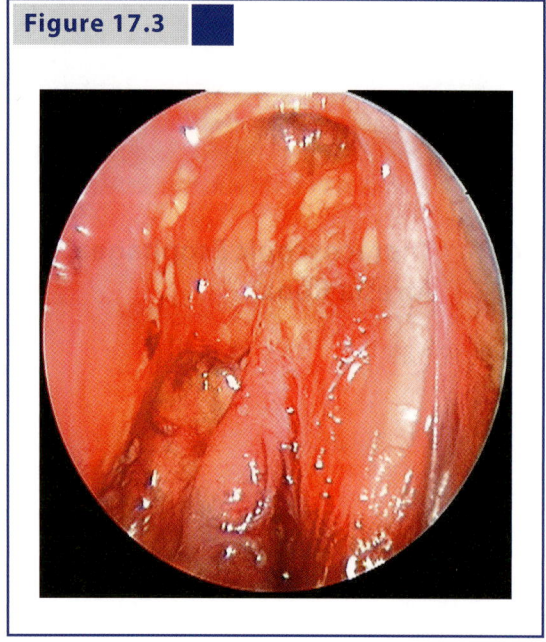

The proximal pouch as well as the distal fistula are visualized

Figure 17.4

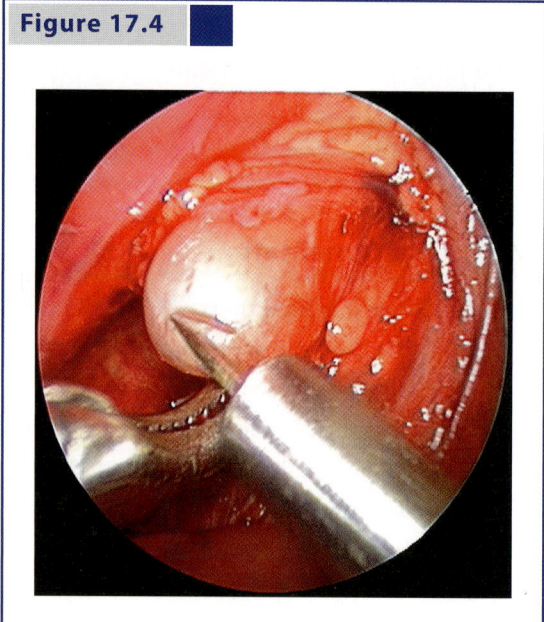

The distal end of the proximal pouch is freed and a wide opening is made right in the center

Figure 17.5

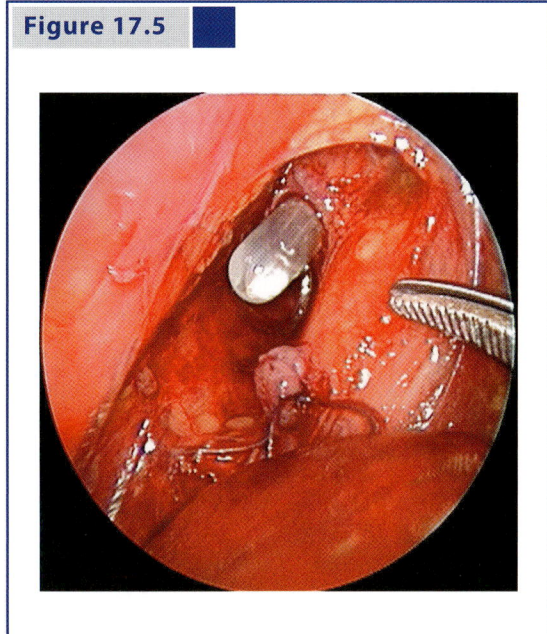

Figure 17.6

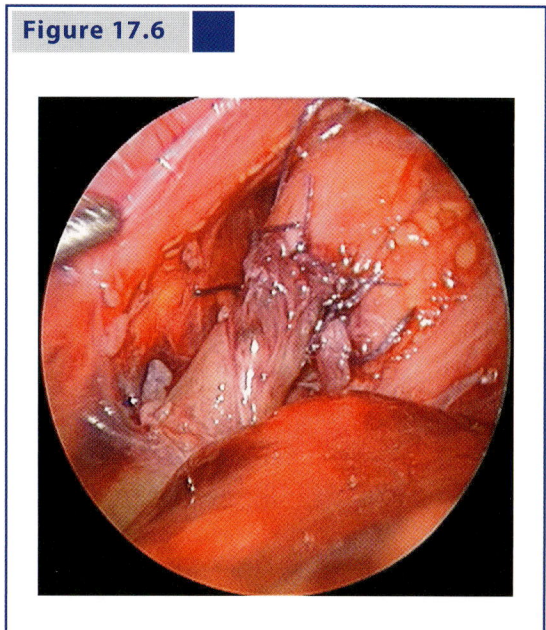

View of the suture-ligated tracheal side of the divided distal fistula and the emergence of the Replogle from the opened proximal pouch

The anastomosis is started in the middle of the left side of the esophagus and completed using 5-0 absorbable suture (Vicryl™; Ethicon, Somerville, NJ, USA). A transanastomotic 6-Fr or 8-Fr nasogastric tube is left in situ

Recommended Literature

1. Aziz GA, Schier F (2005) Thoracoscopic ligation of a tracheoesophageal H-type fistula in a newborn. J Pediatr Surg 40:e35–36
2. Bax KM, van der Zee DC (2002) Feasibility of thoracoscopic repair of esophageal atresia with distal fistula. J Pediatr Surg 37:192–196
3. Holcomb GW 3rd, Rothenberg SS, Bax KM, Martinez-Ferro M, Albanese CT, Ostlie DJ, van der Zee DC, Yeung CK (2005) Thoracoscopic repair of esophageal atresia and tracheoesophageal fistula: a multi-institutional analysis. Ann Surg 242:422–428

18 Congenital Diaphragmatic Hernia Repair

François Becmeur

18.1 Operation Room Setup

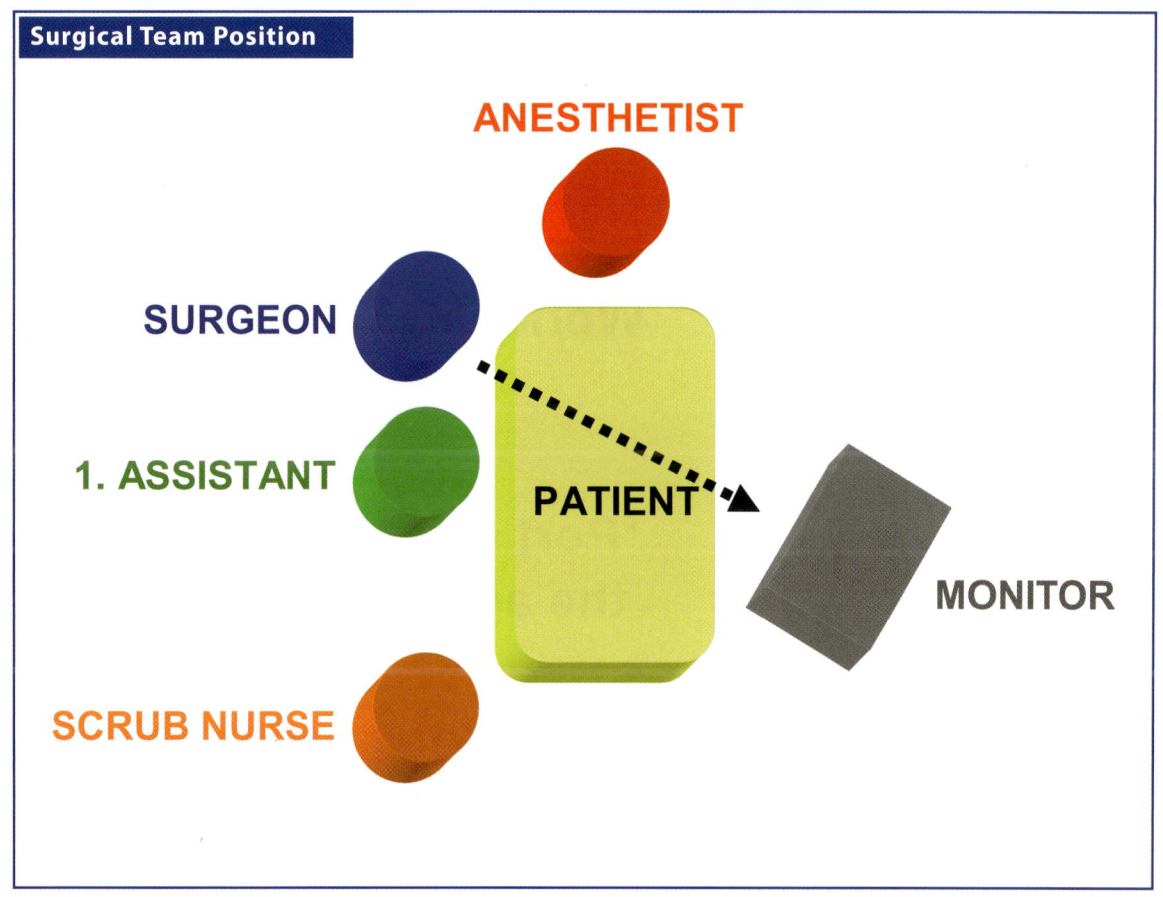

18.2   Patient Positioning

Right lateral decubitus with the left upper extremity left free and supported by the patient's head to permit 360° motion of the ports.

18.3   Special Instruments

- Gore-Tex® (WL Gore & Associates, Flagstaff, AZ, USA)
- Patches for large defects

18.4   Location of Access Points

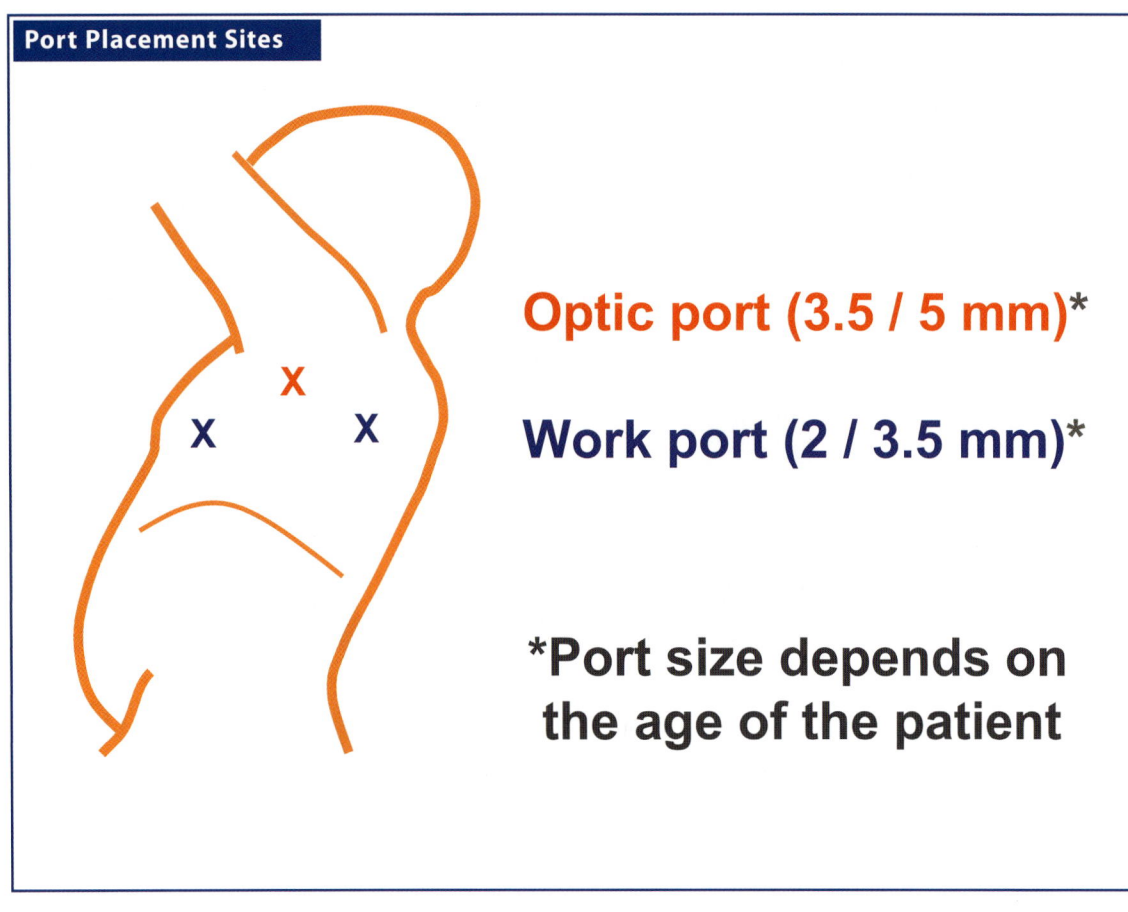

Port Placement Sites

Optic port (3.5 / 5 mm)*

Work port (2 / 3.5 mm)*

***Port size depends on the age of the patient**

18.5 Indications

1. Delayed congenital diaphragmatic hernia (CDH).
2. Incarcerated diaphragmatic hernia
3. CDH in neonates who are stabilized and present with a small defect.
4. Recurrent CDH.

18.6 Contraindications

1. Left-sided CDH with stomach and liver herniation.
2. Right-sided CDH with liver herniation.
3. Cardiopulmonary instability.

18.7 Preoperative Considerations

1. In the operating room, each patient receives perioperative antibiotics.
2. An arterial line and adequate intravenous access is established.
3. Pre- and postductal oxygen saturation monitors are placed.
4. Main stem intubation is not required. Patients are ventilated using pediatric ventilators with a pressure-limited mode of ventilation.

18.8 Technical Notes

1. Insufflation is started with low pressure (4 mmHg) and low flow (1.5 l/min).
2. Reduce contents with gentle manipulation.
3. Open the peritoneal posterior fold.
4. Remove the sac if present.
5. The defect is closed from medial to lateral.
6. Use nonabsorbable sutures (3-0 or 2-0).
7. Apply anchored rib sutures and/or pledgetted sutures at the lateral side of the defect.
8. A chest tube is not required.

18.9 Procedure Variations

1. In case of incarcerated delayed CDH, begin with a thoracoscopic approach.
2. If the hernia contents can not be reduced, continue with a laparoscopic approach (the abdomen prepped for this eventuality).
3. For the laparoscopic approach (in case of a left CDH), the optic port is passed through the umbilicus and the work port is placed in the left upper quadrant.
4. When the hernia contents are reduced, revert back to thoracoscopy to suture the diaphragmatic defect.

18.10 Thoracoscopic Congenital Diaphragmatic Hernia Repair

Please see Figs. 1–14.

Figure 18.1

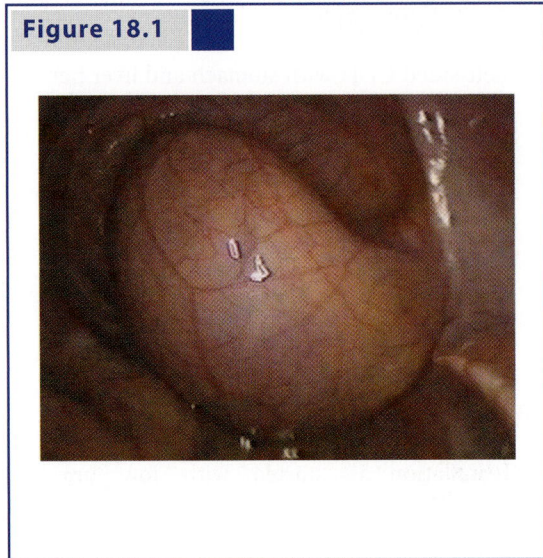

Delayed left congenital diaphragmatic hernia (CDH) presenting with herniation of the left kidney covered by a sac

Figure 18.2

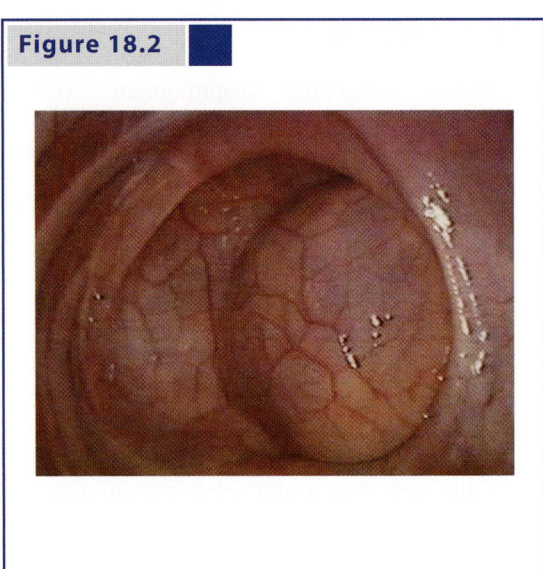

After 5 min of insufflation the contents can be reduced and the defect repaired

Figure 18.3

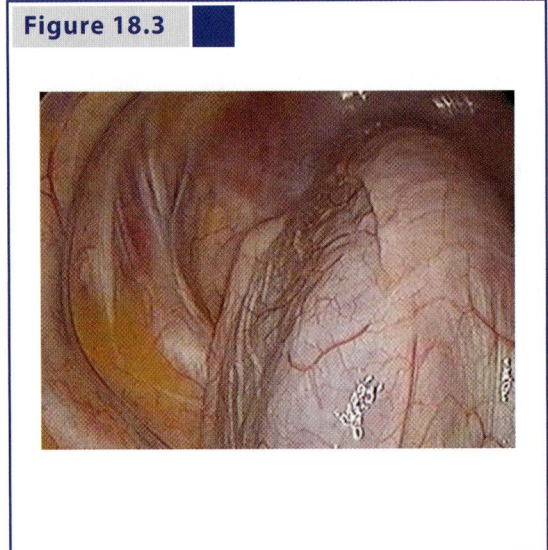

Thoracoscopic view of a delayed left CDH showing the herniated contents covered with a sac

Figure 18.4

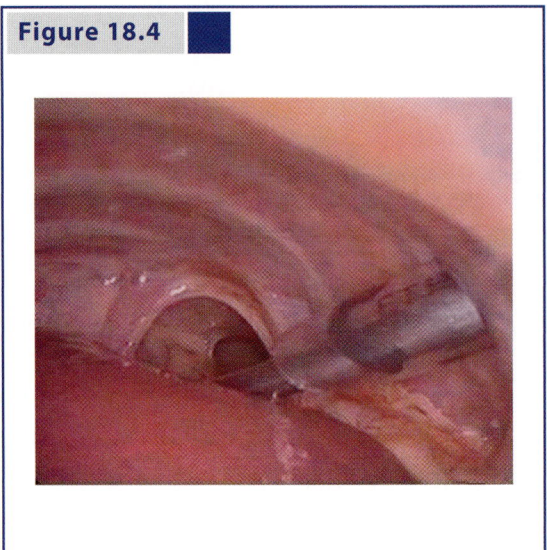

Delayed left CDH with the herniation of the entire spleen in the thoracic cavity

Figure 18.5

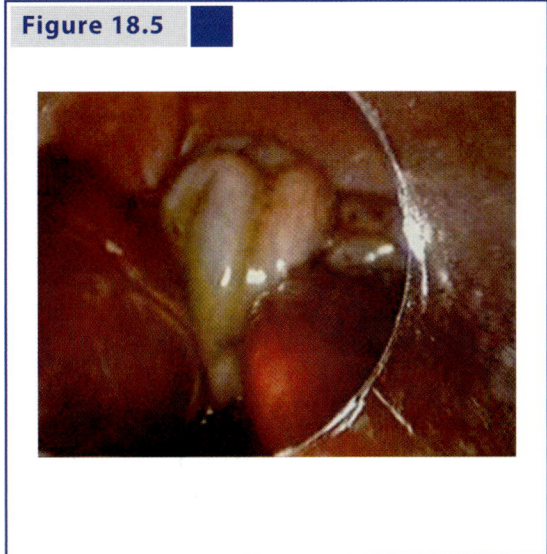

Atraumatic graspers are used to gently reduce the herniated contents

Figure 18.6

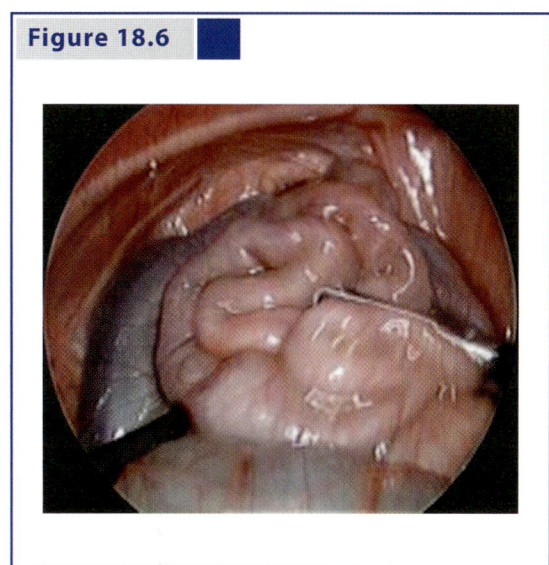

Two atraumatic graspers are employed to successively reduce the herniated intestines

Figure 18.7

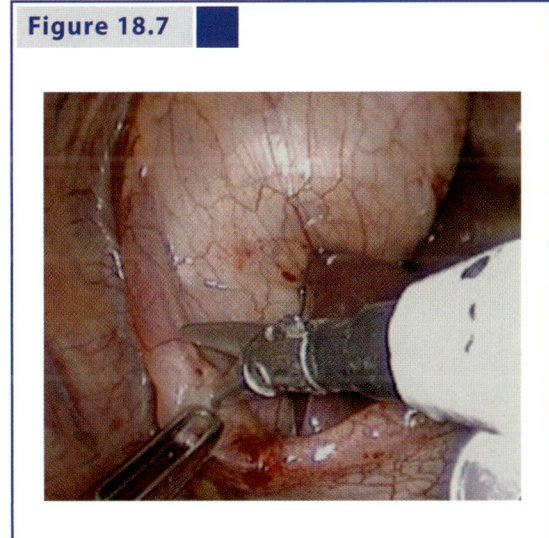
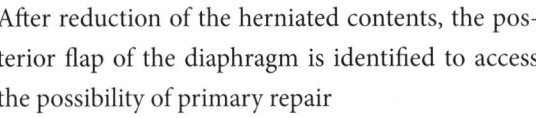

After reduction of the herniated contents, the posterior flap of the diaphragm is identified to access the possibility of primary repair

Figure 18.8

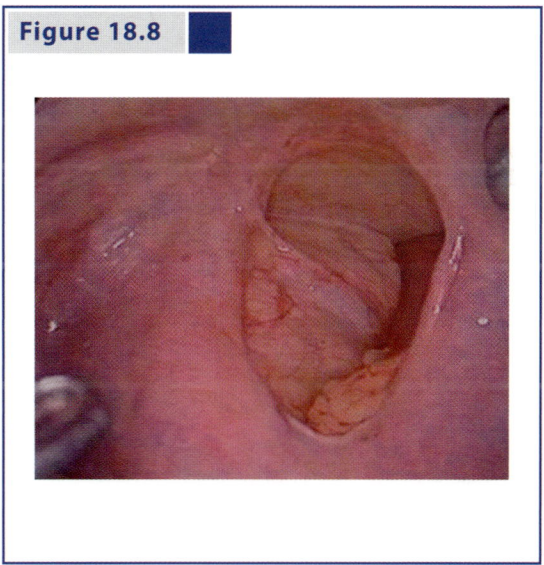

Diaphragmatic hernias may occur without the presence of a sac around the defect

Figure 18.9

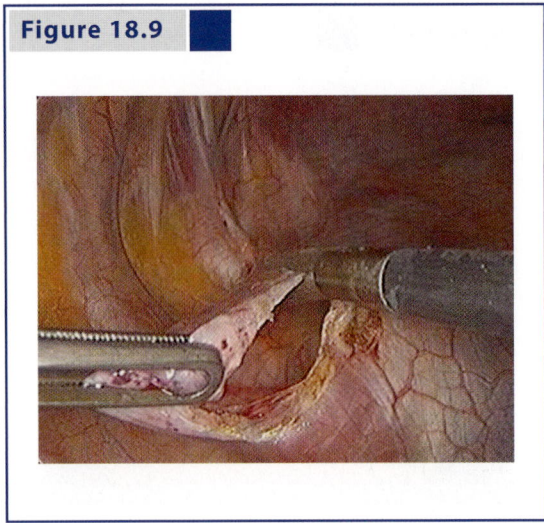

If a sac is present, it is removed by excision using electrosurgical instruments

Figure 18.10

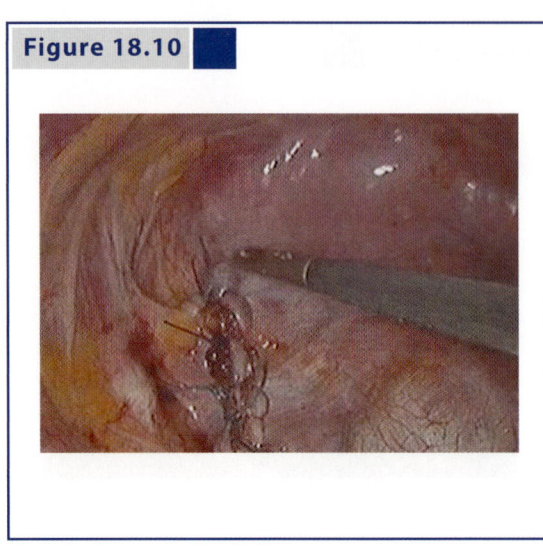

Primary closure with interrupted sutures is possible when sufficient muscle is present

Figure 18.11

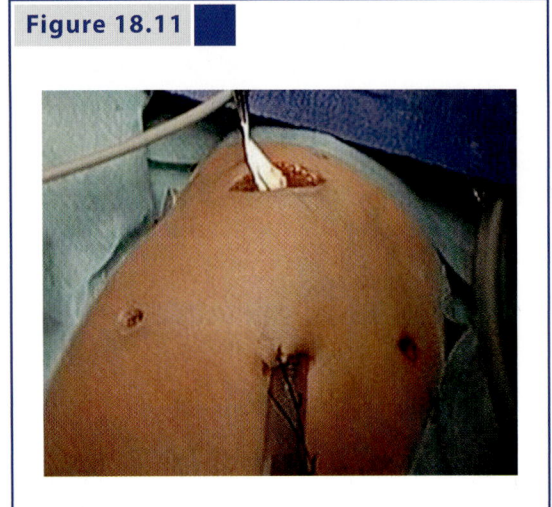

In large defects, the port site incision is increased to facilitate the insertion of a Gore-Tex® patch

Figure 18.12

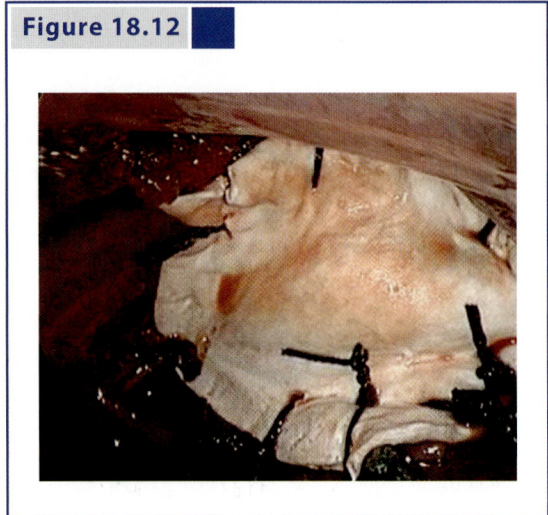

The Gore-Tex® patch is sutured along the brim of the diaphragm using interrupted sutures

Figure 18.13

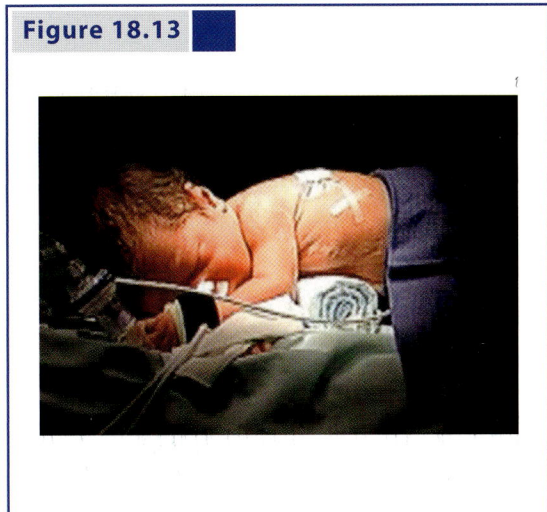

On completion of the procedure, incisions are closed using skin sutures and Steristrips

Figure 18.14

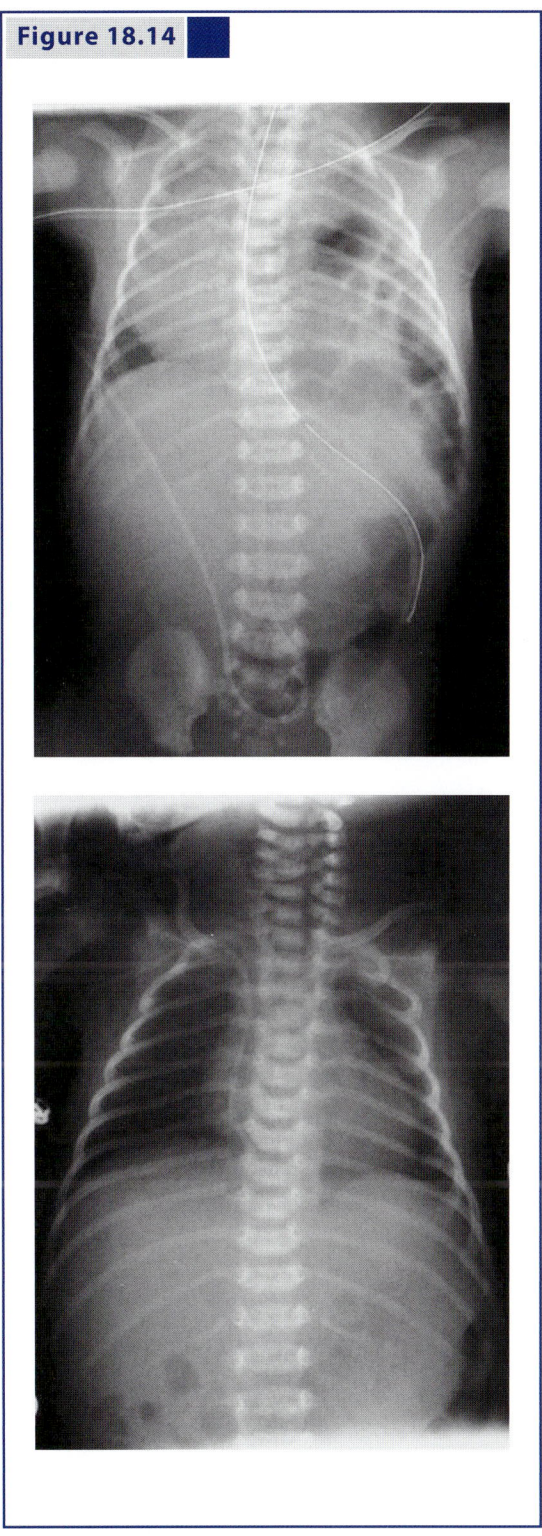

Left-sided CDH closure in a neonate. Preoperative (*above*) and postoperative (*below*) chest films

Recommended Literature

1. Becmeur F, Reinberg O, Dimitriu C, Mooq R, Philippe P (2007) Thoracoscopic repair of congenital diaphragmatic hernia in children. Semin Pediatr Surg 16:238–244

2. Nguyen TL, Le AD (2006) Thoracoscopic repair for congenital diaphragmatic hernia: lessons from 45 cases. J Pediatr Surg 41:1713–1715

3. Yang EY, Allmendinger M, Johnson SM, Chen C, Wilson JM, Fishman SJ (2005) Neonatal thoracoscopic repair of congenital diaphragmatic hernia: selection criteria for successful outcome. J Pediatr Surg 40:1369–1375

19 Thymectomy

MICHAEL E. HÖLLWARTH

19.1 Operation Room Setup

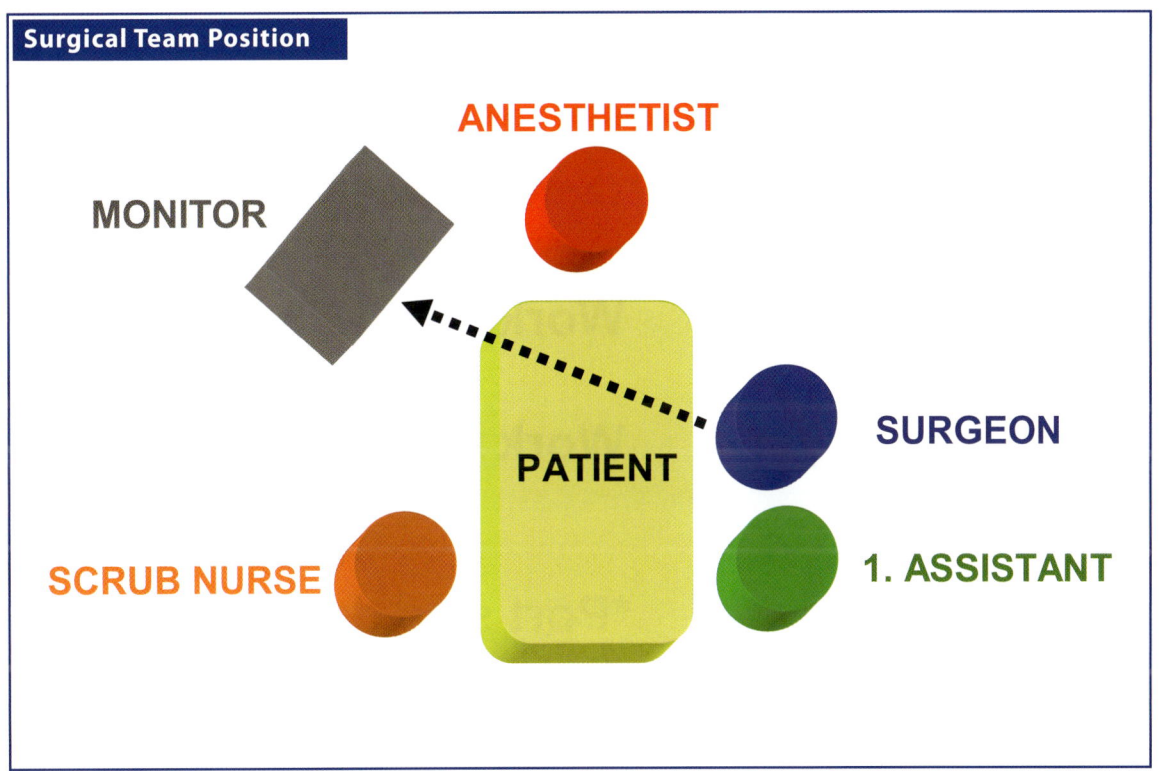

Surgical Team Position

ANESTHETIST

MONITOR

PATIENT

SURGEON

SCRUB NURSE

1. ASSISTANT

19.2   Patient Positioning

A 30° right lateral decubitus position.

19.3   Special Instruments

- Ultracision® harmonic scalpel (Johnson & Johnson Medical Products, Ethicon Endo-Surgery, Cincinnati, OH, USA)
- Endoscopic clip applicator
- Specimen retrieval bag

19.4   Location of Access Points

Port Placement Sites

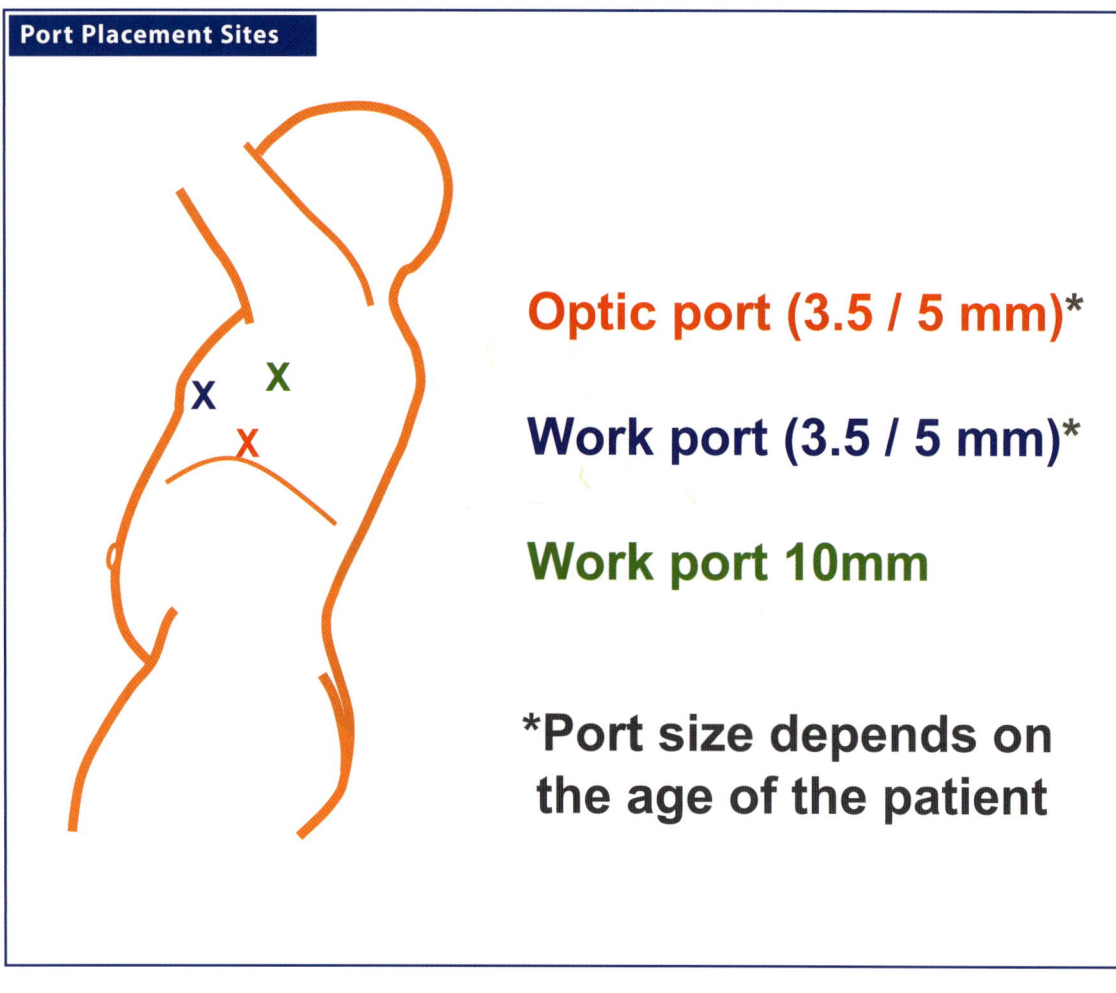

Optic port (3.5 / 5 mm)*

Work port (3.5 / 5 mm)*

Work port 10mm

***Port size depends on the age of the patient**

19.5   Indications

1. Tumors of the thymus gland.
2. Myasthenia gravis.
3. Nonatrophic thymic glands.
4. Thymic cysts.

19.6   Contraindications

1. Neonatal type of myasthenia gravis.
2. Caution in immunocompromised and immunosuppressed patients.

19.7   Preoperative Considerations

1. Admit the patient 48 h prior to surgery.
2. Pulmonary function tests to recognize impending respiratory failure due to general muscle weakness.
3. Adjustment of cholinesterase inhibitors and steroid if indicated.
4. Chest physiotherapy is started.

19.8   Technical Notes

1. Extensive removal of perithymic adipose tissue must be always pursued.
2. Use harmonic scalpel to minimize the risks of electrically induced arrhythmias.
3. Major vascular injuries cannot be controlled thoracoscopically.
4. Care must be taken to avoid phrenic nerve injury during dissection of perithymic adipose tissue and injury to the left recurrent nerve while dissecting in the aortopulmonary window.

19.9   Procedure Variations

1. Video-assisted thoracoscopic thymectomy can be performed through left or right approaches. The left side is preferred.
2. A right-sided approach is preferred in patients with a history of pleurodesis in the left pleural cavity or those with severe cardiomegaly.

19.10   Thoracoscopic Thymectomy

Please see Figs. 1–6.

Figure 19.1

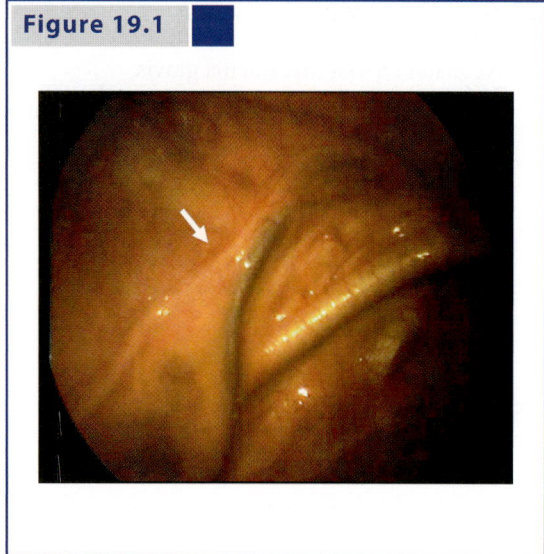

The left anterior phrenic nerve is identified (*arrow*). The mediastinal pleura is incised anterior to the nerve using the harmonic scalpel

Figure 19.2

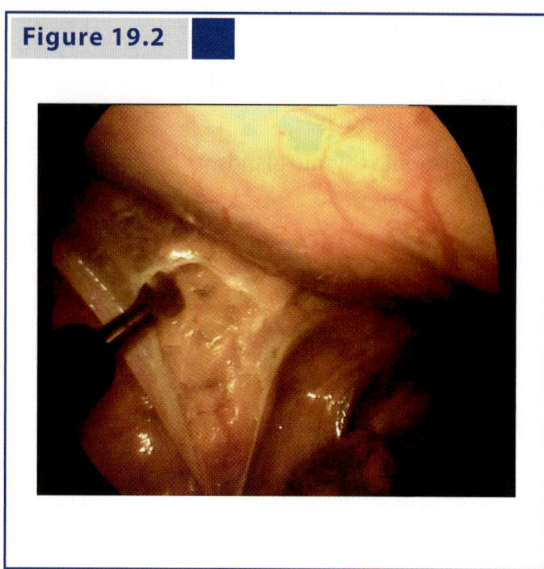

The inferior part of the thymus along with mediastinal fat is dissected. The thymus and mediastinal fat is swept off the pericardium

Figure 19.3

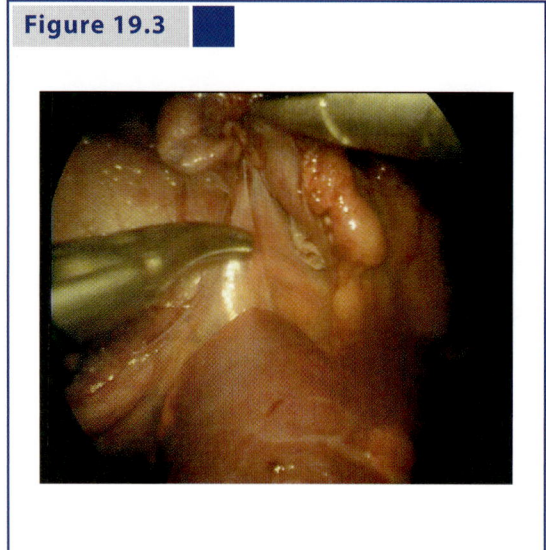

Dissection continues cephalad until the innominate vein is identified

Figure 19.4

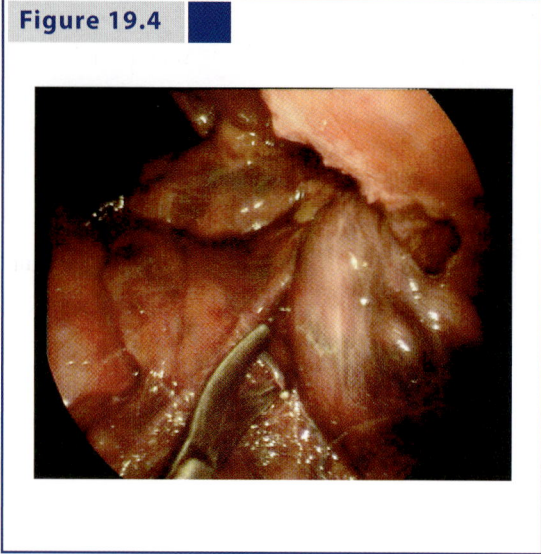

The vessels draining the thymus are ligated using titanium endoscopic clips and dissected using Metzenbaum scissors

Figure 19.5

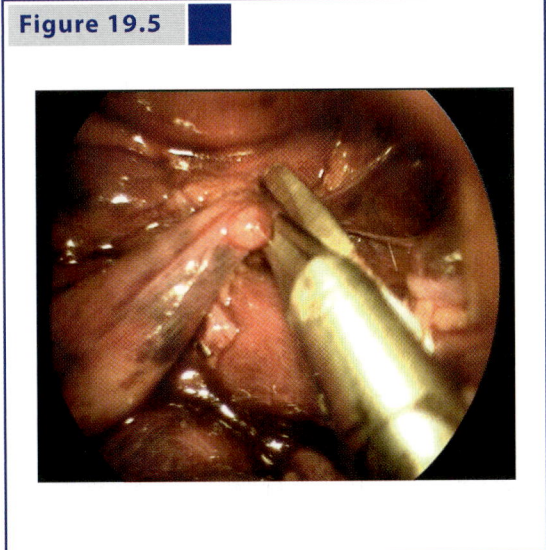

Figure 19.6

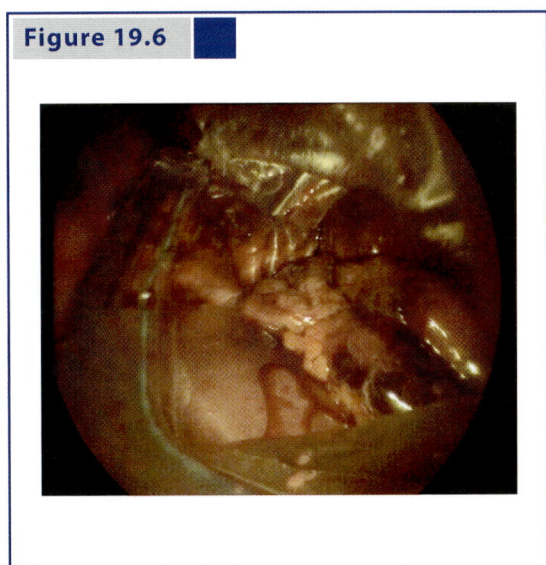

All visible fat should be removed as it may contain remnants of thymic tissue. The cranial part of the thymus is retracted into the thorax and dissected free

A specimen retrieval bag is passed through the 10-mm port. The thymus is placed inside the bag and removed from the thorax

Recommended Literature

1. Shiono H, Inoue A, Tomiyama N, Shigemura N, Ideguchi K, Inoue M, Minami M, Okumura M (2006) Safer video-assisted thoracoscopic thymectomy after location of thymic veins with multidetector computed tomography. Surg Endosc 20:1419–1422

2. Tomulescu V, Ion V, Kosa A, Sqarbura O, Popescu I (2006) Thoracoscopic thymectomy mid-term results. Ann Thorac Surg 82:1003–1007

3. Wagner AJ, Cortes R, Strober J, Grethel E, Clifton M, Harrison M, Farmer D, Nobuhara K, Lee H (2006) Long-term follow-up after thymectomy for myasthenia gravis: thoracoscopic vs open. J Pediatr Surg 41:50–54

20 Aortopexy

Timothy D. Kane

20.1 Operation Room Setup

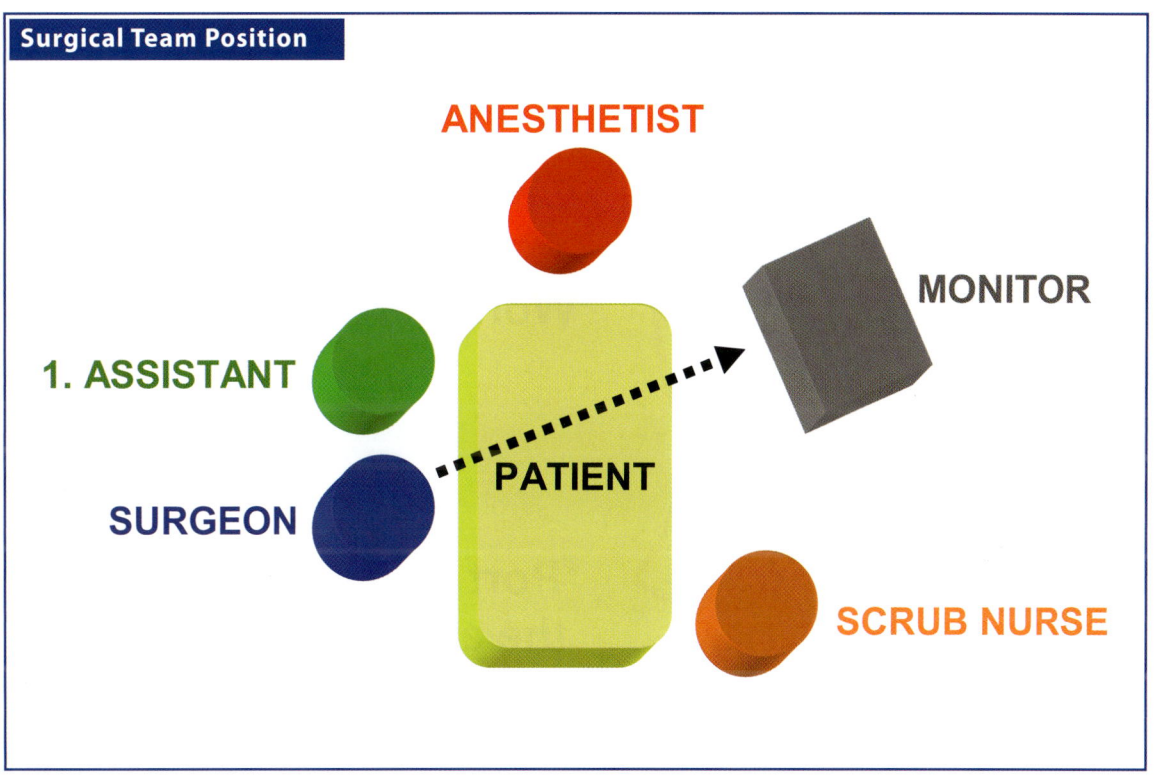

20.2   Patient Positioning

Supine position with arms tucked to the side. Right side (or left side) elevated 30°.

20.3   Special Instruments

- 3.5-mm needle holder
- 2-0 or 3-0 nonabsorbable sutures
- 4-mm 30° angled scope

20.4   Location of Access Points

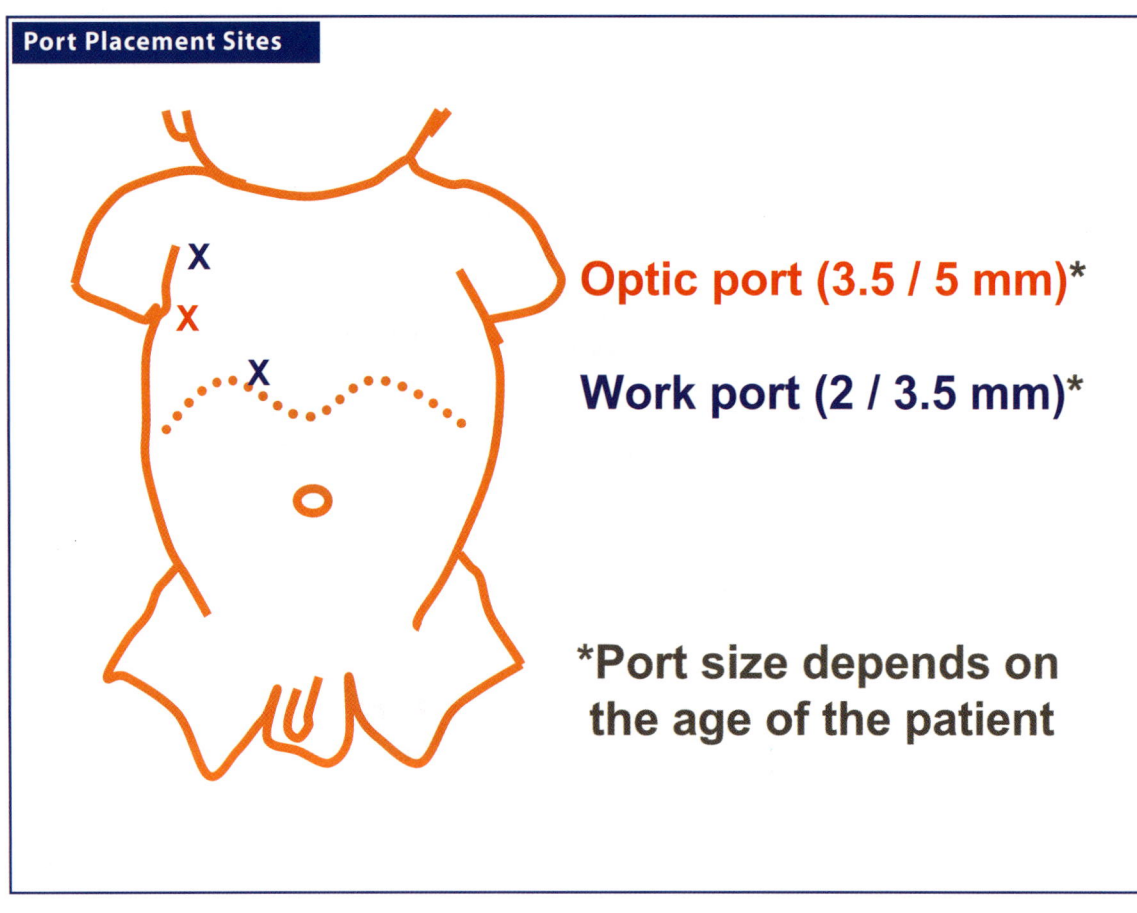

Port Placement Sites

Optic port (3.5 / 5 mm)*

Work port (2 / 3.5 mm)*

*Port size depends on the age of the patient

20.5   Indications

1. Primary or secondary tracheal compression.
2. Aberrant innominate artery takeoff.
3. Anterior tracheal compression with "dying spells" (life-threatening apnea with cyanosis and hypoxia), frequent respiratory infections, stridor, or bradycardia.

20.6   Contraindications

Inability of the patient to tolerate thoracoscopy due to other reasons.

20.7   Preoperative Considerations

1. Assess tracheal compression by magnetic resonance imaging or computed tomography scan if necessary.
2. Evaluate and treat gastroesophageal reflux and esophageal strictures in esophageal atresia patients with esophageal dysmotility, which may exacerbate tracheomalacia.
3. Perform preoperative bronchoscopy during spontaneous respiration to document tracheal compression and intraoperative bronchoscopy to document relief of compression (in addition to intraoperative postaortopexy bronchoscopy).

20.8   Technical Notes

1. Besides port sites, make a 1-cm incision in the second intercostal space near the sternum.
2. Use 4–6 mmHg of carbon dioxide.
3. Dissect the thymus from the aorta.
4. Place three or four sutures transsternally via a sternal incision medial to the mammary vessels. Sutures traverse the pericardium ± aortic adventitial layer, are passed back out through the sternum, and tied extracorporeally.

20.9   Procedure Variations

1. A fourth 3.5-mm port may be added for additional exposure or aortic stabilization during suture placement.
2. A left-sided thoracoscopic approach can be utilized with mirror-image placement of port sites to that described for approach from the right.
3. Thymectomy may be required during the left-sided approach.

20.10   Right Thoracoscopic Aortopexy for Tracheomalacia

Please see Figs. 1–9.

Figure 20.1

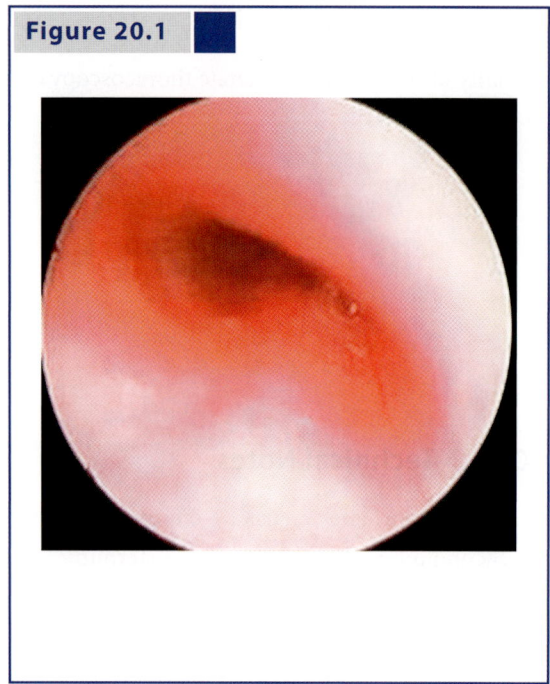

Preoperative bronchoscopic view demonstrating over 50% anterior compression of the trachea by the aorta

Figure 20.2

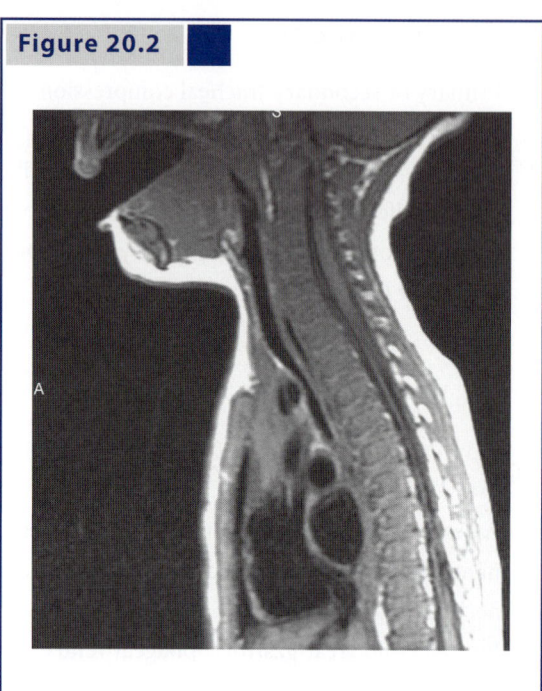

Magnetic resonance image reveals midtracheal compression by the aorta and innominate artery

Figure 20.3

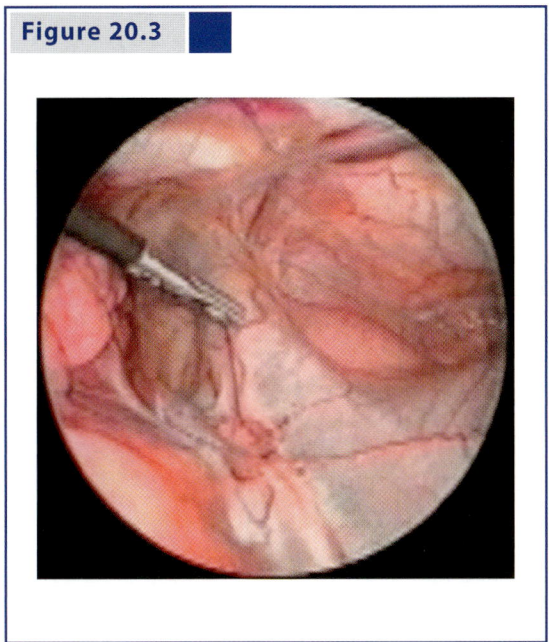

Right thoracoscopic view of the superior vena cava, thymus, retracted right lung, phrenic nerve, and internal mammary vessels (at the top of the picture)

Figure 20.4

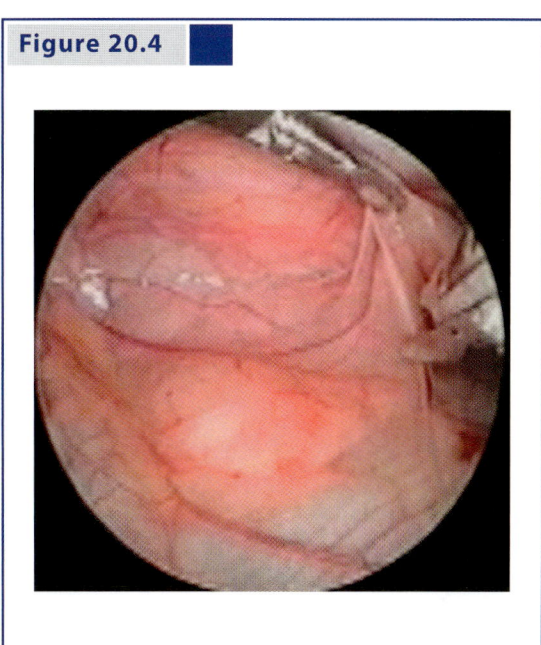

The thymus is mobilized by sharp dissection from the pericardium and aorta

Figure 20.5

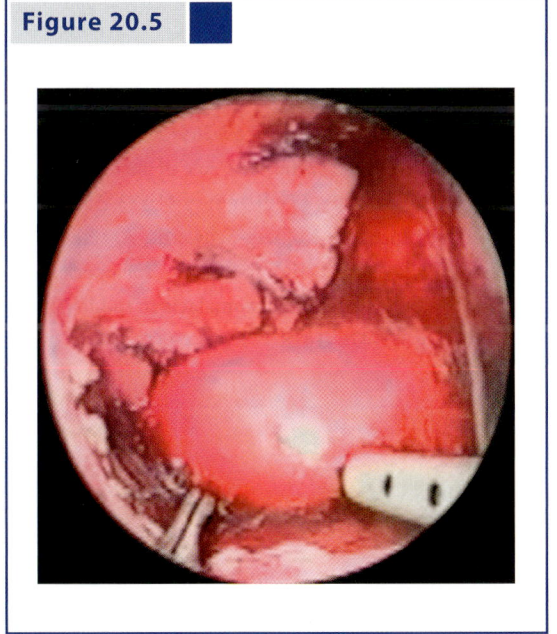

The aorta and overlying pericardium is exposed near the root of the aorta

Figure 20.6

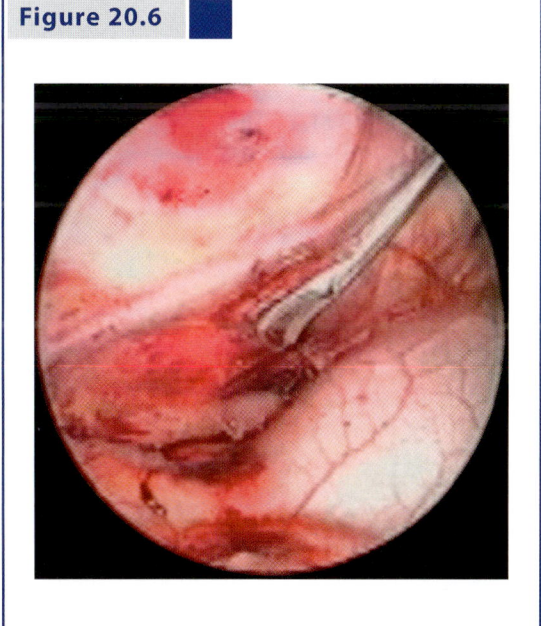

The first suture is passed into the chest through a parasternal incision, medial to the mammary vessels

Figure 20.7

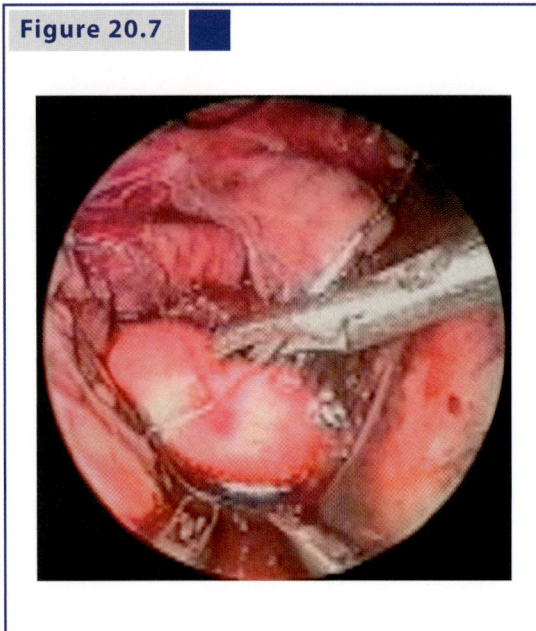

The suture is passed into the pericardium and adventitial wall of the aorta

Figure 20.8

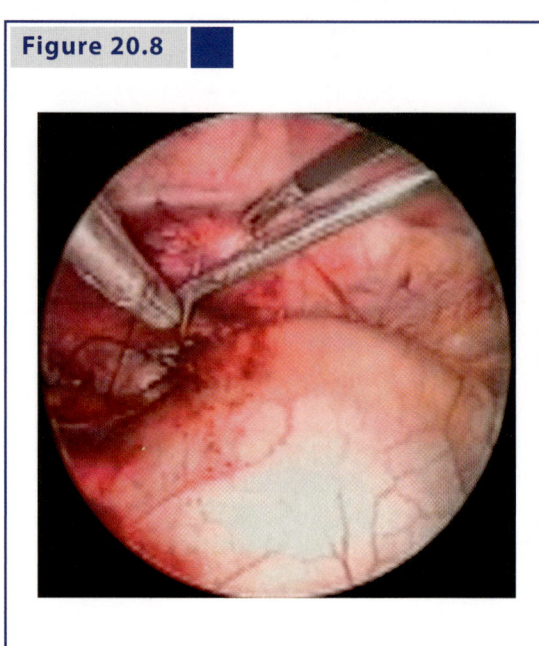

The same suture (as in Fig. 7) is passed back through sternum to be tied extracorporeally

Figure 20.9

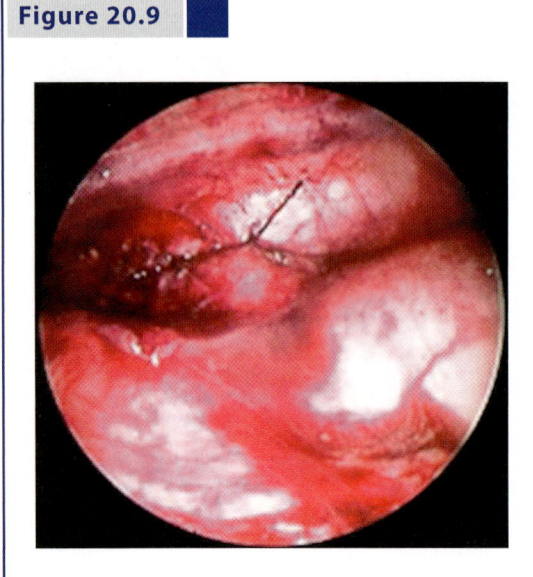

Bronchoscopy should be performed to determine whether the number of sutures placed is sufficient. Final thoracoscopic view of the aorta pexied to the undersurface of the sternum after tying all sutures

Recommended Literature

1. Corbally MT, Spitz L, Kiely E, Brereton RJ, Drake DP (1993) Aortopexy for tracheomalacia in oesophageal anomalies. Eur J Pediatr Surg 3:264–266
2. Dave S, Currie BG (2006) The role of aortopexy in severe tracheomalacia. J Pediatr Surg 41:533–537
3. Schaarschmidt K, Kolberg-Schwerdt A, Pietsch L, Bunke K (2002) Thoracoscopic aortopericardiosternopexy for severe tracheomalacia in toddlers. J Pediatr Surg 37:1476–1478

21 Closure of a Patent Ductus Arteriosus

Kari Vanamo

21.1 Operation Room Setup

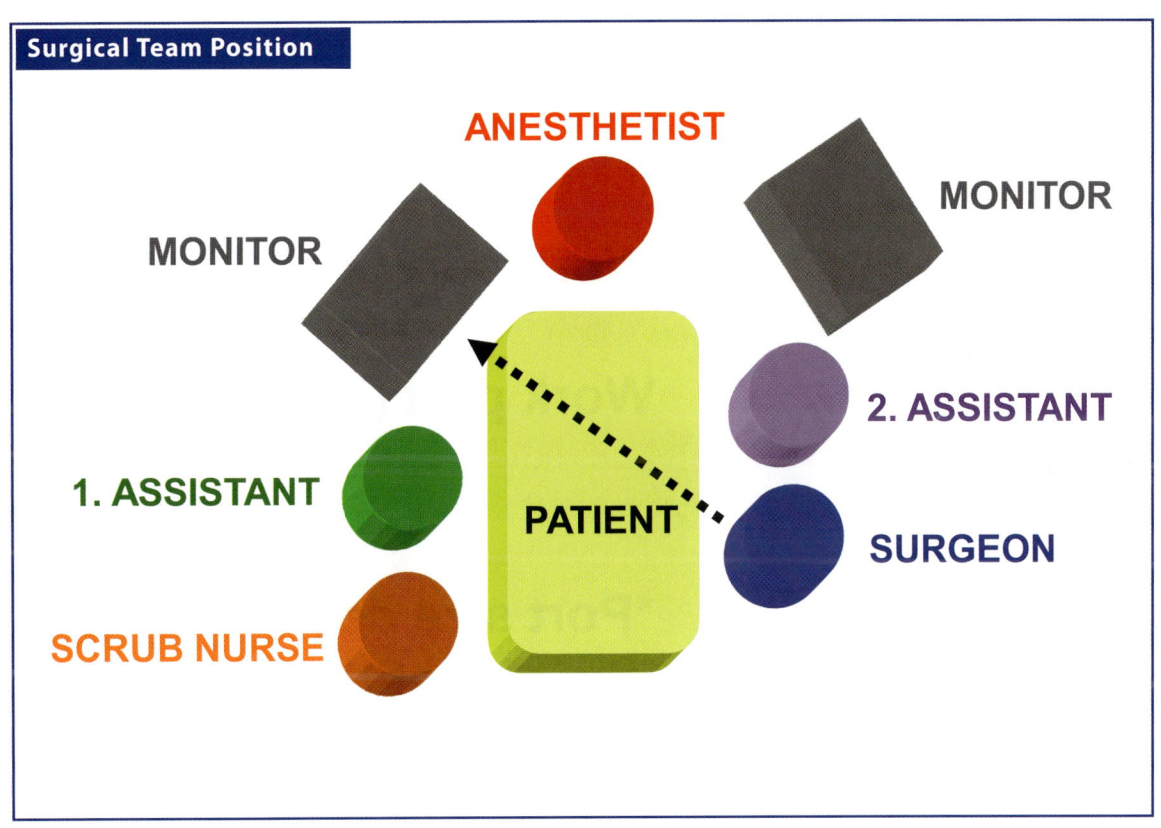

21.2   Patient Positioning

Right lateral position with bent table/support under the right chest to open the left intercostals spaces; left shoulder in 90° of flexion and freely movable.

21.3   Special Instruments

- Cotton swabs
- Nerve hooks
- Dissection hook
- Endoscopic clip applicator

21.4   Location of Access Points

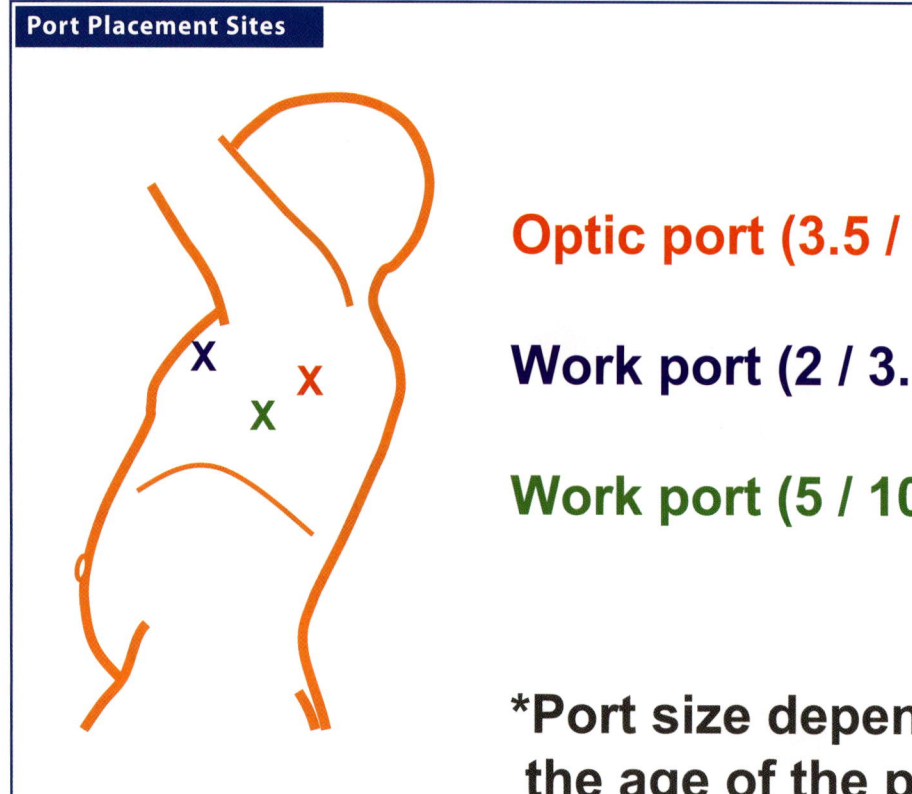

Port Placement Sites

Optic port (3.5 / 5 mm)*

Work port (2 / 3.5 mm)*

Work port (5 / 10 mm)*

*Port size depends on the age of the patient

21.5   Indications

1. Isolated symptomatic patent ductus arteriosus (PDA) after failure of indomethacin treatment.
2. PDA with contraindications to medical therapy.
3. Asymptomatic PDA in older infants with the aim of preventing infective endocarditis.

21.6   Contraindications

1. High-pressure open PDA.
2. PDA associated with other congenital heart defects requiring surgery.
3. Prematurity or small size (relative contraindication).
4. Inability to withstand lung retraction.

21.7   Preoperative Considerations

1. Care should be taken to ensure that the clip is in the clip applicator because the empty applicator can act as a pair of scissors if the clip has fallen out.
2. Normothermia and proper attention to ventilation are imperative, especially in neonatal patients.
3. For PDA repair in the infant, either an operating room or a portable operating room in the neonatal intensive care unit may be sufficient to perform the procedure.

21.8   Technical Notes

1. Single-lung ventilation or carbon dioxide insufflation is not used routinely. A fourth incision anteriorly may be required for additional retraction of the lung to increase visibility.
2. The vagus and recurrent laryngeal nerves should be handled with extreme care and manipulation avoided if possible
3. Two clips are preferred. Inappropriate clip application could cause injury to the recurrent laryngeal nerve or the ductus wall.
4. Chest drain is not necessary; if placed it could be removed once the pleural cavity has been evacuated.

21.9   Procedure Variations

1. Bimanual dissection is feasible. However, this usually requires a fourth incision.
2. In the presence of a large ductus, ligation may be preferred prior to clip application.
3. Monitoring the left laryngeal nerve is feasible and advocated.
4. In older children, transesophageal echocardiography can be utilized to demonstrate the complete interruption of ductal flow in real time during the procedure.

21.10   Thoracoscopic Closure of a Patent Ductus Arteriosus

Please see Figs. 1–6.

Figure 21.1

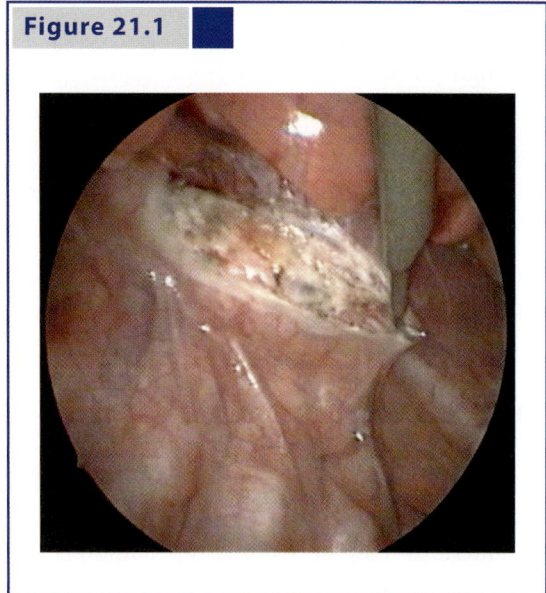

The posterior pleura overlying the aorta is incised with an electrocautery hook from the base of the left subclavian artery toward the ductus arteriosus

Figure 21.2

The medial pleural leaf is retracted with nerve hooks and separated from the aorta using blunt dissection and electrocautery

Figure 21.3

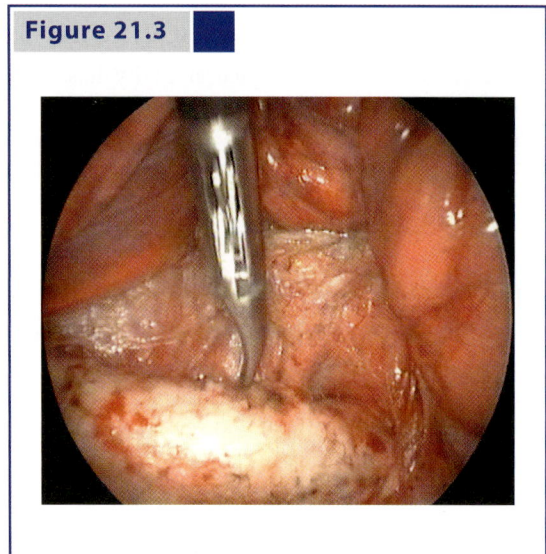

The upper and lower margins of the duct are dissected free, but no attempt is made to circumvent the ductus

Figure 21.4

The port below the scapular angle is removed and the incision extended bluntly to accommodate the endoscopic clip applicator. The ductus is clipped with one or two metal clips

Figure 21.5

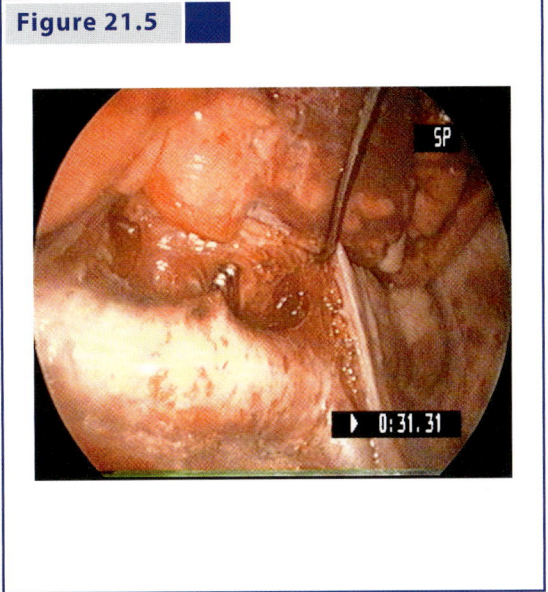

Figure 21.6

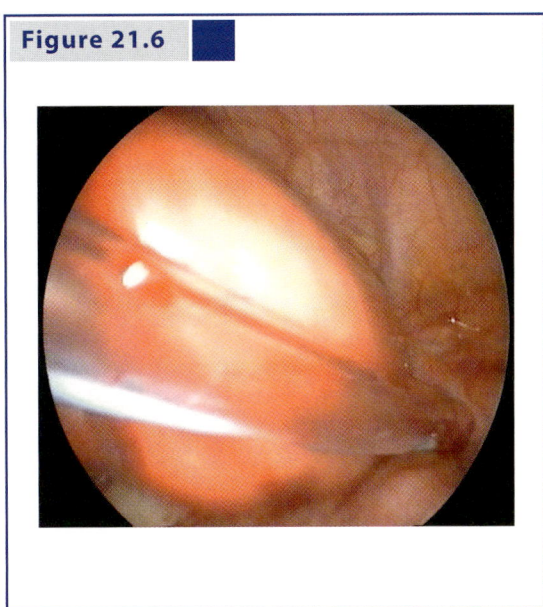

The field is checked for correct placement of the clip(s) and to rule out bleeding or chylous leak

The pleural cavity is drained, the lung expanded, and the incisions closed with absorbable sutures

Recommended Literature

1. Burke RP, Wernovsky G, van der Velde M, Hansen D, Castaneda A (1995) Video-assisted thoracoscopic surgery for congenital heart disease. J Thorac Cardiovasc Surg 109:499–507
2. Laborde F, Noirhomme P, Karam J, Batisse A, Bourel P, Saint Maurice O (1993) A new video-assisted thoracoscopic surgical technique for interruption of patent ductus arteriosus in infants and children. J Thorac Cardiovasc Surg 105:278–280
3. Vanamo K, Berg E, Kokki H, Tikanoja T (2006) Video-assisted thoracoscopic versus open surgery for persistent ductus arteriosus. J Pediatr Surg 41:1226–1229

22 Endoscopic Transthoracic Sympathectomy

Sergey Keidar and Itzhak Vinograd

22.1 Operation Room Setup

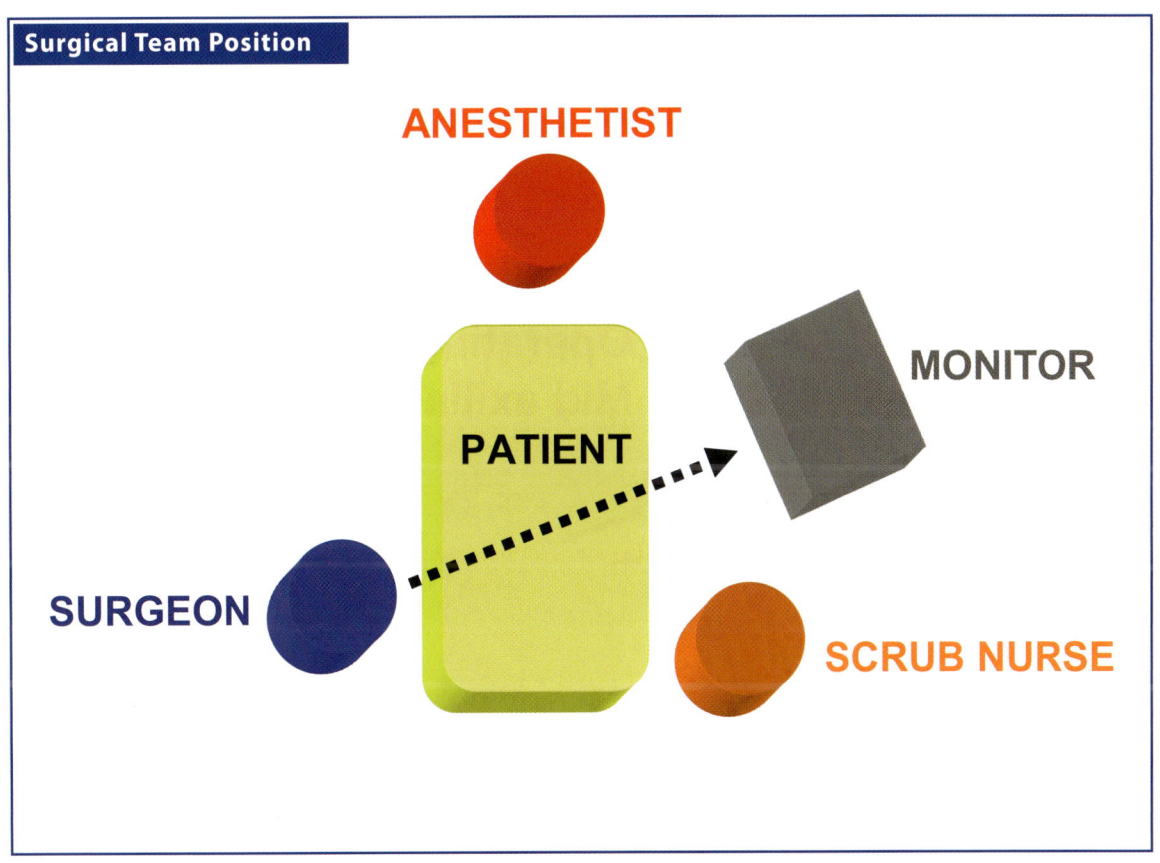

22.2   Patient Positioning

Semisitting position with hands abducted to a 90° angle providing exposure of both axillae. This set-up is for right-side sympathectomy. For the left side, a mirror image of the set-up is preferred.

22.3   Special Instruments

- 10-mm, 0° operating scope with a 5-mm central working channel
- Monopolar hook cautery

22.4   Location of Access Points

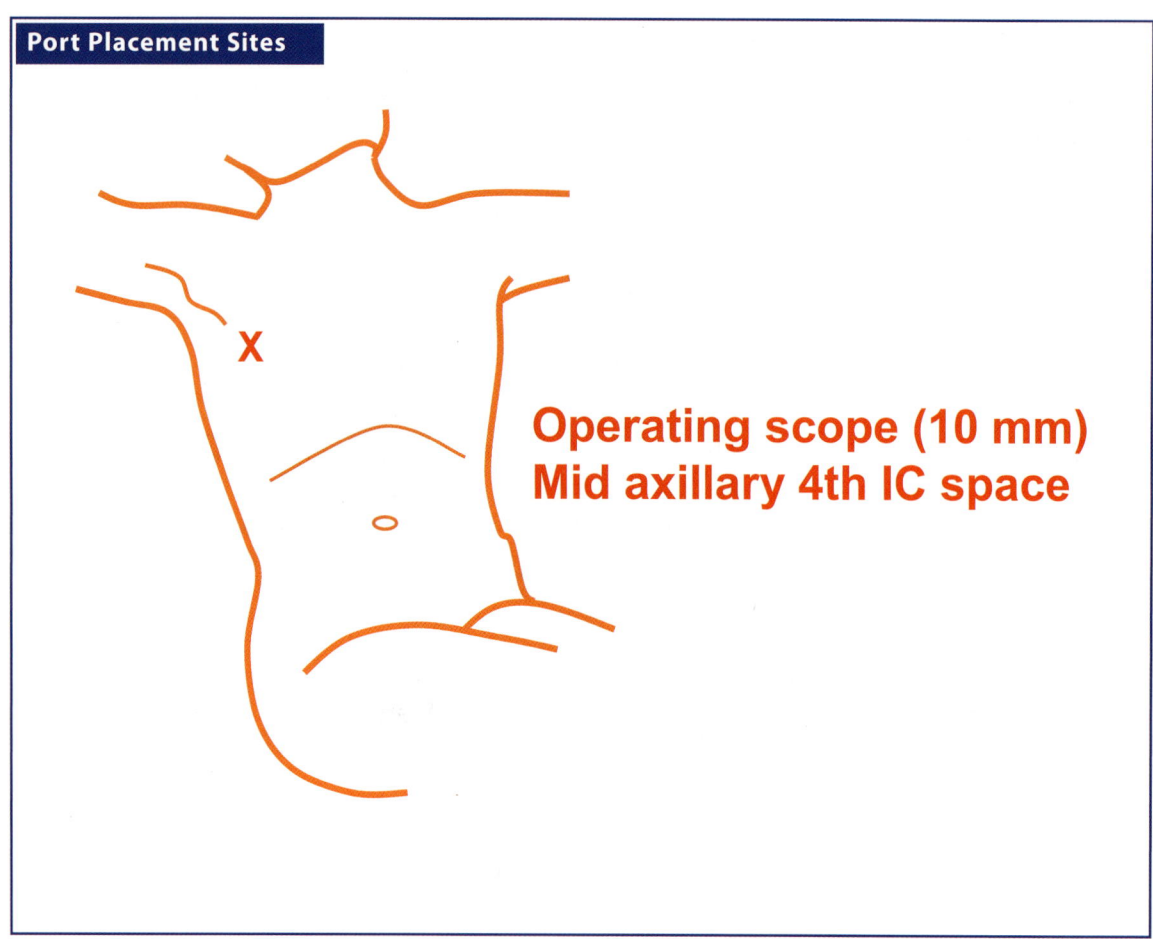

Port Placement Sites

X

Operating scope (10 mm) Mid axillary 4th IC space

22.5 Indications

1. Palmar and axillary hyperhidrosis causing psychological, social, and occupational problems.
2. Failure of conservative treatment.
3. Upper extremity pain syndromes.
4. Early surgery will rescue children from excessive physical discomfort.

22.6 Contraindications

Previous lung surgery, empyema.

22.7 Preoperative Considerations

1. Explain possible complications such as Horner's syndrome, intercostal neuralgia, and compensatory sweating.
2. It is advisable to begin on the right to avoid arrhythmia, since the severance of the left stellate ganglion increases the threshold for arrhythmia.
3. Imaging with computed tomography or magnetic resonance imaging of the cervical and thoracic spine and brachial plexus may be indicated in selected cases when the normal anatomy is in doubt.

22.8 Technical Notes

1. T2–T4 sympathectomy for axillary hyperhidrosis.
2. T2–T3 sympathectomy for palmar hyperhidrosis.
3. Avoid T1 stellate ganglion.
4. Electrocautery ablation of the sympathetic segment; strictly coagulate above the rib surface.
5. Upon completion on one side, sympathectomy is then performed on the opposite side.
6. Lung reinflation under visual control with positive pressure.

22.9 Procedure Variations

1. Biportal procedure (two 5-mm ports, one for optics and the other for instrument).
2. Laser or harmonic scalpel to cauterize the sympathetic ganglia.
3. Depending on the number of ports employed, a 0° or 30° endoscope option may be used for visualization.
4. Either the double-lumen endotracheal tube or the 8- 10-mmHg insufflation pressure pneumothorax option may be chosen.

22.10 Technique of Endoscopic Transthoracic Sympathectomy

Please see Figs. 1–6.

Figure 22.1

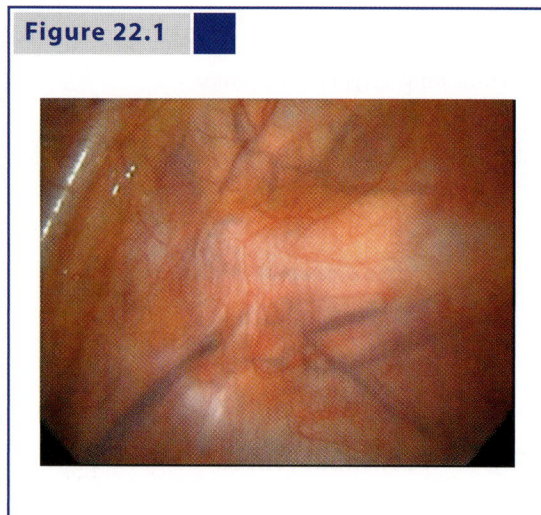

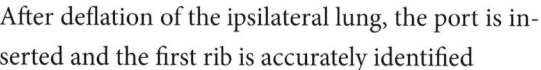

After deflation of the ipsilateral lung, the port is inserted and the first rib is accurately identified

Figure 22.2

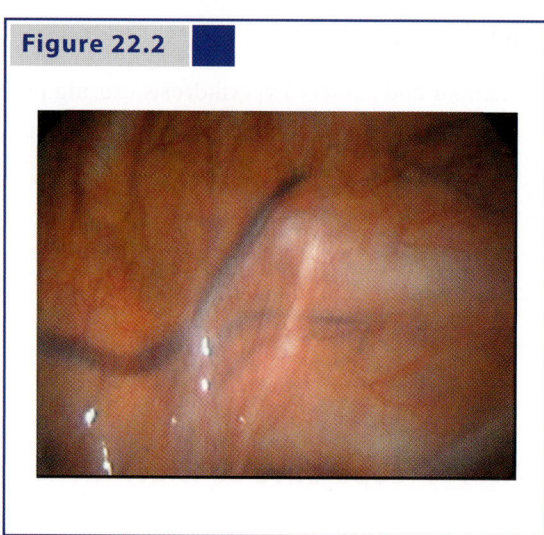

The second and third ribs are then identified. The sympathetic chain courses over the rib and heads close to costovertebral junction

Figure 22.3

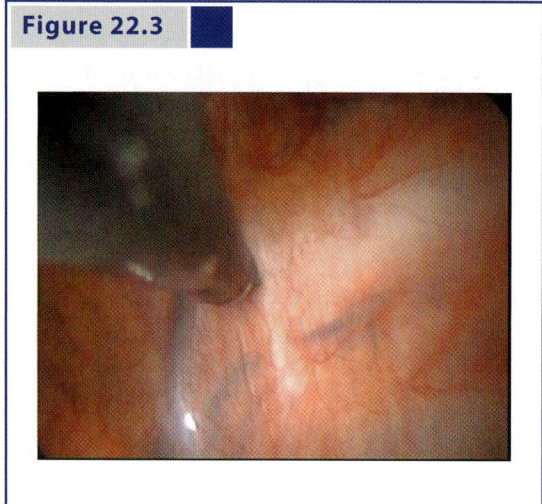

The sympathetic chain location is confirmed visually and manually by palpating it with the back of the monopolar hook cautery

Figure 22.4

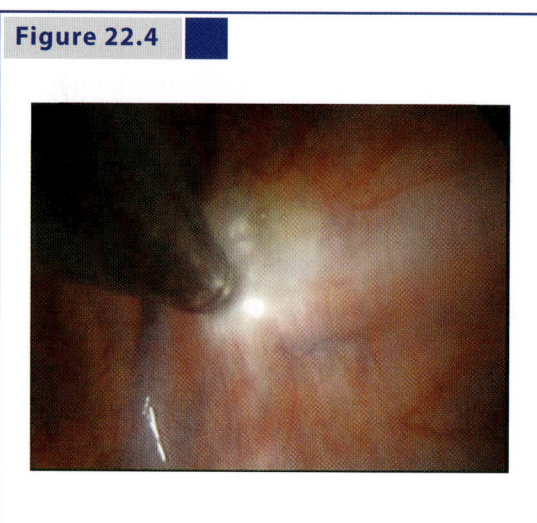

The T2 ganglia is cauterized after opening the pleura from both sides of the nerve and elevating it by the hook

Figure 22.5

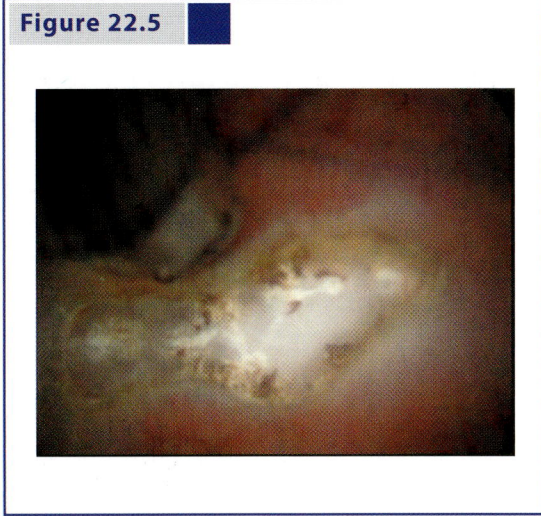

Figure 22.6

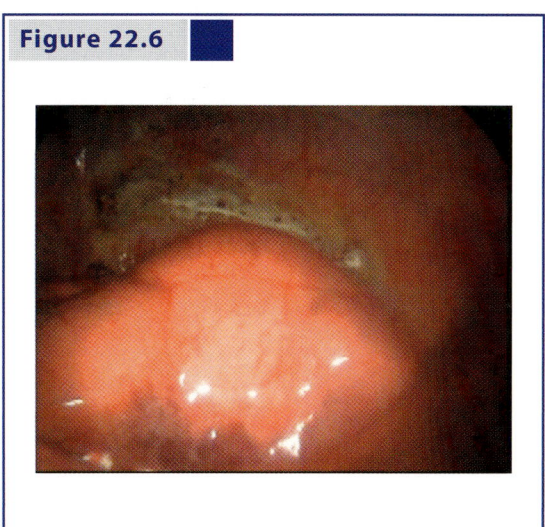

Extension of cauterization over the second and third rib provides complete denervation of T2 and T3, wich also includes the division of Kuntz nerve

The port is removed and expansion of the lung is visualized through the endoscope. Skin is closed under the Valsalva maneuver

Recommended Literature

1. Gossot D, Galetta D, Pascal A, Debrosse D, Caliandro R, Girard P, Stern JB, Grunenwald D (2003) Long-term results of endoscopic thoracic sympathectomy for upper limb hyperhidrosis. Ann Thorac Surg 75: 1075–1079

2. Lin TS, Fang HY (1999) Transthoracic endoscopic sympathectomy in the treatment of palmar hyperhidrosis – with emphasis on perioperative management (1,360 case analyses) Surg Neurol 52:453–457

3. Lin TS, Kuo SJ, Chou MC (2002) Uniportal endoscopic thoracic sympathectomy for treatment of palmar and axillary hyperhidrosis: analysis of 2000 cases. Neurosurgery 51:84–87

23 Anterior Discectomy and Hemivertebrectomy

Jerry Kieffer

23.1 Operation Room Setup

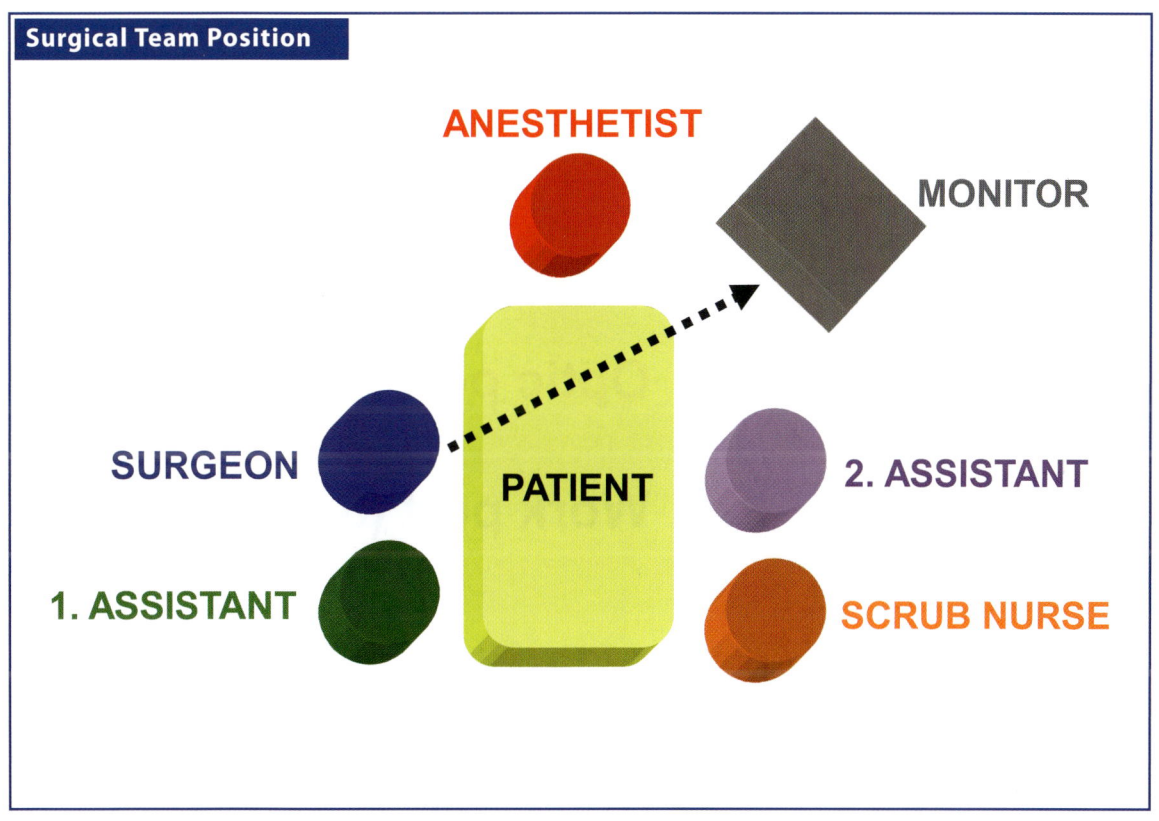

Surgical Team Position

ANESTHETIST

MONITOR

SURGEON

PATIENT

2. ASSISTANT

1. ASSISTANT

SCRUB NURSE

23.2   Patient Positioning

Lateral decubitus position with the convexity side up, the upper arm resting on a raised arm board.

23.3   Special Instruments

1. Orthopedic endoscopic instruments
   - rongeurs
   - forceps
   - elevators
   - curettes
   - osteotomes
2. Endoscopic fan retractor
3. High-speed bur for bone resections
4. Hemostatic agents

23.4   Location of Access Points

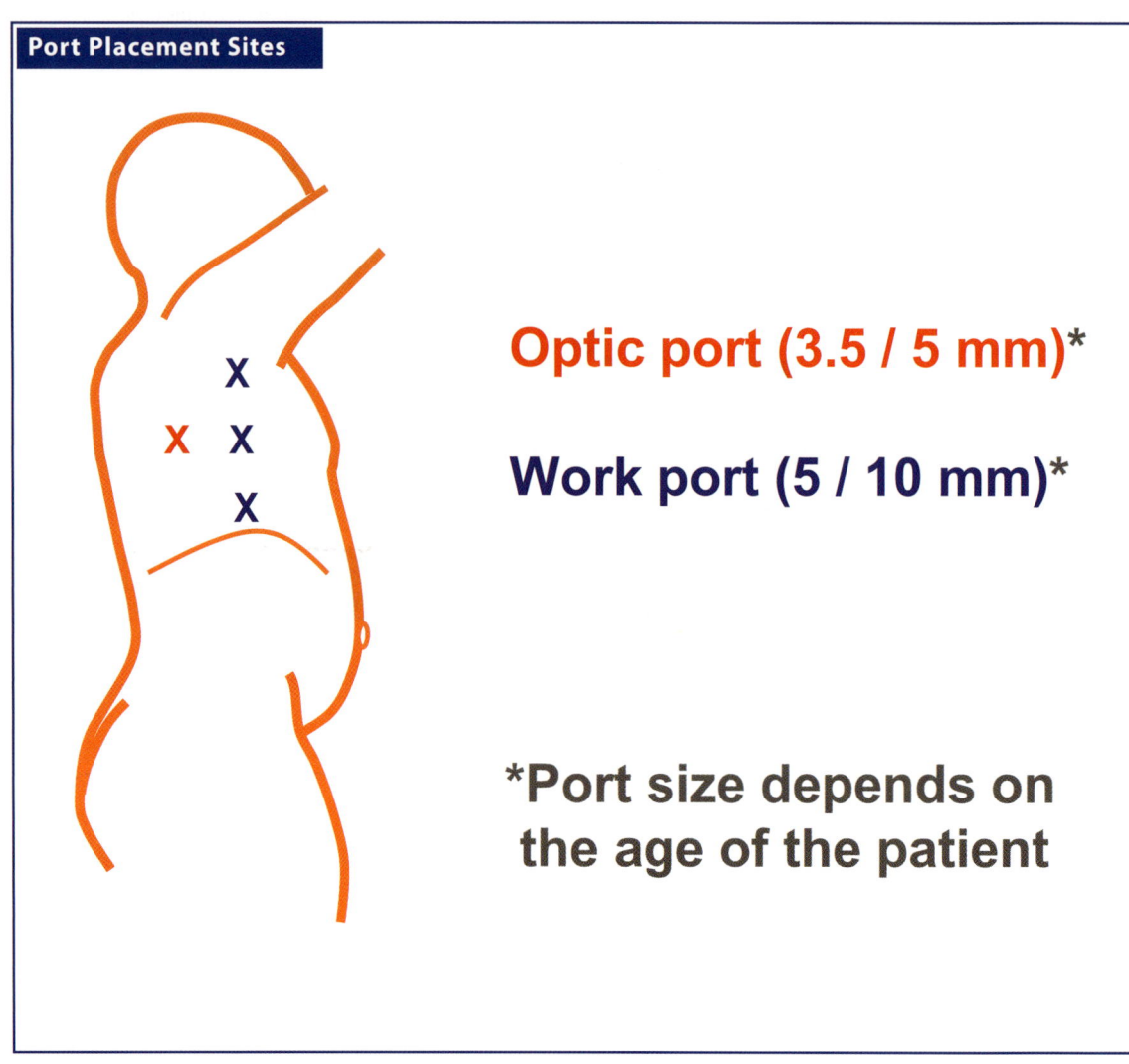

Port Placement Sites

Optic port (3.5 / 5 mm)*

Work port (5 / 10 mm)*

*Port size depends on the age of the patient

23.5 Indications

1. Deformity correction: anterior discectomy and fusion with or without instrumentation, hemi-vertebrectomy.
2. Trauma: anterior fusion with or without instrumentation.
3. Infection: abscess evacuation and curettage.
4. Tumor: biopsy.

23.6 Contraindications

Intolerance to single-lung ventilation.

23.7 Preoperative Considerations

1. Double-lumen intubation is mandatory for ipsilateral lung collapse in thoracoscopic procedures. If total lung collapse is not possible, use a fan retractor.
2. Somatosensory and motor-evoked potentials are monitored during the whole procedure.
3. Use a fluoroscopic C-arm to determine the disc levels and mark them directly onto the patient's skin, as well as the entry points of the ports.

23.8 Technical Notes

1. In severe deformity with contact between the spine and the rib cage, a chest wall suspension is used to create working space.
2. Incisions for ports are made over the rib, allowing harvesting of a 2-cm rib segment to be used as an autologous bone graft.
3. Ligation of segmental vessels is not necessary in anterior discectomy.

23.9 Procedure Variations

1. Anterior thoracic discectomy and fusion is completed by anterior endoscopic instrumentation and correction in a single-staged procedure or by posterior instrumentation and correction in a single- or double-staged procedure.
2. Thoracoscopic hemivertebrectomy is completed by posterior instrumentation and correction in a single-staged procedure.
3. If the hemivertebra wears a surplus rib, its head and proximal part are also removed endoscopically.

23.10 Thoracoscopic Anterior Discectomy and Fusion

Please see Figs. 1–12.

Figure 23.1

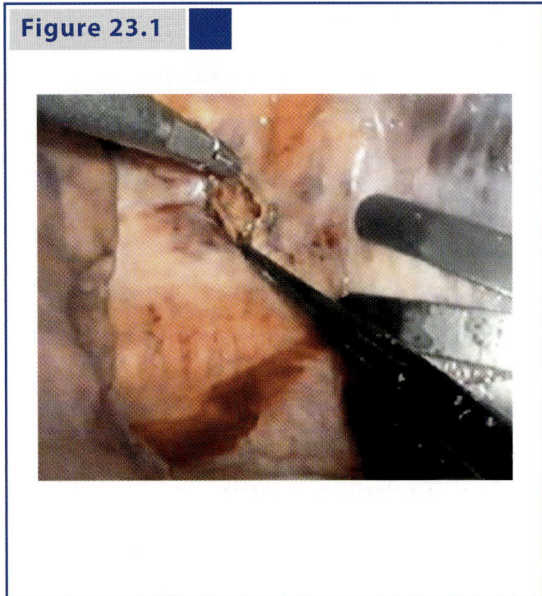

The pleura is lifted with a forceps and incised with electrocautery

Figure 23.2

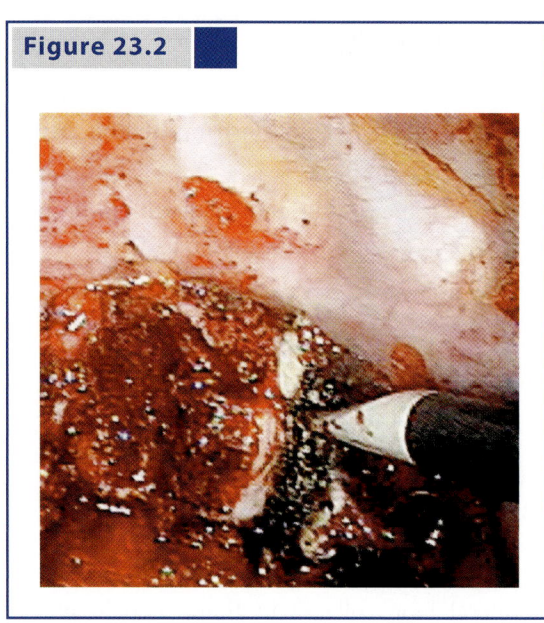

The superior and inferior margins of the disc are incised with electrocautery

Figure 23.3

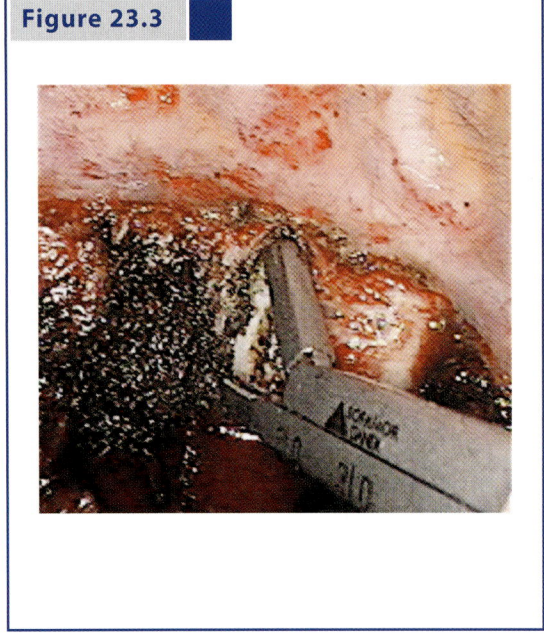

The discectomy goes down to the posterior margin of the annulus using a graduated endoscopic rongeur. The disc space created (to the left of the rongeur in picture) is filled with hemostatic gauze

Figure 23.4

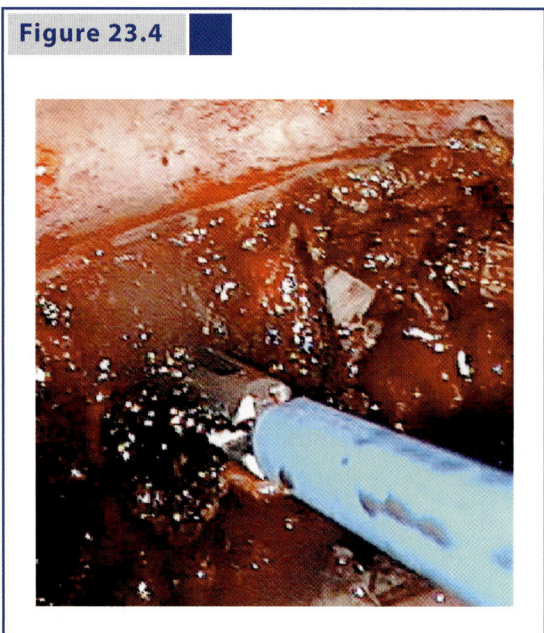

The growth plates are curetted

Figure 23.5

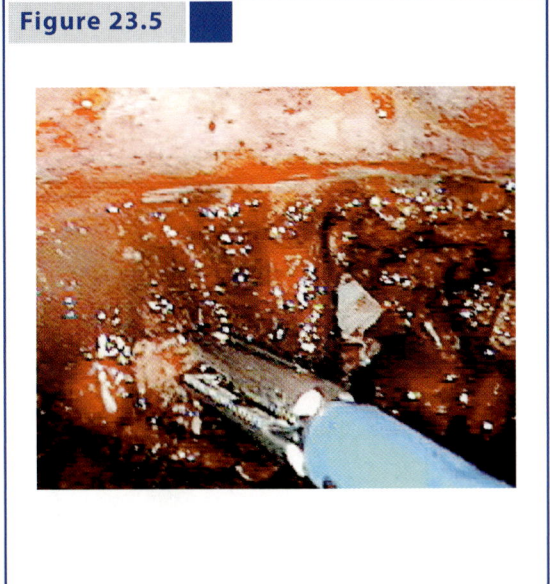

Figure 23.6

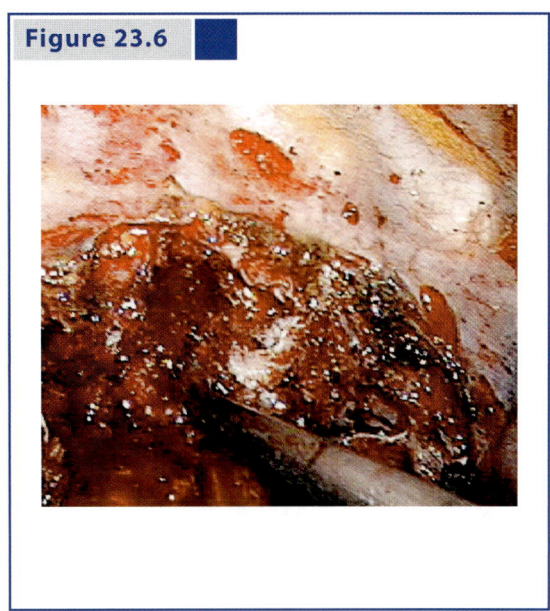

The hemostatic gauzes are removed prior to grafting

The gap created by the discectomy is filled with bone chips

23.11   Thoracoscopic Hemivertebrectomy

Figure 23.7

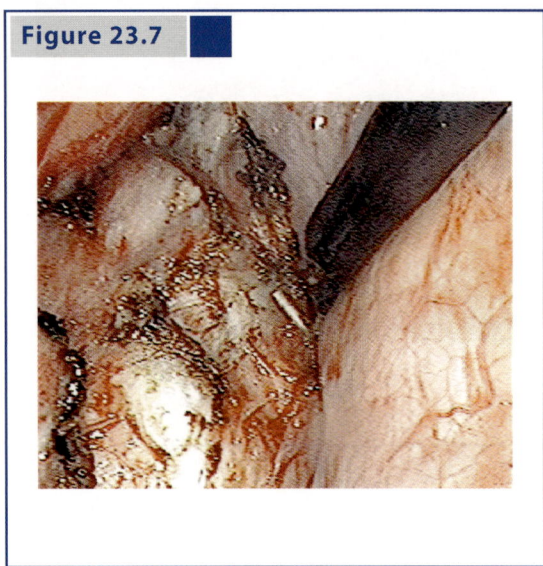

The pleura is incised with electrocautery over the hemivertebra and the superior and inferior adjacent vertebra

Figure 23.8

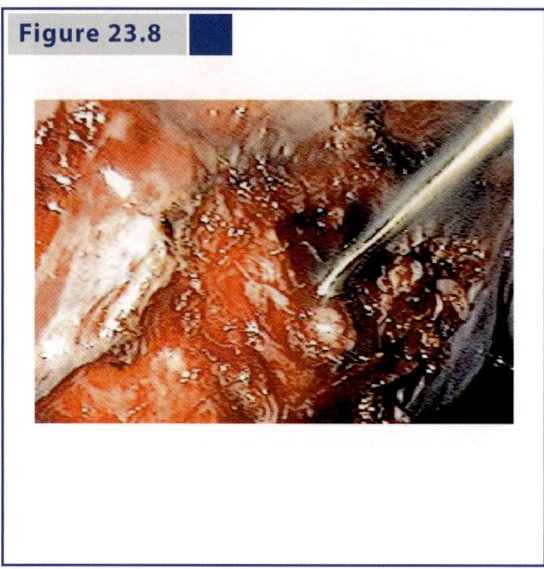

The growth cartilages above and below the hemivertebra are curetted

Figure 23.9

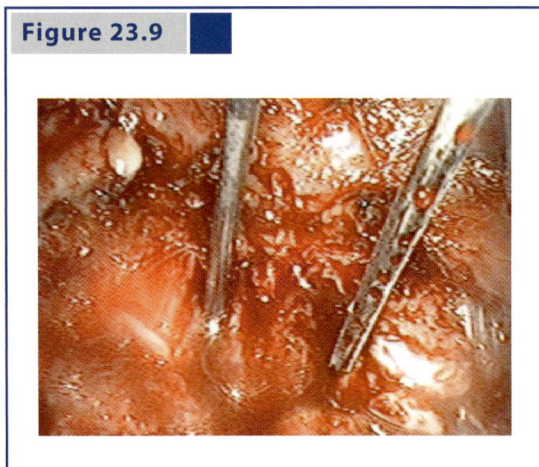

Two needles are placed at the estimated superior and inferior margins of the hemivertebra and their position is checked with fluoroscopy

Figure 23.10

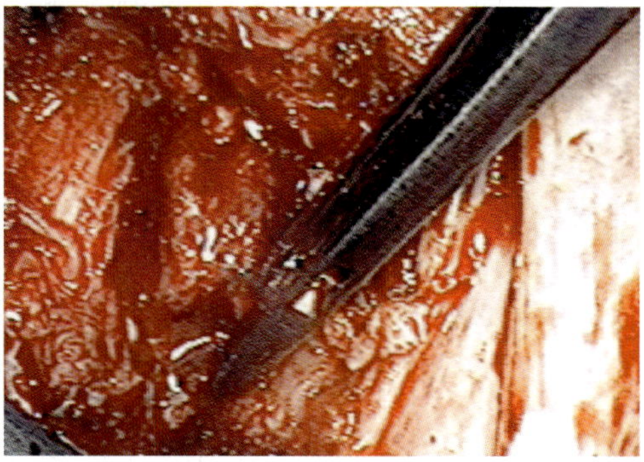

Growth-plate removal is completed with a standard rongeur

Figure 23.11

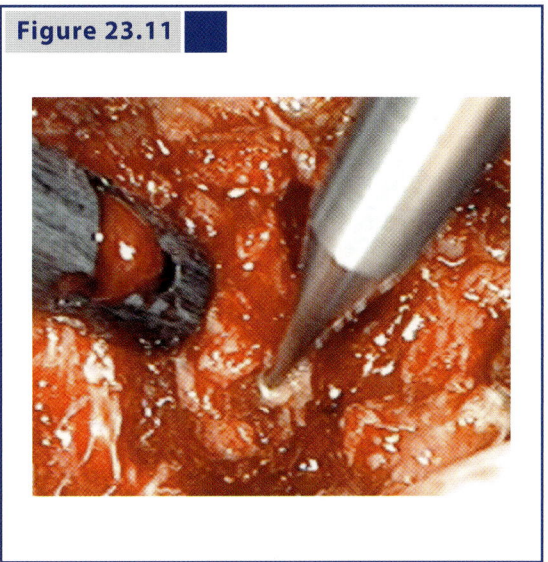

Figure 23.12

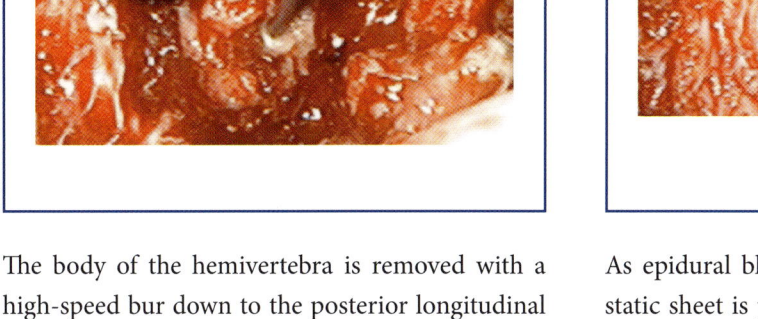

The body of the hemivertebra is removed with a high-speed bur down to the posterior longitudinal ligament

As epidural bleeding is not uncommon, a hemostatic sheet is placed at the bottom of the gap created by the hemivertebrectomy

Recommended Literature

1. Benazet JP (2000) Chirurgie Endoscopique du Rachis, Cahiers d'Enseignement de la SOFCOT (75). Elsevier, Paris, ISBN 978-2-84299-222-4
2. Lenke L, Betz R, Harms J (eds) (2004) Modern Anterior Scoliosis Surgery. Quality Medical Publishing, St. Louis, ISBN-10 1-57626-134-4
3. Regan JJ, Lieberman IH (2002) Atlas of Minimal Access Spine Surgery, 2nd edn. Quality Medical Publishing, St. Louis, ISBN-10 1-57626-100-X

24 Pectus Excavatum Repair

Michael E. Höllwarth

24.1 Operation Room Setup

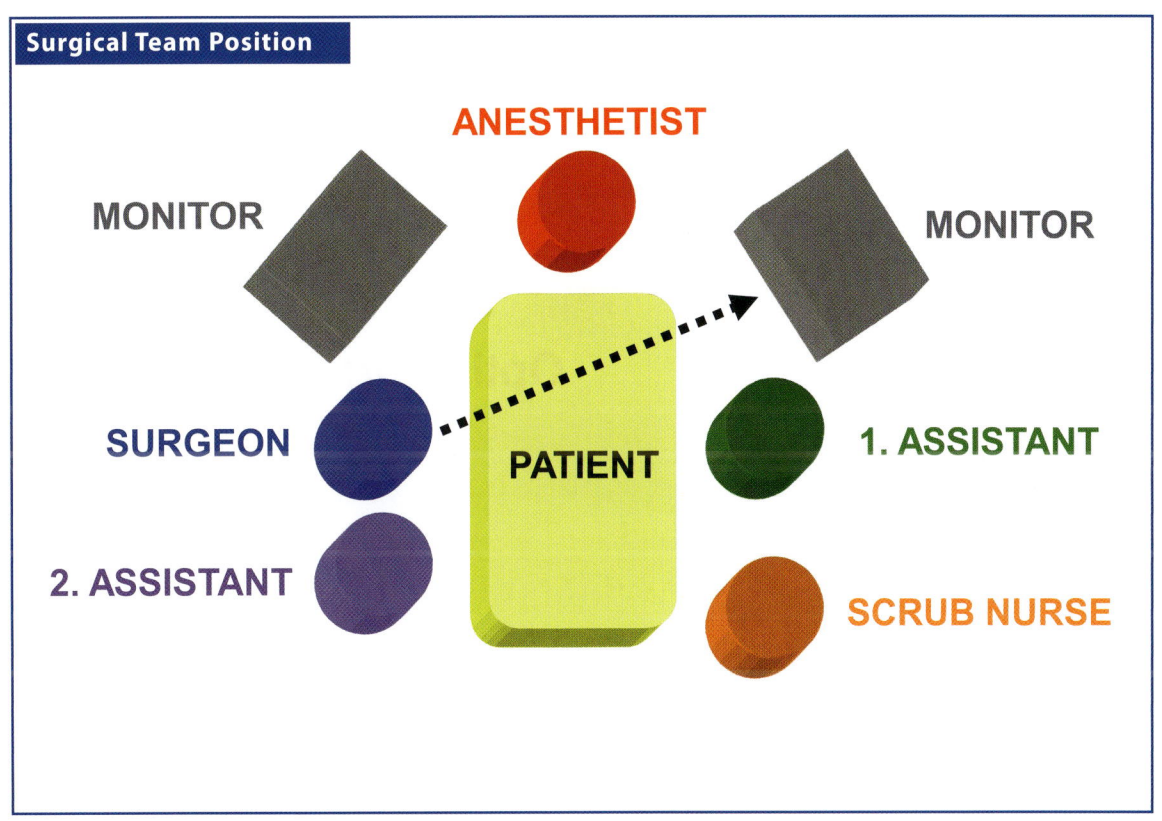

Surgical Team Position

ANESTHETIST

MONITOR

MONITOR

SURGEON

PATIENT

1. ASSISTANT

2. ASSISTANT

SCRUB NURSE

24.2   Patient Positioning

Supine position with both arms extended at 90° to the body.

24.3   Special Instruments

- Pectus bar
- Bar stabilizer plate
- Introducer
- Flexible template
- Pectus bar bender
- Pectus bar flipper

24.4   Location of Access Points

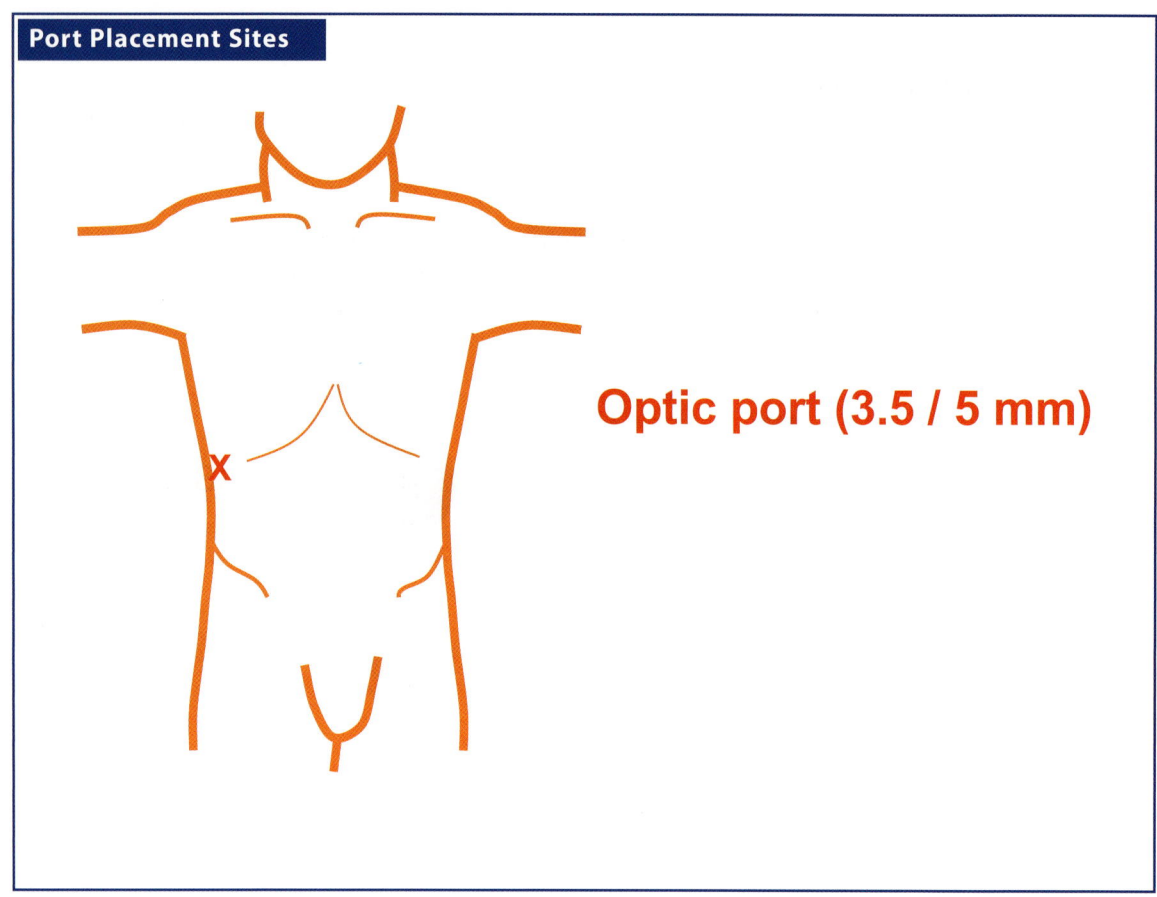

Port Placement Sites

Optic port (3.5 / 5 mm)

24.5 Indications

1. Improvement of chest-wall appearance.
2. Pulmonary compromise with activity.
3. Chest-wall pain.
4. Psychosocial impairment.

24.6 Contraindications

1. There are no absolute contraindications for pectus excavatum
2. Combined pectus carinatum and excavatum deformities.

24.7 Preoperative Considerations

1. Intravenous antibiotic cefuroxime (30 mg/kg; max 1.5 g) is administered at the time of anesthesia induction.
2. Drapes are placed so as to provide complete exposure of the chest wall as well as the lateral thorax.
3. Evaluate chest films with regard to the level of the diaphragm, which is important to determine the level of port insertion and avoid injury to the liver.

24.8 Technical Notes

1. Careful evaluation of the diaphragm on chest films to avoid trocar-related injuries to the diaphragm or liver.
2. The pectus bar is placed under the lowest part of the sternal depression.
3. In the case of severe deformities a second pectus bar may be required
4. Postoperative evacuation of the insufflated gas through the port is important to minimize morbidity due to residual pneumothorax. For this, the patient is placed in a left semilateral, head-down position.
5. The bar must enter and exit the thoracic cavity close to the right and left ridge of the depression.

24.9 Procedure Variations

1. Substernal incision to elevate the sternum in older patients with a deep and rigid chest wall
2. Use of bilateral thoracoscopy.
3. Use of bilateral stabilizer plates.
4. Extrapleural placement of the pectus bar.

24.10 Minimal-Access Repair of Pectus Excavatum

Please see Figs. 1–12.

Figure 24.1

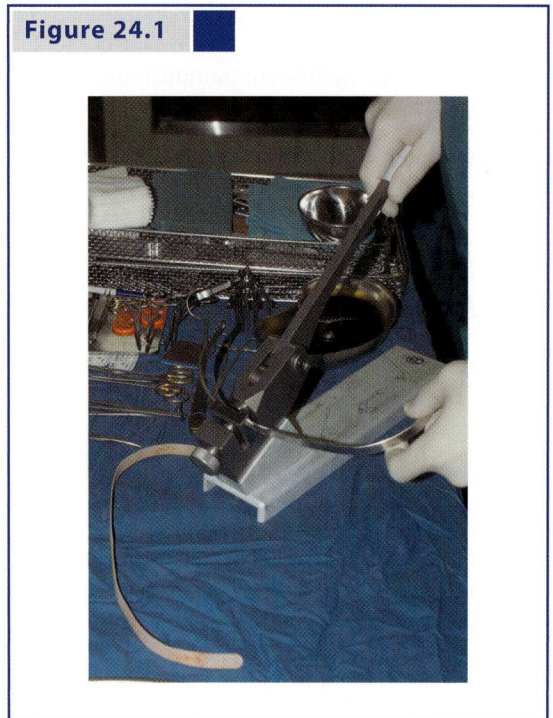

The thoracic contours are marked with a flexible template and the pectus bar is bent to the desired shape

Figure 24.2

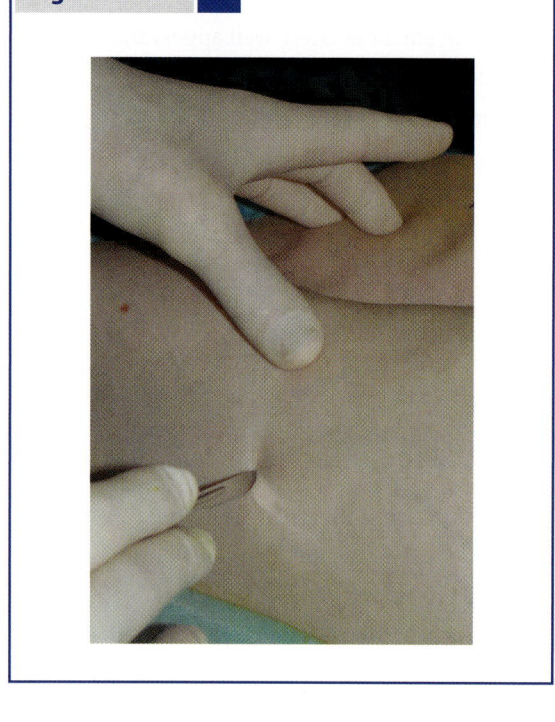

Bilateral horizontal thoracic skin incisions are placed at the predetermined point of pectus bar insertion and exit. The muscles are incised along their fibers and a space is created between the ribs and the muscle layers towards the edge of the pectus

Figure 24.3

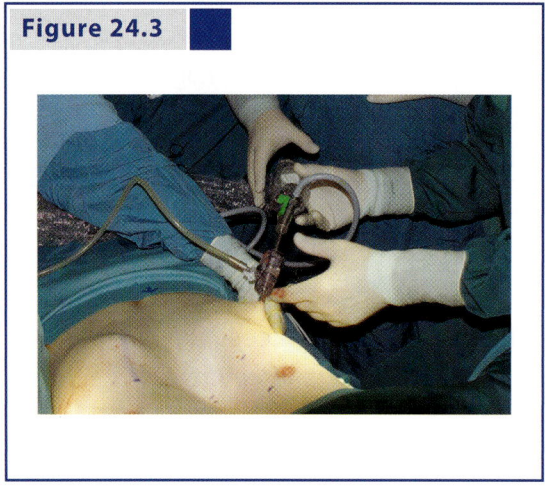

A 30° scope is introduced into the optic port placed in the anterior axillary line in the right lower rib margin and above the level of the diaphragm

Figure 24.4

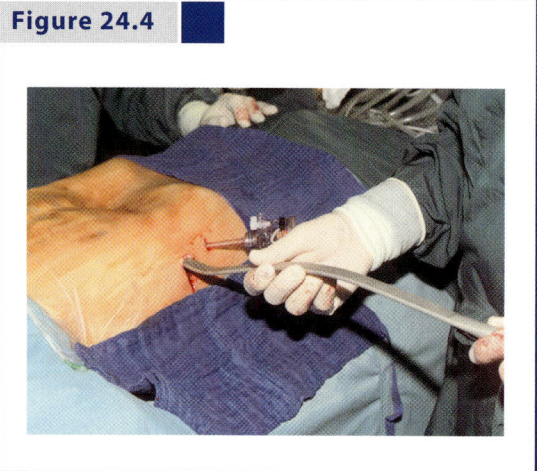

The introducer is inserted through the right incision into the thoracic cavity

Figure 24.5

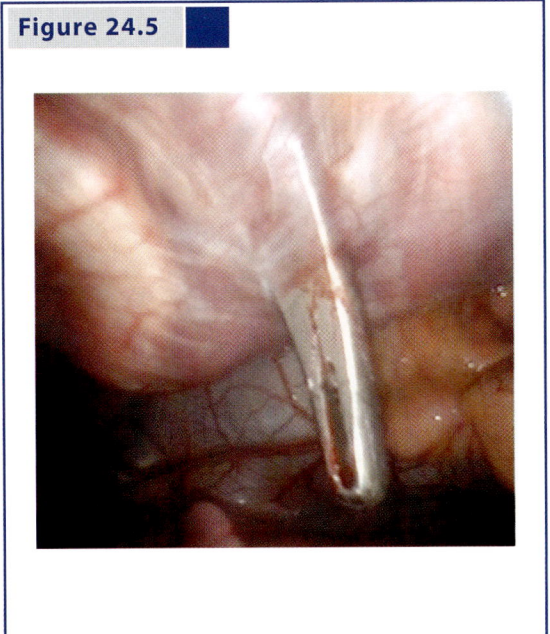

The introducer tip is passed through the intercostal muscles medial to the rim of the pectus and inserted into the right thoracic cavity

Figure 24.6

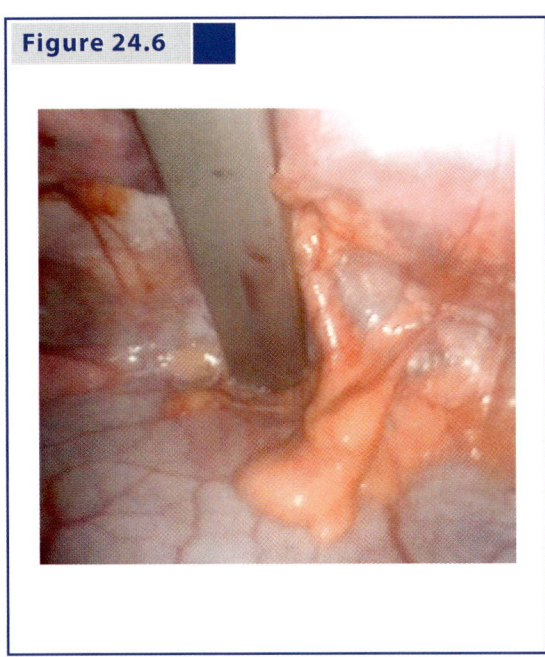

The introducer tip is slowly advanced through the retrosternal and prepericardial plane under visual control, and exits again medial to the pectus rim

Figure 24.7

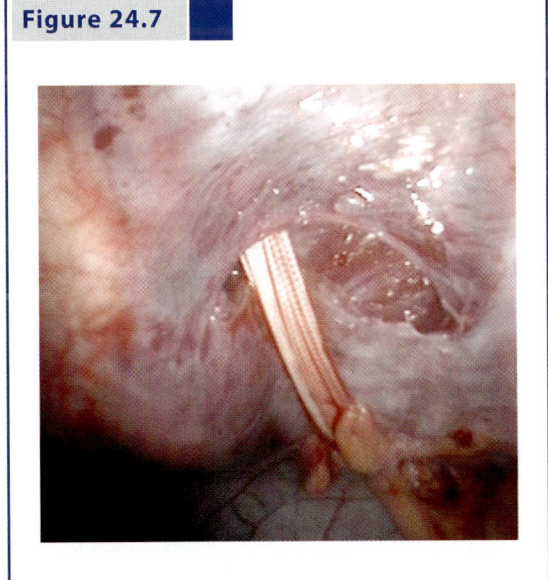

Two umbilical tapes are knotted to the introducer tip on the contralateral side and retrieved

Figure 24.8

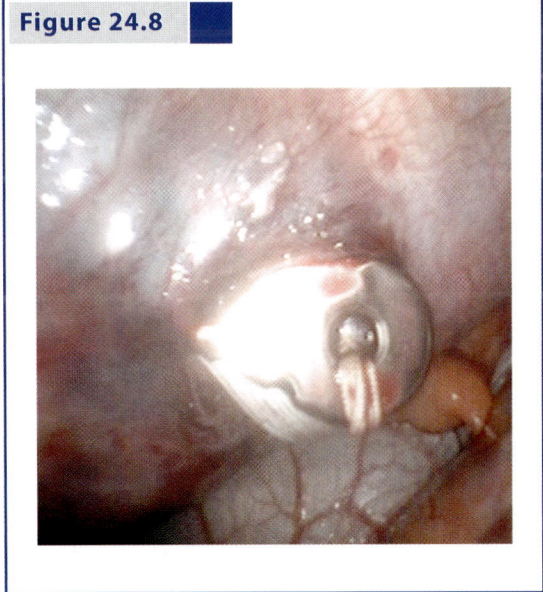

The pectus bar is then knotted to the tape and introduced into the right thorax

Figure 24.9

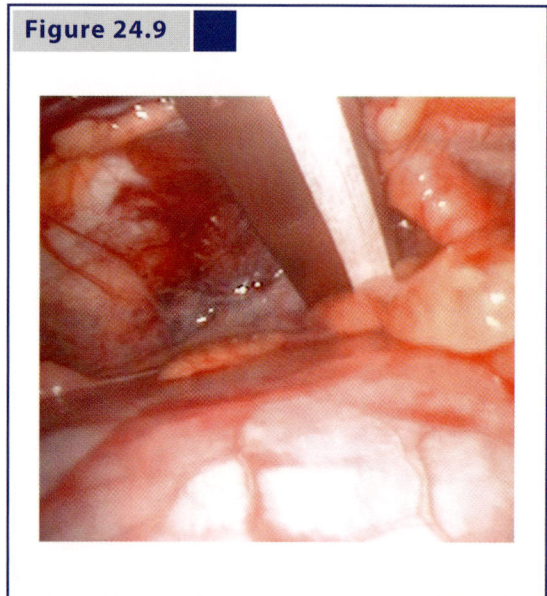

Using the umbilical tape as a guide, the pectus bar is advanced to the contralateral side and flipped

Figure 24.10

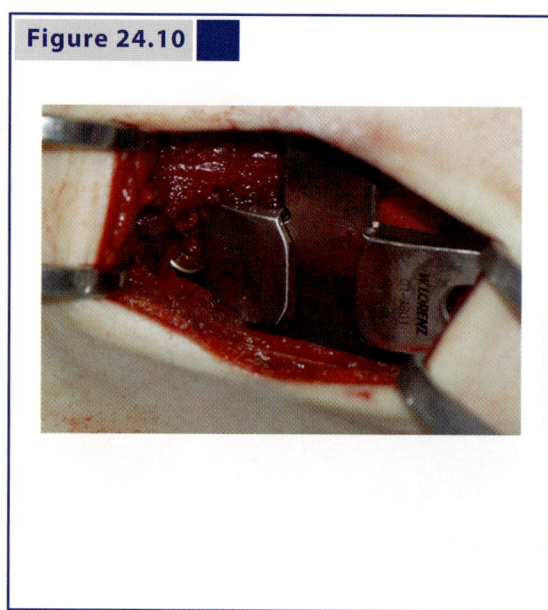

A single stabilizer plate is used on the right side and slid over the free end of the pectus bar

Figure 24.11

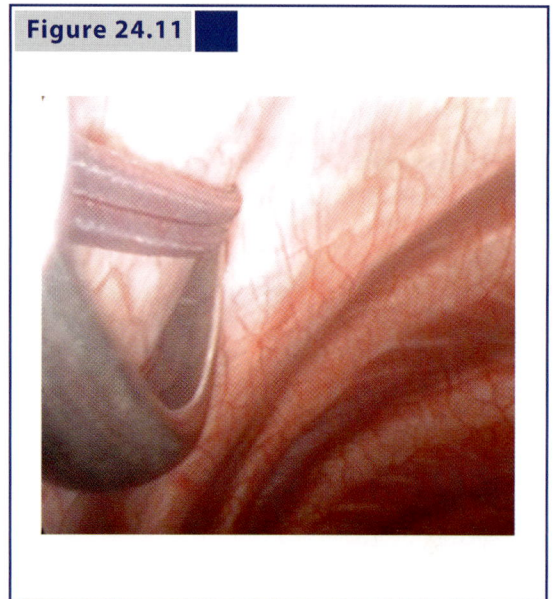

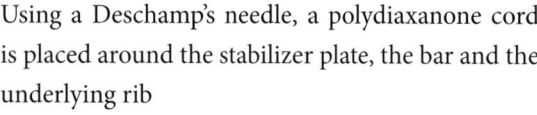

Using a Deschamp's needle, a polydiaxanone cord is placed around the stabilizer plate, the bar and the underlying rib

Figure 24.12

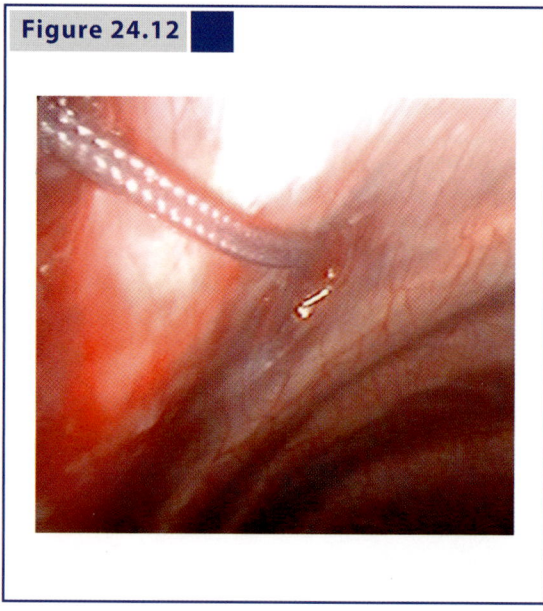

The polydioxanone cord is tied to secure the pectus bar and stabilizer plate to the underlying rib

Recommended Literature

1. Nuss D, Croitoru DP, Kelly RE Jr, Goretsky MJ, Nuss KJ, Gustin TS (2002) Review and discussion of the complications of minimally invasive pectus excavatum repair. Eur J Pediatr Surg 12:230–234

2. Saxena AK, Castellani C, Hollwarth ME (2007) Surgical aspects of thoracoscopy and efficacy of right thoracoscopy in minimally invasive repair of pectus excavatum. J Thorac Cardiovasc Surg 133:1201–1205

3. Schalamon J, Pokall S, Windhaber J, Hoellwarth ME (2006) Minimally invasive correction of pectus excavatum in adult patients. J Thorac Cardiovasc Surg 132:524–529

Section 3
Gastrointestinal Procedures

25 Diagnostic Laparoscopy

Atsuyuki Yamataka and Tadaharu Okazaki

25.1   Operation Room Setup

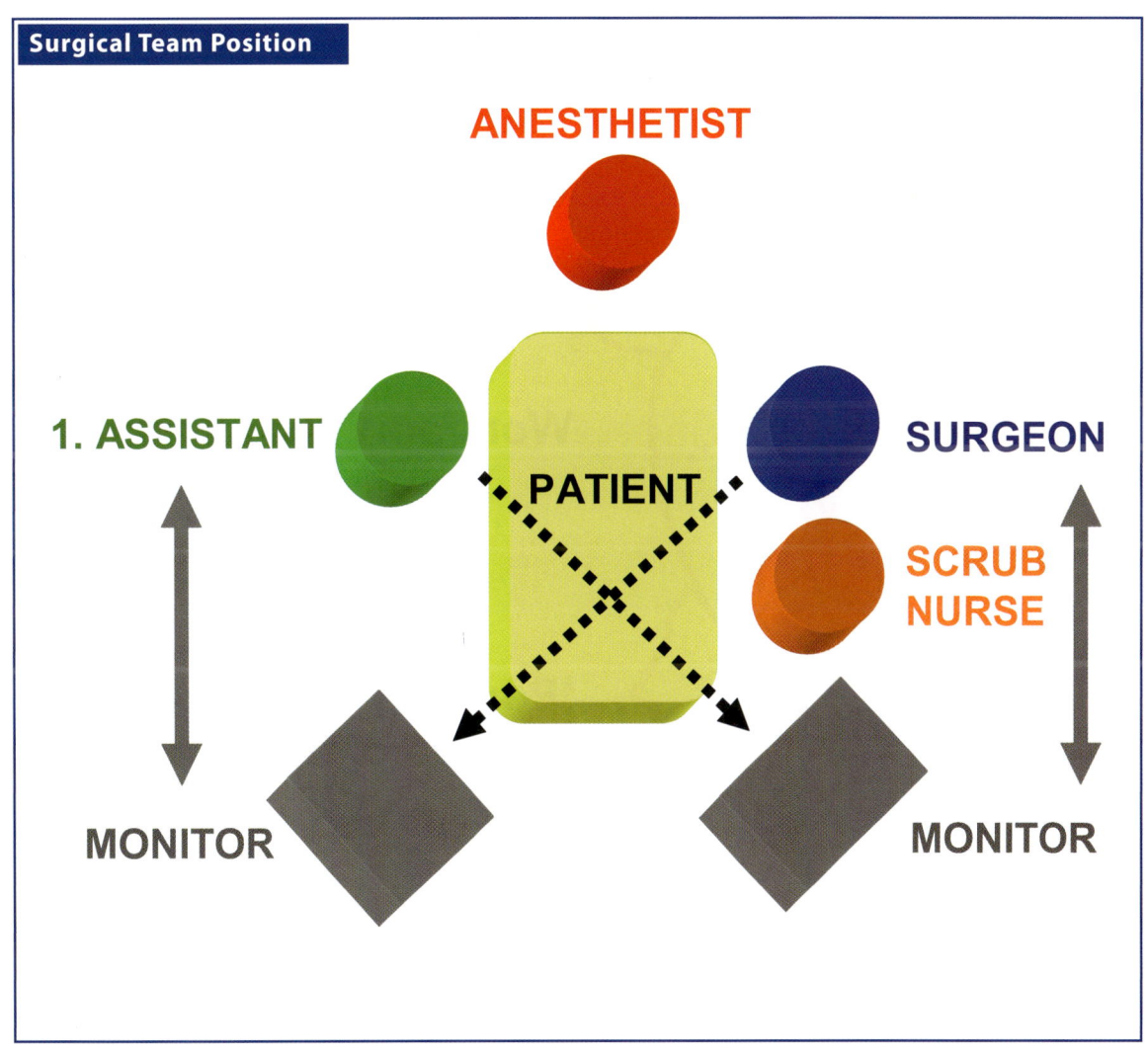

25.2   Patient Positioning

Supine and secured to allow tilting of the operating table intraoperatively to facilitate examination of the peritoneal cavity.

25.3   Special Instruments

- Endoscopic retractors
- Babcock forceps
- Specimen retrieval bag
- Ultracision® shears (Johnson & Johnson Medical Products, Ethicon Endo-Surgery, Cincinnati, OH, USA)
- Cholangiogram needles

25.4   Location of Access Points

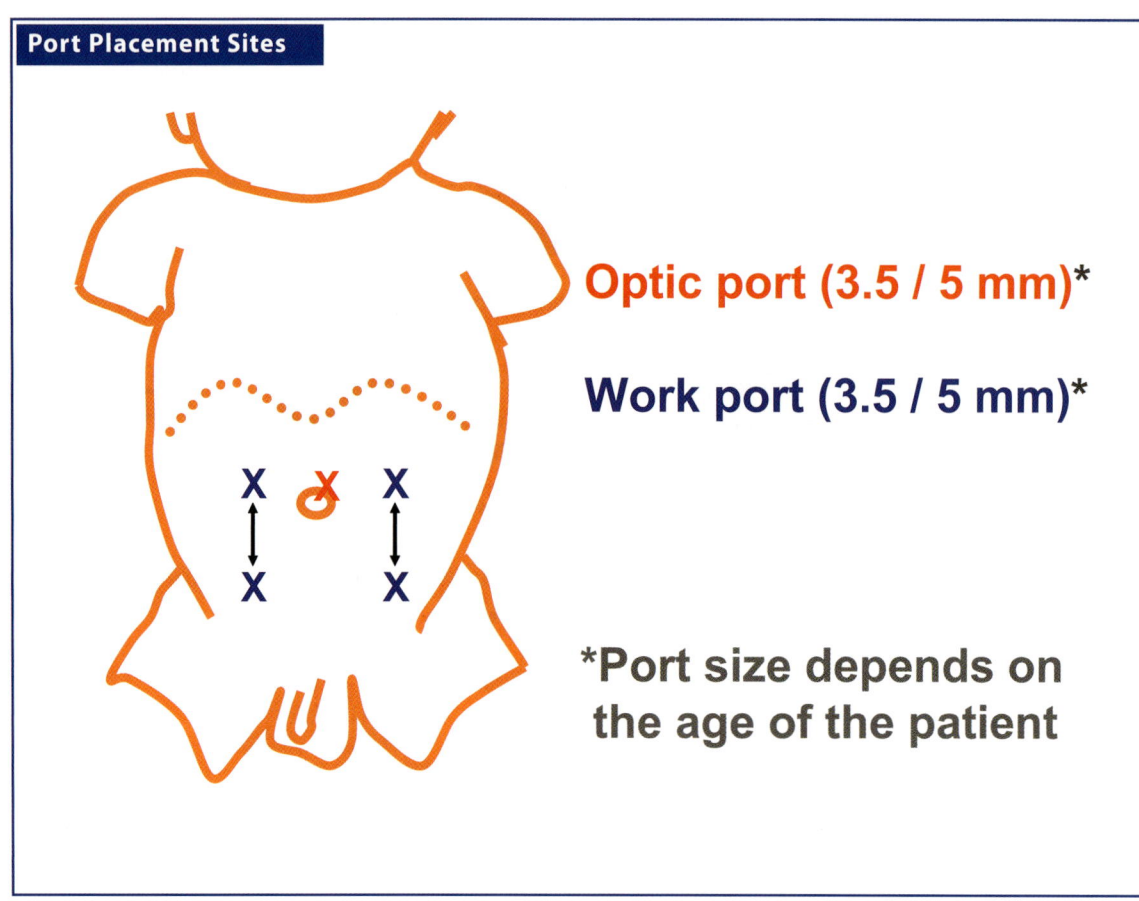

Port Placement Sites

Optic port (3.5 / 5 mm)*

Work port (3.5 / 5 mm)*

*Port size depends on the age of the patient

25.5   Indications

1. Acute abdominal pain including intestinal obstruction.
2. Recurrent or chronic abdominal pain.
3. Meckel's diverticulum diagnosis.
4. Antenatally diagnosed intestinal atresia.
5. Evaluation of abdominal masses – including malignant tumor, appendiceal mass, duplication cyst, and mesenteric cyst.
6. Hirschsprung's disease – colon biopsies.
7. Evaluation of impalpable testes and intersex states.
8. Investigation of pelvic mass.
9. Blunt and penetrating visceral trauma.

25.6   Contraindications

1. Uncorrected hypotension, hypoxia, and bleeding disorders.
2. Severe bowel obstruction with dilated bowel loops.

25.7   Preoperative Considerations

1. Patients should be prepared for general anesthesia. Blood grouping and crossmatching should be undertaken if clinically indicated.
2. General anesthesia with optimal muscle relaxation.
3. Place a nasogastric tube and urinary catheter.
4. Indications for preoperative antibiotics are the same as for the open procedure.
5. Liaison with histopathology services if biopsies are planned.

25.8   Procedure Variations

1. The viscera should be examined using a consistent routine starting with a clockwise inspection from the cecum and appendix, right colon, gallbladder, liver, stomach, spleen, left colon, pelvic organs, internal inguinal rings, gonadal vessels, and back to the ileocecal region.
2. The entire small bowel can be inspected using two pairs of atraumatic grasping forceps until the duodenojejunal junction is reached.
3. Two linked monitors are ideal to avoid difficulties with parallax.

25.9   Appendiceal Mass

Please see Figs. 1 and 2.

Figure 25.1

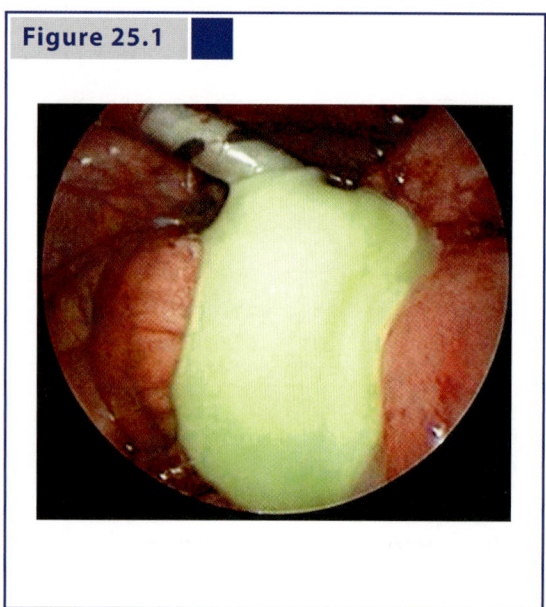

Figure 25.2

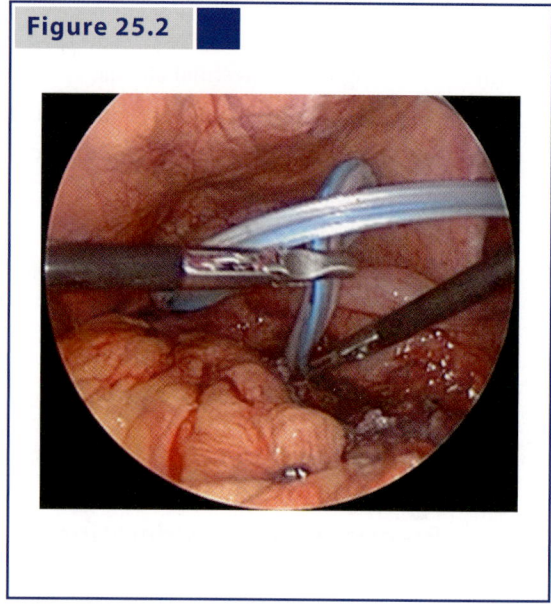

An appendiceal mass is carefully opened and the purulent exudate is aspirated completely using a suction/irrigation device

A J-VAC (Ethicon, Somerville, NJ, USA) drainage tube is placed within the abscess cavity. Laparoscopic appendectomy is planned several months later

25.10 Stoma Closure

Please see Figs. 3 and 4.

Figure 25.3

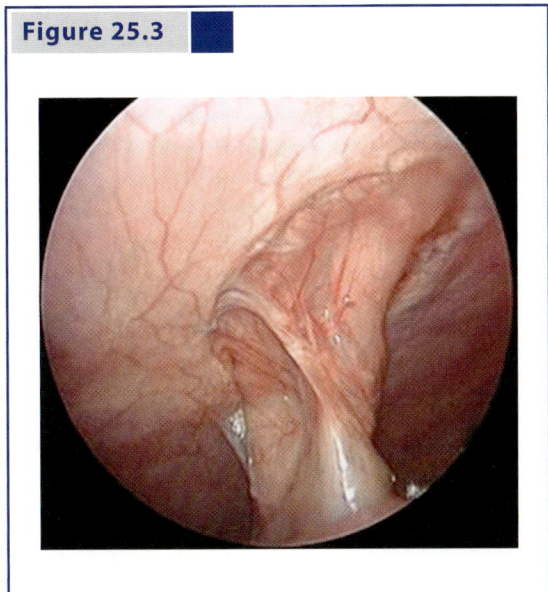

Figure 25.4

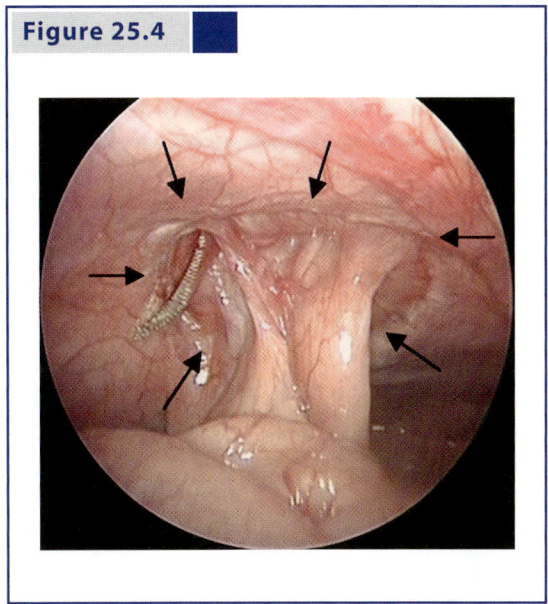

The bowel loop of the stoma is clearly visualized under laparoscopic control

A stoma can be removed under laparoscopic control (*arrowheads*). This is less traumatic to the abdominal wall and prevents bowel injury

25.11   Laparoscopic-Assisted Cholangiography

Please see Figs. 5–8.

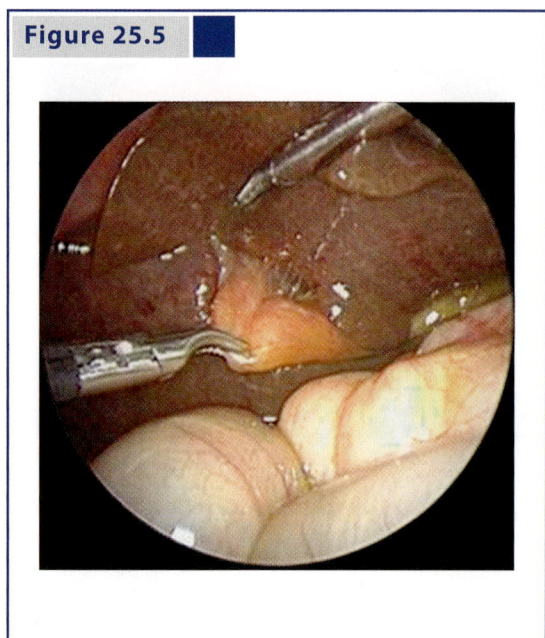

Figure 25.5

Figure 25.6

In patients with biliary atresia, the gallbladder is usually atretic and direct insertion of a catheter is technically difficult

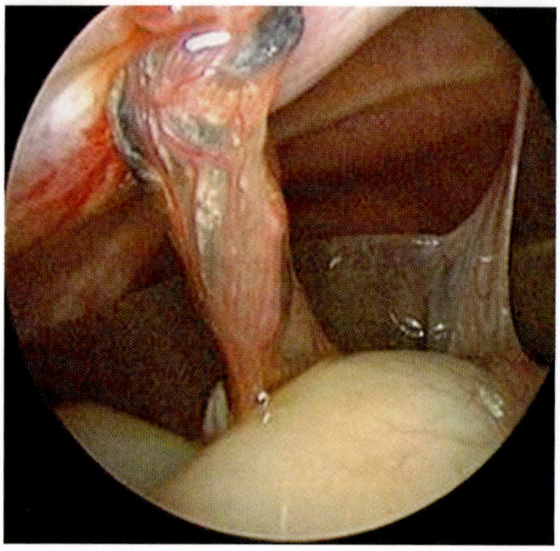

If the gallbladder is of reasonable size, the fundus can be exteriorized through a small right subcostal incision following partial laparoscopic dissection from the liver bed

Figure 25.7

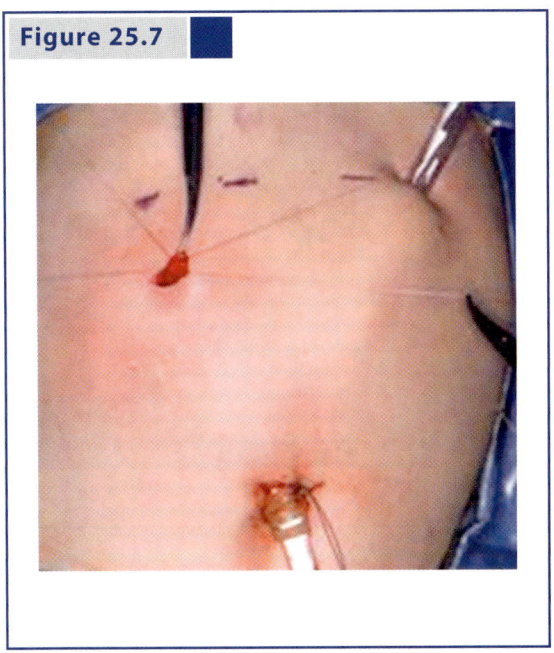
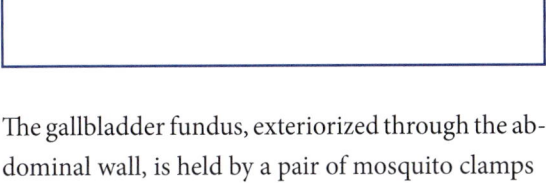

Figure 25.8

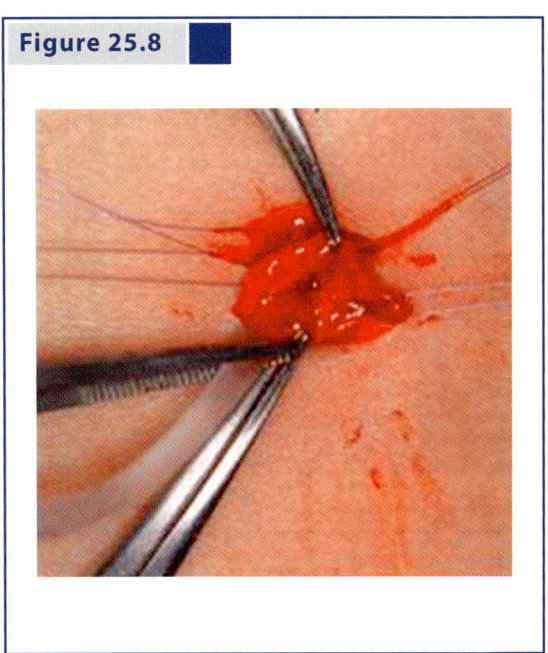

The gallbladder fundus, exteriorized through the abdominal wall, is held by a pair of mosquito clamps

A 5-Fr feeding tube is inserted into the gallbladder for cholangiography

25.12   Antenatally Diagnosed Small-Bowel Atresia

Please see Figs. 9 and 10.

Figure 25.9

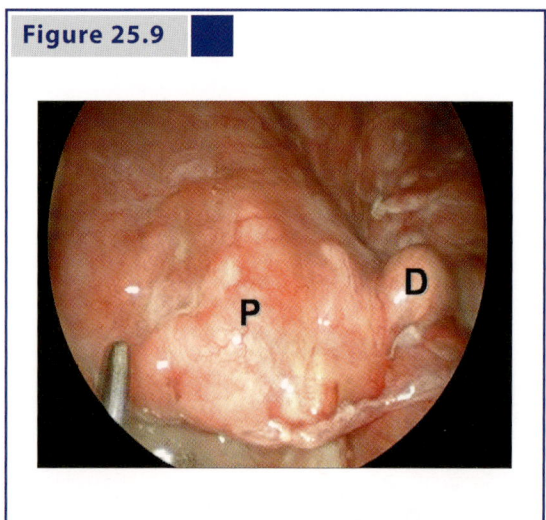

Figure 25.10

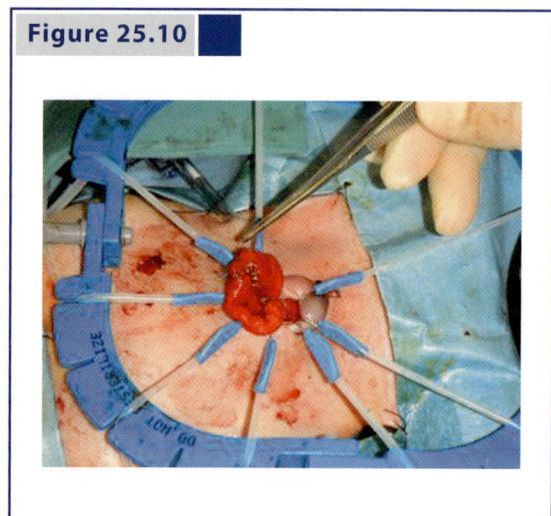

A 0° laparoscope is introduced through the umbilical port and both the proximal (**P**) and distal (**D**) bowel ends are identified

Both the proximal and distal bowel ends are exteriorized via the umbilical port wound, which is expanded by using a wound retractor, and anastomosis is performed

Recommended Literature

1. Okazaki T, Miyano G, Yamataka A, Kobayashi H, Koga H, Lane GJ, Miyano T (2006) Diagnostic laparoscopy-assisted cholangiography in infants with prolonged jaundice. Pediatr Surg Int 22:140–143
2. Marusasa T, Miyano G, Kato Y, Yanai T, Okazaki T, Ichikawa S, Lane GJ, Yamataka A (2007) New primary management for appendiceal masses in children: laparoscopic drainage. J Laparoendosc Adv Surg Tech 17:497–500
3. Yamataka A, Koga H, Shimotakahara A, Urao M, Yanai M, Kobayashi H, Lane G, Miyano T (2004) Laparoscopy-assisted surgery for prenatally diagnosed small bowel atresia: simple, safe, and virtually scar free. J Pediatr Surg 39:1815–1818

26 Thal Fundoplication

Jürgen Schleef and Gloria Pelizzo

26.1 Operation Room Setup

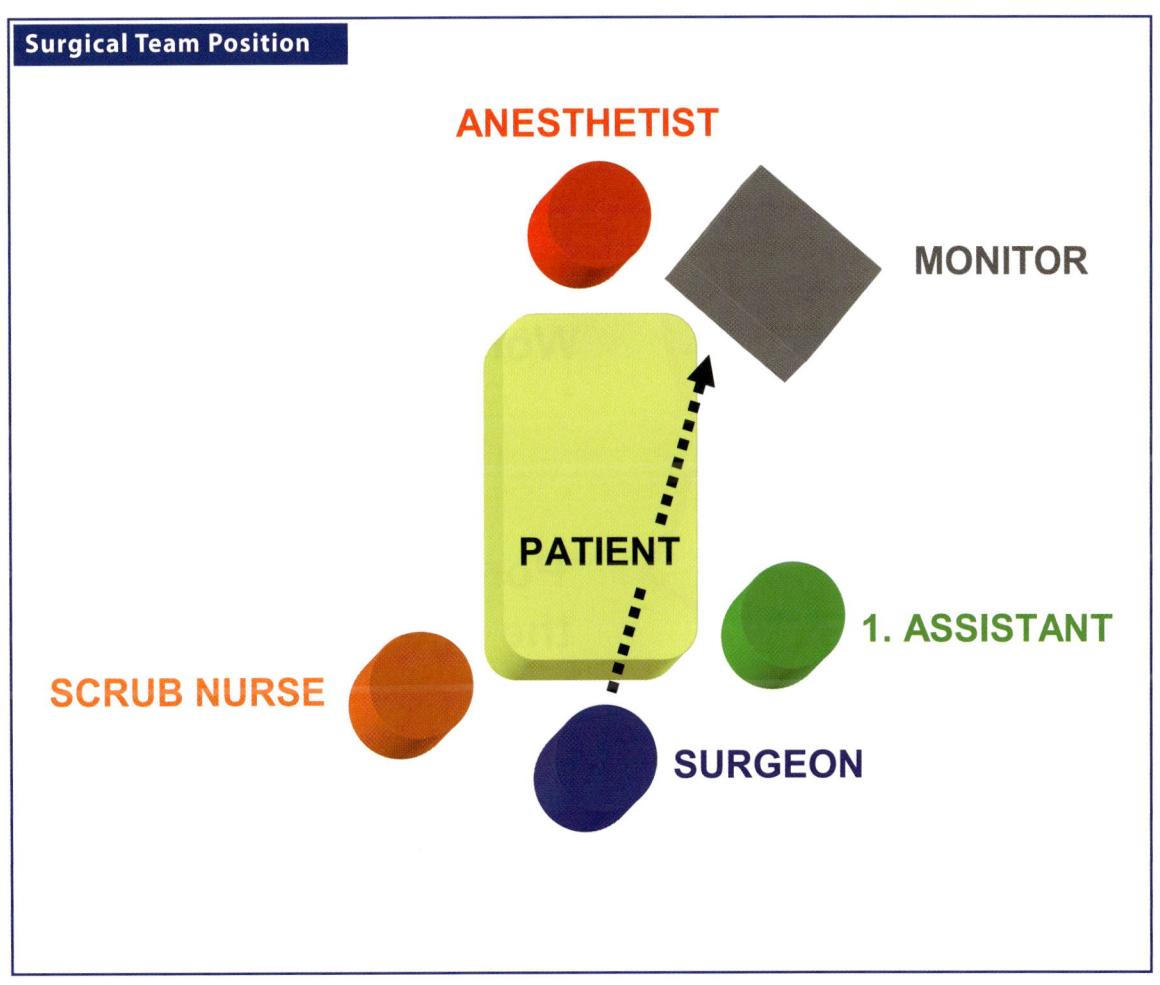

Surgical Team Position

ANESTHETIST

MONITOR

PATIENT

1. ASSISTANT

SCRUB NURSE

SURGEON

26.2   Patient Positioning

Supine with both arms tucked to the sides. Frog-leg position in small children, while in adolescents the legs are opened to allow the surgeon to stand in between.

26.3   Special Instruments

Esophageal retractor.

26.4   Location of Access Points

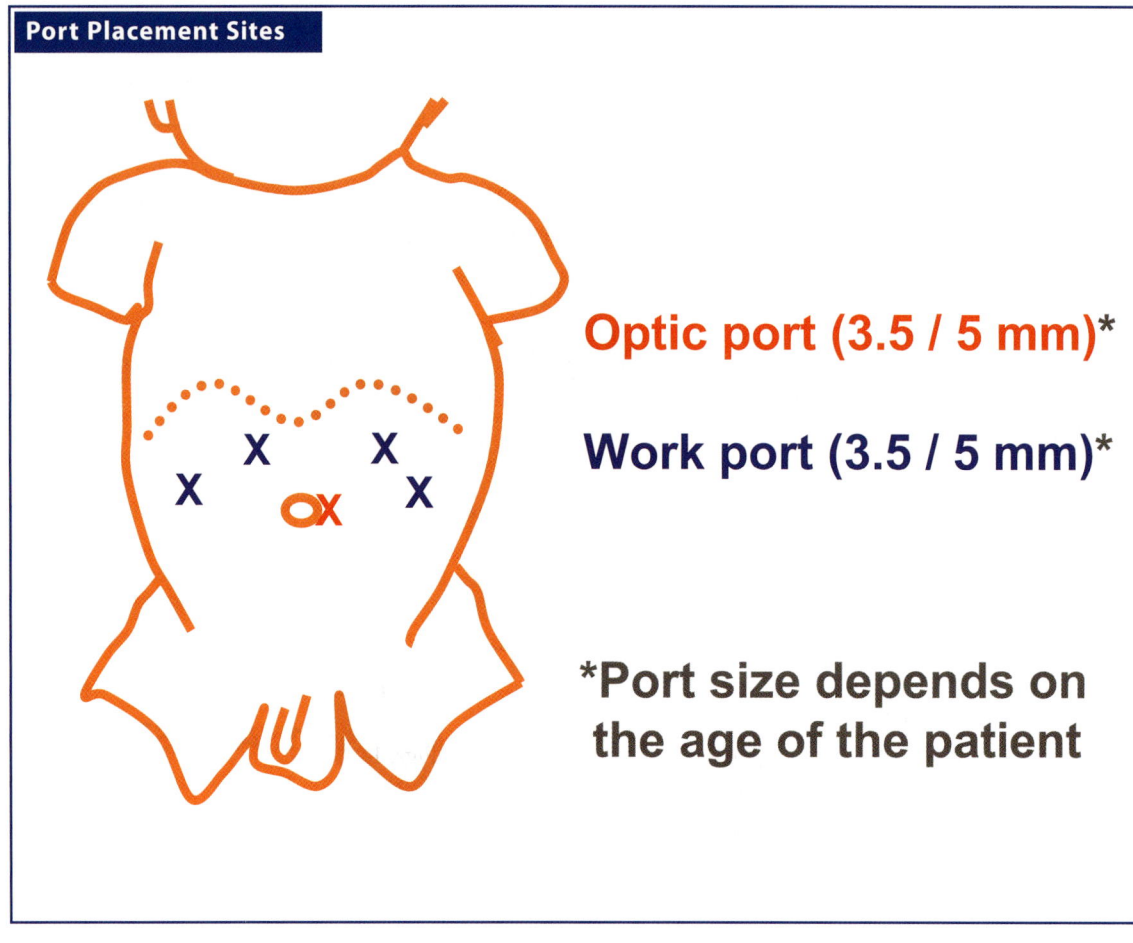

Port Placement Sites

Optic port (3.5 / 5 mm)*

Work port (3.5 / 5 mm)*

*Port size depends on the age of the patient

26.5   Indications

Gastroesophageal reflux:

1. Refractory to medical treatment.
2. With aspiration pneumonia.
3. Failure to thrive.

26.6   Contraindications

1. Severe respiratory distress associated with any of the aforementioned indications.
2. Severe scoliosis (relative contraindication).
3. Prior abdominal surgery with adhesions (relative contraindication).

26.7   Preoperative Considerations

1. The bladder has to be emptied before the procedure with the Crede maneuver or the placement of a Foley catheter.
2. Neurological patients should be positioned according to the severity of scoliosis. Sufficient support should be provided to the body of to stabilize it during the procedure.
3. The size of nasogastric tube or bougie should be decided upon before the procedure commences; and sufficient access of the head area should be provided to the anesthetist.

26.8   Technical Notes

1. The liver can be retracted using a three-finger liver retractor. Otherwise, a simple grasper can be introduced from the right side to grasp the diaphragm, thereby raising the liver.
2. Suturing of the fundus to the esophagus is done with the first line of sutures. This is followed by a second suture line, which sutures the fundus to the diaphragm and the right crus.
3. Port placements have to be adjusted in children with severe scoliosis.

26.9   Procedure Variations

1. Umbilical tapes can be used to retract the esophagus instead of the esophageal retractor.
2. Short gastric vessels may have to be mobilized to facilitate mobilization of the fundus.
3. In patients with a percutaneous endoscopic gastrostomy, it is not necessary to take down the stoma for fundoplication.
4. LigaSure™ (Valleylab, Boulder, CO, USA) or Ultracision® (Johnson & Johnson Medical Products, Ethicon Endo-Surgery, Cincinnati, OH, USA) shears may be used in older children.

26.10   Laparoscopic Thal Fundoplication

Please see Figs. 1–6.

Figure 26.1

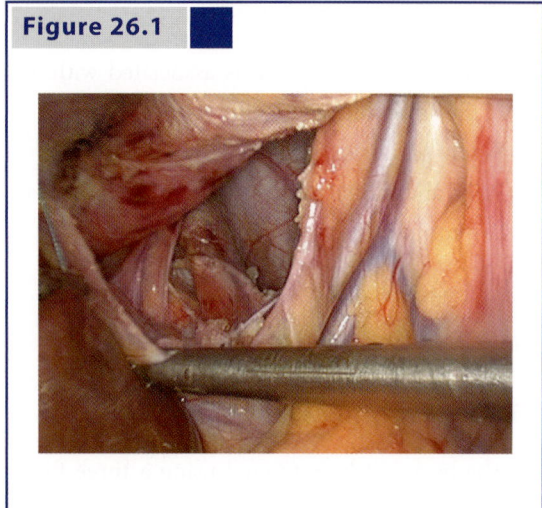

The avascular window of the gastrohepatic ligament is opened with monopolar hook cautery and the peritoneum around the hiatus is dissected. The esophagus is held retracted during the dissection

Figure 26.2

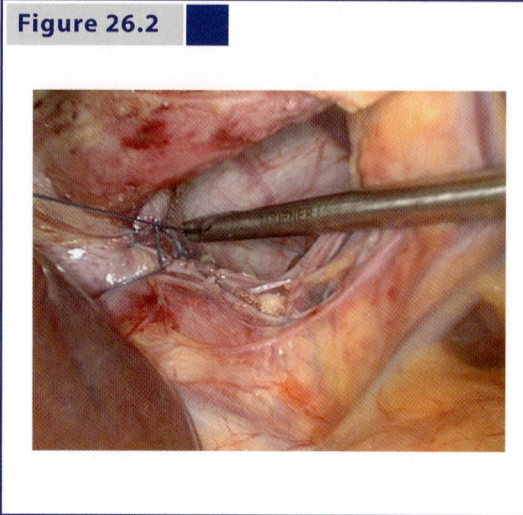

A bougie is placed in the esophagus. The left and the right crus of the diaphragm are sufficiently exposed and nonabsorbable sutures are used to close the esophageal hiatus

Figure 26.3

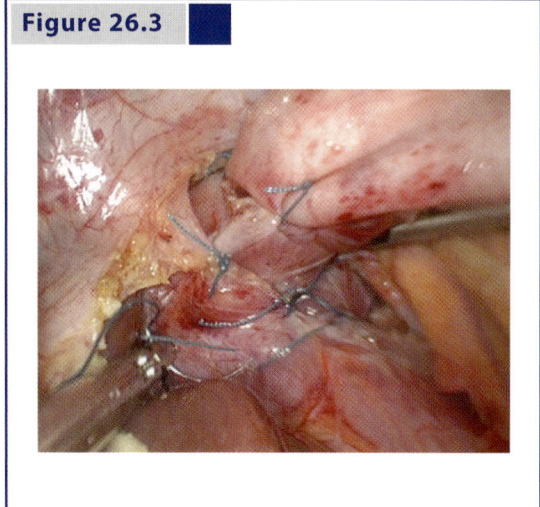

Stay sutures are used on either side of the esophagus to secure it to the diaphragm. The fundus is mobilized anteriorly and is sutured on the right side of the esophagus

Figure 26.4

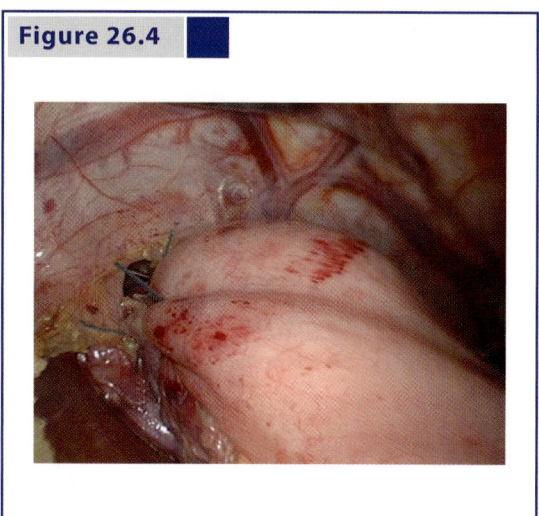

The first row of sutures is used to suture the fundus to the esophagus. Sutures are places on the anterior side of the esophagus and along the right edge of the esophagus

Figure 26.5

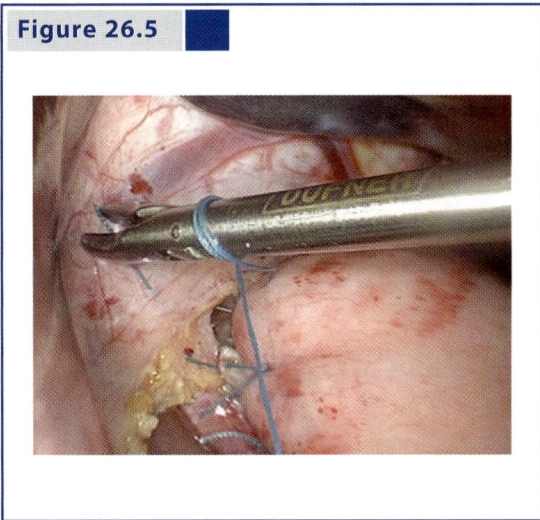

Figure 26.6

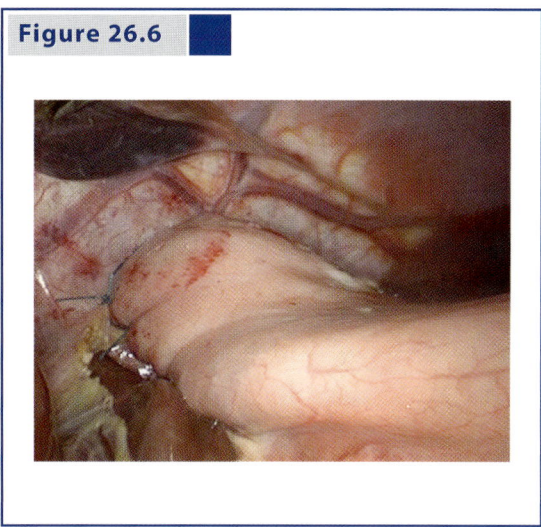

A second row of sutures is placed along the line of the first row to further secure the fundus to the diaphragm and the right crus of the diaphragm. The second row reinforces the first row of sutures

The final view of the anterior wrap before closure of the abdomen. The bougie is removed by the anesthetist under visual aid

Recommended Literature

1. Garzi A, Valla JS, Molinaro F, Amato G, Messina M (2007) Minimally invasive surgery for achalasia: combined experience of two European centers. J Pediatr Gastroenterol Nutr 44:587–591

2. Martinez-Frontanilla LA, Sartorelli KH, Hasse GM, Meagher DP Jr (1996) Laparoscopic Thal fundoplication with gastrostomy in children. J Pediatr Surg. 31:275–276

3. Van der Zee DC, Bax KN, Ure BM, Besselink MG, Pakvis DF (2002) Long-term results after laparoscopic Thal procedure in children. Semin Laparosc Surg 9:168–171

27 Nissen Fundoplication

SHAWN D. ST PETER AND GEORGE W. HOLCOMB III

27.1   Operation Room Setup

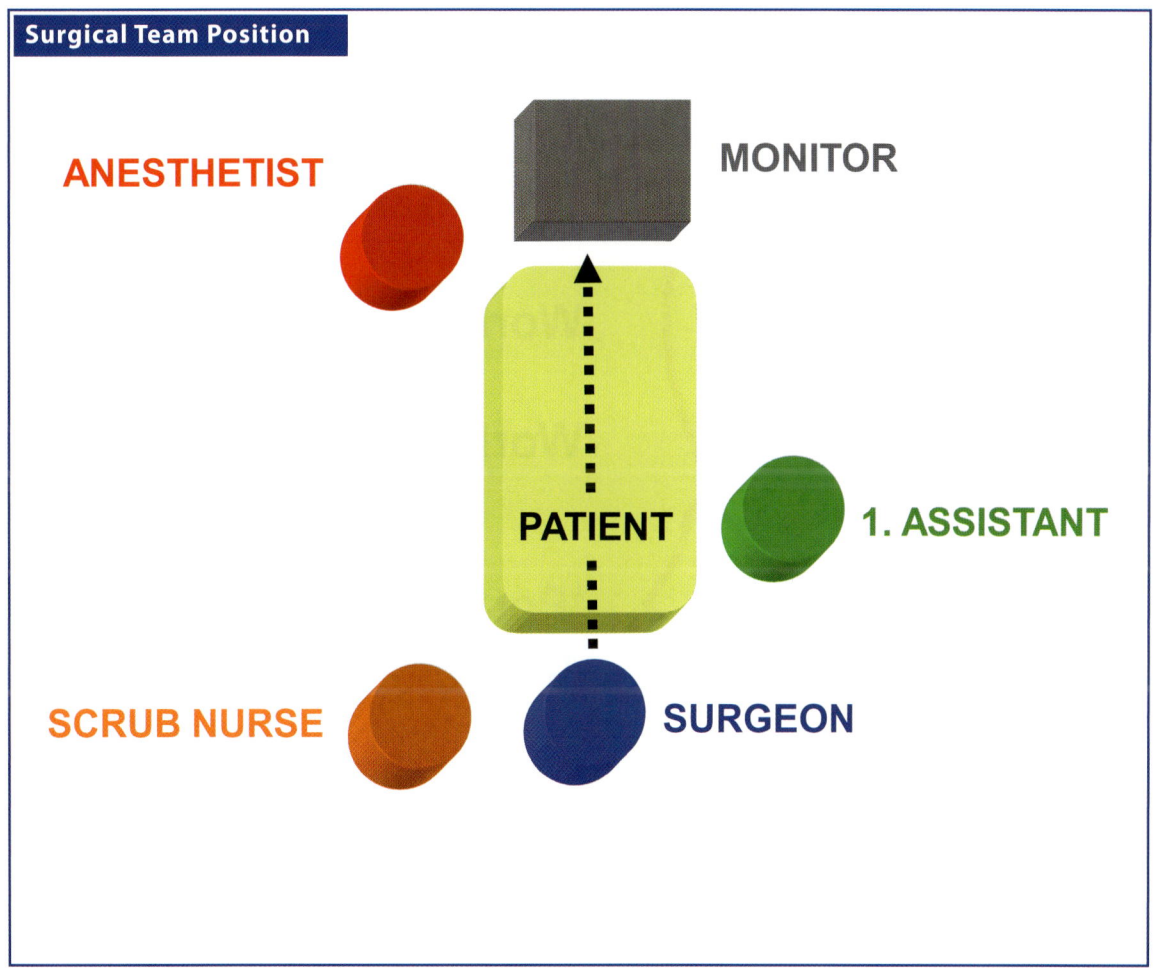

Surgical Team Position

ANESTHETIST

MONITOR

PATIENT

1. ASSISTANT

SCRUB NURSE

SURGEON

27.2   Patient Positioning

Frog-leg position at the end of the table with arms tucked for infants and small children. Older children require stirrups.

27.3   Special Instruments

- Endoscopic liver rectractor
- Patients over 5 years age require one of the following devices to divide short gastric vessels:
    - Ultracision® shears (Johnson & Johnson Medical Products, Ethicon Endo-Surgery, Cincinnati, OH, USA) or
    - LigaSure™ (Valleylab, Boulder, CO, USA) or
    - EnSeal® (SurgRx, Redwood City, CA, USA)

27.4   Location of Access Points

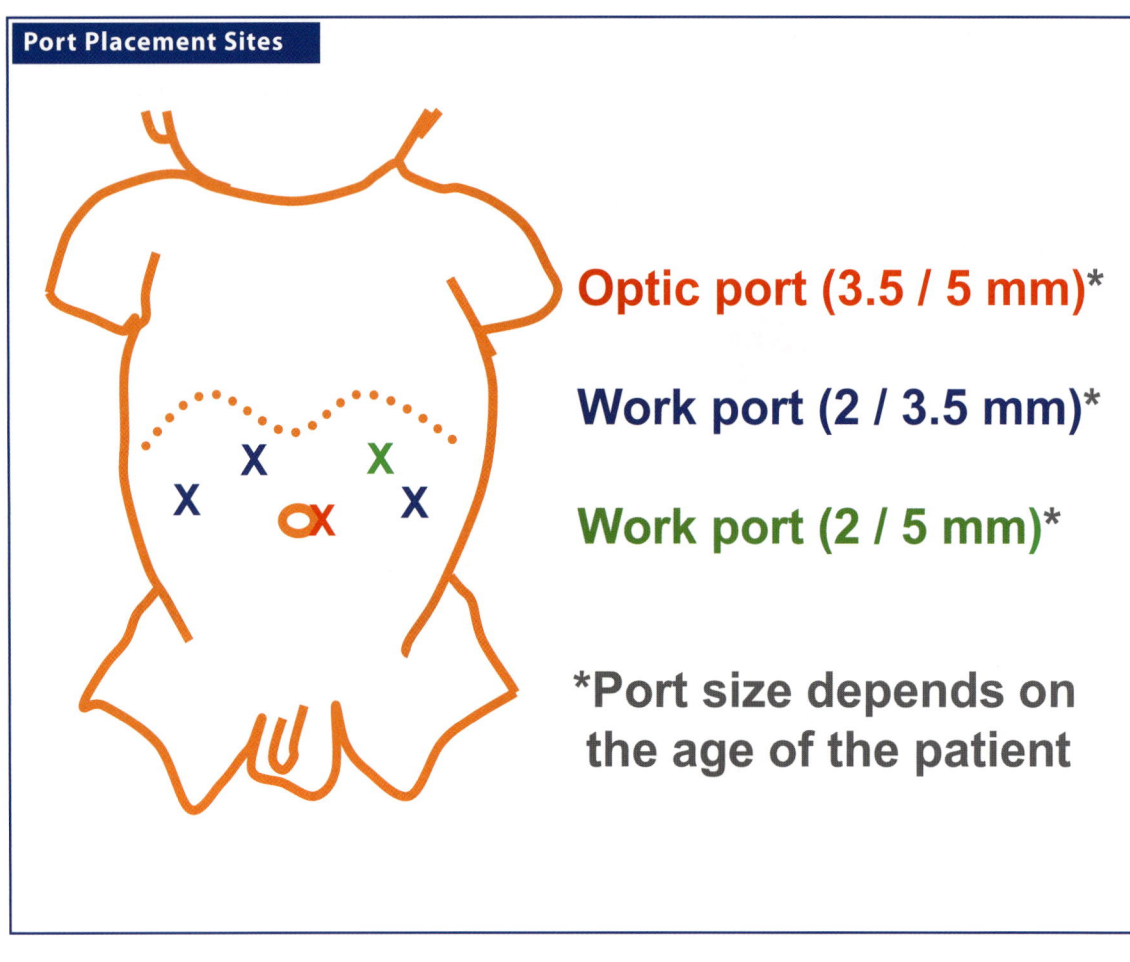

Port Placement Sites

Optic port (3.5 / 5 mm)*

Work port (2 / 3.5 mm)*

Work port (2 / 5 mm)*

*Port size depends on the age of the patient

27.5   Indications

Gastroesophageal reflux causing one or more of the following problems:

1. Failure to thrive.
2. Aspiration pneumonia.
3. Apparent life-threatening event.
4. Esophagitis, persistent vomiting or severe symptoms refractory to medical therapy.

27.6   Contraindications

Severe cardiac or pulmonary diseases and severe musculoskeletal malformations.

27.7   Preoperative Considerations

1. Place a nasogastric tube and have bougie available for the anesthesiologist to place.
2. Place foot pedals for hemostatic devices at the end of the bed.
3. Choose the length of sutures to be prepared by the scrub nurse.
4. Prep to the nipples as the skin will be drawn inferiorly by insufflation.
5. Drape in a manner that will provide easy access to the mouth for the anesthesiologist.
6. Place the drape in reverse direction. So the head portion, which is shorter, is not in the way of the surgeon's feet.

27.8   Technical Notes

1. If a gastrostomy button is to be placed, identify the spot on the abdomen prior to insufflation and this will serve as the port used by the surgeon's operating right hand.
2. Place a 2-0 nonabsorbable suture in the crus posteriorly, tie a knot, then secure it to the posterior esophagus.
3. Place four interrupted 3-0 nonabsorbable sutures between the crus and the esophagus circumferentially (7, 11, 2, and 5 o'clock).
4. Identify the portion of fundus to be brought around the esophagus, then push it back through to the left side while the bougie is inserted.

27.9   Procedure Variations

1. A 5-mm port for the surgeon's right hand allows vessel sealing devices to be used.
2. The esophagophrenic attachments can be completely mobilized or left in place laterally and anteriorly.
3. Pledgets may be employed to buttress the fundoplasty sutures.
4. A liver retractor can be a locking grasping forcep secured onto the right crus of the diaphragm
5. A table-mounted device can be used to hold the liver retractor in place.

27.10   Laparoscopic Nissen Fundoplication

Please see Figs. 1–6.

Figure 27.1

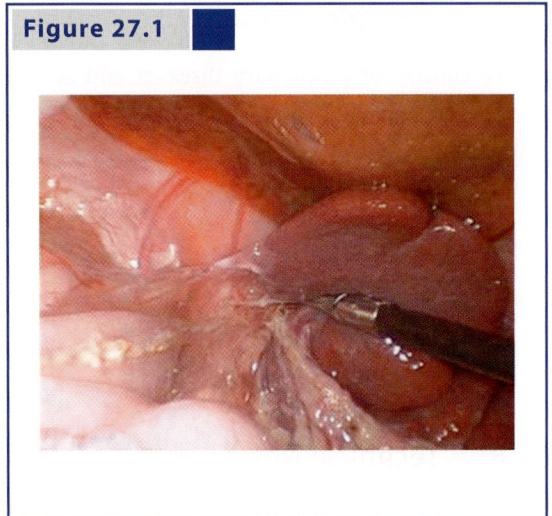

Dissection is commenced beyond the short gastric vessels toward the left crus, and the spleen is separated from the stomach

Figure 27.2

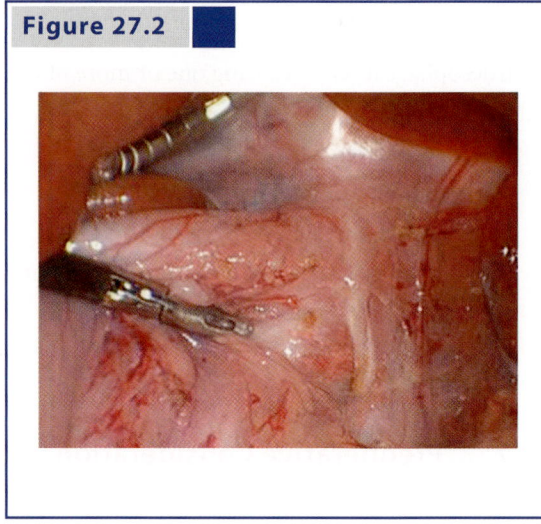

The left crus is identified and a retro-esophageal window is created

Figure 27.3

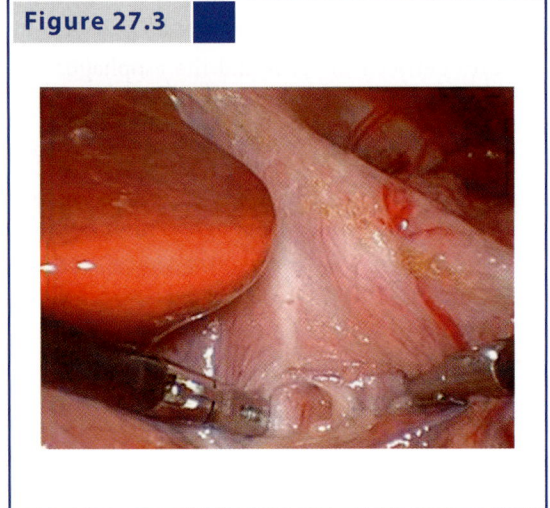

The right crus is identified and communication of the retroesophageal window is matured

Figure 27.4

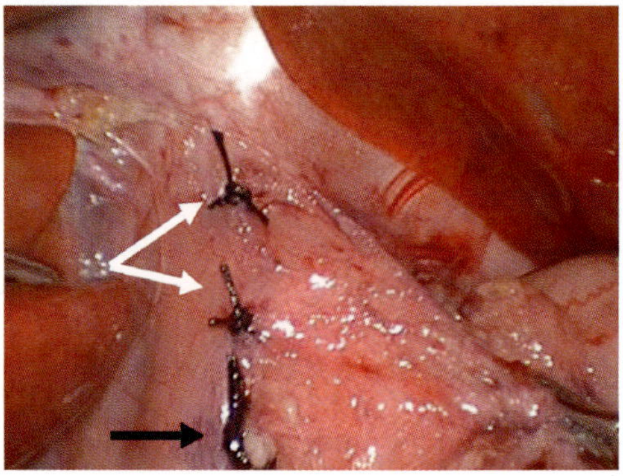

A posterior crural suture (2–0 nonabsorbable suture) is secured to the esophagus (**black arrow**) Two 3-0 nonabsorbable sutures are placed between the crus and esophagus on the right side (**white double arrow**)

Figure 27.5

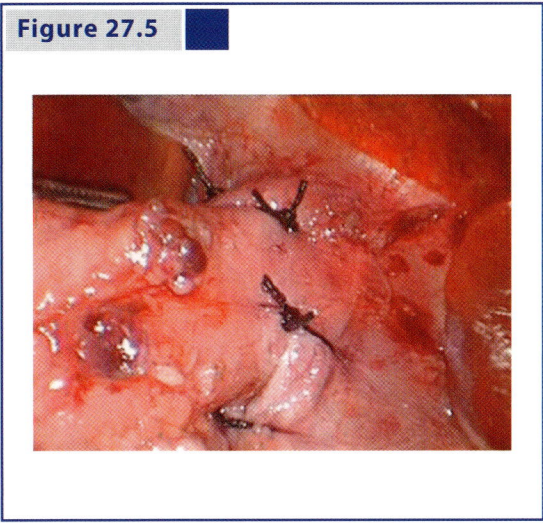

Figure 27.6

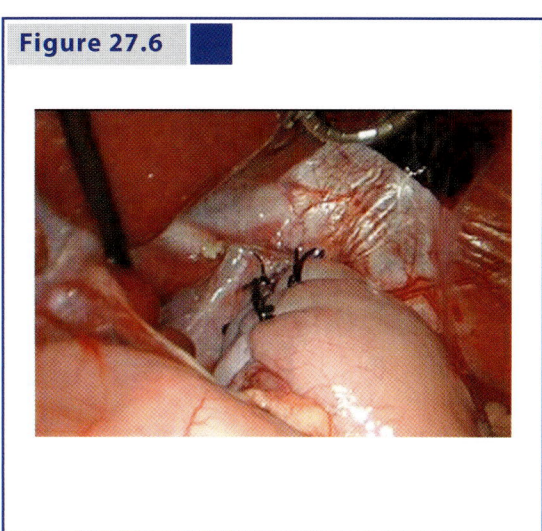

As on the right, two 3-0 nonabsorbable esophago-crural sutures are placed on the left side

Nissen fundoplication is formed with three interrupted 2–0 nonabsorbable sutures, the superior of which incorporates the anterior esophagus

Recommended Literature

1. St Peter SD, Holcomb GW III (2008) Gastroesophageal reflux disease and fundoplication in infants and children. Ann Pediatr Surg (in press)

2. St Peter SD, Valusek TA, Calkins CM, Shew SB, Ostlie DJ, Holcomb GW III (2007) Use of esophagocrural sutures and minimal esophageal dissection reduces the incidence of postoperative transmigration of laparoscopic Nissen fundoplication wrap. J Pediatr Surg 42:25–29

3. St Peter SD, Valusek TA, Ostlie DJ, Holcomb GW III (2007) The use of biosynthetic mesh to enhance hiatal repair at the time of redo Nissen fundoplication. J Ped Surg 42:1298–1301

28 Toupet Fundoplication

PHILIPPE MONTUPET AND AMULYA K. SAXENA

28.1 Operation Room Setup

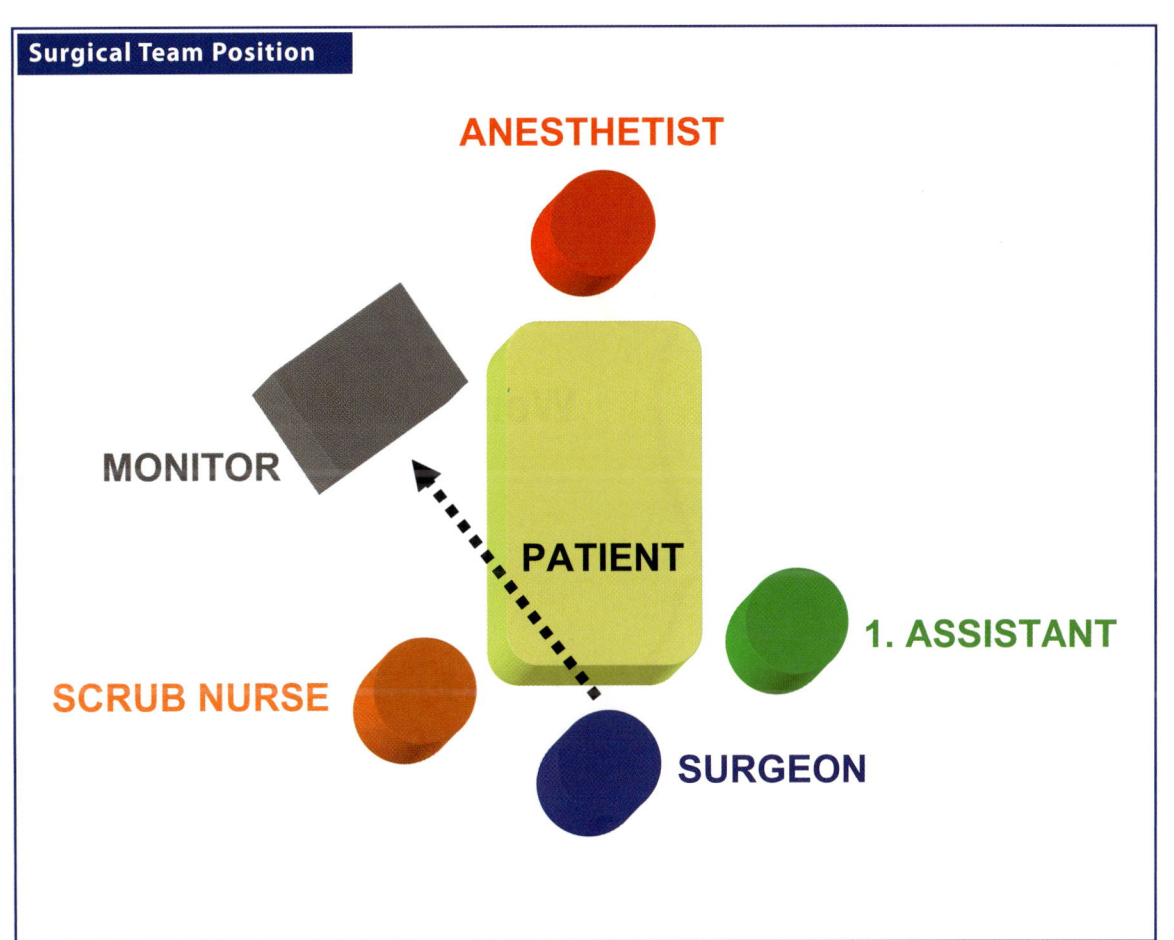

Surgical Team Position

ANESTHETIST

MONITOR

PATIENT

1. ASSISTANT

SCRUB NURSE

SURGEON

28.2   Patient Positioning

Reverse Trendelenburg with folded legs wrapped and fixed at the table.

28.3   Special Instruments

- Endoscopic liver retractor (three fingers) or snake retractor
- Monopolar hook or scissors
- LigaSure™ (Valleylab, Boulder, CO, USA) or
- Ultracision® harmonic scalpel (Johnson & Johnson Medical Products, Ethicon Endo-Surgery, Cincinnati, OH, USA).

28.4   Location of Access Points

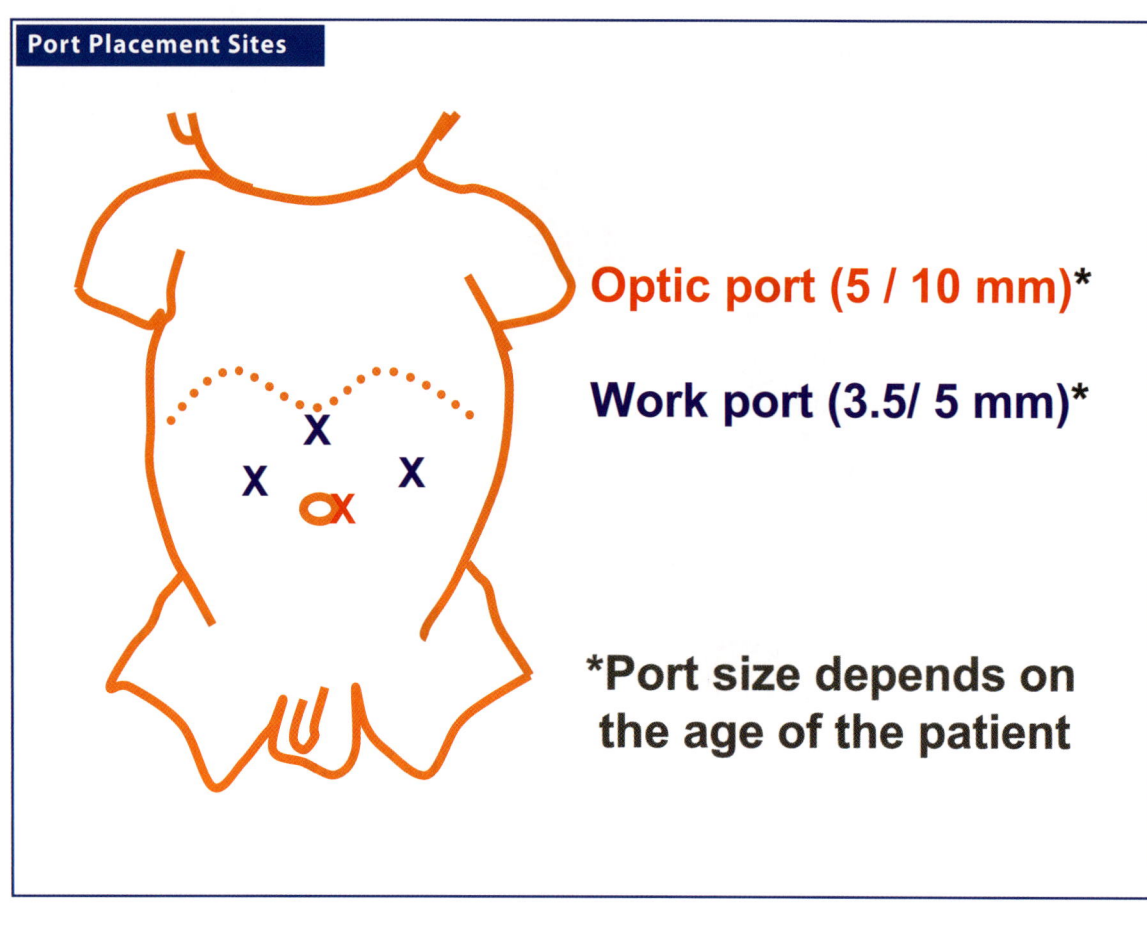

Port Placement Sites

Optic port (5 / 10 mm)*

Work port (3.5/ 5 mm)*

*Port size depends on the age of the patient

28.5   Indications

1. Severe gastroesophageal reflux.
2. Esophageal dysmotility.
3. Esophageal peptic stricture.
4. Heller procedure's complement.

28.6   Contraindications

Severe cachexia (delay surgery).

28.7   Preoperative Considerations

1. Discuss outcomes with parents regarding transient dysphagia, controls, and preserved ability to belch.
2. Upper gastrointestinal studies to evaluate gastric emptying.
3. Avoid nitrous oxide anesthesia to prevent bowel dilatation.
4. Intracorporeal knotting is recommended for suturing of the wrap.

28.8   Technical Notes

1. The posterior vagus nerve is a valuable landmark during hiatal dissection.
2. The esophagus is pulled down to expose a wide retrocardial window.
3. Two stitches should be used to tack the posterior wrap to the right pillar after the fundus has been widely drawn.
4. Use two rows of stitches along the sides of the esophagus after encircling the fundus on three-quarters of its girth.

28.9   Procedure Variations

1. A temporary frame-stitch can tack the both sides of the fundus encircling the esophagus.
2. The number of stitches on each row has to be increased in case of neurologically impaired patients.
3. In a redo procedure, care should be taken to separate the liver from the wrap. This can be challenging.
4. Intracorporeal knotting ensures a suitable tightness. A final picture is a useful routine.

28.10   Laparoscopic Toupet Fundoplication with Three-Port Technique

Please see Figs. 1–6.

Figure 28.1

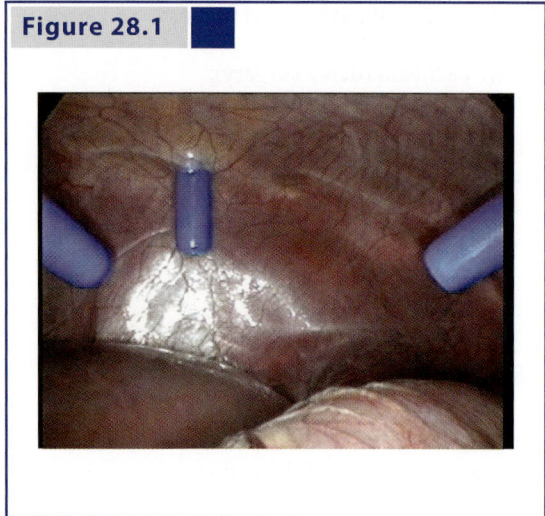

Three ports are placed in the upper abdomen

Figure 28.2

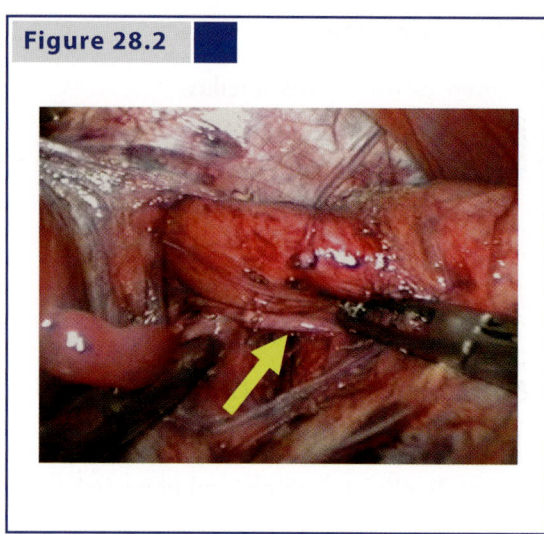

The posterior vagus nerve is identified as a landmark and a large retrocardial window is created

Figure 28.3

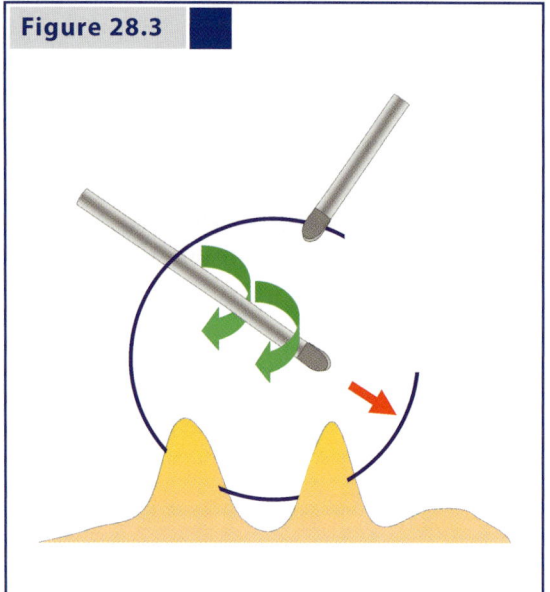

The intracorporeal knotting technique is favorable during this procedure

Figure 28.4

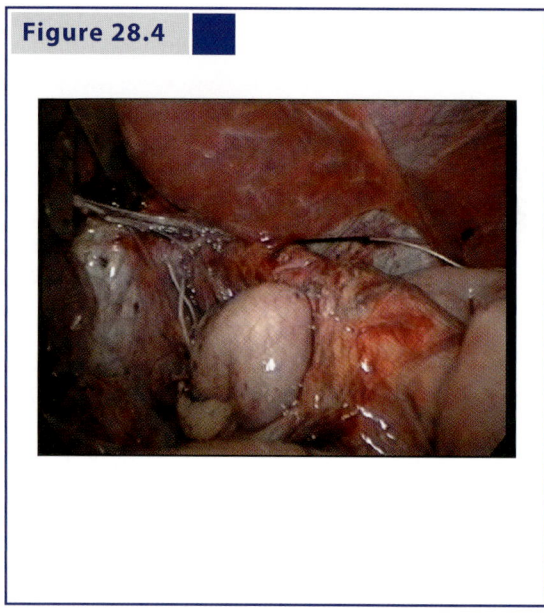

The fundus wrap has to be drawn bulging in front of the pillar and three sutures tack both together

Figure 28.5

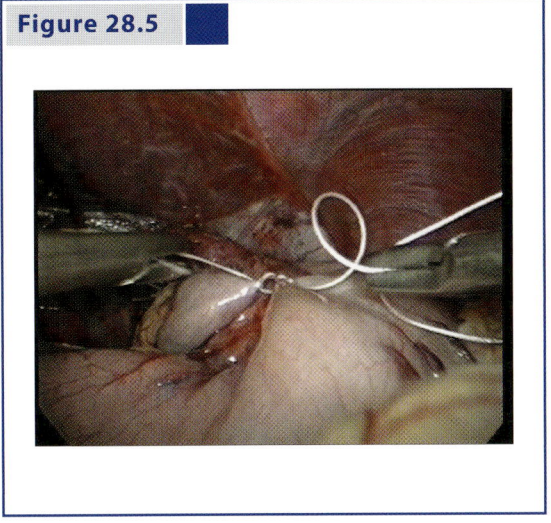

Placement of a frame-stitch facilitates the montage

Figure 28.6

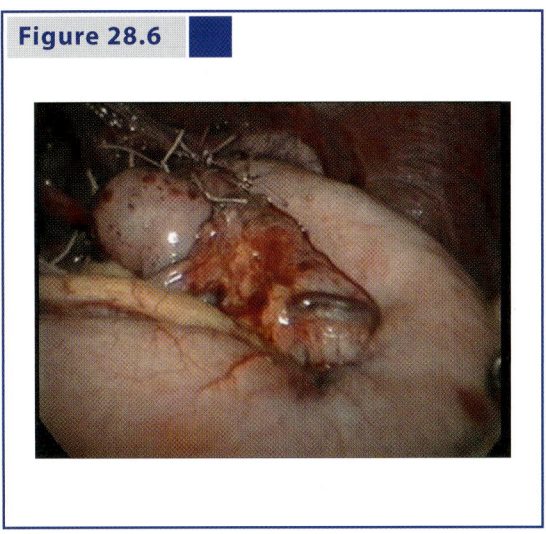

Final aspects to be checked are (a) no torsion and (b) no tightness in the wrap

28.11 Laparoscopic Toupet Fundoplication with Four-Port Technique

28.11.1 Port Placement Sites

Please see Figs. 7–14.

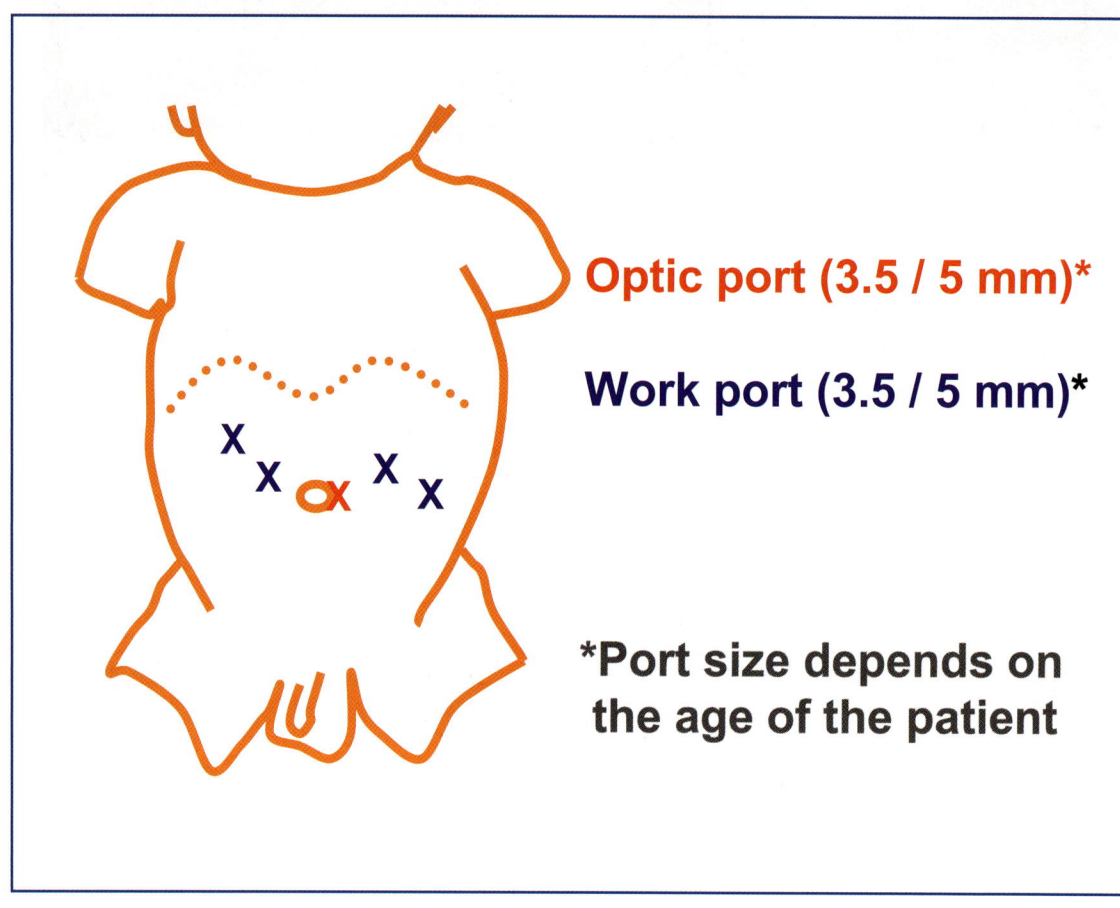

Optic port (3.5 / 5 mm)*

Work port (3.5 / 5 mm)*

*Port size depends on the age of the patient

Figure 28.7

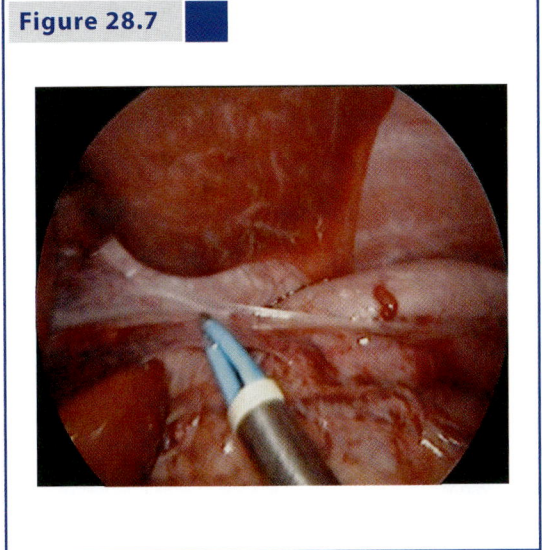

The hepatogastric ligaments are dissected to gain access to the diaphragmatic crura

Figure 28.8

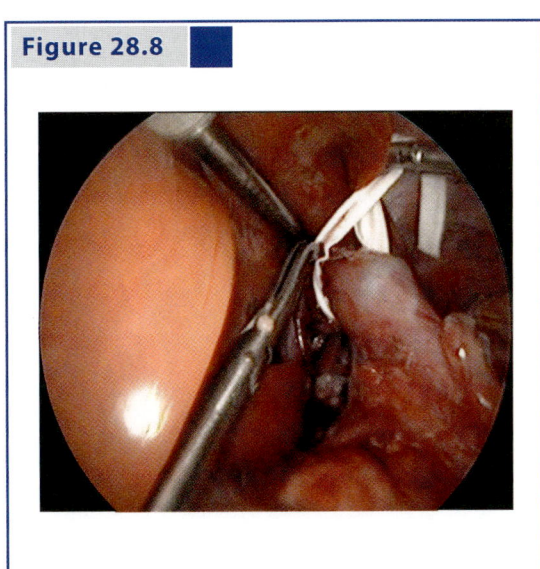

An umbilical tape is passed behind the esophagus with its ends held by a grasper in the fourth port (inserted into the left hypochondriac region just below the level of the rib cage)

Figure 28.9

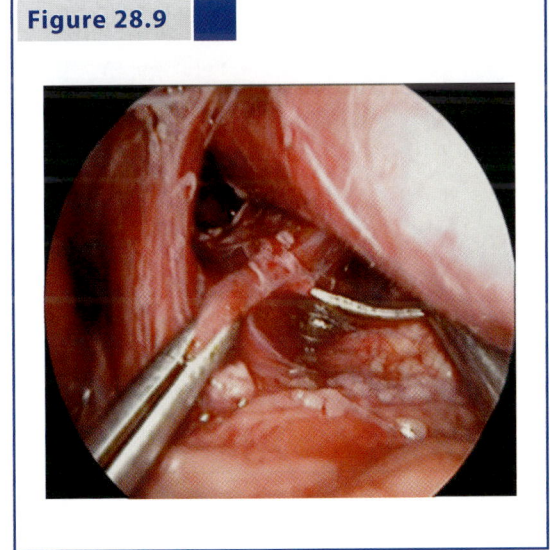

A nasogastric tube of desired size is now passed into the stomach

Figure 28.10

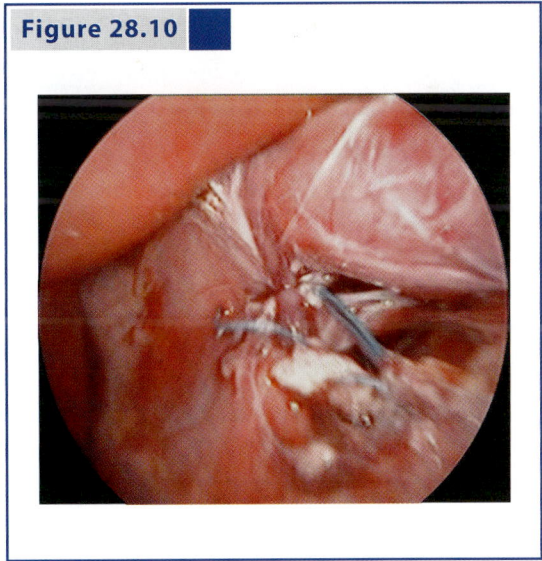

Approximation of the diaphragmatic crura is completed using nonabsorbable suture material

Figure 28.11

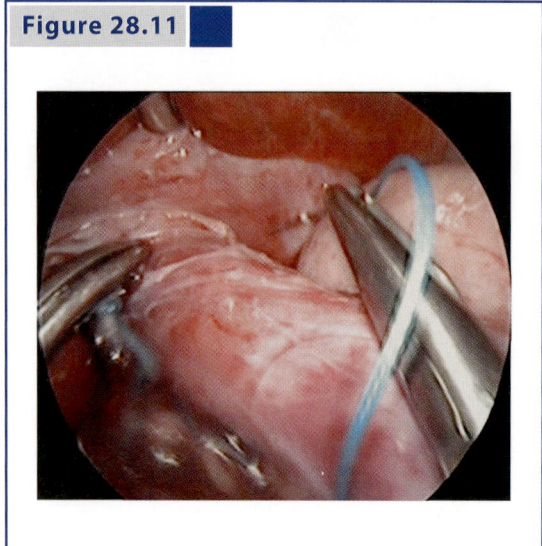

Sutures are placed on the left and right side of the esophagus to secure it to the diaphragm

Figure 28.12

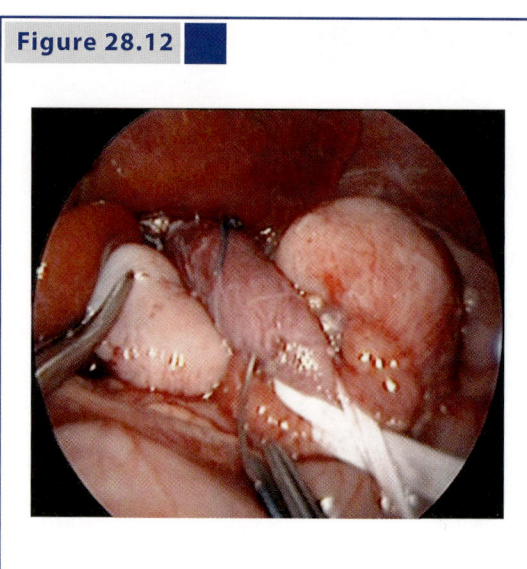

The fundus is then passed behind the esophagus and positioned for the wrap

Figure 28.13

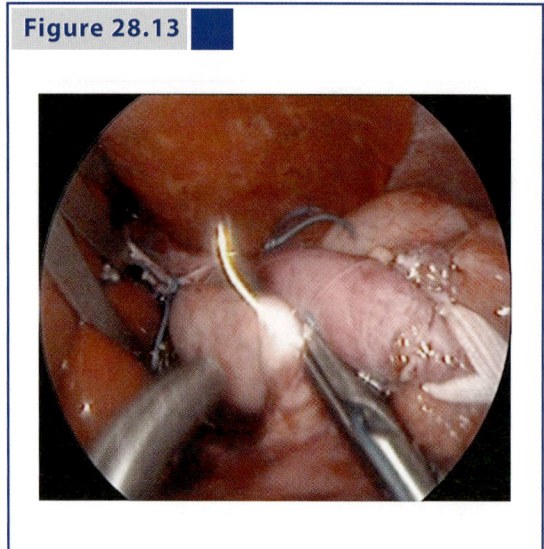

The left side is sutured initially with a line of three sutures, which are tied intracorporeally. The uppermost suture of the wrap is also secured to the diaphragm

Figure 28.14

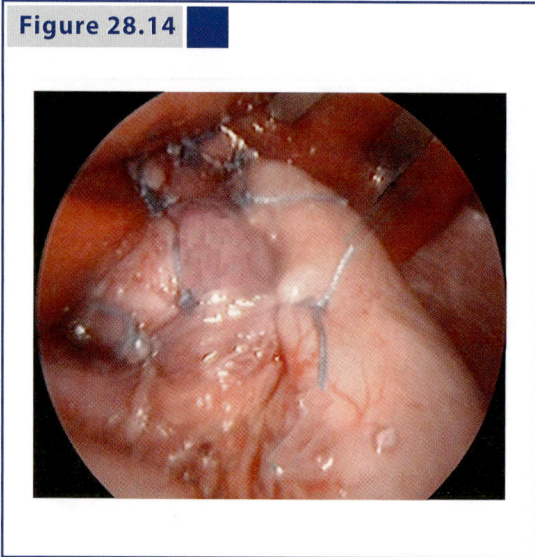

The 270° wrap is completed with left-side suturing, and is checked for torsion and tightness

Recommended Literature

1. Bensoussan AL, Yazbeck S, Carceller-Blanchard A (1994) Results and complications of Toupet's partial posterior wrap: 10 years experience. J Pediatr Surg 29:1215–1217
2. Esposito C, Montupet P, Amici G (2000) Complications of laparoscopic antireflux surgery in childhood. Surg Endosc 14:658–660
3. Montupet P (2002) Laparoscopic Toupet's fundoplication in children. Semin Laparosc Surg 9:163–167

29 Cardiomyotomy for Esophageal Achalasia

Luigi Bonavina

29.1 Operation Room Setup

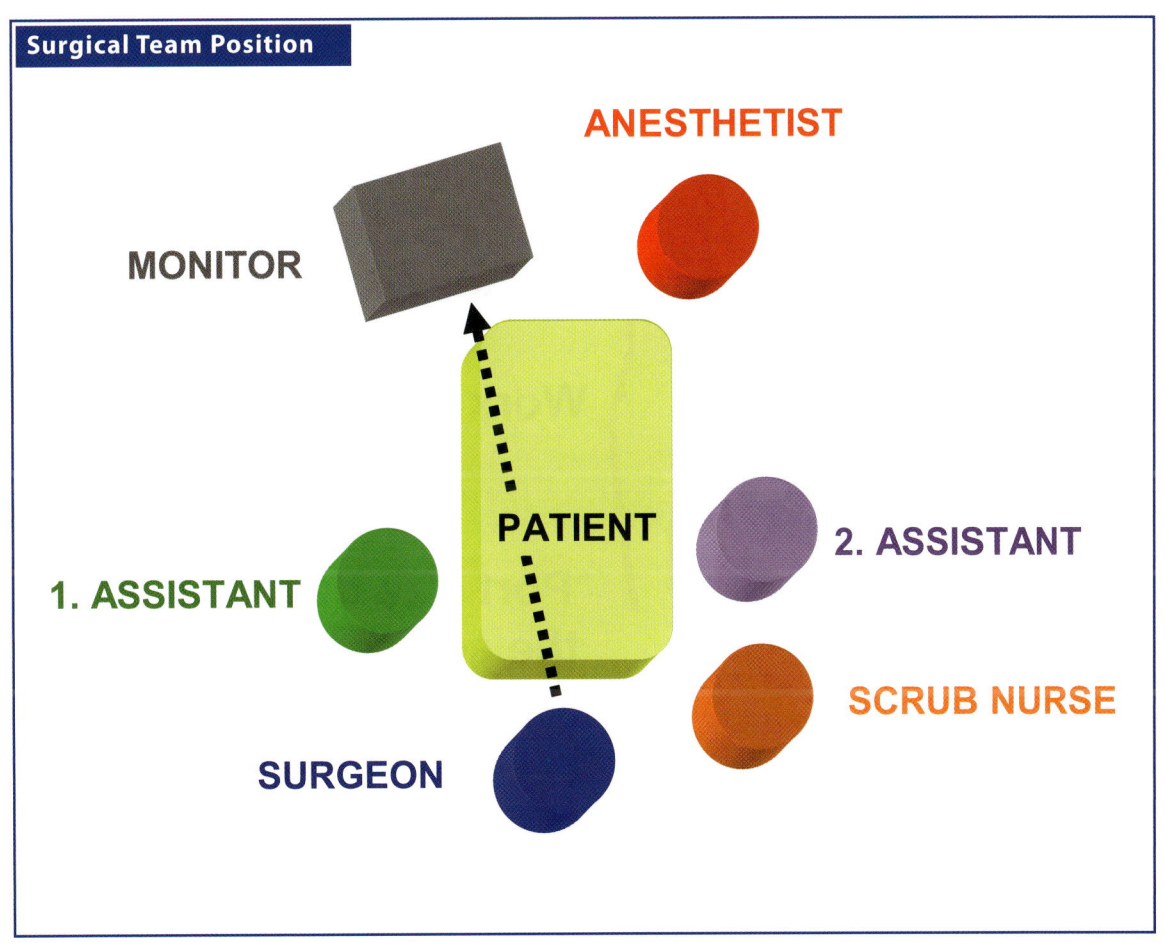

Surgical Team Position

ANESTHETIST

MONITOR

PATIENT

1. ASSISTANT

2. ASSISTANT

SCRUB NURSE

SURGEON

29.2   Patient Positioning

Patient is in 20–30° reverse Trendelenburg lithotomy position with arms tucked to the side.

29.3   Special Instruments

Ultracision® harmonic scalpel. (Johnson & Johnson Medical Products, Ethicon Endo-Surgery, Cincinnati, OH, USA)

29.4   Location of Access Points

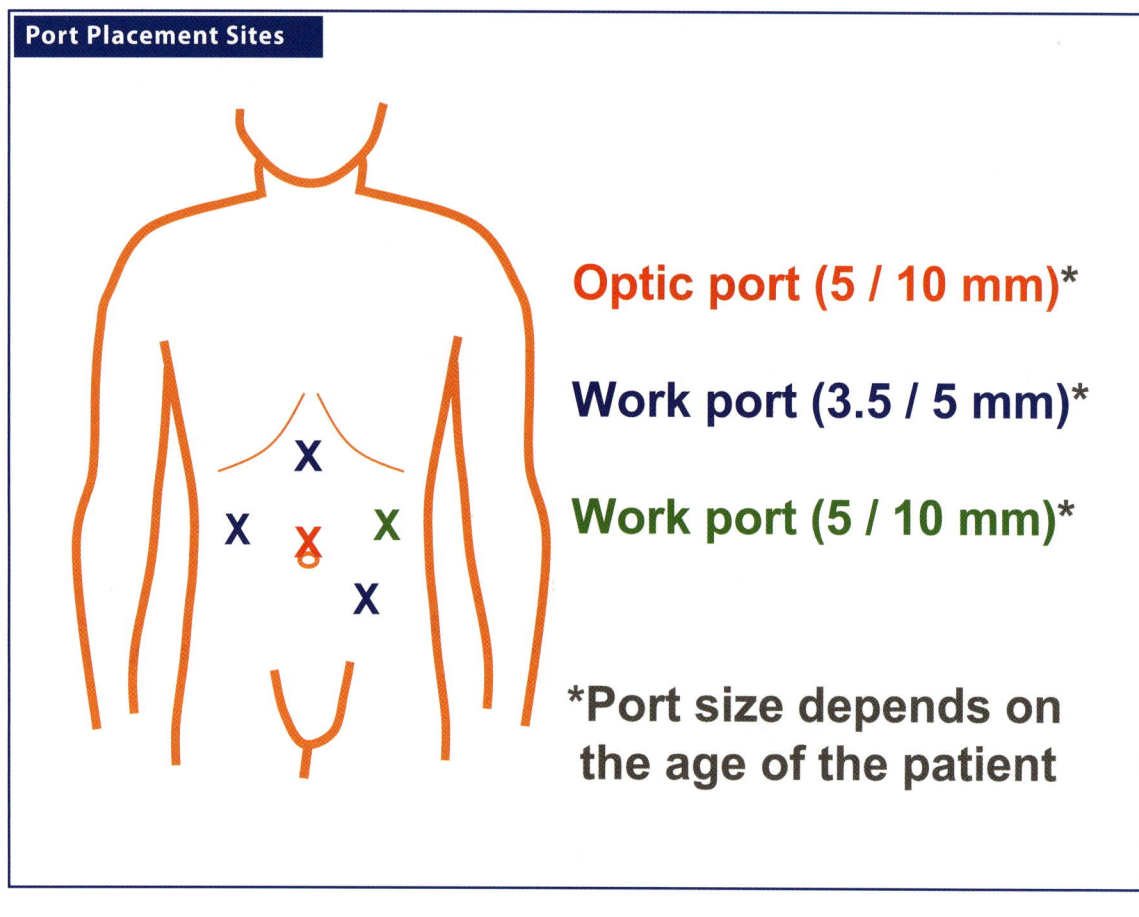

Port Placement Sites

Optic port (5 / 10 mm)*

Work port (3.5 / 5 mm)*

Work port (5 / 10 mm)*

*Port size depends on the age of the patient

29.5   Indications

During the past two decades, laparoscopic cardio-myotomy combined with an anterior (Dor) fundo-plication has emerged as the initial approach of choice in the treatment of esophageal achalasia. The operation is indicated to provide symptomatic relief of dysphagia and food regurgitation, and to prevent aspiration pneumonia and weight loss.

29.7   Preoperative Considerations

1. Insert a double-lumen nasogastric tube before surgery to wash and clean the esophageal lumen from food debris.
2. Give short-term antibiotic prophylaxis.

29.9   Procedure Variations

1. The esophagus should be encircled only in se-lected patients with sigmoid-type redundancy, associated hiatal hernia, or previous failed myo-tomy; in such circumstances the crura should be approximated posteriorly with interrupted stitches.
2. Intraoperative endoscopy may help to identify the cardia during the learning curve of this op-eration and during redo surgery. An endoscop-ically placed Rigiflex balloon dilator (Meditech-Boston Scientific, Natick, MA, USA) can be used to distend the cardia and facilitate the di-vision of residual muscle fibers. Air insufflation through the endoscope provides testing for oc-cult mucosal perforations.

29.6   Contraindications

Extensive adhesions after previous abdominal sur-gery (relative contraindication).

29.8   Technical Notes

1. Avoid extensive dissection of the esophagogas-tric junction to prevent postoperative gastro-esophageal reflux.
2. Bleeding from the muscle edges of the myotomy is self-limiting; excessive electrocoagulation must be avoided.
3. Pay attention to the geometry of the Dor fundo-plication to avoid undue tension and to provide a uniform patch over the esophageal mucosa; in most patients there is no need to divide the short gastric vessels.

29.10   Laparoscopic Cardiomyotomy for Esophageal Achalasia

Please see Figs. 1–6.

Figure 29.1

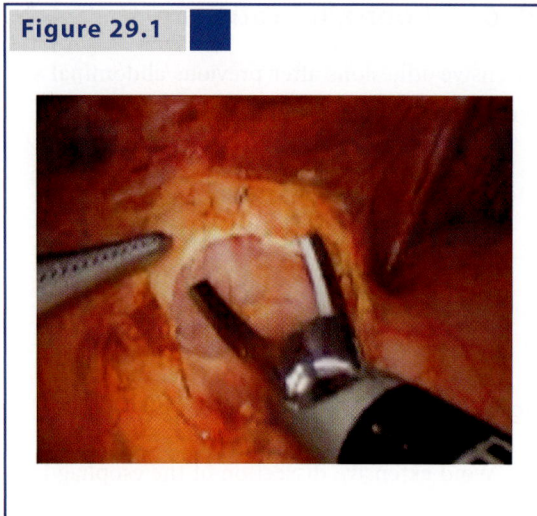

The anterior surface of the esophagus is exposed

Figure 29.2

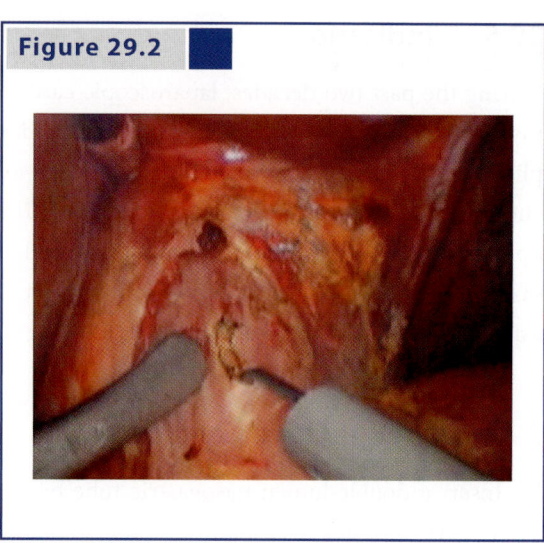

The Heller myotomy is started on the distal esophagus, on the left of the anterior vagus nerve, using an L-shaped electrocoagulating hook, until the submucosal plane is identified

Figure 29.3

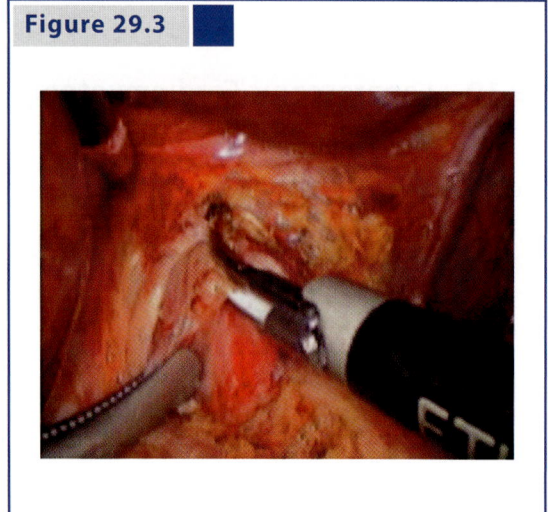

The myotomy is extended proximally for about 6 cm using the ultrasonic scissors with the active blade positioned upward

Figure 29.4

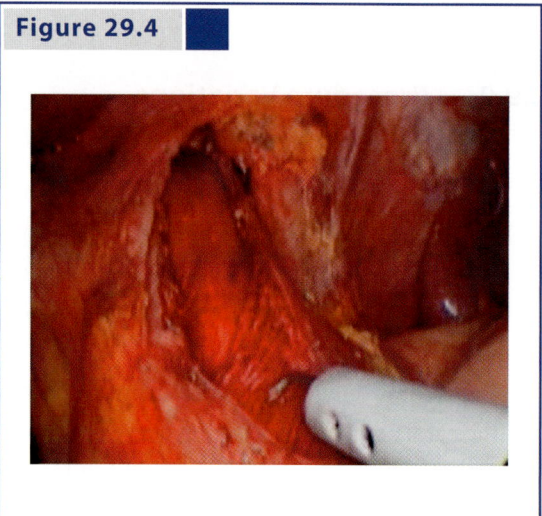

The myotomy is extended on the gastric side for about 2 cm to divide the oblique muscle fibers

Figure 29.5

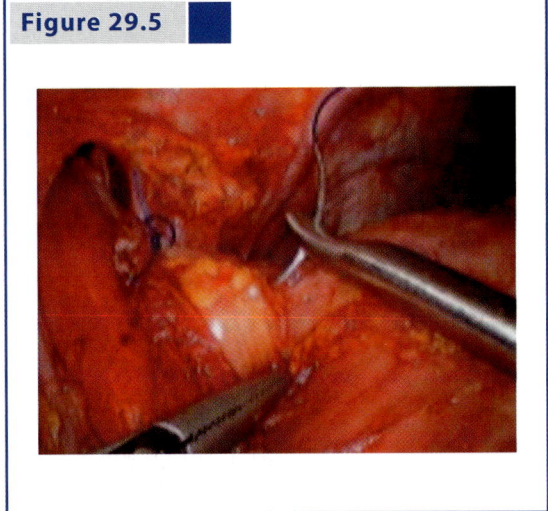

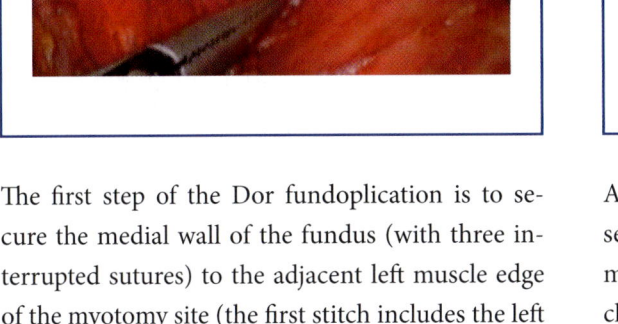

Figure 29.6

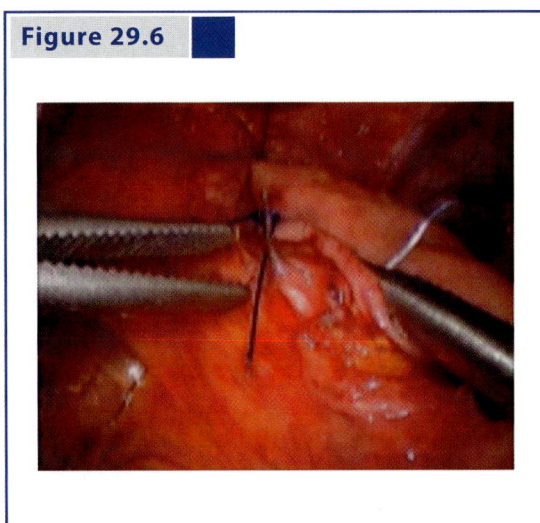

The first step of the Dor fundoplication is to secure the medial wall of the fundus (with three interrupted sutures) to the adjacent left muscle edge of the myotomy site (the first stitch includes the left diaphragmatic crus)

A more lateral portion of the anterior fundus wall is secured with three interrupted sutures to the right muscle edge of the myotomy site (the first stitch includes the right diaphragmatic crus)

Recommended Literature

1. Bonavina L (2006) Minimally invasive surgery for esophageal achalasia. World J Gastroenterol 12:5921–5925
2. Patti MG, Albanese CT, Holcomb GW III, Molena D, Fisichella PM, Perretta PM, Way LW (2001) Laparoscopic Heller myotomy and Dor fundoplication for esophageal achalasia in children. J Pediatr Surg 36:1248–1251
3. Rakita S, Villadolid D, Kalipersad C, Thometz D, Rosemurgy A (2007) Outcomes promote reoperative Heller myotomy for symptoms of achalasia. Surg Endosc 21:1709–1714

30 Gastric Banding

Amulya K. Saxena

30.1 Operation Room Setup

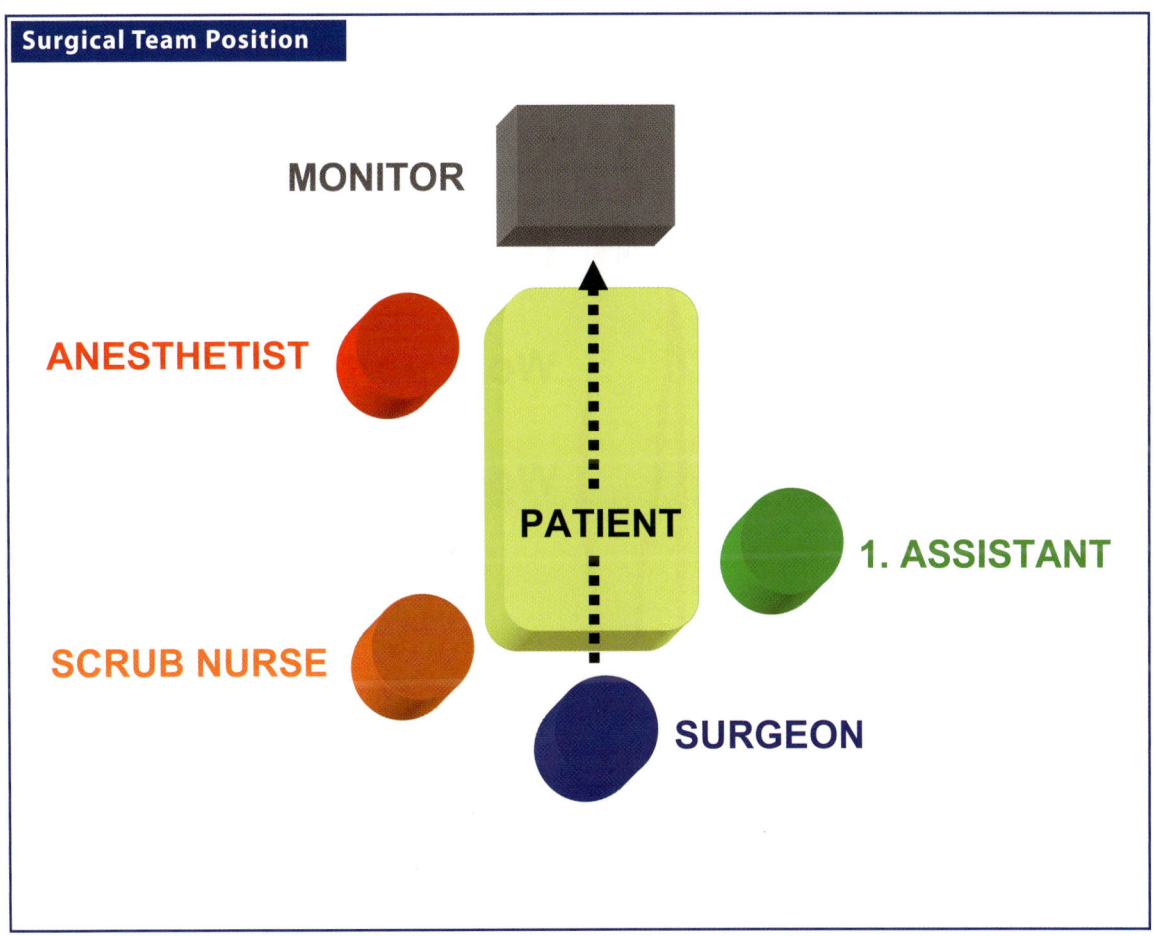

30.2   Patient Positioning

Modified lithotomy position. The surgeon stands between the spread legs of the patient.

30.3   Special Instruments

- Swedish adjustable gastric band (SAGB) (Obtech, Ethicon Endo-Surgery, Cincinnati, OH, USA)
- LigaSure™ (Valleylab, Boulder, CO, USA)
- Goldfinger® dissector (Johnson & Johnson Medical Products, Ethicon Endo-Surgery, Cincinnati, OH, USA)

30.4   Location of Access Points

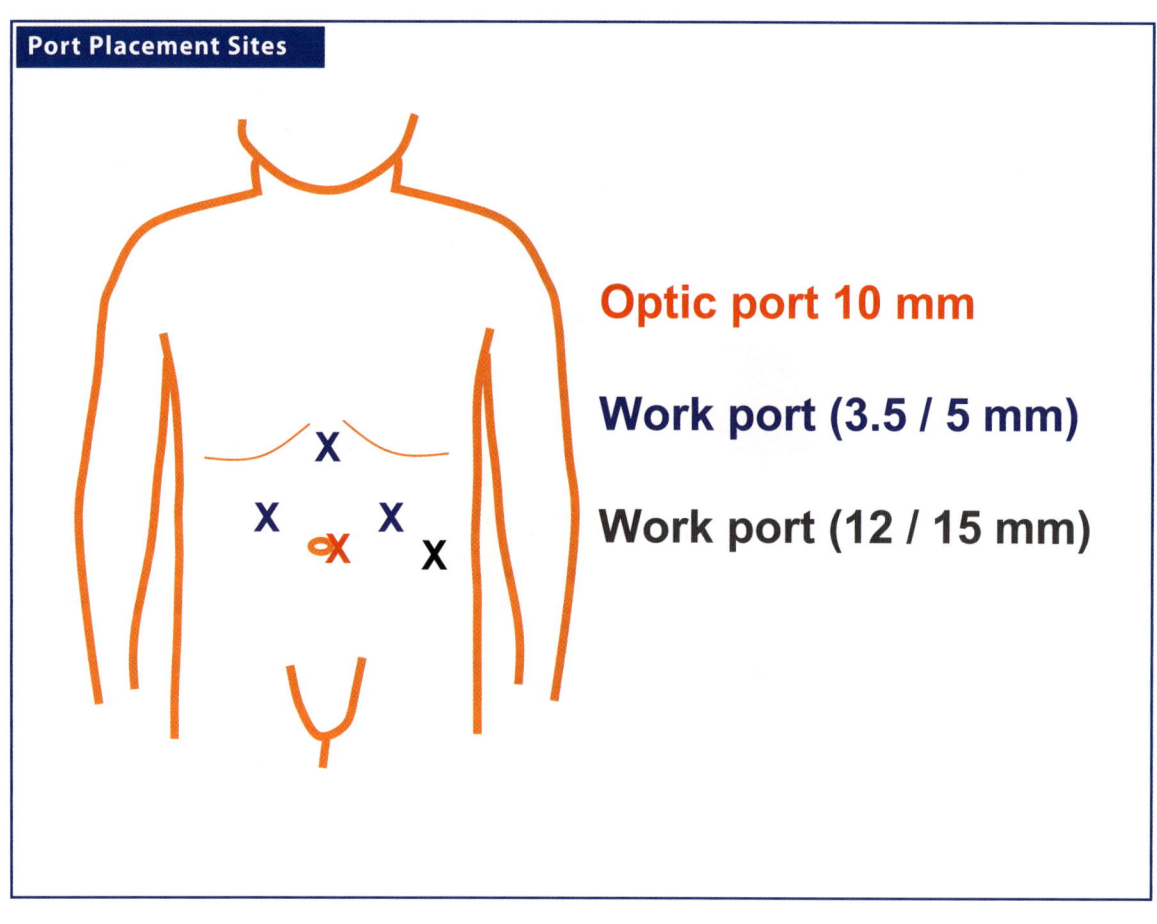

Port Placement Sites

Optic port 10 mm

Work port (3.5 / 5 mm)

Work port (12 / 15 mm)

30.5   Indications

1. Body mass index above 40.
2. Age between 12 and 55 years.
3. Failure of dietary or weight-loss drug therapy for more than 1 year.
4. Willingness to comply with the substantial life-long dietary restrictions required.
5. Acceptable operative risk.

30.6   Contraindications

1. Untreated glandular diseases.
2. Inflammatory gastrointestinal tract diseases.
3. Severe cardiopulmonary disease.
4. Dependency on alcohol or drugs.
5. Mental retardation or emotional instability.
6. Serious concerns about the compliance of the patient

30.7   Preoperative Considerations

1. The large body size and associated serious co-morbidities make patients who are morbidly obese high-risk surgical candidates.
2. Additional padded safety belts, gel or foam pads, and large elastic bandages are needed to prevent injury and movement of the extremities during surgery.
3. Gastric pH blockers are administered because of the increased incidence of gastroesophageal reflux disease and hiatal hernia in this patient population.

30.8   Technical Notes

1. Intra-abdominal access can be achieved by either an open technique using the Hasson cannula, or a closed technique using the Veress needle.
2. One 15-mm trocar also is placed for introduction of the laparoscopic adjustable gastric band into the peritoneal cavity.
3. The tubing is removed from the abdominal cavity through the subxiphoidal incision and connected to the reservoir placed and secured on the lowest part of the sternum.

30.9   Procedure Variations

1. Perigastric technique: dissection begins at the lesser curve behind the stomach and proceeds toward the angle of His.
2. Pars flaccida technique: dissection starts directly in the avascular space of the pars flaccida toward the right crus and finally the left crus muscles.
3. Two-step technique: this begins with the pars flaccida technique, followed by a second dissection near the stomach until the perigastric dissection intercepts the pars flaccida dissection.

30.10   Laparoscopic "Swedish Adjustable Gastric Band" Procedure

Please see Figs. 1–6.

Figure 30.1

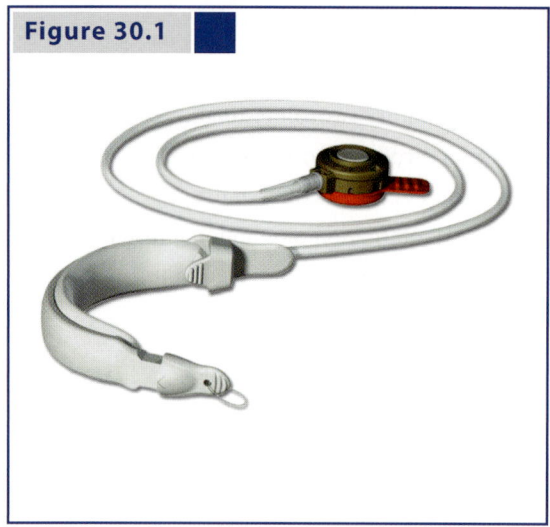

Swedish adjustable gastric band (SAGB) system (Courtesy of Johnson & Johnson Medical Products, Ethicon Endo-Surgery, Vienna, Austria)

Figure 30.2

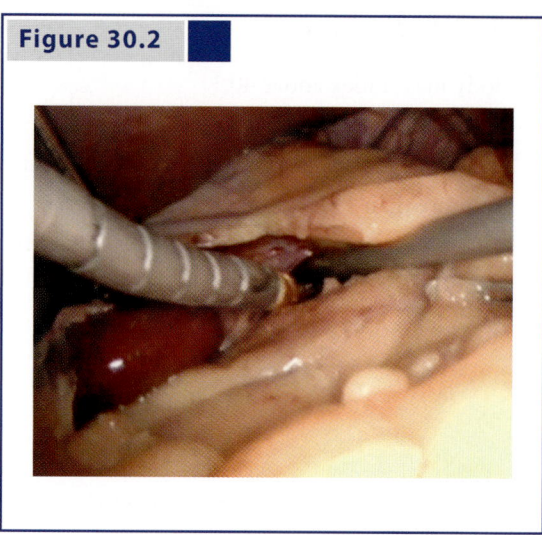

The lesser omentum is dissected with the LigaSure® device and a retrogastric tunnel is created with the Goldfinger® dissector

Figure 30.3

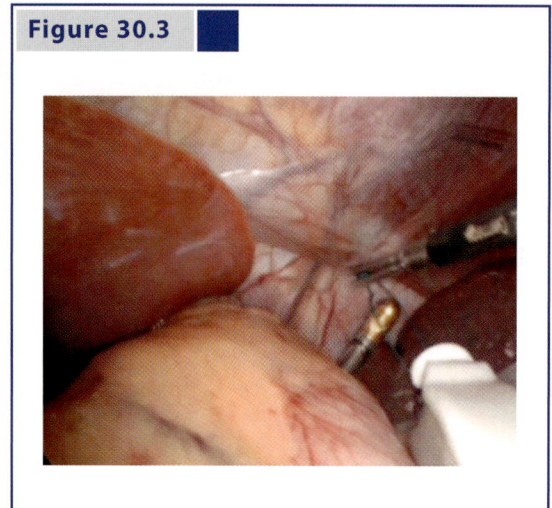

The SAGB system is introduced into the abdomen and its cord is secured to the tip of the Goldfinger® dissector to facilitate its placement

Figure 30.4

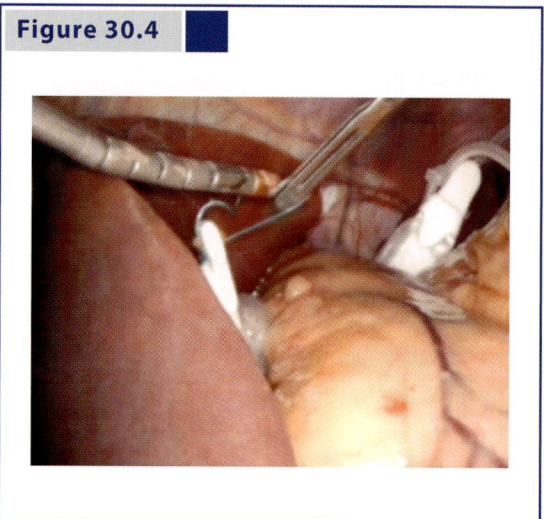

The band is positioned behind the stomach with the inflatable part directly in contact with the stomach wall

Figure 30.5

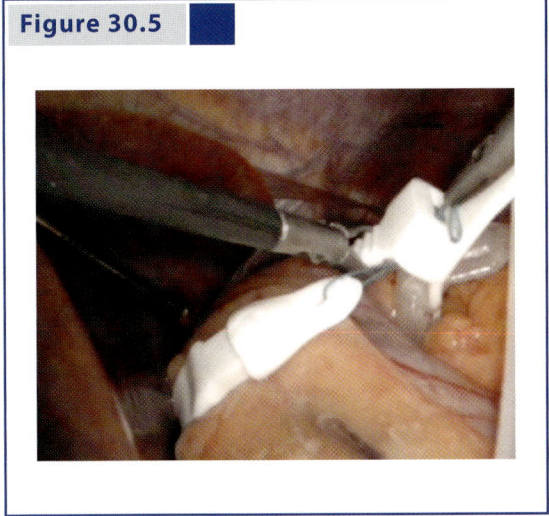

Figure 30.6

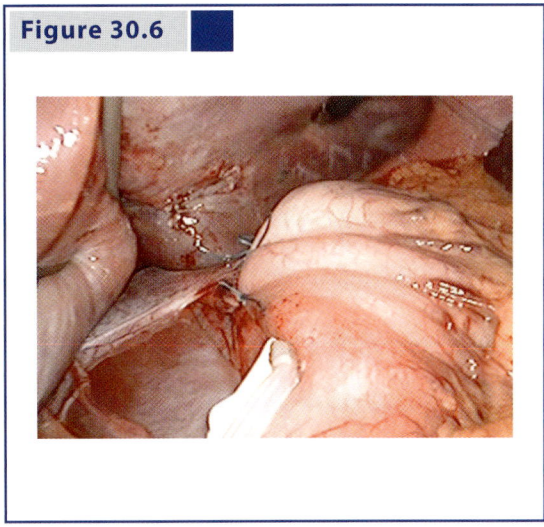

The band is locked into place at the chosen location on the stomach (almost at the level of the cardia), creating a 20-ml gastric pouch

The stomach is sutured over the band with nonabsorbable sutures. The tubing is brought out through the subxiphoidal incision where it is connected to the reservoir, which is placed on the distal sternum and secured to the fascia with sutures

Recommended Literature

1. Ponce J, Fromm R, Paynter S (2006) Outcomes after laparoscopic adjustable gastric band repositioning for slippage or pouch dilation. Surg Obes Relat Dis 2:627–31
2. Mizrahi S, Avinoah E (2007) Technical tips for laparoscopic gastric banding: years' experience in 2800 procedures by a single surgical team. Am J Surg 193:160–5
3. Yitzhak A, Mizrahi S, Avinoah E (2006) Laparoscopic gastric banding in adolescents. Obes Surg 16:1318–22

31 Pyloromyotomy

Celeste M. Hollands and Sani Yamout

31.1   Operation Room Setup

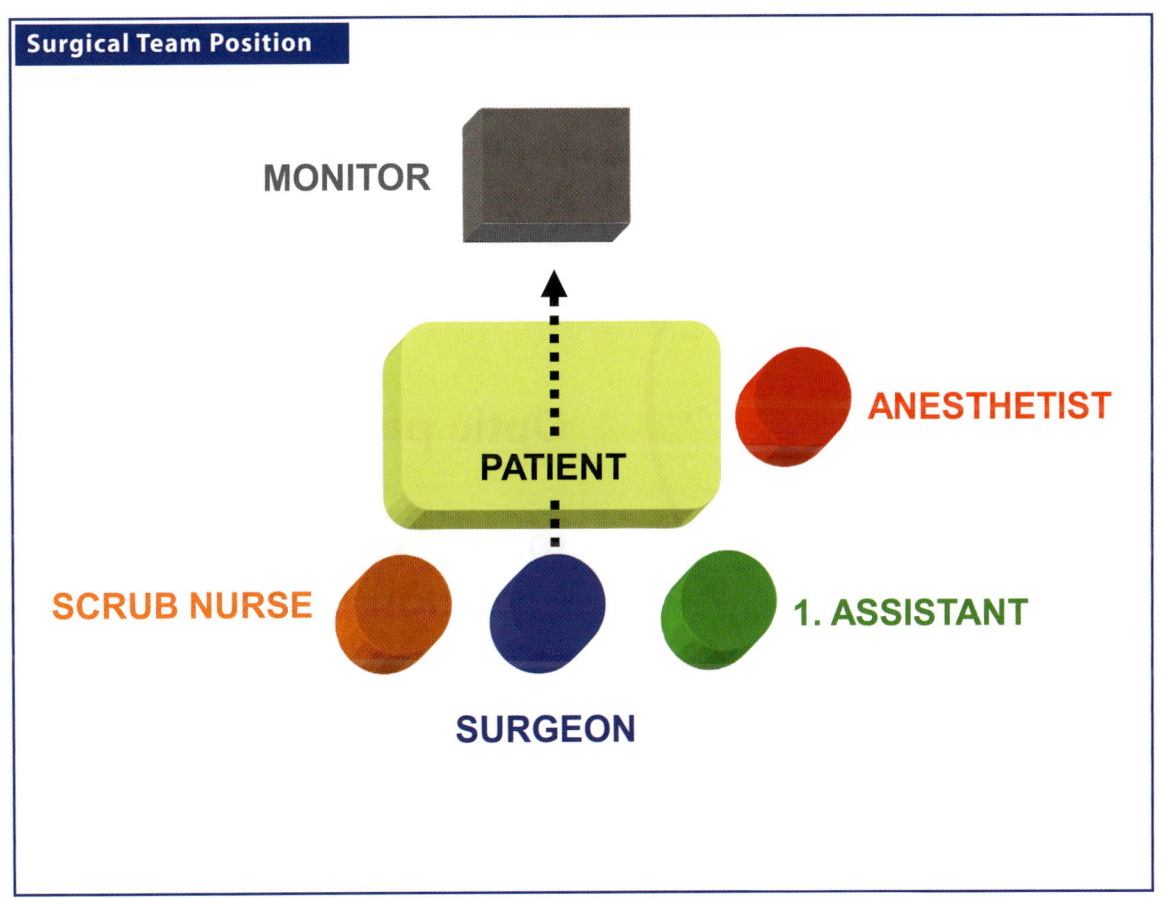

31.2   Patient Positioning

Infant placed horizontally across operating table in the supine position with arms by his/her side

31.3   Special Instruments

- Lefthand – 3-mm single action atraumatic bowel grasper
- Right hand – arthroscopy knife
- Tan pyloric spreader (Karl Storz, Tuttlingen, Germany)
- 5-mm Step trocar (VersaStep™; Auto Suture, Norwalk, CT, USA) as optic port
- 4-mm 30° scope

31.4   Location of Access Points

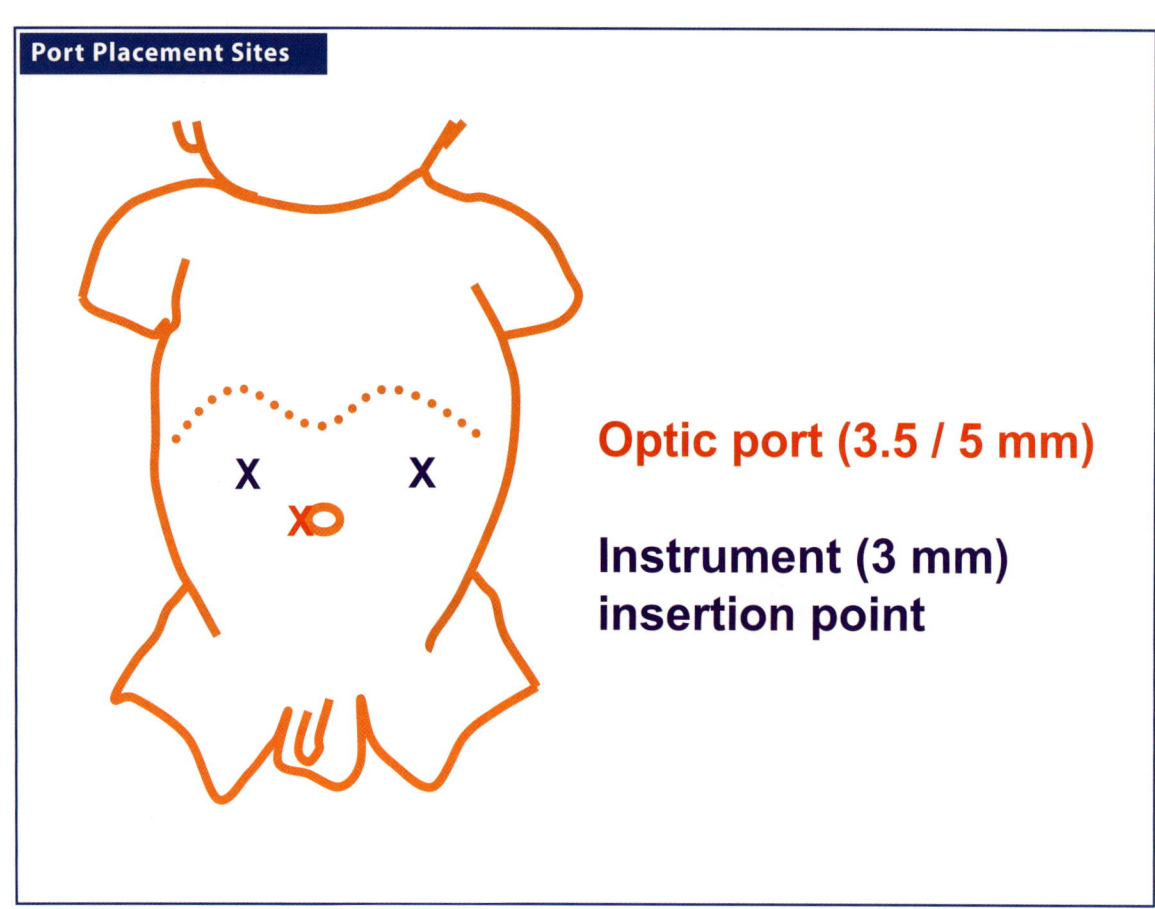

Port Placement Sites

Optic port (3.5 / 5 mm)

Instrument (3 mm) insertion point

31.5 Indications

Hypertrophic pyloric stenosis.

31.6 Contraindications

1. Failed prior pyloromyotomy.
2. Prior upper abdominal surgery with dense adhesions.

31.7 Preoperative Considerations

1. Appropriate fluid resuscitation and correction of electrolyte abnormalities.
2. Preoperative antibiotics in case of a nonhealed umbilical stump.
3. Preoperative resuscitation should be performed if there are signs of peritonitis.
4. Evacuate the gastric contents via the orogastric (OG) tube prior to induction of anesthesia. Leave the OG tube in place for the operation.

31.8 Technical Notes

1. Gently grasp the entire circumference of the duodenum with the bowel grasper to avoid injury.
2. Expose a flat portion of pylorus by lifting up and rotating it towards you.
3. Test for leakage at the myotomy: occlude the duodenum, inject the tube with 30 ml crystalloid and 30 ml of air. Depress the stomach.
4. Evacuate the gastric contents at the end of the procedure.
5. Close the fascia at all instrument sites.

31.9 Procedure Variations

Start the myotomy with arthroscopy knife then complete it with (1) a Tan pyloric spreader, (2) a single-action bowel grasper, or (3) a Maryland dissector.

31.10 Laparoscopic Pyloromyotomy

Please see Figs. 1–8.

Figure 31.1

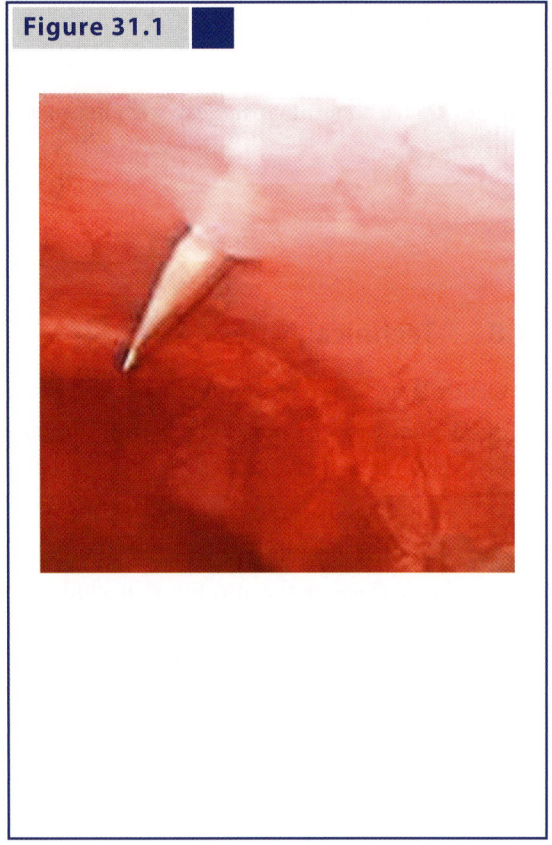

Figure 31.2

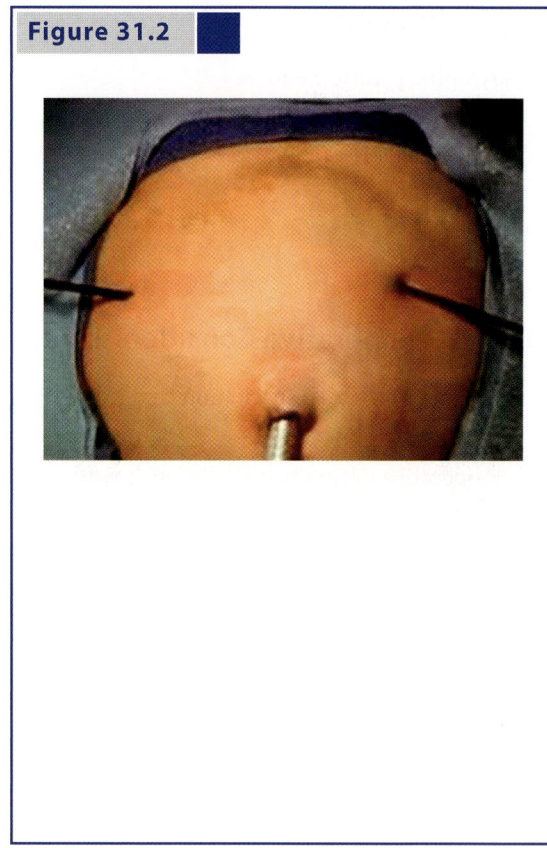

The right- and left-hand working instruments are inserted directly through the abdominal wall after making a stab incision with a no. 11 blade inserted just to the widest portion of the blade

Working instruments shown inserted directly through the abdominal wall in the right and left upper abdominal quadrants. The 5-mm Step trocar is inserted through the umbilicus

Figure 31.3

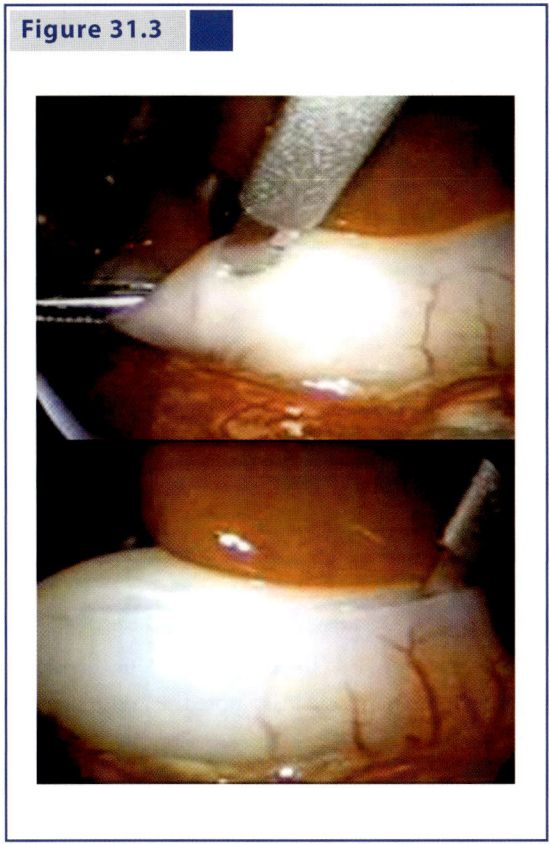

Figure 31.4

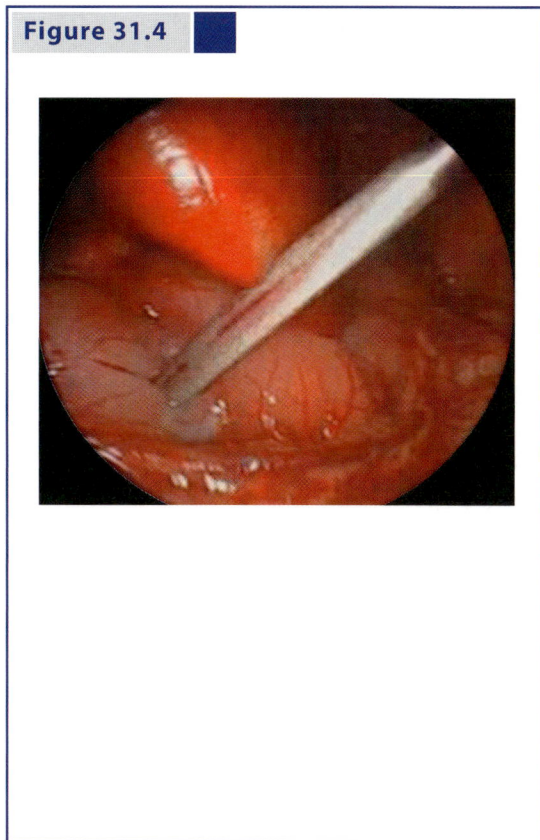

The arthroscopy knife is used to make a 1-mm-deep incision along the flat portion of pylorus starting on the gastric side of the vein of Mayo and extending onto the stomach

The knife blade is retracted into the sheath. The sheath is then introduced into the myotomy site and rotated to make enough space to insert the pyloric spreader

Figure 31.5

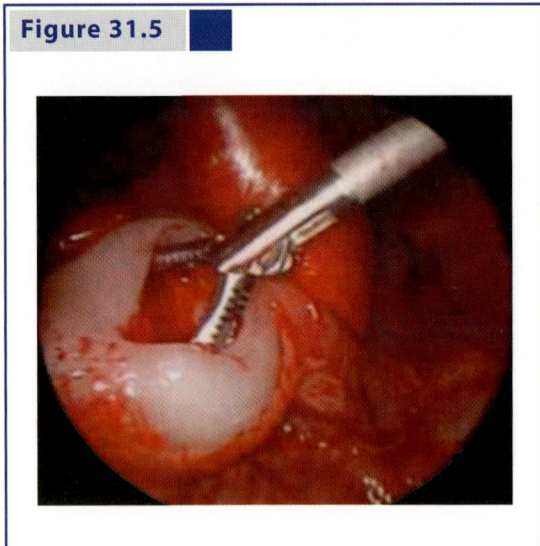

The pyloric spreader is inserted until it touches the mucosa (this will avoid bleeding complication) and opened with a slow and steady motion to spread the myotomy

Figure 31.6

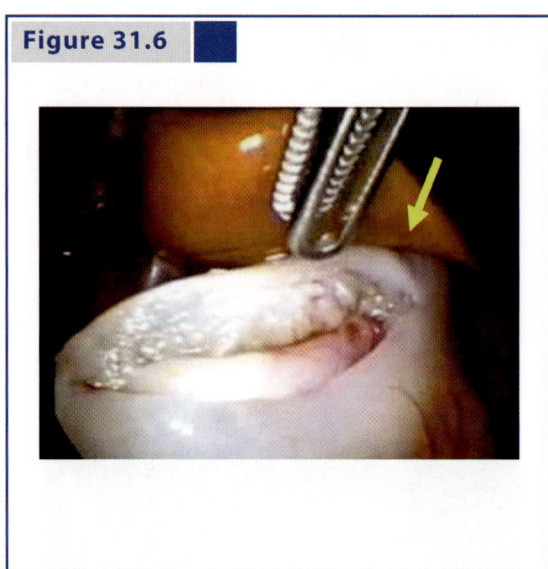

Note the circular muscle is visible on the gastric side of the myotomy, as is the transition from the thickened to normal muscle. Also note the asymmetry of a complete myotomy, which is most pronounced on the superior gastric border (***arrow***)

Figure 31.7

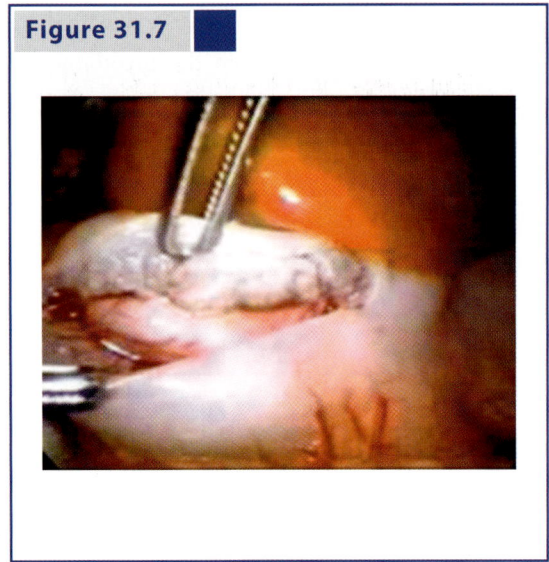

The "shoeshine" maneuver confirms that both sides of the myotomy move independently, confirming a complete myotomy Again, note the asymmetry on the gastric side

Figure 31.8

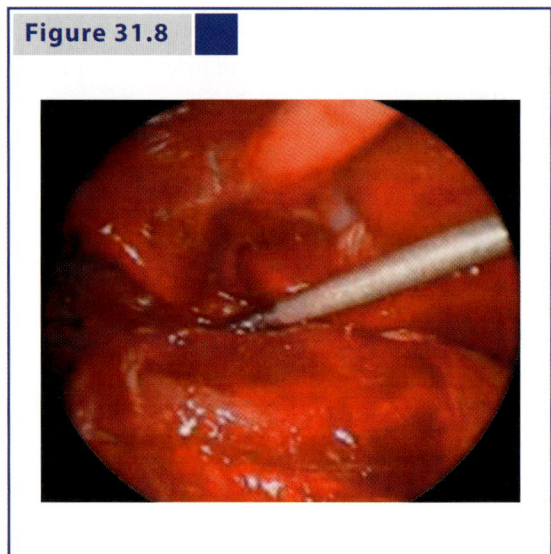

The omentum is placed over the myotomy after confirming there is no leak

Recommended Literature

1. Adibe OO, Nichol PF, Flake AW, Mattei P (2006) Comparison of outcomes after laparoscopic and open pyloromyotomy at a high-volume pediatric teaching hospital. J Pediatr Surg 41:1676–1678

2. Greason KL, Thompson WR, Downey EC, La Sasso B (1995) Laparoscopic pyloromyotomy for infantile hypertrophic pyloric stenosis: a report of 11 cases. J Pediatr Surg 30:1571–1574

3. St Peter SD, Holcomb GW III, Calkins CM, Murphy JP, Andrews WS, Sharp RJ, Snyder CL, Ostlie DJ (2006) Open versus laparoscopic pyloromyotomy for pyloric stenosis: a prospective, randomized trial. Ann Surg 244:363–3670

32 Laparoscopic-Assisted Jejunostomy

Ciro Esposito and Chiara Grimaldi

32.1 Operation Room Setup

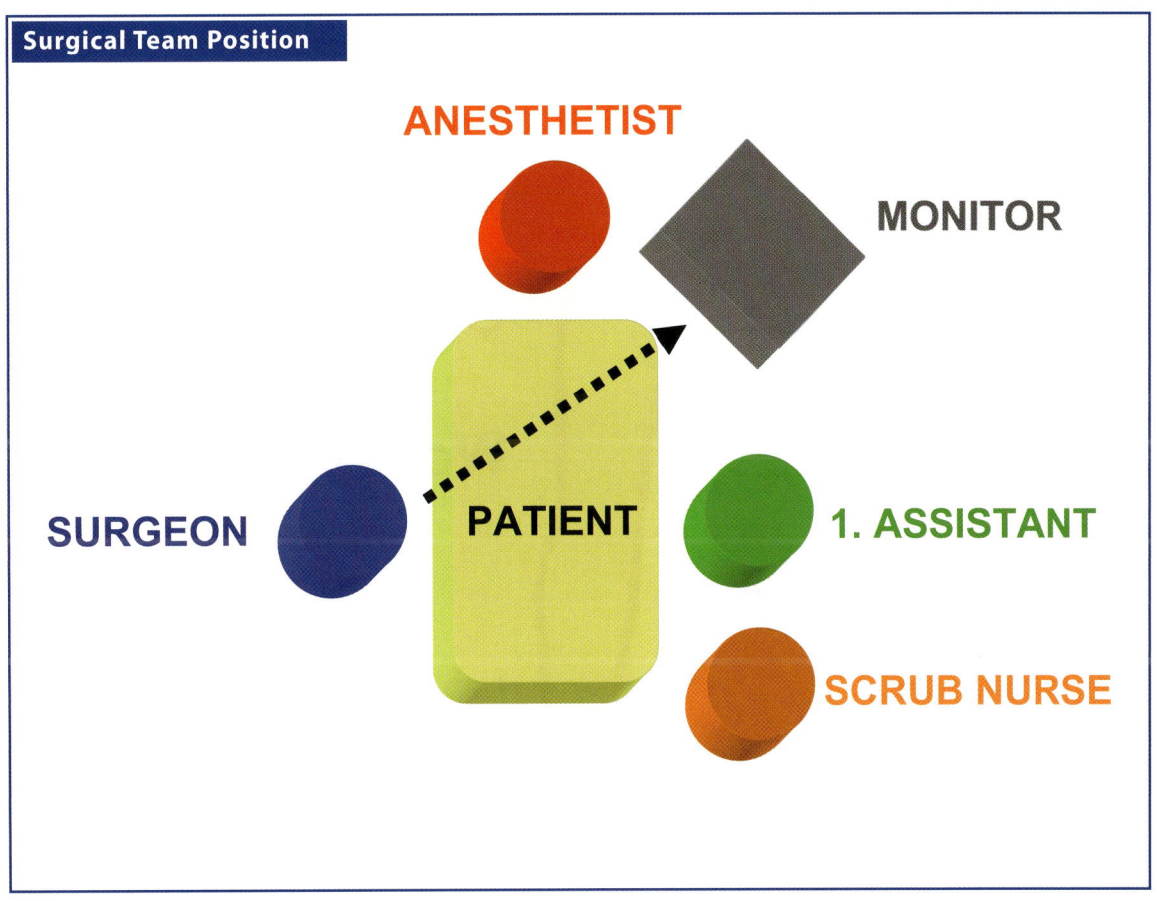

32.2   Patient Positioning

Supine position with the arms tucked to the side.

32.3   Special Instruments

Feeding tube for jejunal placement.

32.4   Location of Access Points

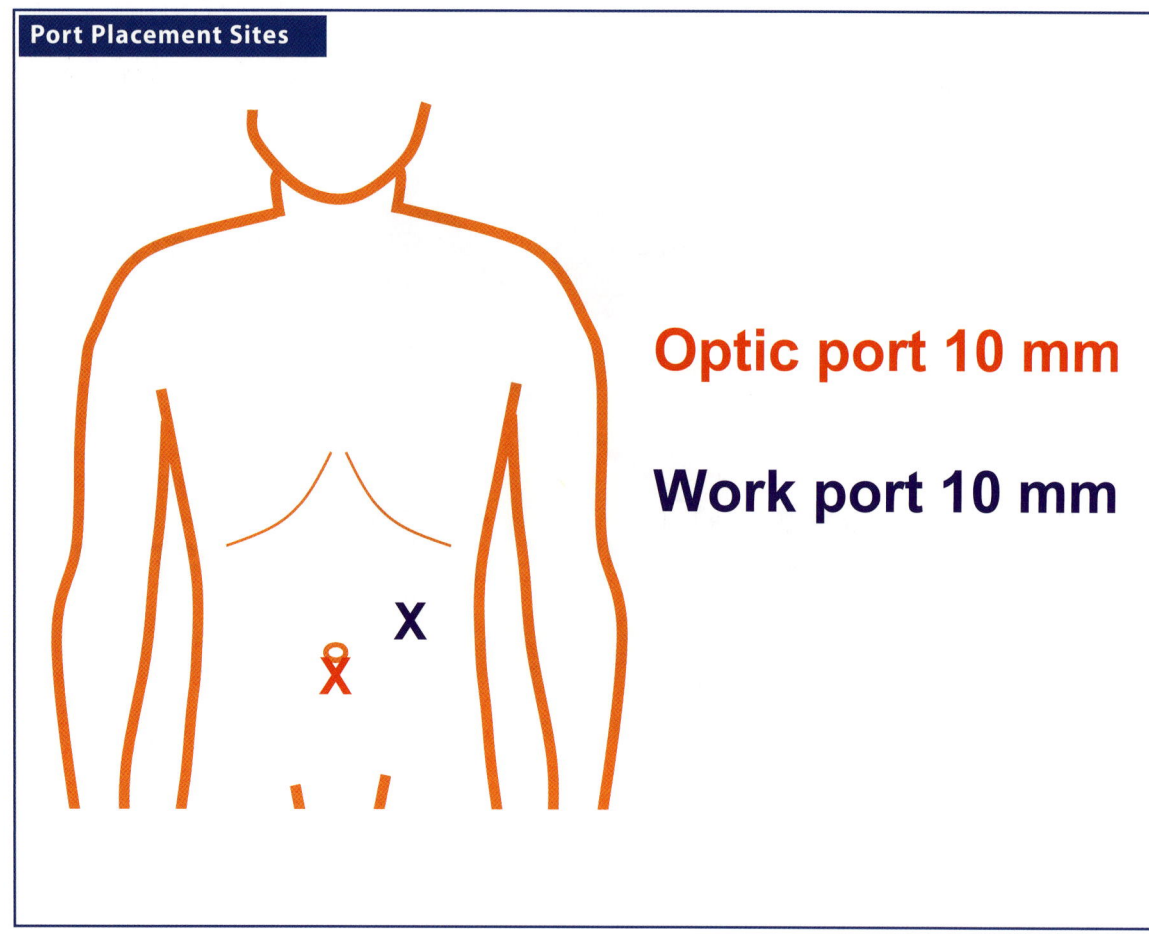

Port Placement Sites

Optic port 10 mm

Work port 10 mm

32.5 Indications

Laparoscopy-assisted jejunostomy (LAJ) is a technique used to assure a correct nutritional intake to neurologically impaired children with gastroesophageal reflux disease (GERD), who are affected by feeding problems associated to delayed gastric emptying. These children are at high risk for aspiration pneumonia when fed by gastrostomy; jejunal feeding significantly reduces this risk.

32.7 Technical Notes

1. LAJ is a two-port technique where two 10-mm ports are used. The first is positioned infraumbilically for the insertion of a 10-mm 0° optic; the other is positioned in the left abdominal quadrant at the site where the jejunostomy has to be created.
2. To facilitate the identification of the first jejunal loop, the great omentum and the transverse colon have to be moved up
3. The jejunal loop is grasped 20–30 mm down from the Treitz ligament with a fenestrated atraumatic forceps.
4. Under visual guidance, the antimesentric side of the loop is exteriorized through the port site.
5. The fixation of the intestinal loop to the abdominal wall is performed by six diamond-shaped stitches.
6. A purse-string suture on the jejunum is performed before inserting the jejunostomy feeding tube.
7. The status of the jejunostomy is verified outside and inside using the umbilical optics.

32.6 Preoperative Considerations

1. Preoperatively, GERD has to be confirmed by a 24-h-pHmetry and a barium swallow.
2. Ultrasonography or scintigraphy is then performed to evaluate gastric emptying.
3. The majority of children in which LAJ is performed are neurologically impaired with a spastic tetraparesis and a severe kyphoscoliosis; they are positioned on the operative table according to their particular anatomic condition.

32.8 Laparoscopic-Assisted Jejunostomy

Please see Figs. 1–6.

Figure 32.1

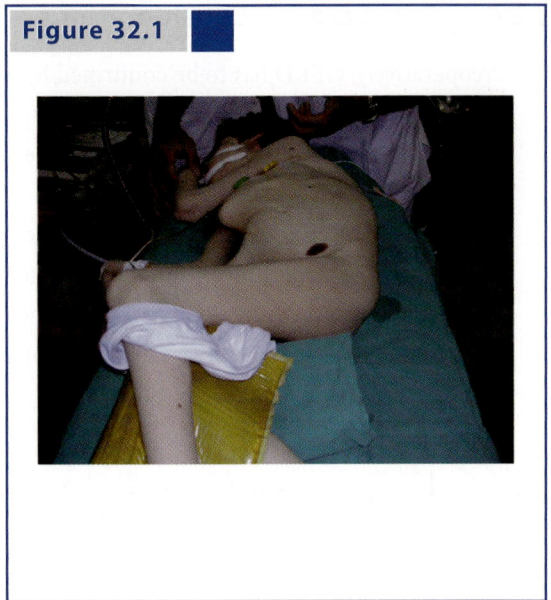

Due to their musculoskeletal deformities, the children are positioned on the table according to their anatomic condition

Figure 32.2

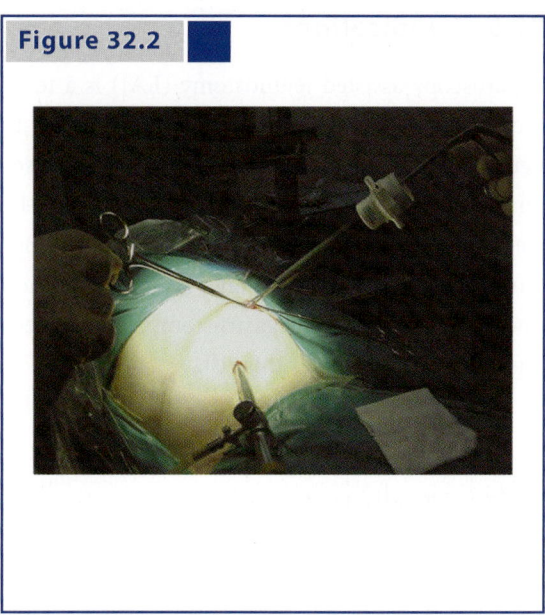

The jejunal loop is exteriorized through the port site located in left quadrant together with the port

Figure 32.3

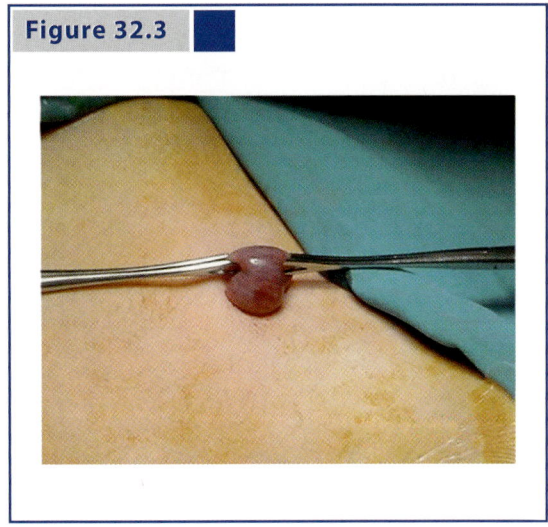

Before fixing it to the aponeurosis, the jejunal loop is grasped with two atraumatic grasping forceps to avoid its retraction into the abdominal cavity

Figure 32.4

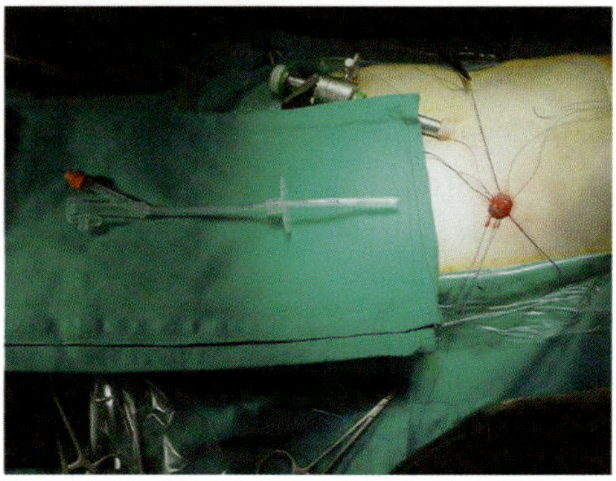

The operative field shows the umbilical port, the jejunostomy site with the "diamond-shape" stitches, and the feeding tube before its placement

Figure 32.5

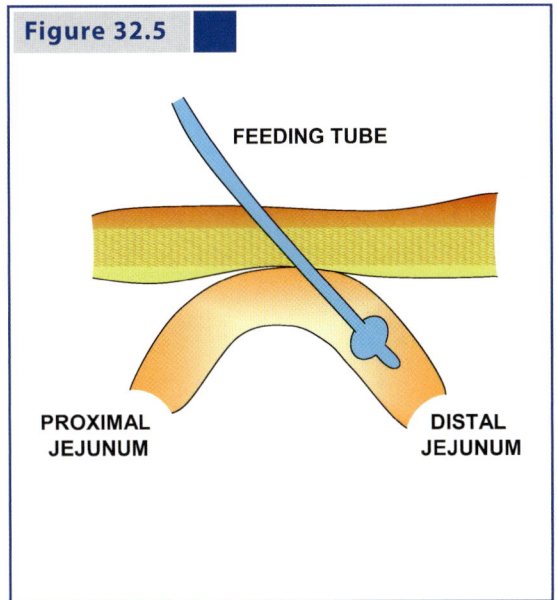

FEEDING TUBE

PROXIMAL JEJUNUM

DISTAL JEJUNUM

Figure 32.6

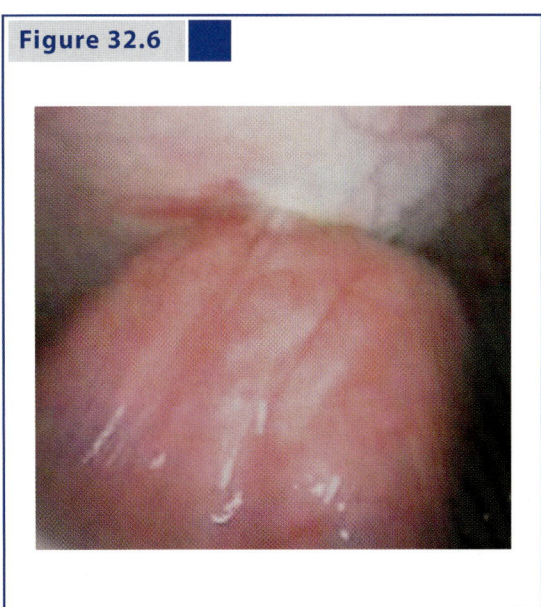

At the end of procedure the "balloon" of the feeding tube is positioned in the distal part of the jejunum

The exact position of the loop after insertion of the feeding tube is monitored before closure

Recommended Literature

1. Esposito C, Settimi A, Centonze A, Capano G, Ascione G (2005) Laparoscopic-assisted jejunostomy. An effective procedure for the treatment of neurologically impaired children with feeding problems and gastroesophageal reflux. Surg Endosc 19:501–504

2. Murayama KM, Johnson T, Thompson J (1996) Laparoscopic gastrostomy and jejunostomy are safe and effective for obtaining enteral access. Am J Surg 172: 591–594

3. Wales PW, Diamond IR, Dutta S, Muraca S, Chait P, Connolly B, Langer JC (2002) Fundoplication and gastrostomy versus image-guided gastrojejunal tube for enteral feeding in neurologically impaired children with gastroesophageal reflux. J Pediatr Surg 37:407–412

33 Resection of Meckel's Diverticulum

Felix Schier

33.1 Operation Room Setup

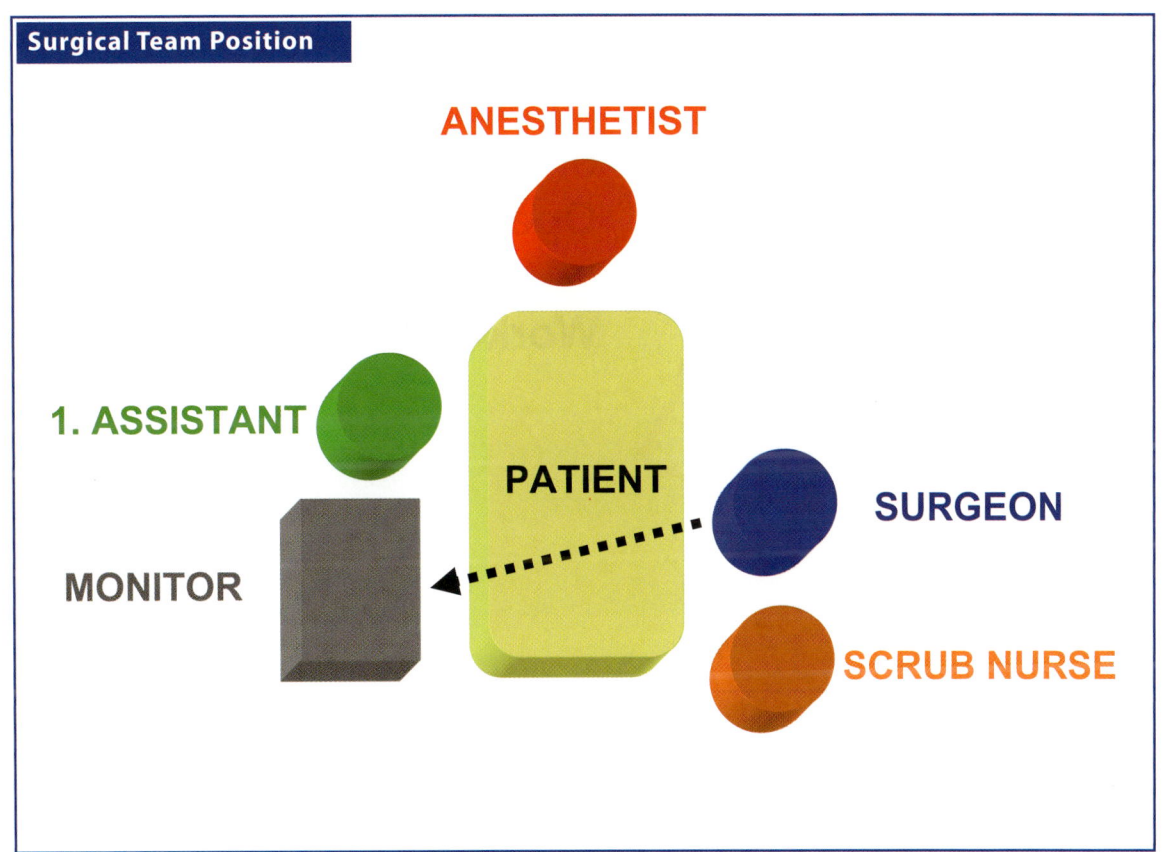

33.2　Patient Positioning

Supine position with the arms tucked to the side.

33.3　Special Instruments

- Endoscopic stapler
- Endoscopic loop suture
- Operating scope

33.4　Location of Access Points

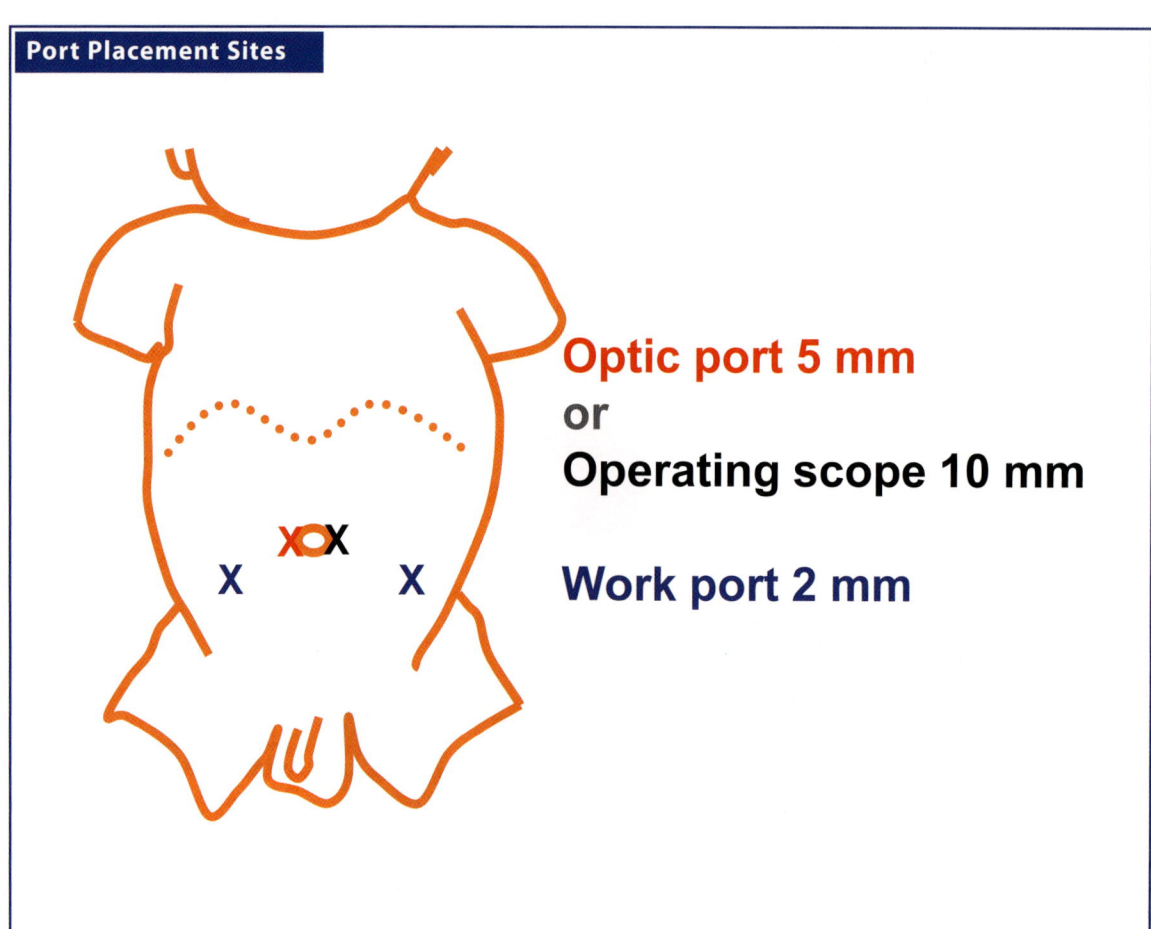

Port Placement Sites

Optic port 5 mm
or
Operating scope 10 mm

Work port 2 mm

33.5　Indications

Proven or suspected Meckel's diverticula (MD). Indications are identical to the traditional indications for "Meckel scans" (which became obsolete with the advent of laparoscopy, since they cause considerable radiation, detect only a fraction of MDs, and require a subsequent operation anyway in case an MD is identified).

33.6　Contraindications

General contraindications to laparoscopy.

33.7   Preoperative Considerations

1. The most efficient approach to MD is "laparoscopy-assisted" (i.e., the MD is identified or confirmed by laparoscopy and thereafter exteriorized via the umbilicus for resection outside the abdomen).

2. Pure laparoscopic resections of MDs are unnecessarily complicated when executed by intra-abdominal suturing and are expensive when performed with endoscopic staplers, which in turn require 12-mm trocars, resulting in a total length of incision similar to the conventional "open" approach.

33.8   Technical Notes

Two laparoscopy-assisted techniques are favorable for MD resection:

1. The 5-mm optic port technique: this requires two additional work ports placed in the middle or lower abdomen.

2. The 10-mm operating scope technique: this requires a 10-mm port at the umbilicus (for a double-barreled laparoscope with coaxial 5-mm working channel) and one or two additional 2-mm ports at the middle or lower abdomen.

33.9   Procedure Variations

1. Stapler excision: beside the umbilical optic port, a 12-mm port for the endoscopic stapler and two work ports for additional instruments are required in order to hold the small bowel in position while transecting the MD. The expense of endoscopic staplers, added size of the incision, and metal staples left behind are disadvantages of this technique.

2. Endoscopic loop suture removal: this requires an optic port and two additional work ports. Endoscopic loop sutures leave behind a slightly exposed mucosa, as in appendectomy. This can be used for small-based MDs.

33.10   Laparoscopic-Assisted Resection Using a 10-mm Operating Scope

1. A 10-mm port is inserted at the umbilicus. An optic with a coaxial working channel (both of 5 mm diameter) is introduced into the abdomen through this port. These instruments are used for thoracoscopic sympathectomies.

2. Occasionally, an additional 2-mm trocar is required for manipulation of the MD.

3. A 5-mm forceps is inserted via the working channel and the tip of the MD is pulled back into the trocar until it becomes visible from the outside.

4. Again, translucent ports are best suited for this procedure.

5. The MD is fully exteriorized and resected outside as in open surgery

Please see Figs. 1–3.

Figure 33.1

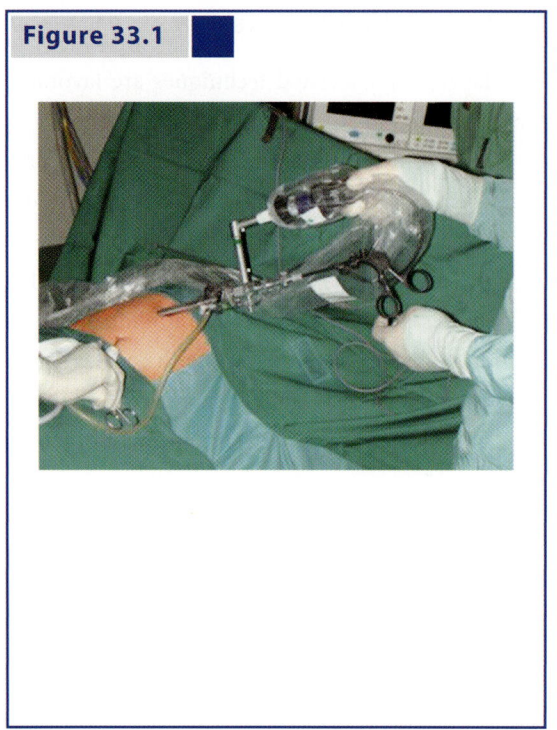

A coaxial operating scope is used; occasionally, an additional 2-mm port can be used at the left lower abdominal wall to manipulate the intestines

Figure 33.2

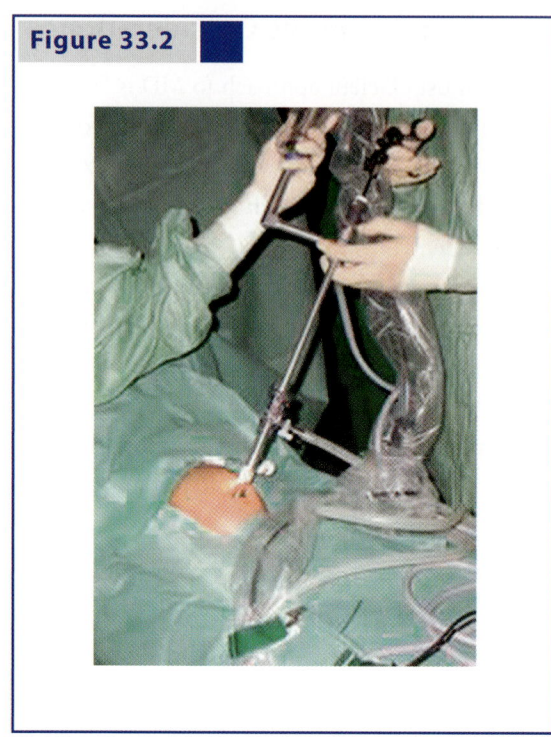

A 5-mm forceps is passed through the working channel and the MD is grasped back into the translucent port shaft until it is visualized and grabbed from outside

Figure 33.3

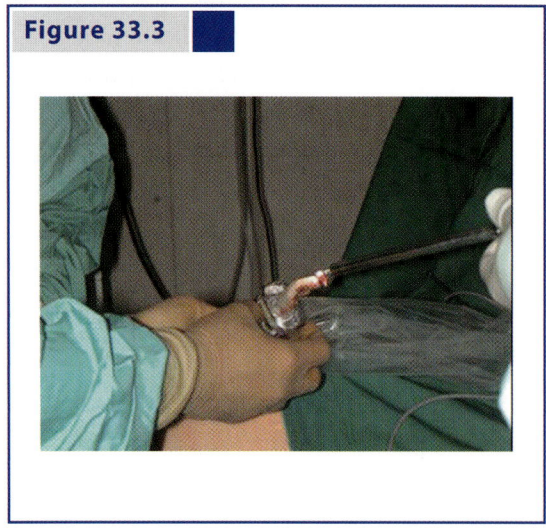

The shaft is removed and the MD is resected as in the "open" technique

33.11 Laparoscopic-Assisted Resection Using a 5-mm Optic Port

1. A 5-mm port and scope are inserted at the umbilicus.

2. A suture is attached to the tip of the MD.

3. The suture is retracted into the 5-mm umbilical port (this technique works best with translucent ports).

4. The port is withdrawn, the suture grabbed from outside, and the MD pulled outside the abdominal cavity for open resection.

5. In certain cases a single port might be sufficient.

6. At the end of the resection, the bowel might be congested and it may become unexpectedly difficult to reduce it into the abdominal cavity – almost like an incarceration. It therefore is advisable not to pull out too much bowel and, if in doubt, the incision should be enlarged in time.

7. In some cases, a 5-mm forceps can be inserted via the working channel and the tip of the MD pulled back into the port until it is becomes visible from outside.

Please see Figs. 4–6.

Figure 33.4

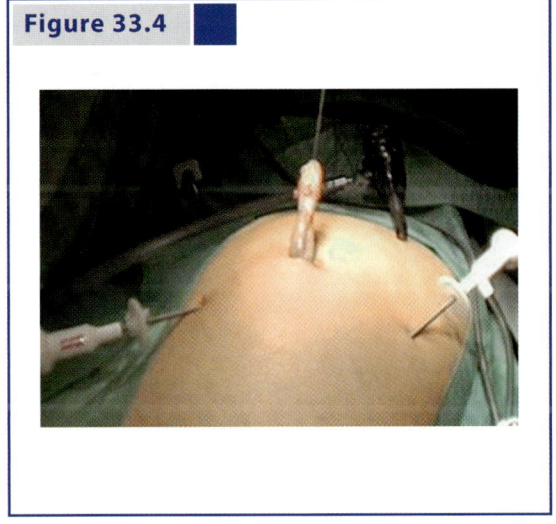

A suture is placed at the tip of the MD via the two 2-mm ports, after which the 5-mm port at the umbilicus is removed

Figure 33.5

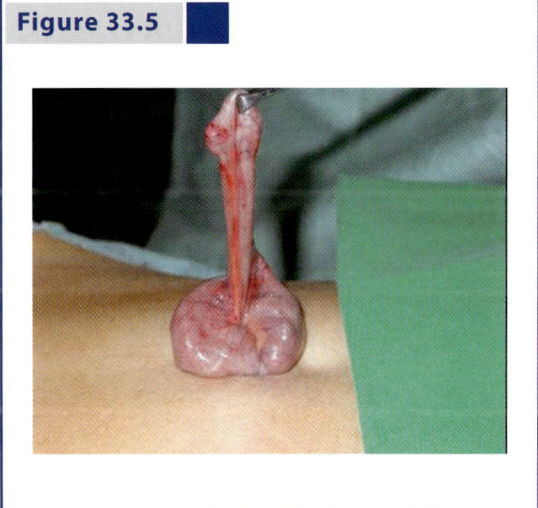

The MD is exposed

Figure 33.6

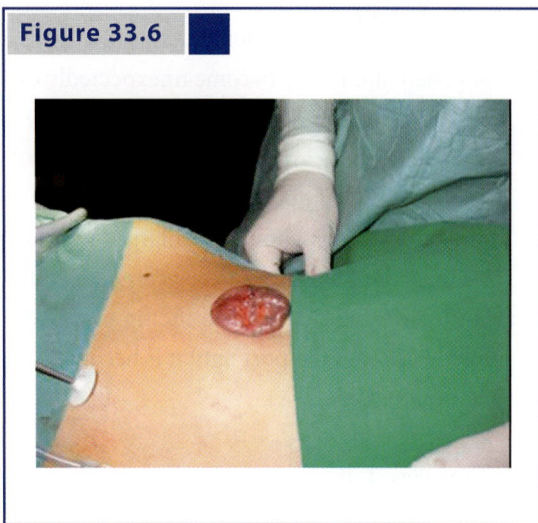

The MD is resected. The 2-mm port is kept in place in order to assist the reduction of the bowel into the abdominal cavity

Recommended Literature

1. Lee KH, Yeung CK, Tam YH, Ng WT, Yip KF (2000) Laparoscopy for definitive diagnosis and treatment of gastrointestinal bleeding of obscure origin in children. J Pediatr Surg 35:1291–1293

2. Martino A, Zamparelli M, Cobellis G, Mastroianni L, Amici J (2001) One-trocar surgery: a less invasive video surgical approach in childhood. J Pediatr Surg 36:811–814

3. Schier F, Hoffmann K, Waldschmidt J(1996) Laparoscopic removal of Meckel's diverticula in children. Eur J Pediatr Surg 6:38–39

34 Intussusception Treatment

J. Duncan Phillips

34.1   Operation Room Setup

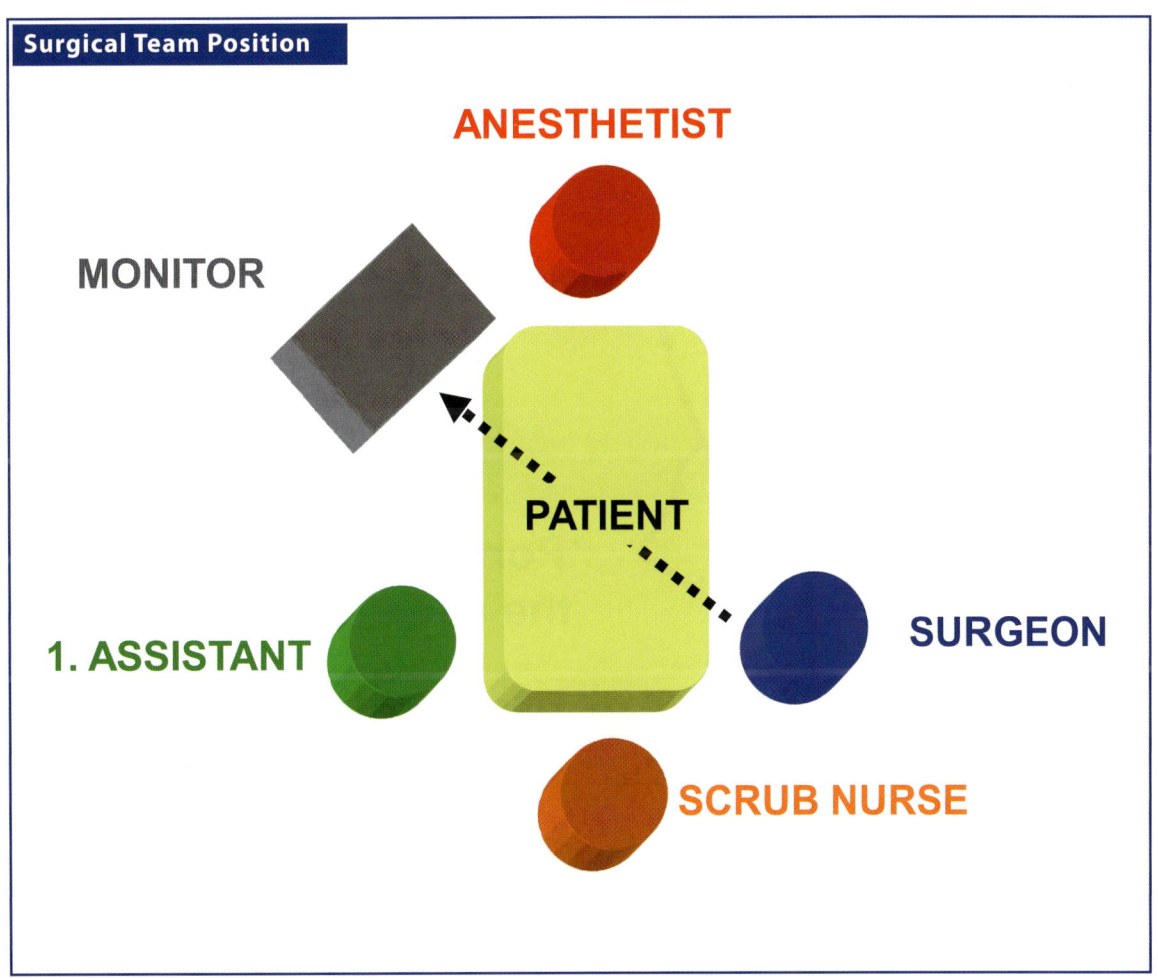

34.2   Patient Positioning

Supine position, body elevated on towels or pads, and arms straight out to the sides.

34.3   Special Instruments

- Hunter (or other similar) non-traumatic bowel graspers
- Endoscopic loop sutures

34.4   Location of Access Points

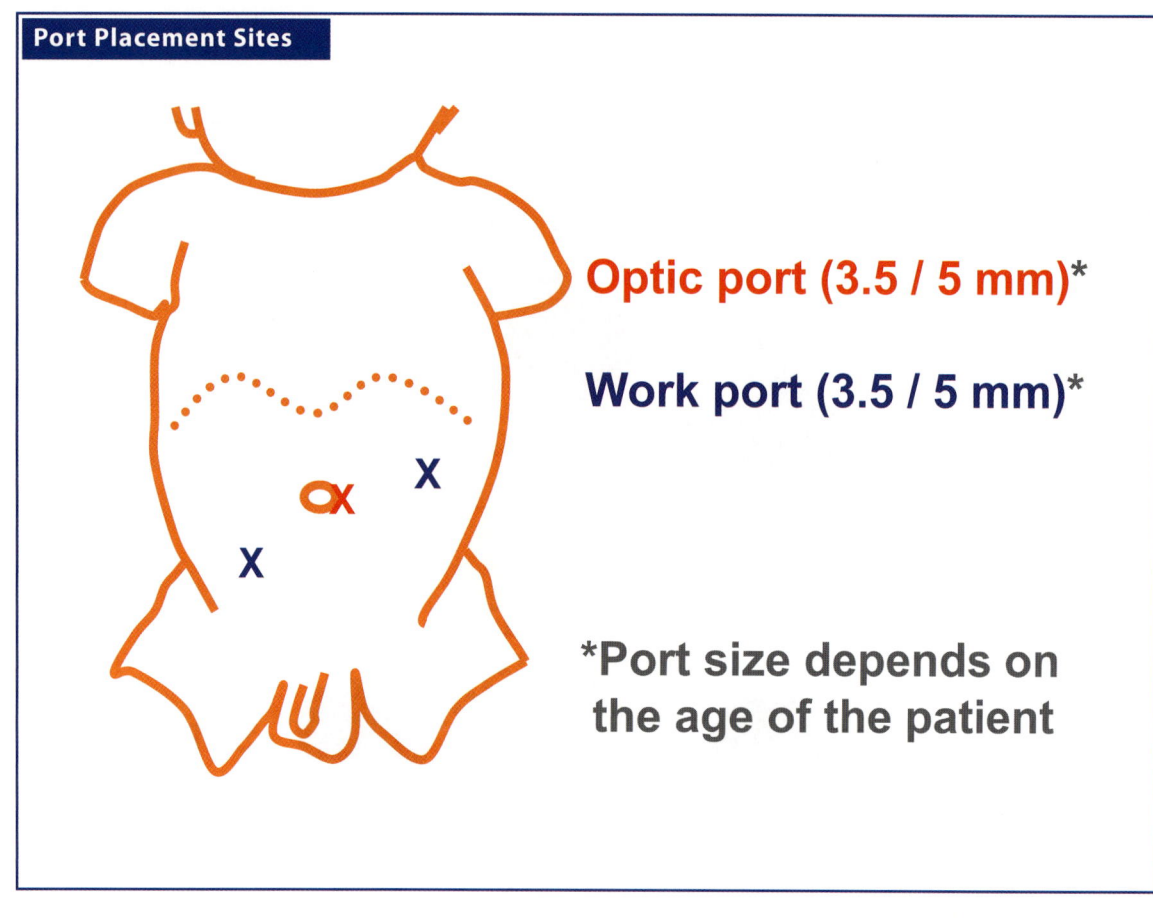

Port Placement Sites

Optic port (3.5 / 5 mm)*

Work port (3.5 / 5 mm)*

*Port size depends on the age of the patient

34.5   Indications

1. Nonreduced intussusception.
2. Suspected incompletely reduced intussusception.
3. Suspected intussusception.
4. Recurrent intussusception.

34.6   Contraindications

Long-standing intussusception with complete small-bowel obstruction resulting in massive small-bowel distension with subsequent severely limited free space.

34.7   Preoperative Considerations

1. Attempt reduction with air or liquid contrast enema (if no evidence of peritonitis). Even "partial" reduction of intussusception is helpful.
2. Resuscitation with intravenous fluids and antibiotics if dehydrated.
3. Decompress stomach with nasogastric or orogastric tube.
4. Decompress urinary bladder after induction of anesthesia.
5. Prophylactic intravenous antibiotics (if not already given).

34.8   Technical Notes

1. Diagnostic laparoscopy may disclose that complete reduction was successful by contrast enema (or may have occurred upon induction of general anesthesia), thus avoiding laparotomy.
2. Even proof of "partial" reduction is helpful, since this decreases the size of the incision necessary for "open" reduction.
3. Complete reduction may require both antegrade squeezing of the intestine ("pushing") and retrograde "pulling" of the intussuscepted intestine.

34.9   Procedure Variations

1. Laparoscopic verification of incompletely reduced intussusception, followed by laparotomy for reduction.
2. Laparoscopic verification of infarcted intestine, followed by laparotomy for resection.
3. Laparoscopic-assisted transumbilical reduction and/or resection.
4. Laparoscopic-assisted air (or liquid contrast) enema reduction.
5. Intra-abdominal or extra-abdominal (via port site) appendectomy.

34.10   Laparoscopic Approach to Intussusception

Please see Figs. 1–8.

Figure 34.1

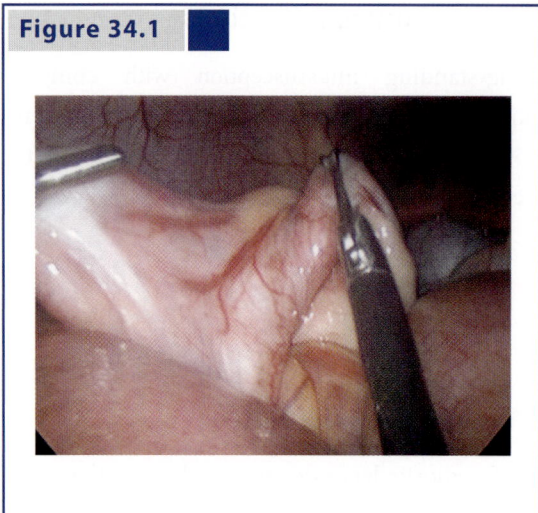

The cecum and terminal ileum are grasped, confirming preoperative suspicion of nonreducible small-bowel-to-small-bowel intussusception

Figure 34.2

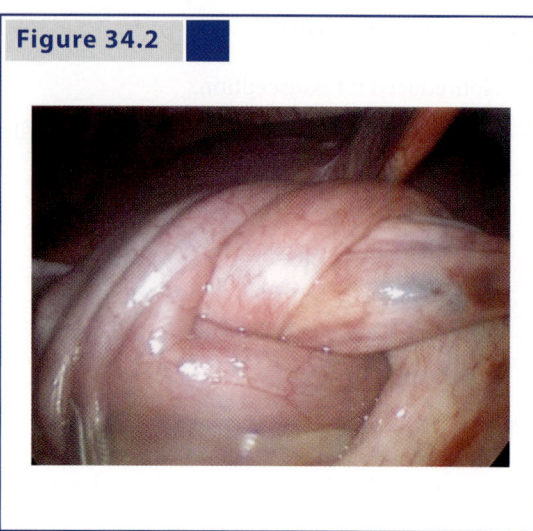

Small-bowel-to-small-bowel intussusception is identified in the right upper quadrant. The mesentery typically has multiple enlarged lymph nodes and may have areas of mild hemorrhage

Figure 34.3

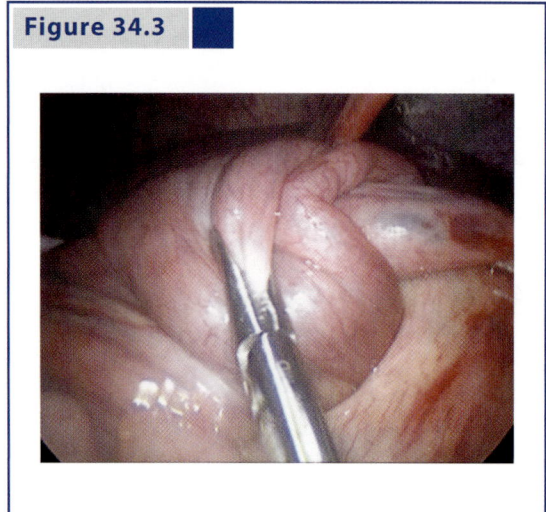

Reduction is begun by gently pulling on the intussuscepted small intestine (grasper not seen in this photo) and pushing backward on the distal intestine to "unfold" the accepting intestine

Figure 34.4

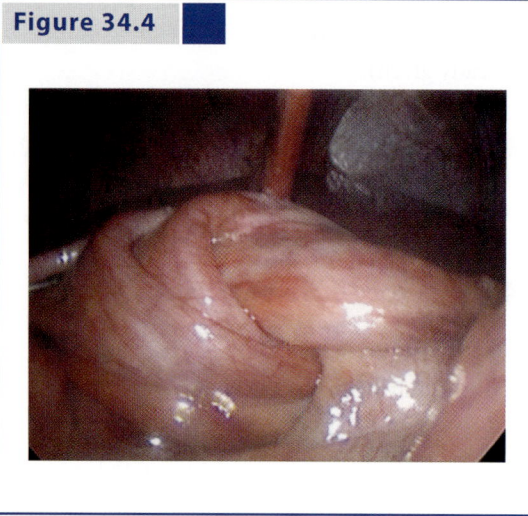

Continued gentle traction on the intussuscepted small intestine and gentle pressure on the edges of the distal intestine allows slow, gradual reduction of the intussusception

Figure 34.5

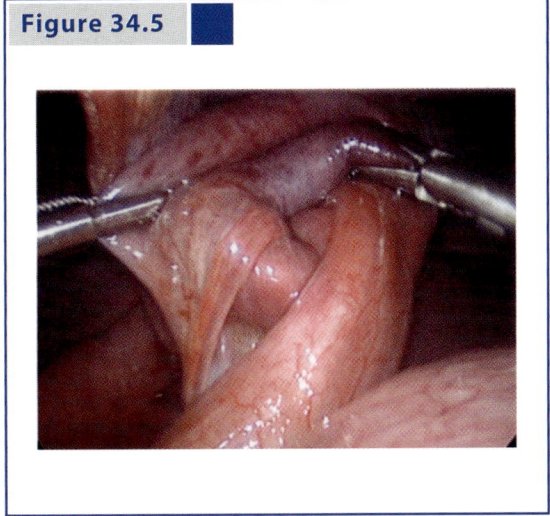

Just prior to complete reduction of the intussusception, continued gentle traction is applied on the intussuscepted intestine

Figure 34.6

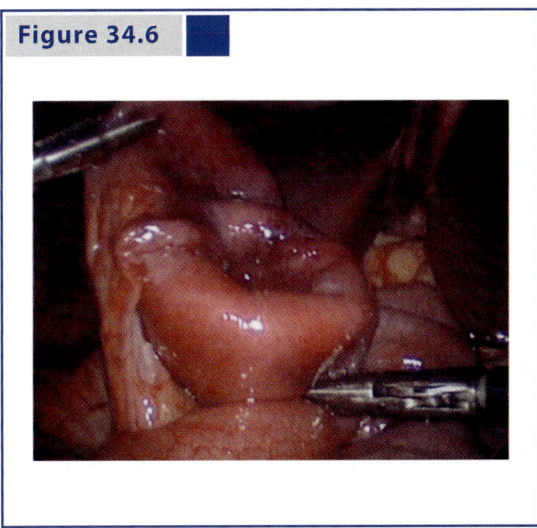

After completed reduction, the segment of intestine is exteriorized through a slightly enlarged umbilical incision

Figure 34.7

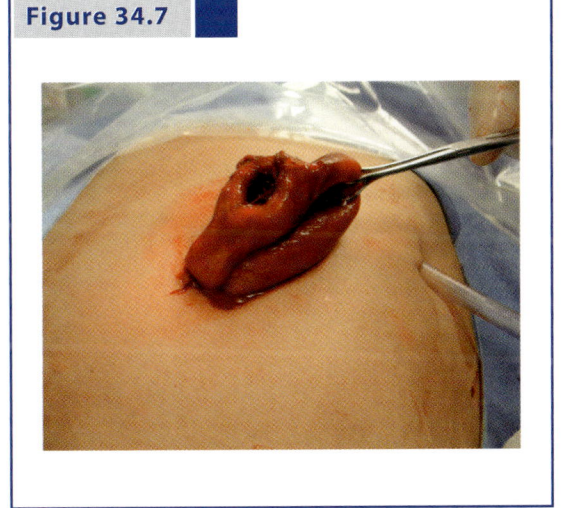

Exteriorization allows manual palpation of the affected intestinal segment and segmental resection of the "lead point"

Figure 34.8

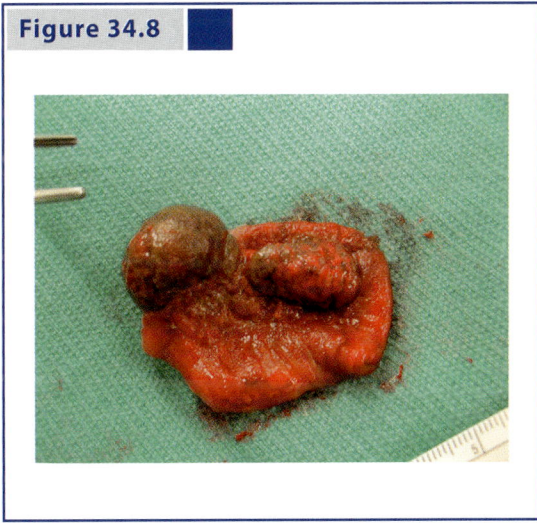

Two benign polyps were identified as the "lead points" in the resected intestinal segment

Recommended Literature

1. Kia KF, Mony V, Drongowski R, Golladay E, Geiger J, Hirschl R, Coran A, Teitelbaum D (2005) Laparoscopic vs open surgical approach for intussusception requiring operative intervention. J Pediatr Surg 40:281–284
2. Poddoubnyi IV, Dronov A, Blinnikov O, Smirnov A, Darenkov I, Dedov K (1998) Laparoscopy in the treatment of intussusception in children. J Pediatr Surg 33:1194–1197
3. van der Laan M, Bax NM, van der Zee DC, Ure BM (2001) The role of laparoscopy in the management of childhood intussusception. Surg Endosc 15:373–376

35 Appendectomy

Amulya K. Saxena

35.1 Operation Room Setup

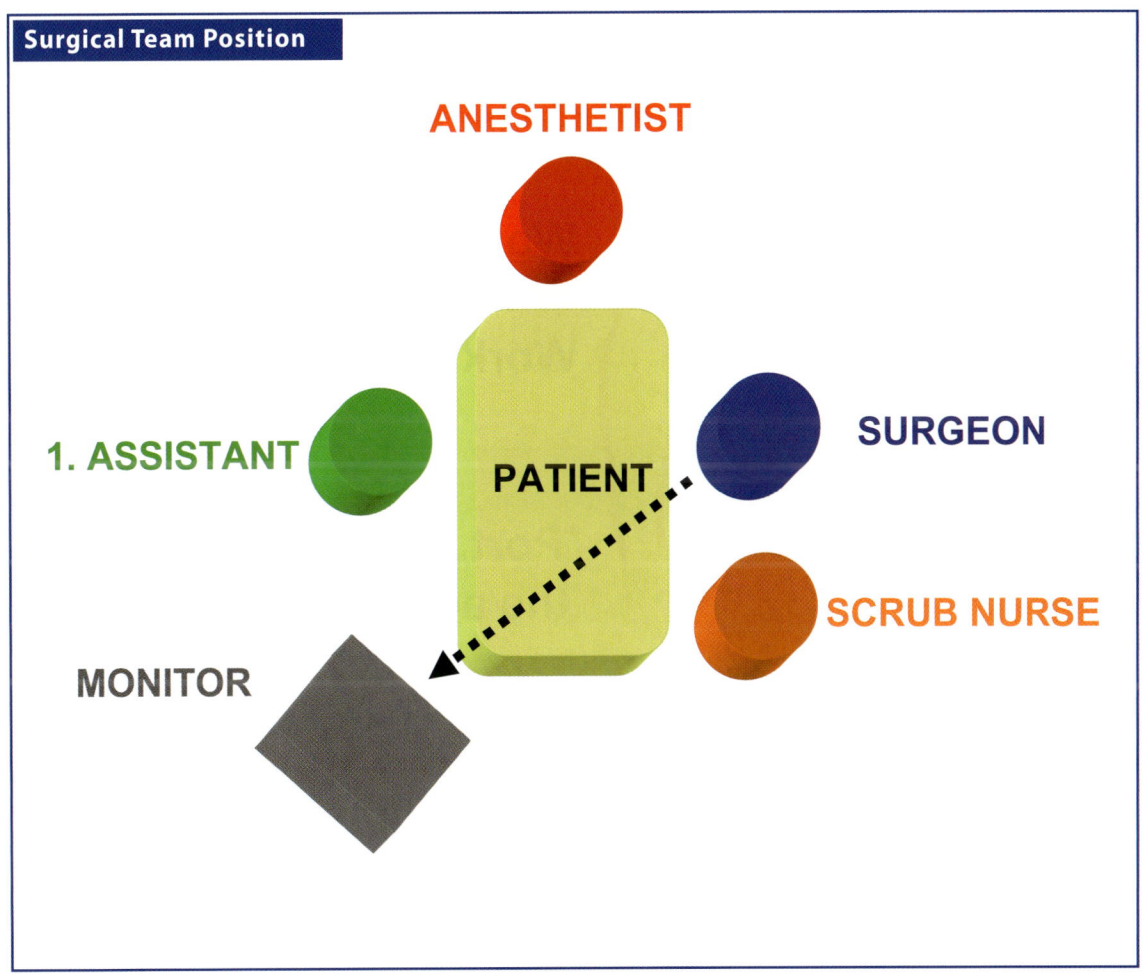

Surgical Team Position

ANESTHETIST

1. ASSISTANT

PATIENT

SURGEON

SCRUB NURSE

MONITOR

35.2   Patient Positioning

Supine position with arms tucked to the side.

35.3   Special Instruments

- Endoscopic loop sutures
- Bipolar forceps
- Specimen retrieval bag

35.4   Location of Access Points

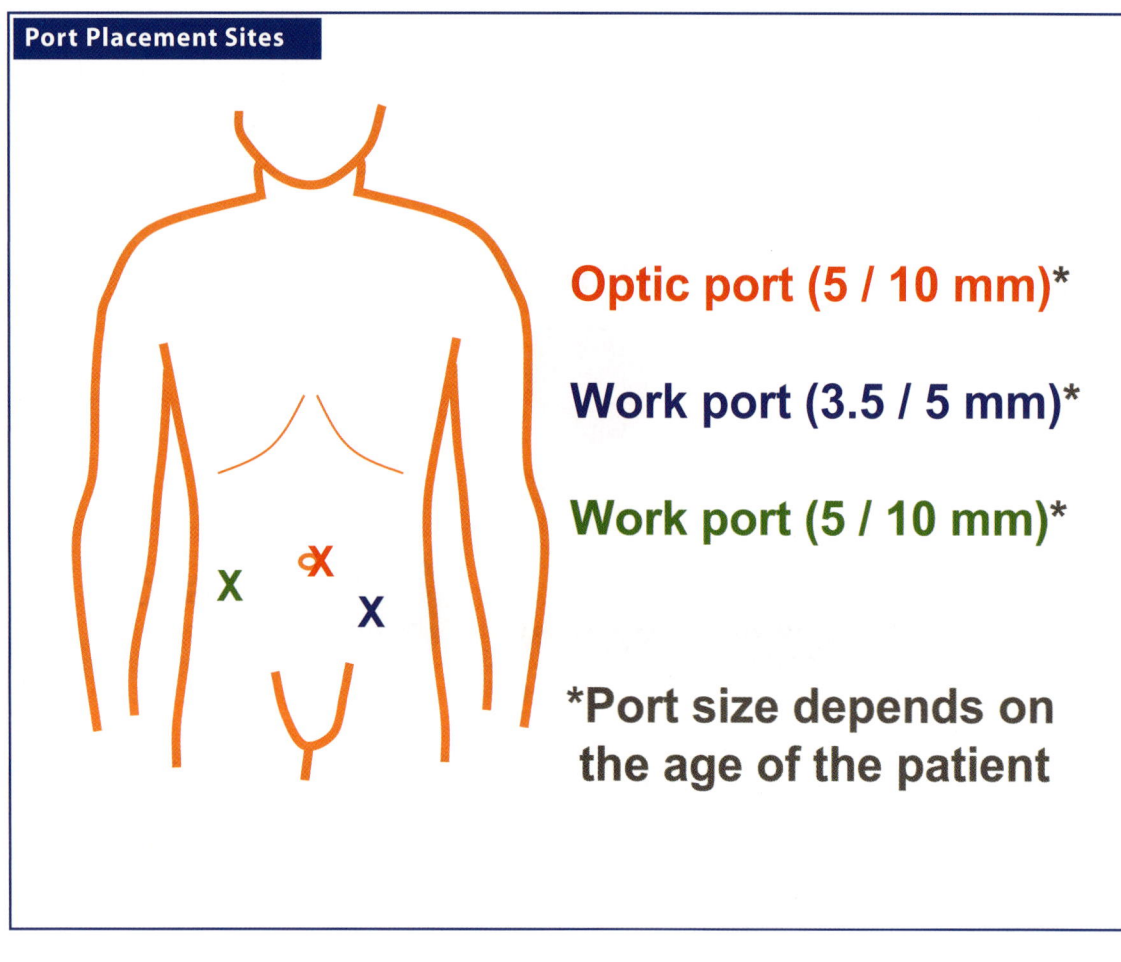

Port Placement Sites

Optic port (5 / 10 mm)*

Work port (3.5 / 5 mm)*

Work port (5 / 10 mm)*

*Port size depends on the age of the patient

35.5   Indications

1. Acute appendicitis.
2. Perforated appendicitis.
3. Appendicitis with coprolith.
4. Retrocecal appendicitis.

35.6   Contraindications

Appendicitis complicated by bowel obstruction with abdominal distension (mesoceliac appendicitis).

35.7   Preoperative Considerations

1. Leave a povidone iodine gauge in the umbilicus until the patient enters the operating room.
2. Place a Foley catheter before the procedure.
3. Preoperative resuscitation should be done if there are signs of peritonitis.
4. In case of suspected perforation, antibiotics should be administered before general anesthesia is induced.

35.8   Technical Notes

1. Manipulate the fragile appendix with care. In this case, manipulation using the mesoappendix is recommended.
2. In cases of localized abscess, care should be taken not to burst the abscess. Pus should be aspirated using a large needle inserted through the abdominal wall under laparoscopic guidance.
3. A preperforative or perforated appendix must be removed from the abdomen in an specimen retrieval bag.

35.9   Procedure Variations

1. Extra-abdominal (laparoscopic-assisted), single-port method (see Chap. 36).
2. Mixed technique (mesoappendix hemostasis performed intra-abdominally and the appendix is ligated extra-abdominally), three-port method.
3. Intra-abdominal techniques with:
   a. Endoscopic stapler.
   b. Intra-/extracorporeal suturing.

35.10   Laparoscopic Appendectomy

Please see Figs. 1–6.

Figure 35.1

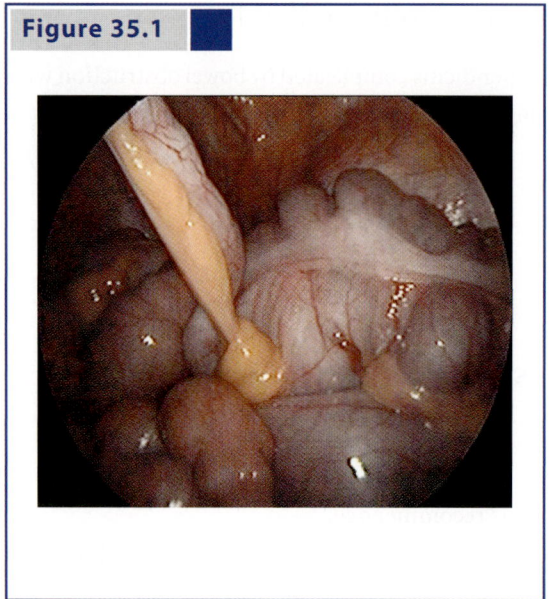

The bowel loops are mobilized and the appendix is lifted using an atraumatic grasper

Figure 35.2

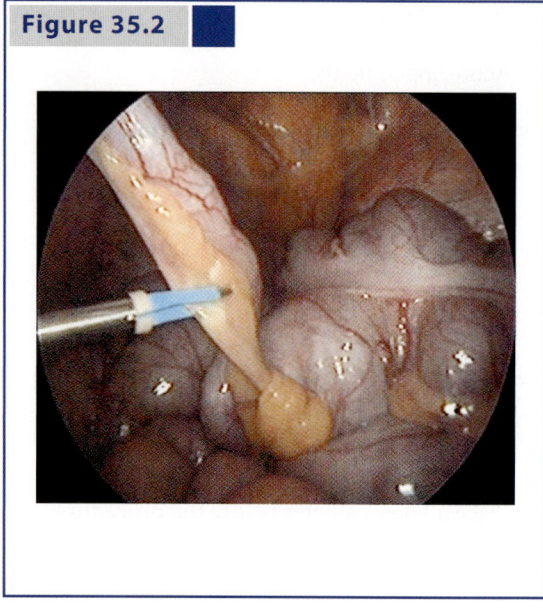

The vessels of the mesoappendix are coagulated using bipolar forceps

Figure 35.3

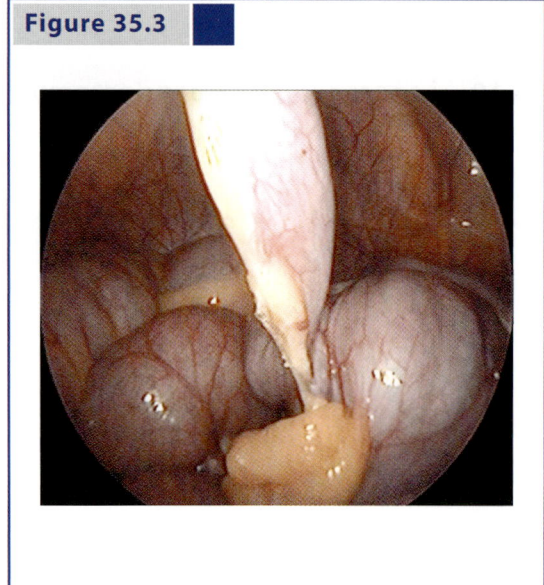

The cauterized mesoappendix is cut using a pair of hooked scissors

Figure 35.4

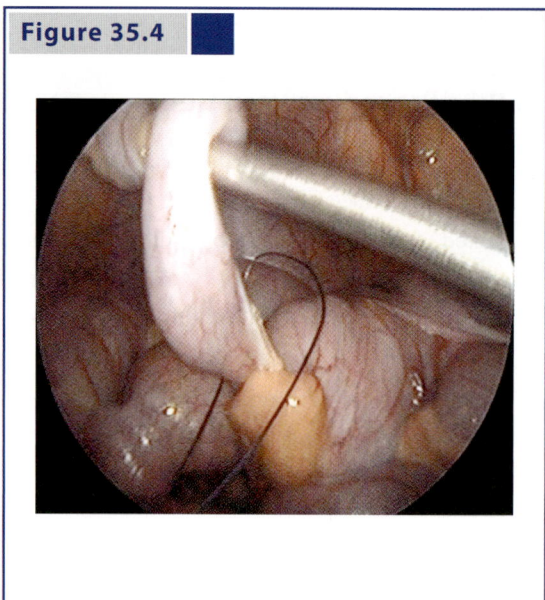

Three endoscopic loop sutures are used and the appendix is ligated toward the base

Figure 35.5

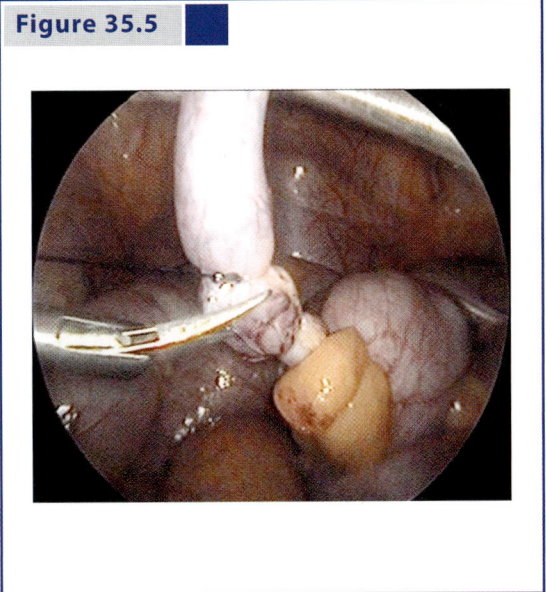

Figure 35.6

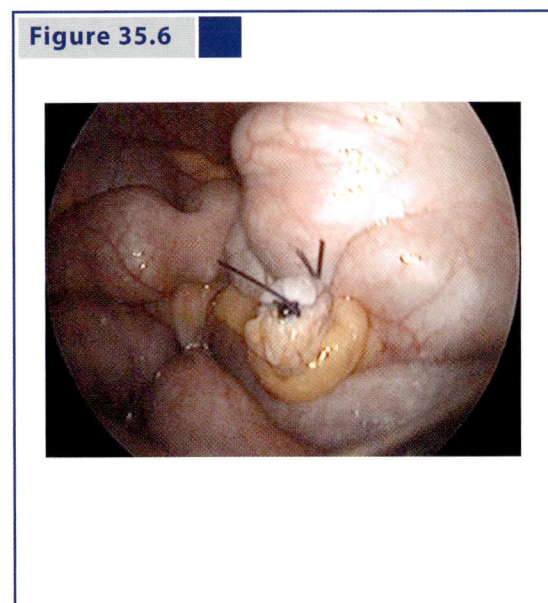

The distal endoscopic loop suture is left uncut and the appendix is cut between it and the two proximal sutures

The distal endoscopic loop suture is used to extract the dissected appendix through the (5-/10-mm) port. Postoperative view of the appendix stump with the two sutures

Recommended Literature

1. Gauderer MW (2007) An individualized approach to appendectomy in children based on anatomico-laparoscopic findings. Am Surg 73:814–817
2. Saxena AK, Springer A, Tsokas J, Willital GH (2004) Laparoscopic appendectomy in children with *Enterobius vermicularis*. Surg Laparosc Endosc Percutan Tech 11:284–286
3. Schmelzer TM, Rana AR, Walters KC, Norton HJ, Bambini DA, Heniford BT (2007) Improved outcomes for laparoscopic appendectomy compared with open appendectomy in the pediatric population. J Laparoendosc Adv Surg Tech A 17:693–697

36 Single-Port Appendectomy

JOHANNES SCHALAMON

36.1 Operation Room Setup

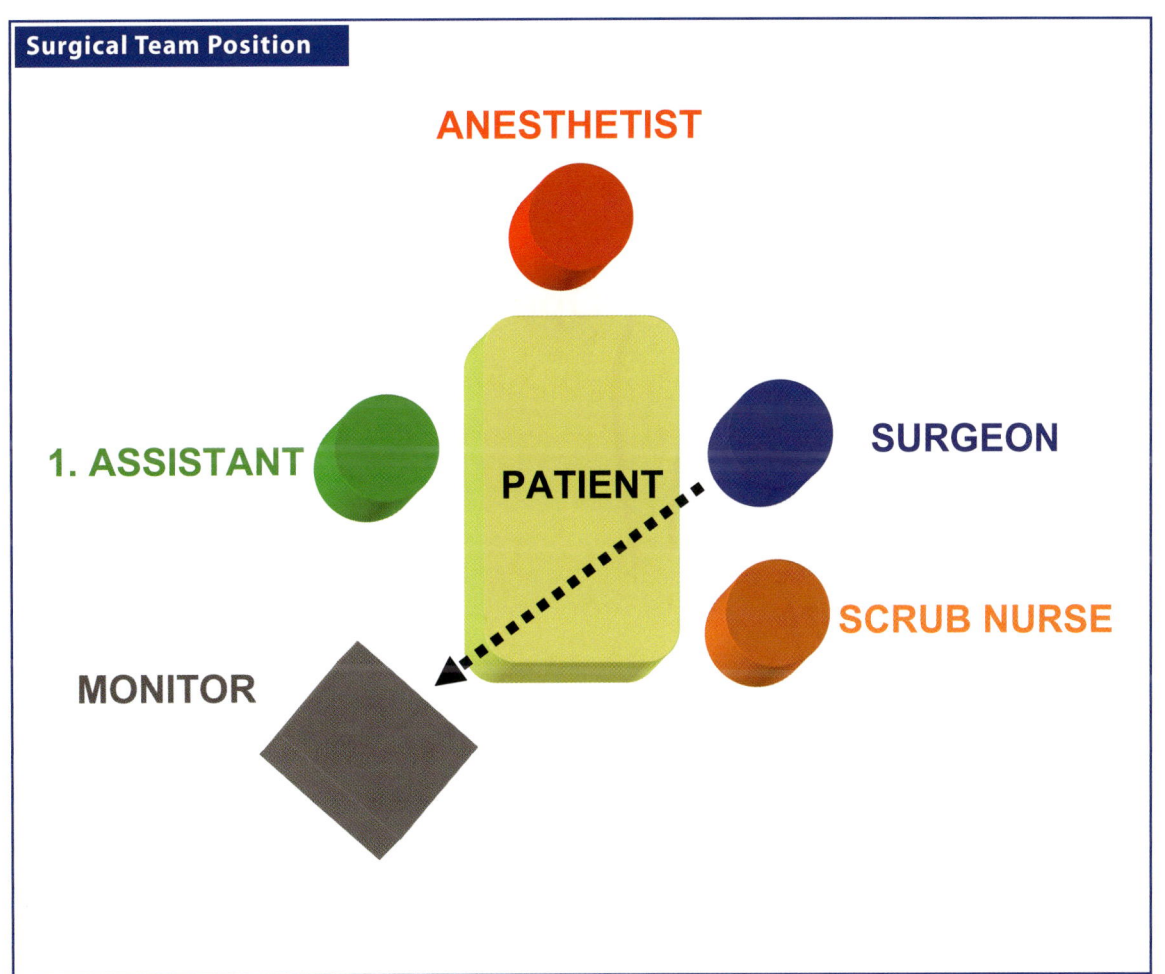

Surgical Team Position

ANESTHETIST

1. ASSISTANT

PATIENT

SURGEON

SCRUB NURSE

MONITOR

36.2   Patient Positioning

Supine position with the arms tucked to the side.

36.3   Special Instruments

10-mm operating scope with a 5-mm working channel.

36.4   Location of Access Points

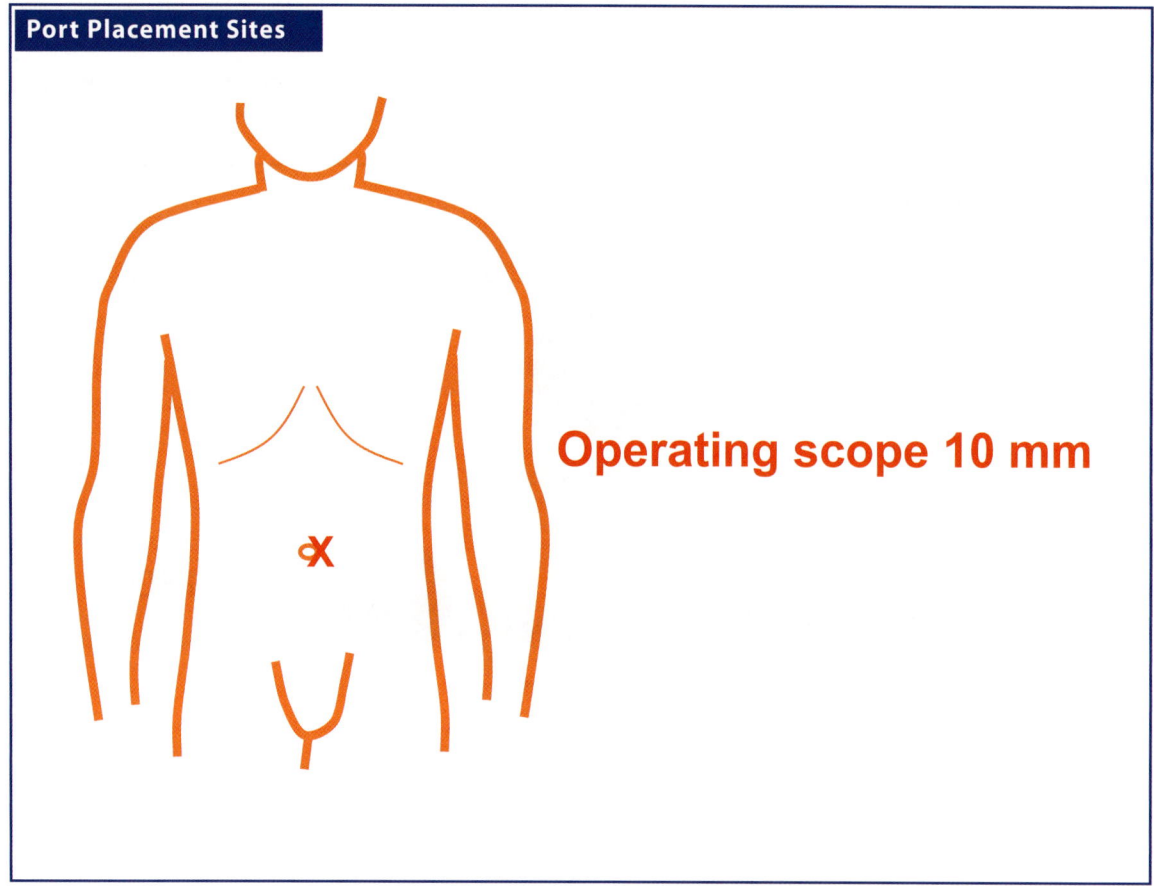

Port Placement Sites

Operating scope 10 mm

36.5 Indications

1. Nonperforated appendicitis.
2. Phlegmonous appendicitis.
3. Appendicitis with impacted stool.
4. Obese patients.

36.6 Contraindications

1. Friable appendix.
2. Generalized peritonitis after perforation.
3. Retrocecal appendicitis.
4. Severe adhesions after prior surgery.

36.7 Preoperative Considerations

1. Place a betadine swab in the umbilicus at the point of port insertion.
2. The patient should be draped so that it may also possible to introduce additional ports if deemed necessary.
3. Antibiotic administration depends upon the condition of the appendix and peritoneal inflammation.
4. The bladder should be drained before commencement of the procedure.

36.8 Technical Notes

1. The single-port technique has its limitations in certain forms of appendicitis, where a two-instrument manipulation may be required.
2. Difficulties arise in the search of Meckel's diverticulum that is not floating and where the intestine has to be manipulated.
3. Single-port appendectomy leaves "no" visible skin scars as the scar is concealed in the umbilical folds.

36.9 Procedure Variations

1. Single-port appendectomy can be conducted intracorporeally with the aid of a transabdominal sling suture.
2. Exteriorization of the inflamed appendix can be performed by insertion of the working scope directly into the right iliac fossa instead of the umbilicus.
3. Right-iliac-fossa appendectomy under local pneumoperitoneum conditions using 12-mm operating scope fitted with a transparent plastic cap.

36.10 Laparoscopic-Assisted Single-Port Appendectomy

Please see Figs. 1–6.

Figure 36.1

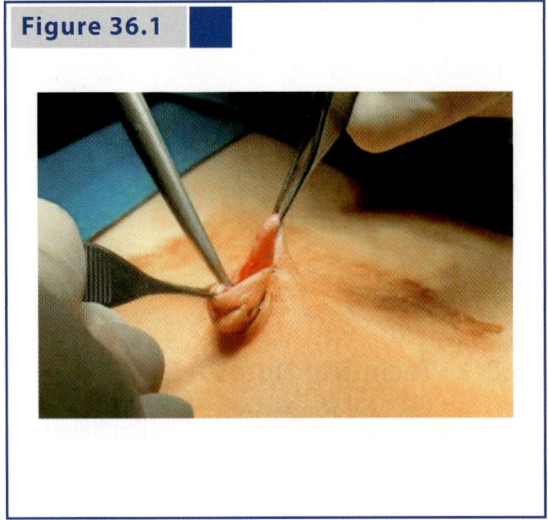

Access is gained into the abdominal cavity using the open-access method

Figure 36.2

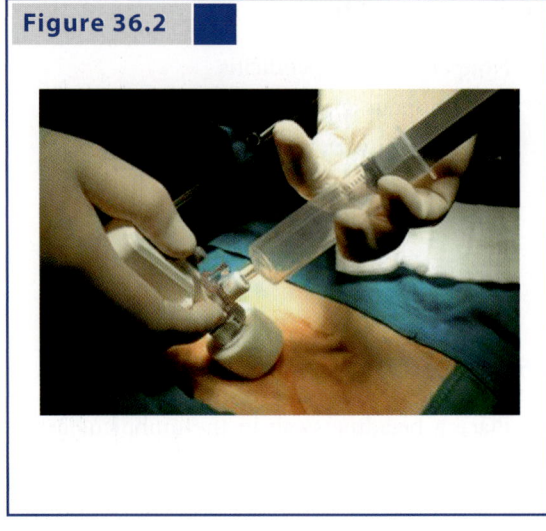

A disposable 10-mm port is inserted and secured to the abdominal wall

Figure 36.3

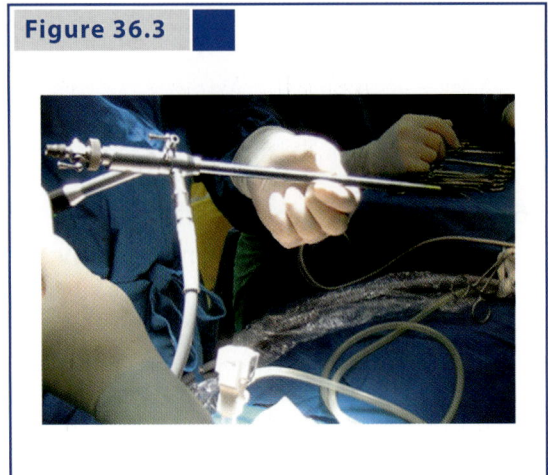

The operating scope used has a 6° angle of view and 5-mm instrument channel

Figure 36.4

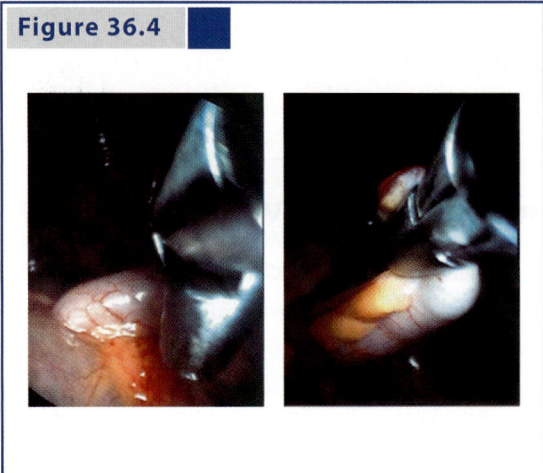

A grasper is introduced (**left**) through the working channel to grasp the appendix (**right**)

Figure 36.5

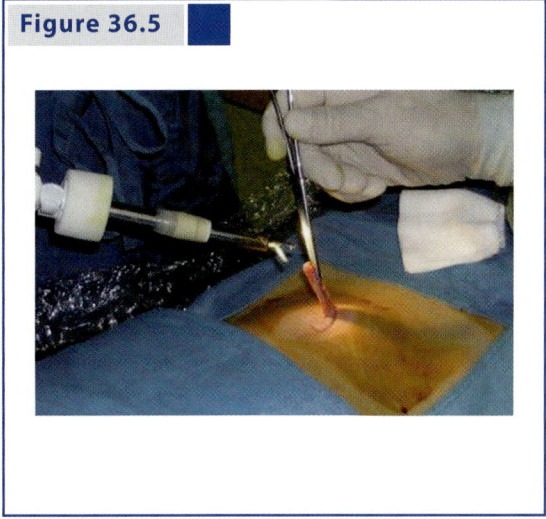

Figure 36.6

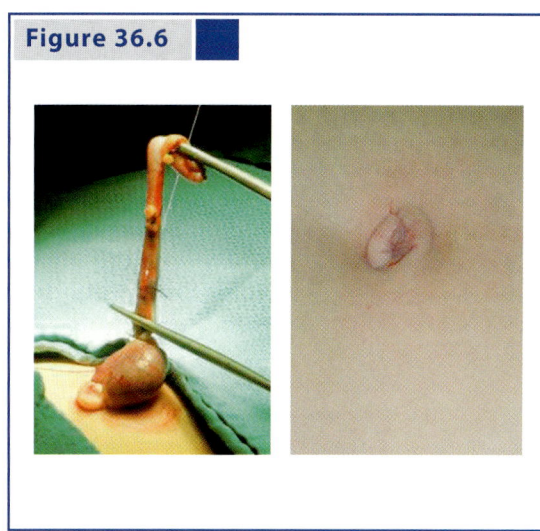

The grasper, scope, and port are removed as a single unit and the appendix is exteriorized

The appendectomy is performed as in open surgery (*left*) with good cosmesis (*right*)

Recommended Literature

1. D'Alessio A, Piro E, Tadini B, Beretta F (2002) One-trocar transumbilical laparoscopic-assisted appendectomy in children: our experience. Eur J Pediatr Surg 12:24–27
2. Koontz CS, Smith L, Burkholder H, Higdon K, Aderhold R, Carr M (2006) Video-assisted transumbilical appendectomy in children. J Pediatr Surg 41:710–712
3. Ates O, Hakguder G, Olguner M, Akgür F (2007) Single-port laparoscopic appendectomy conducted intracorporeally with the aid of a transabdominal sling suture. J Pediatr Surg 42:1071–1074

37 Extramucosal Colon Biopsy

CORNELIA VAN TUIL AND AMULYA K. SAXENA

37.1 Operation Room Setup

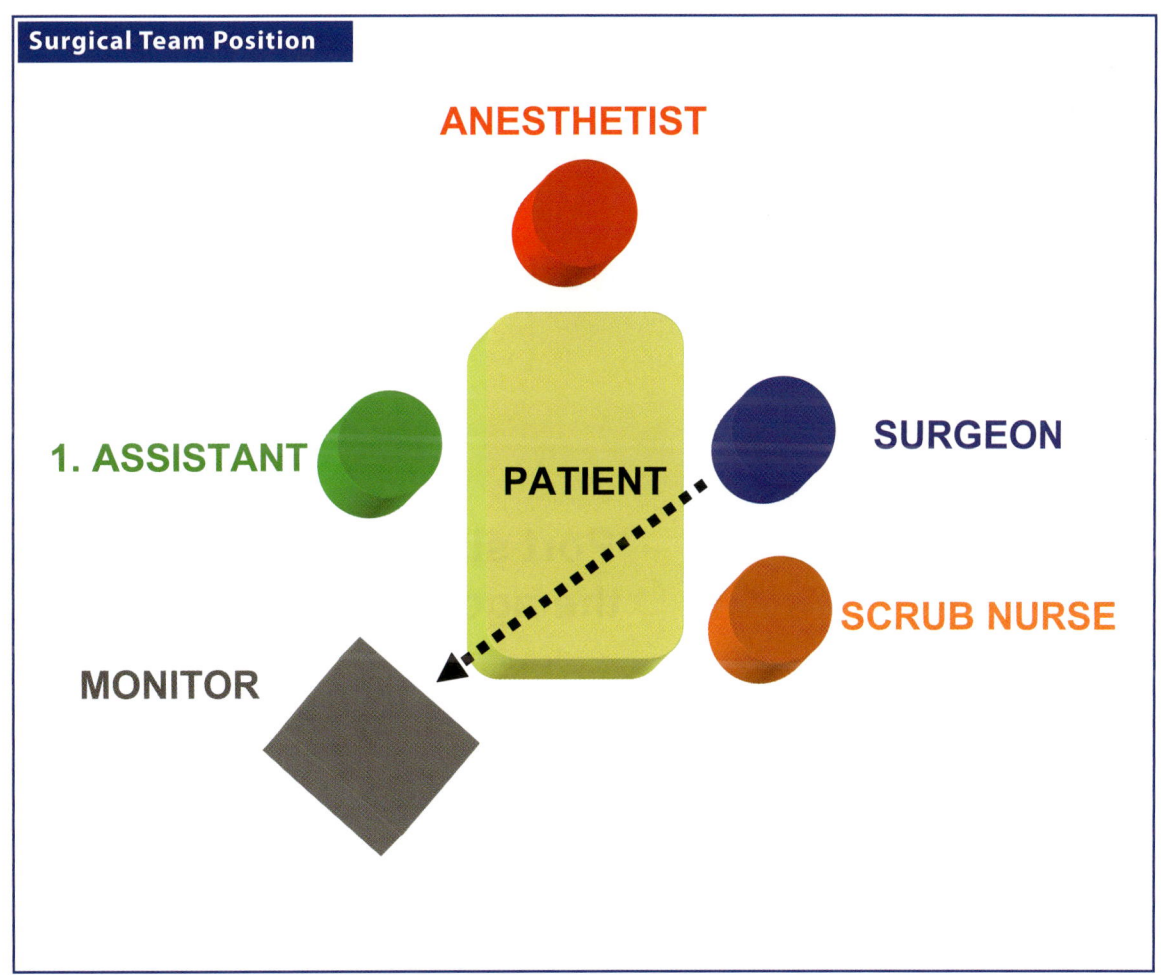

37.2   Patient Positioning

Supine position with the arms tucked to the side.

37.3   Special Instruments

Atraumatic forceps.

37.4   Location of Access Points

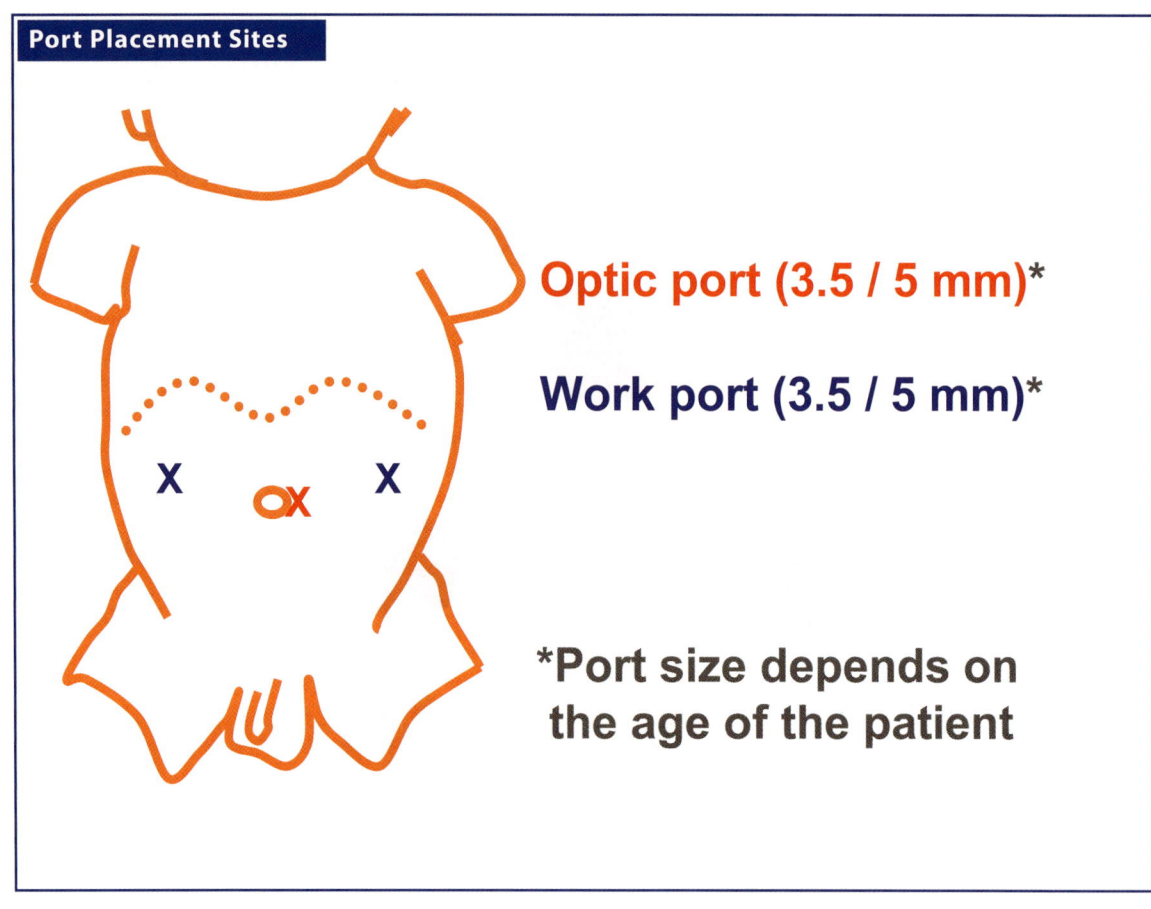

Port Placement Sites

Optic port (3.5 / 5 mm)*

Work port (3.5 / 5 mm)*

*Port size depends on the age of the patient

37.5   Indications

1. Hirschsprung's disease.
2. Neuronal intestinal dysplasia.
3. Dysmotility disorders.
4. Ganglioneuromatosis.
5. Chronic constipation.

37.6   Contraindications

Inflammatory bowel disease is a relative contra-indication.

37.7   Preoperative Considerations

1. Bowel wash outs should be done 24 h before the procedure.
2. Oral laxatives may be necessary in chronic constipation patients.
3. Antibiotics are generally not recommended before the procedure, but should be administered if inflammation is suspected.
4. Metronidazole is the antibiotic of choice in Hirschsprungs's disease.

37.8   Technical Notes

1. The preferred biopsy site is the taenia libera, which is on the antimesenteric side.
2. Grasp only one end and manipulate the specimen from this freed end. Multiple grasping can damage the specimen.
3. After the specimen is retrieved, control the biopsy site for signs of perforation. This finding has to be documented on video for legal reasons, because perforations can be sometimes missed under visual inspection.

37.9   Procedure Variations

1. Full-thickness biopsy procedures can be performed using laparoscopic techniques. If the bowel was not prepared before the procedure, this technique has the risk of abdominal contamination. This technique also requires suturing of the biopsy site.
2. Single-port laparoscopic-assisted biopsy procedures are performed by retracting the bowel through the umbilical incision using a grasper and then performing an open biopsy.

37.10   Laparoscopic Extramucosal Colon Biopsy

Please see Figs. 1–6.

Figure 37.1

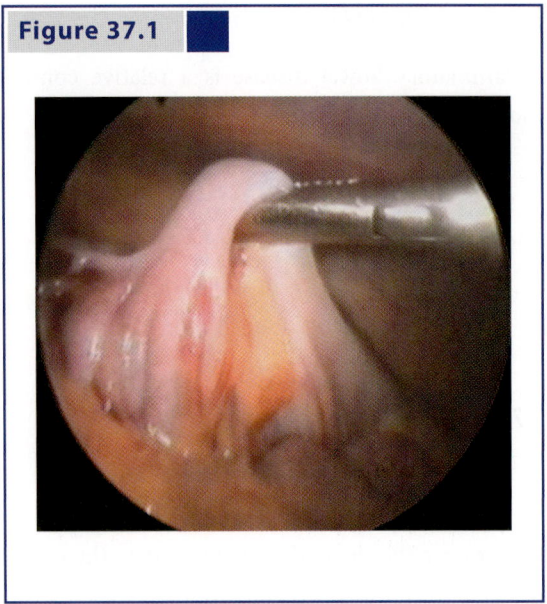

The bowel loops are mobilized and the colon is lifted using an atraumatic grasper

Figure 37.2

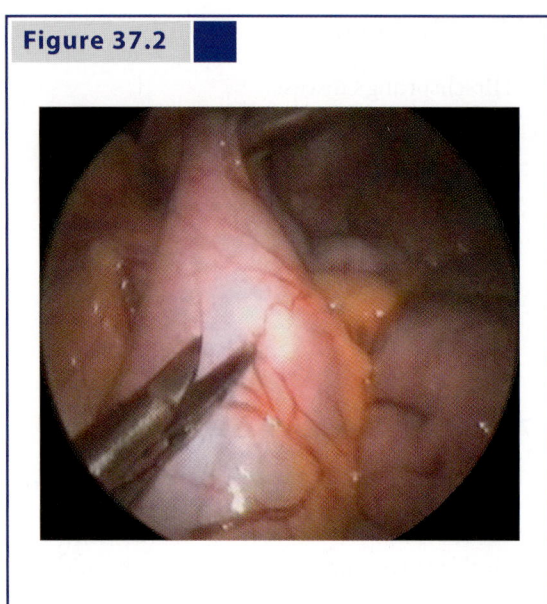

While holding the colon under tension, an incision is made in the serosa using Metzenbaum scissors

Figure 37.3

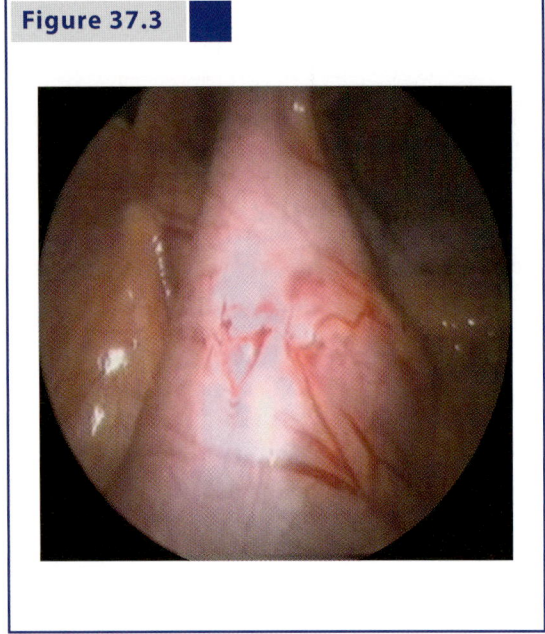

The incision on the antimesenteric side avoids vessels that cross the other two taenia

Figure 37.4

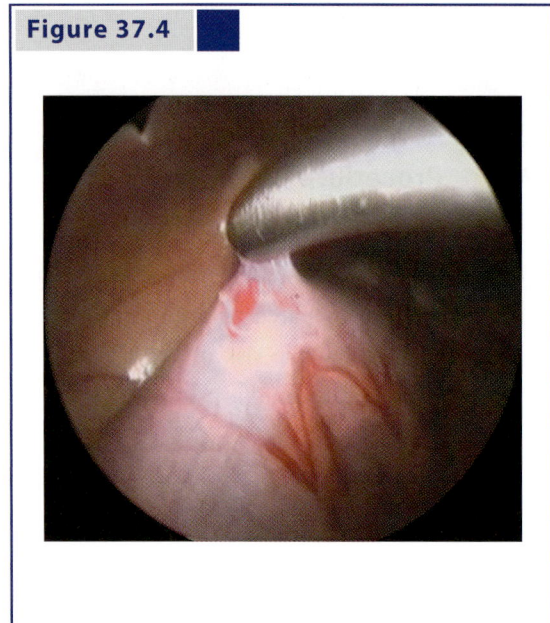

The free end of the biopsy is grasped to expose the plane between the mucosa and serosa

Figure 37.5

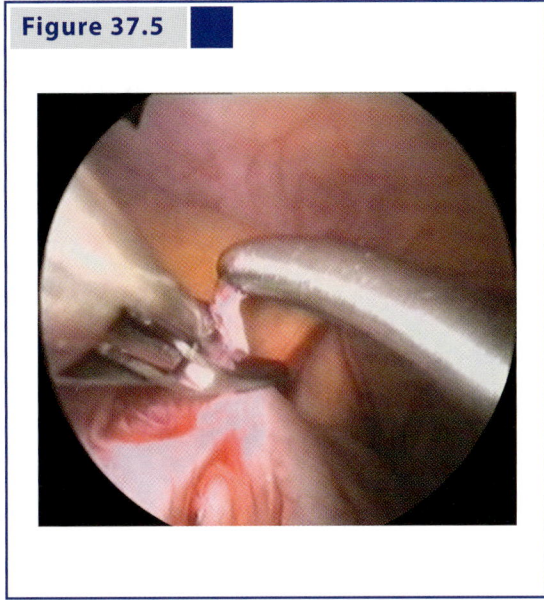

Metzenbaum scissors are used to dissect the biopsy free from the mucosa

Figure 37.6

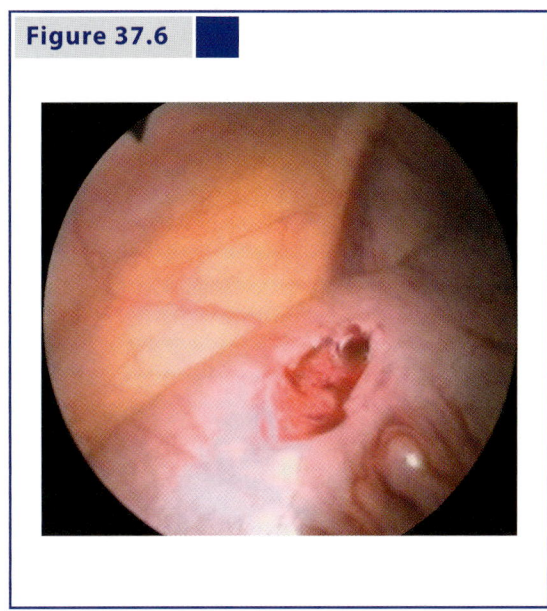

After the specimen is retrieved, the site is controlled to rule out possible perforation

Recommended Literature

1. Imaji R, Kubota Y, Hengel P, Hutson JM, Chow CW (2000) Rectal mucosal biopsy compared with laparoscopic seromuscular biopsy in the diagnosis of intestinal neuronal dysplasia in children with slow-transit constipation. J Pediatr Surg 35:1724–1727
2. King SK, Sutcliffe JR, Hustson JM (2005) Laparoscopic seromuscular colonic biopsies: a surgeon's experience. J Pediatr Surg 40:381–384
3. van Tuil C, Saxena AK, Willital GH (2004) Extramucosal colon biopsies. Eur Surg 36:13

38 Total Colectomy with Pelvic Pouch

Ivan R. Diamond and Jacob C. Langer

38.1   Operation Room Setup

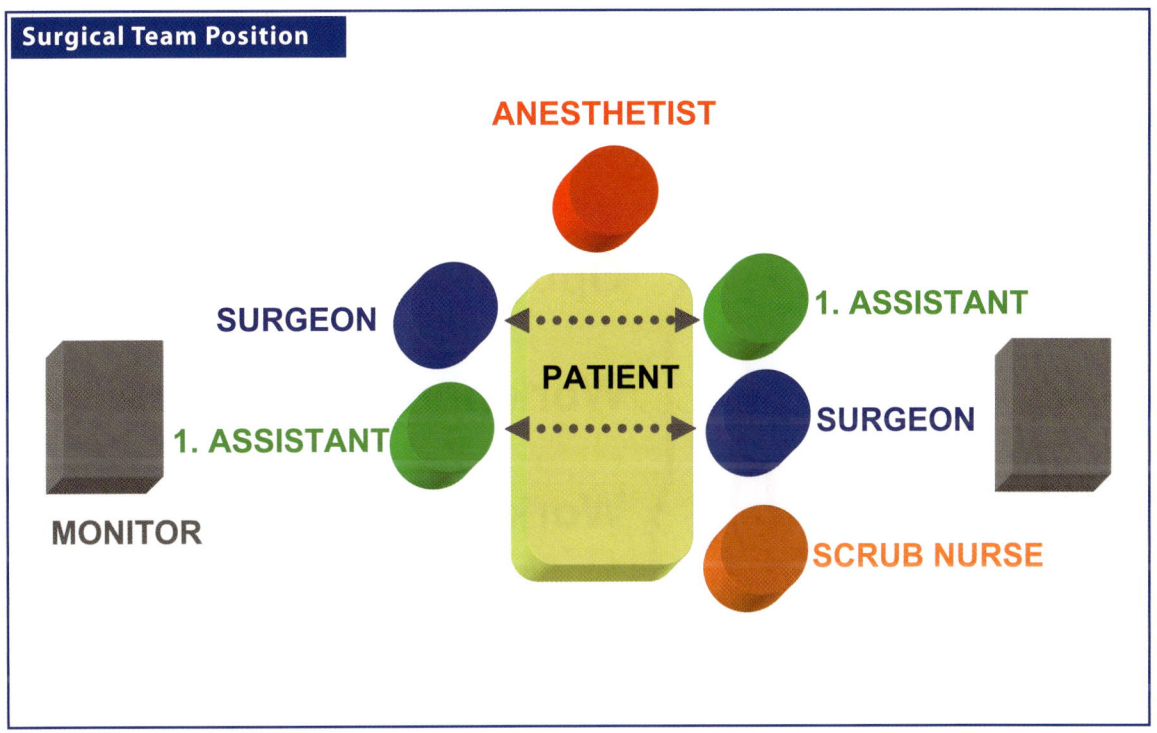

38.2   Patient Positioning

Supine position with arms tucked to the side for the initial portion of the procedure. Move to the lithotomy position at the conclusion of the rectal dissection for pouch–anal anastomosis.

38.3   Special Instruments

- LigaSure™ (Valleylab, Boulder, CO, USA)
- Endo GIA™ stapler (Auto Suture, Norwalk, CT, USA)
- Circular end-to-end anastomosis (EEA) stapler
- Typically 12mm ports are used at umbilicus and in the right lower quadrant at the position determined to be optimal for the ileostomy.

38.4   Location of Access Points

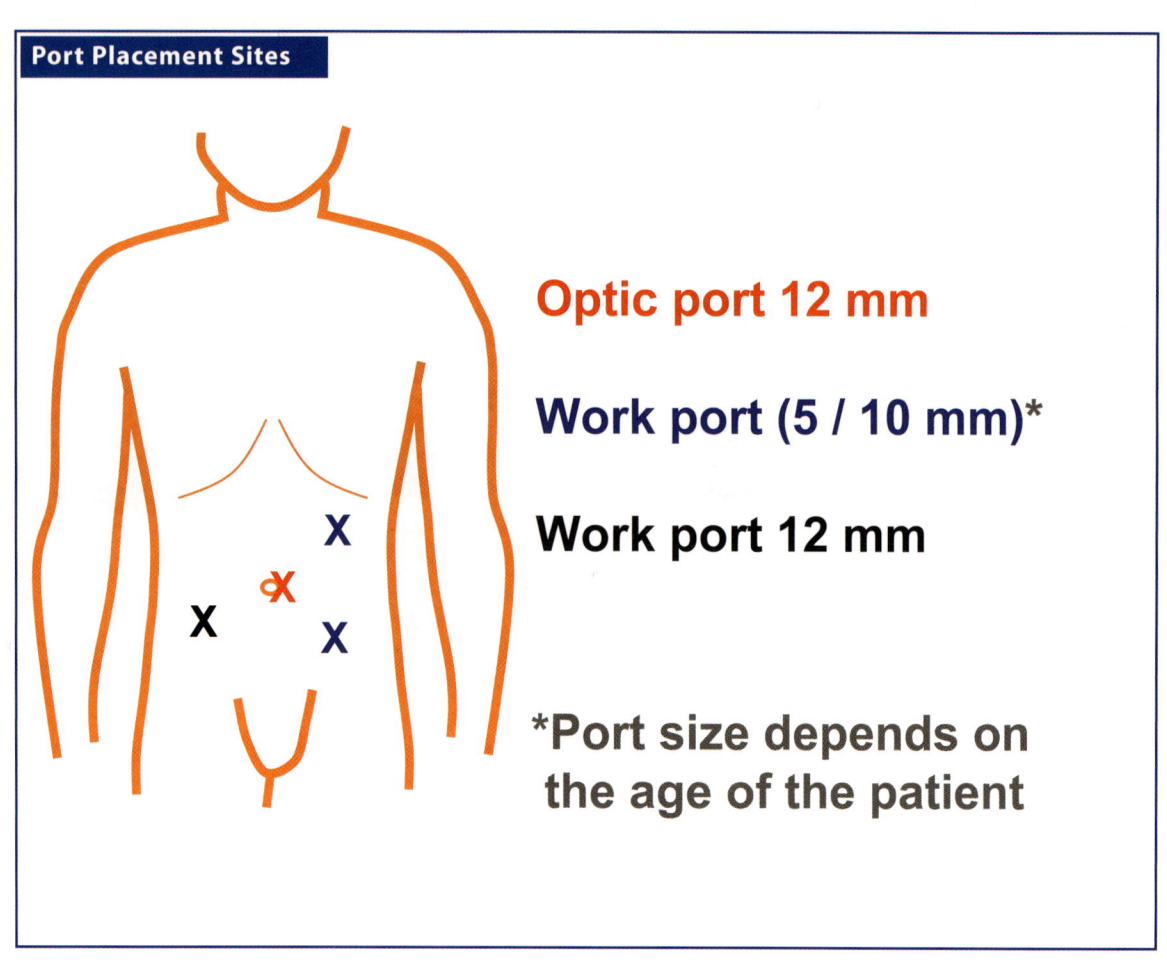

Port Placement Sites

Optic port 12 mm

Work port (5 / 10 mm)*

Work port 12 mm

*Port size depends on the age of the patient

38.5   Indications

1. Ulcerative colitis:
   a. Refractory to medical treatment.
   b. Complication of medical therapy.
   c. Dysplasia/malignancy (rare in children).
2. Familial adenomatous polyposis (FAP).

38.6   Contraindications

1. Absolute contraindication: Crohn's disease
2. Relative contraindication
   a. Very young child.
   b. Indeterminate colitis.
   c. Patient who is sick, malnourished, or on chronic high-dose steroids.

38.7   Preoperative Considerations

1. Bowel preparation in the absence of severe acute colitis.
2. Place a Foley catheter and a nasogastric tube before the procedure.
3. Administer prophylactic antibiotics.
4. Administer steroids perioperatively if the patient is on current or has had recent steroid treatment.

38.8   Technical Notes

1. Perform the initial diagnostic laparoscopy to ensure that there is no evidence of Crohn's disease.
2. Creation of a small (8–10 cm) pouch is optimal to the minimize risk of pouchitis.
3. When anastomosing the pouch, take care to ensure that there is no torsion of the pouch mesentery.
4. Plan to close the loop-ileostomy after 6 weeks or longer, preceded by a contrast study of the pouch.

38.9   Procedure Variations

1. Three-stage procedure consisting of: (a) subtotal colectomy, (b) formation of a pelvic pouch, and (c) ileostomy closure in malnutrition, prolonged steroid use, severe acute colitis, or the very young child. Alternatively, the identical initial operation with two modifications: (a) a more distal division of the sigmoid colon; and (b) temporary end-ileostomy rather than the ileal-pouch.
2. "One-step" procedure without protecting the loop ileostomy in FAP.
3. Laparoscopic-assisted procedure with low transverse incision (Pfannenstiel) for rectal dissection and pouch creation.

38.10   Laparoscopic Total Colectomy with Pelvic Pouch

Please see Figs. 1–12.

Figure 38.1

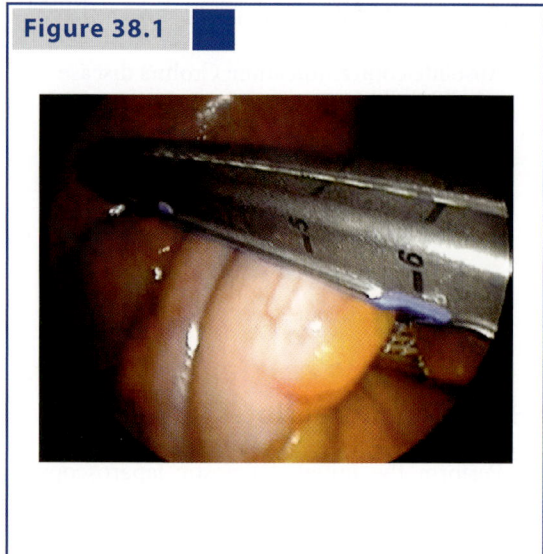

A window is made in the sigmoid mesentery and the sigmoid colon is divided using the EndoGIA™ stapler

Figure 38.2

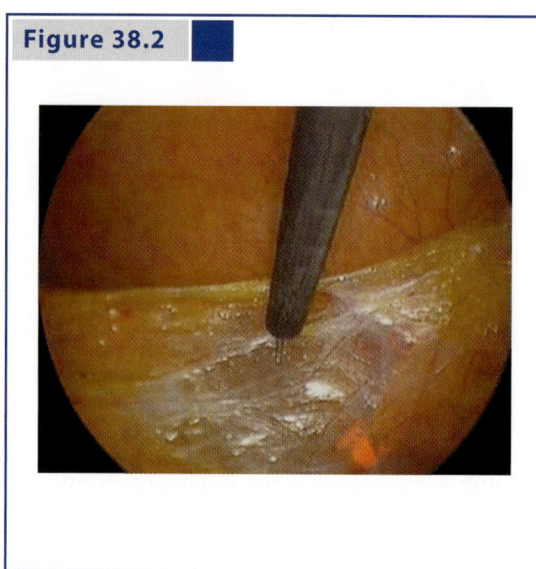

The lateral attachments of the descending colon are mobilized using the electrocautery

Figure 38.3

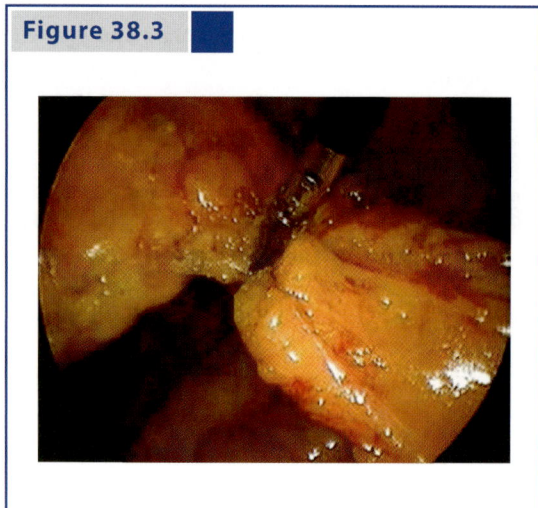

Starting from the sigmoid colon and moving from distal to proximal toward the right colon, the colonic mesentery is divided using the LigaSure™ device

Figure 38.4

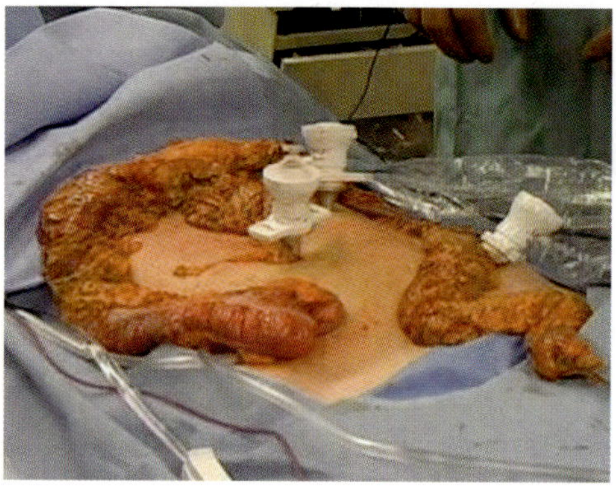

The colon is extracted through the right lower quadrant port site, and resected by using the Endo-GIA™ stapler to divide the ileum. If the pouch is to be created at a second operation, an end-ileostomy is sited at this time

Figure 38.5

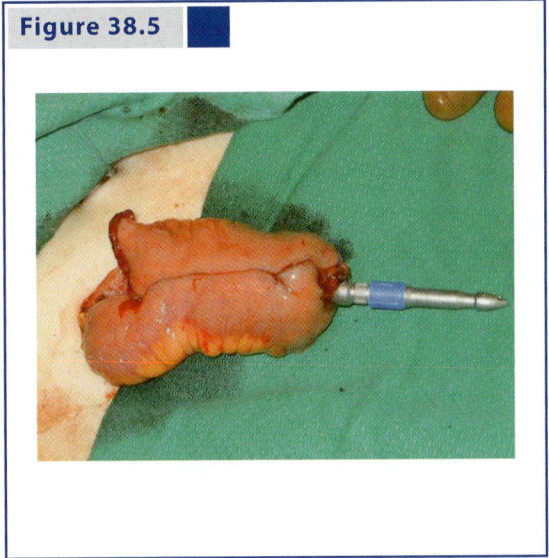

The ileal pouch is created using the EndoGIA™ stapler; the anvil from the EEA stapler is placed using a polypropylene purse-string suture

Figure 38.6

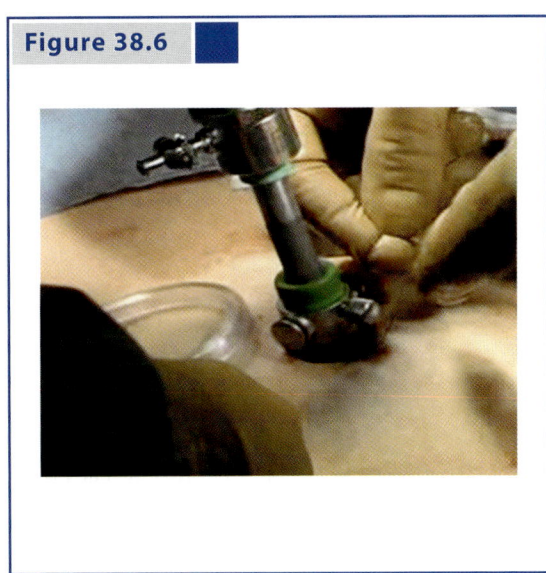

Once the pouch is returned to the abdomen, the right lower quadrant port site is closed by placement of a Hasson trocar

Figure 38.7

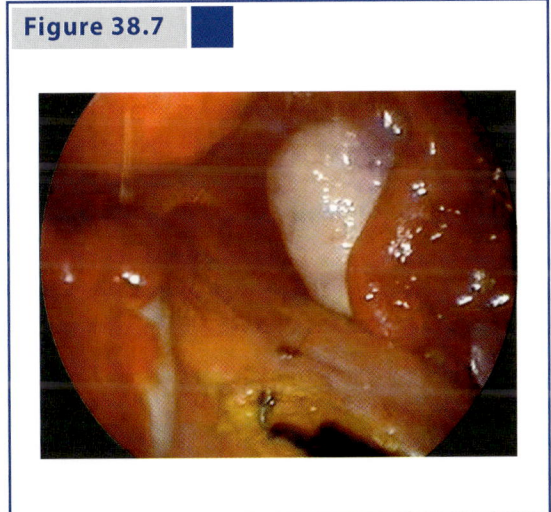

Starting from the sigmoid stump, the dissection of the rectosigmoid is completed using the LigaSure™ for the mesentery, and the electrocautery to divide the peritoneal reflection

Figure 38.8

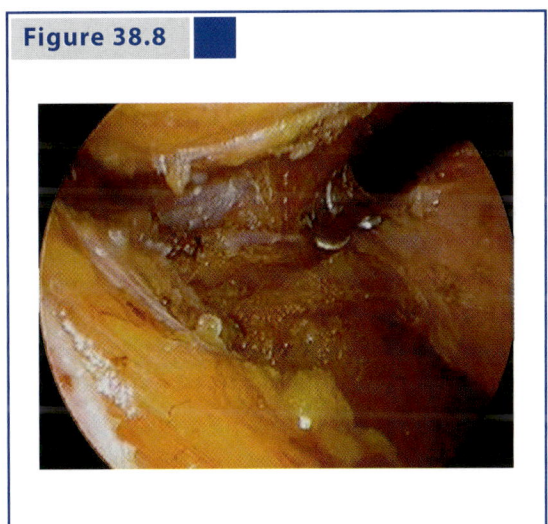

Dissection of the rectum is continued down to the pelvic floor, taking great care to stay immediately on the rectal wall. At this point the patient is placed in the lithotomy position to facilitate pouch–anal anastomosis

Figure 38.9

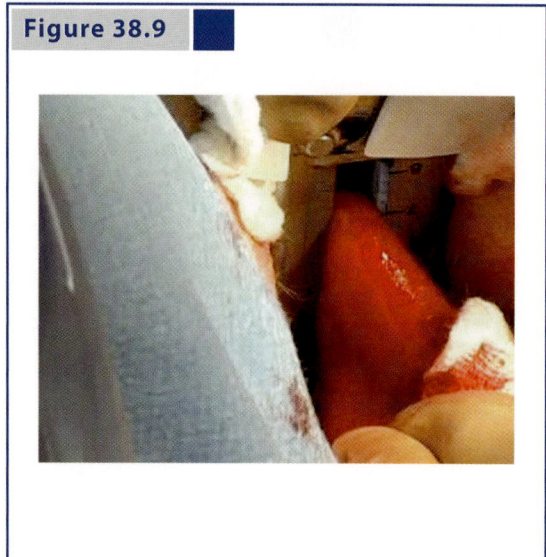

Figure 38.10

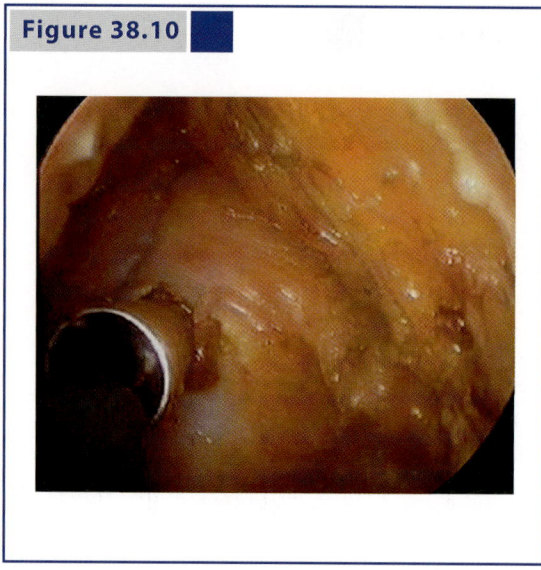

Using a Babcock forceps placed into the rectum, the rectal stump is everted. The specimen is then resected 1 cm above the dentate line using an EndoGIA™ stapler. This avoids interference with the transitional mucosa that is important in maintaining continence, and also avoids leaving an excessive amount of rectal mucosa

The circular EEA stapler is advanced through the anus at the top of the staple line, with laparoscopic visualization

Figure 38.11

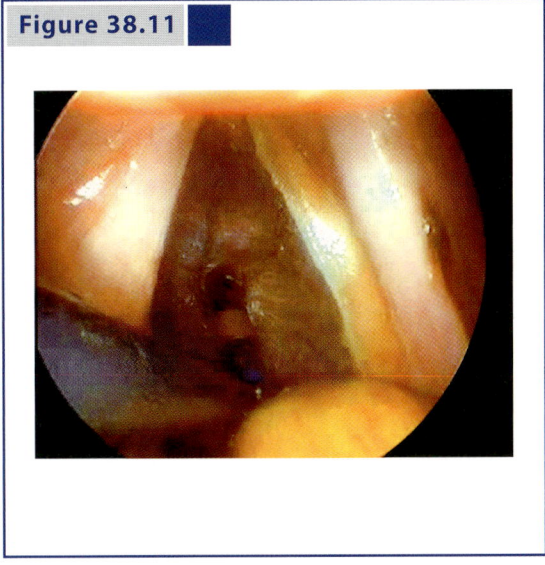

Figure 38.12

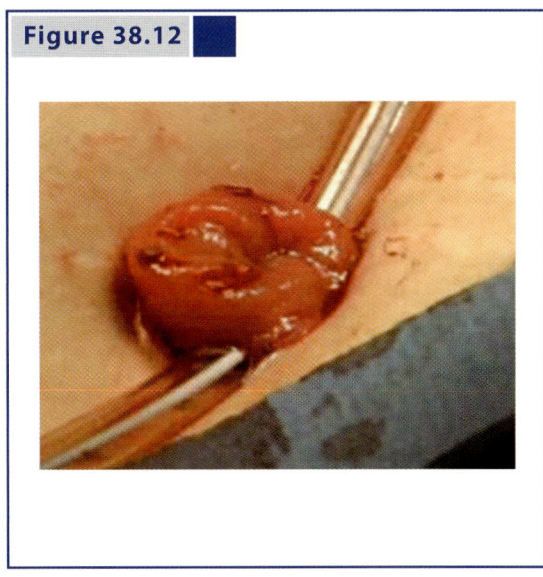

The pouch is advanced to the EEA stapler and anastomosed to the anus under direct laparoscopic visualization. The staple lines can be tested by filling the pelvis with saline and gently blowing air into the pouch. If there is a small leak, a drain can be placed into the pelvis through the left lower quadrant laparoscopic port site

A loop ileostomy is sited at the right lower quadrant port site

Recommended Literature

1. Georgeson KE (2002) Laparoscopic-assisted total colectomy with pouch reconstruction. Semin Pediatr Surg 11:233–236
2. Kienle P, Zgraggen K, Schmidt J, Benner A, Weitz J, Buchler MW (2005) Laparoscopic restorative proctocolectomy. Br J Surg 92:88–93
3. Proctor ML, Langer JC, Gerstle JT, Kim PC (2002) Is laparoscopic subtotal colectomy better than open subtotal colectomy in children? J Pediatr Surg 37:706–708

39 Duhamel-Martin Procedure for Hirschsprung's Disease

David C. van der Zee and Klaas N.M.A Bax

39.1   Operation Room Setup

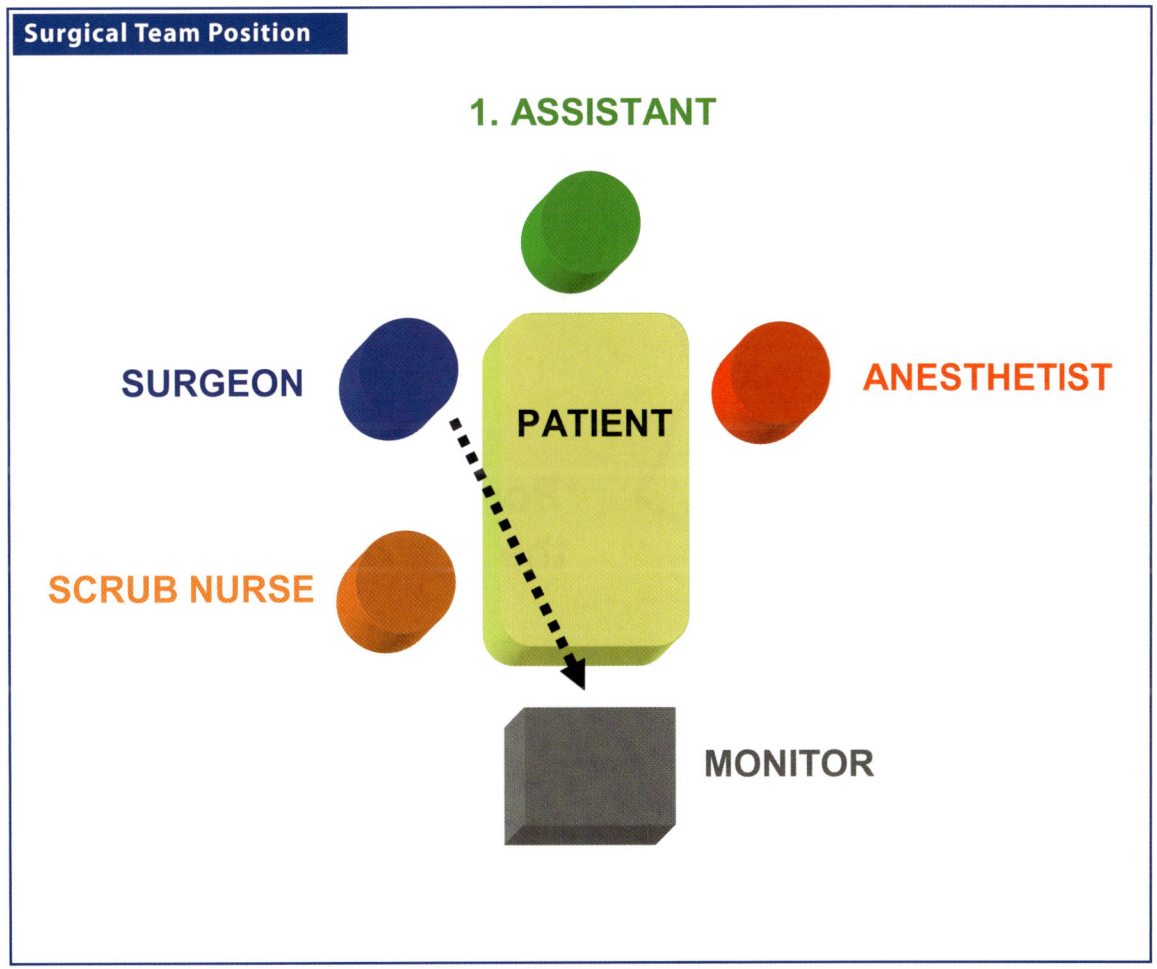

Surgical Team Position

1. ASSISTANT

SURGEON

ANESTHETIST

PATIENT

SCRUB NURSE

MONITOR

39.2   Patient Positioning

Supine position and placed transverse on a short operating table. The surgeon is standing at the upper right side of the patient.

39.3   Special Instruments

Endo GIA™ stapler (Auto Suture, Norwalk, CT, USA).

39.4   Location of Access Points

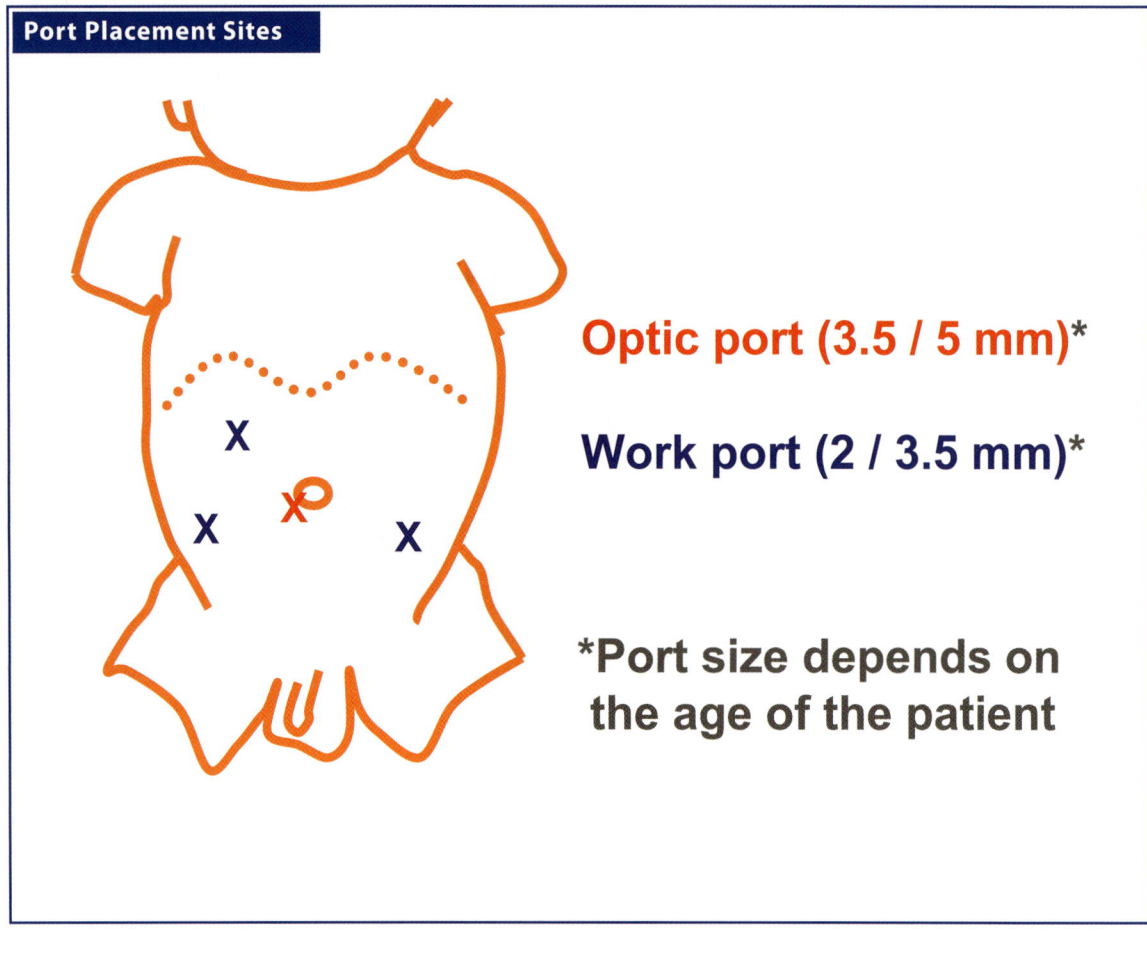

Port Placement Sites

Optic port (3.5 / 5 mm)*

Work port (2 / 3.5 mm)*

*Port size depends on the age of the patient

39.5   Indications

1. Hirschsprung's disease.
2. Extended Hirschsprung's disease.

39.6   Contraindications

None.

39.7   Preoperative Considerations

1. Antegrade intestinal washout should be performed on the day prior to surgery.
2. Repeat the rectal washout on the operating table before commencement of the procedure.
3. Drape the patient in such a way so that his/her legs can be maneuvered up and down.
4. Place a urine catheter after draping.
5. Perioperative antibiotics should be administered.

39.8   Technical Notes

1. Always place a suture over the biopsy site to avoid contamination.
2. When using monopolar diathermy, care should be taken not to cause collateral damage to the intestines and the vas deferens.
3. Precaution should be taken not to twist the intestine when pulling through.
4. Where the patient has an enterostomy, this can be closed during this procedure.

39.9   Procedure Variations

1. Instead of ligating and transecting the colon before pulling through, the intestine can also be exvaginated transanally and transected extracorporeally.
2. In the case of extended Hirschsprung's disease a somewhat longer rectal stump can be left in place with a side-to-side anastomosis, as reported by Duhamel-Martin.

39.10   Laparoscopic Duhamel-Martin Procedure

Please see Figs. 1–11.

Figure 39.1

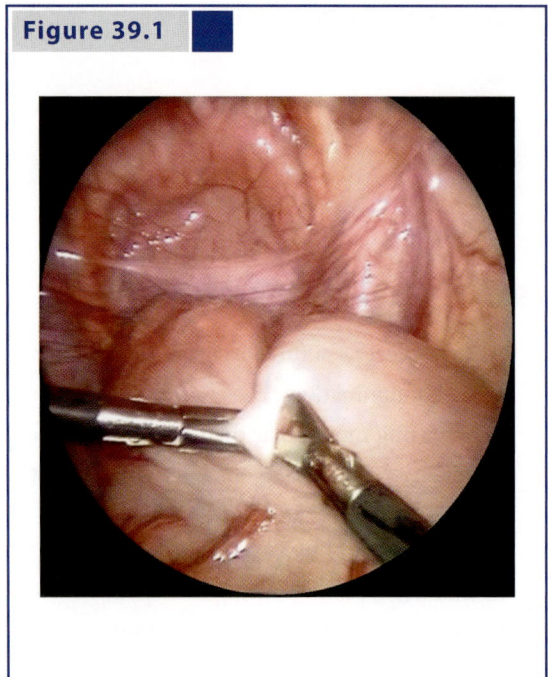

Figure 39.2

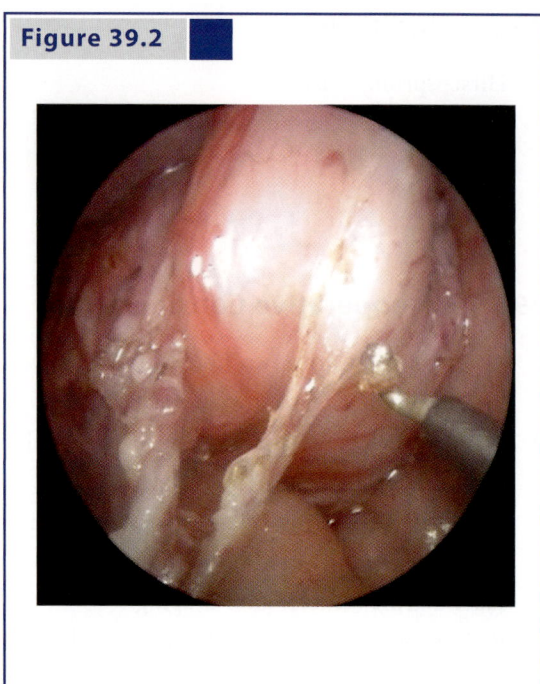

The first step is to take extramucosal biopsy samples and to determine the level of aganglionosis. Usually one sample is taken from the transition zone and one from the more proximal "normal-looking" bowel

After confirmation of the frozen section by the pathologist, the mesentery is dissected close to the bowel, from the pelvic floor up to the site of the most proximal biopsy

Figure 39.3

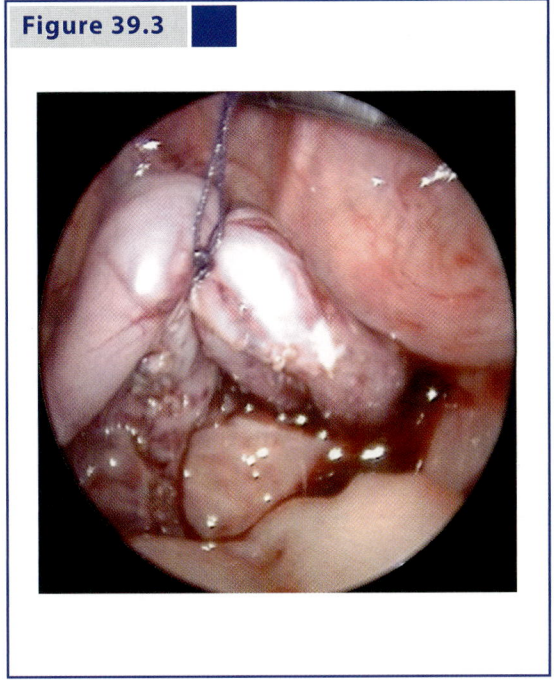

Figure 39.4

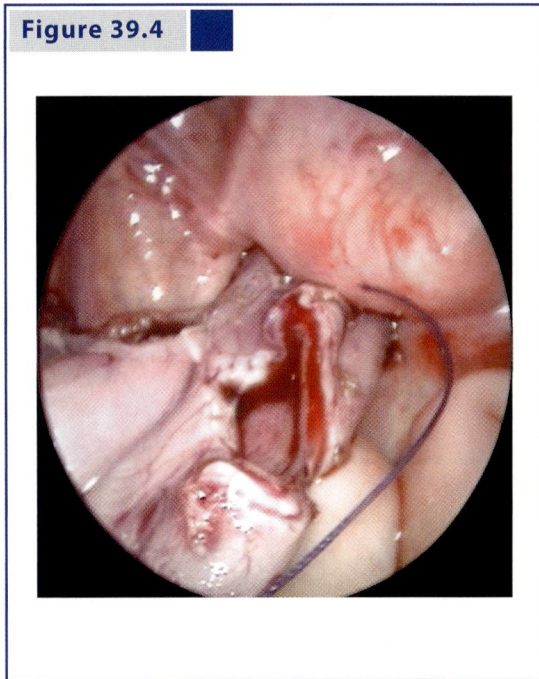

A ligature is placed around the dissected bowel to avoid spillage during the pull-through

The distal rectum is cleaned and residual contents are aspirated again before the bowel is transected

Figure 39.5

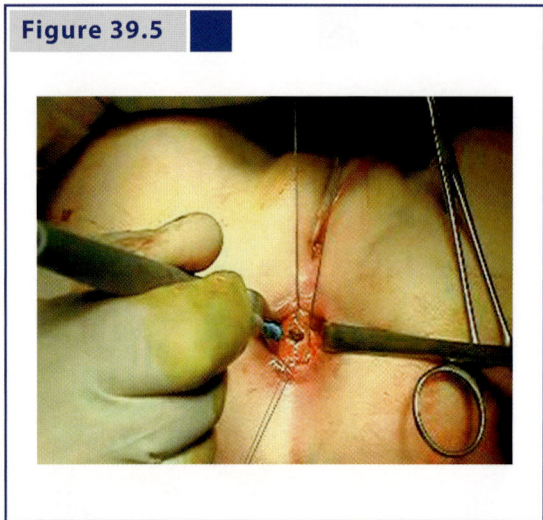

The anal phase is started with incision of the posterior wall of the rectum 0.5 cm proximal to the dentate line. Stay-sutures are placed at the anterior side of the incision and at the lateral corners for traction

Figure 39.6

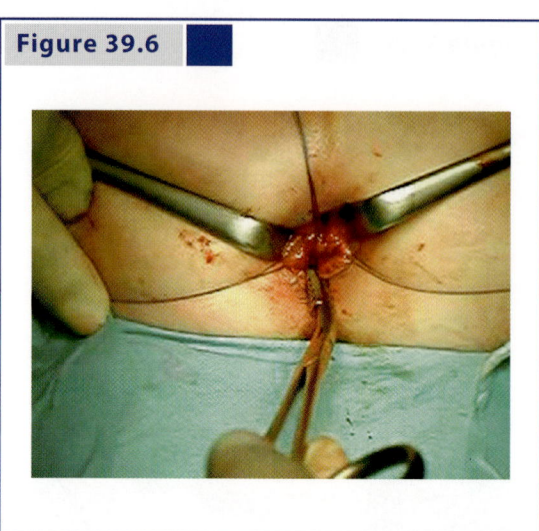

A grasping clamp is attached to a pulled-through endoscopic instrument and introduced into the abdomen

Figure 39.7

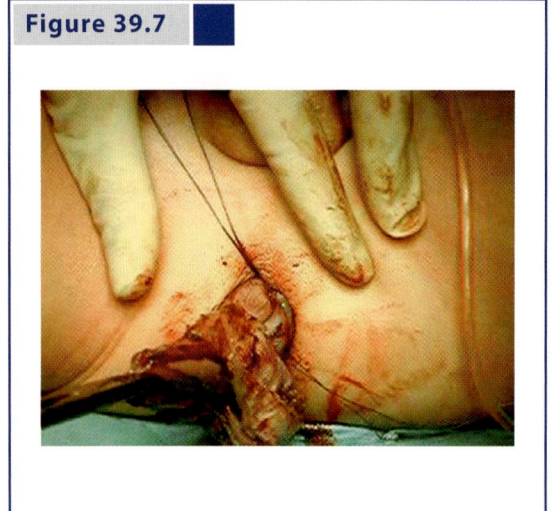

The transected colon (up to the level of the proximal biopsy sampling point) is pulled out through the posterior opening in the anus under close endoscopic control so that the bowel does not twist

Figure 39.8

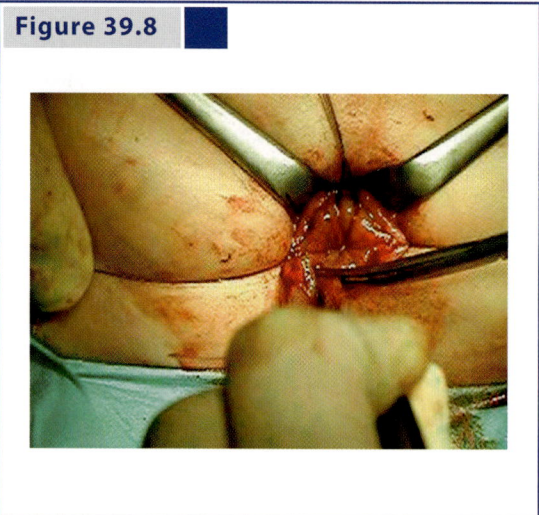

The bowel is resected at this point. After trimming, the pulled-through bowel is anastomosed to the anus

Figure 39.9

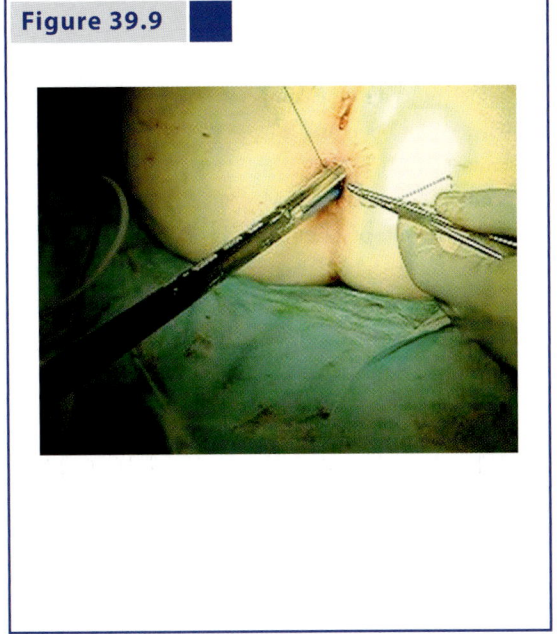

Figure 39.10

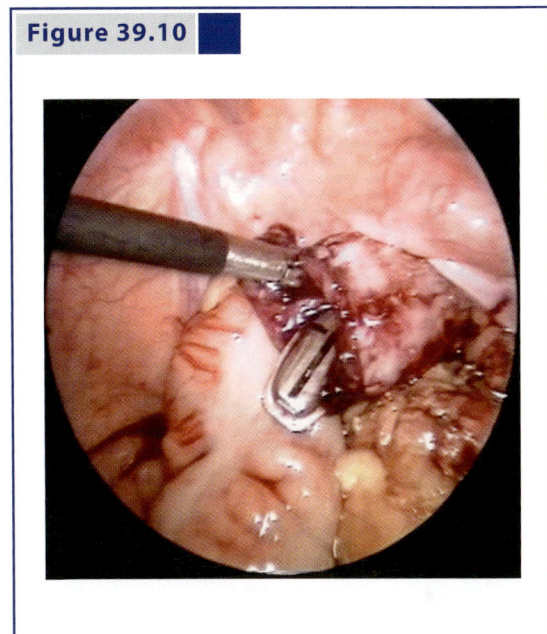

Keeping the stay-sutures under traction, an En-doGIA™ stapler can be introduced with one leg in the "old" rectum and one leg in the pulled-through bowel

Under endoscopic control, the right position of the EndoGIA™ stapler can be determined before firing the device. Usually two cartridges are necessary to complete the side-to-side anastomosis

Figure 39.11

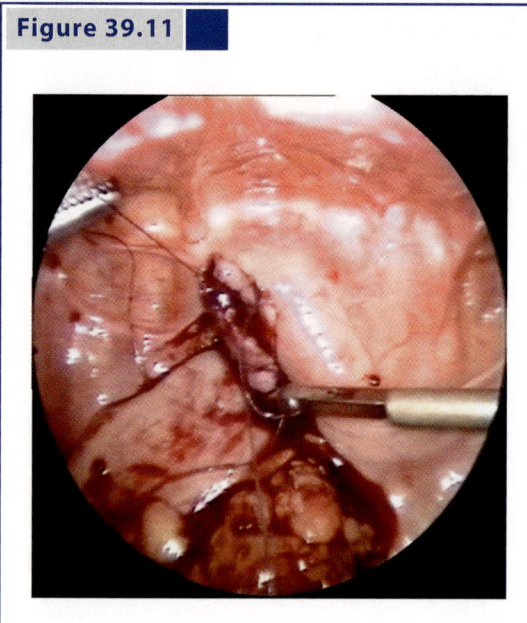

Recommended Literature

1. Travassos DV, Bax NM, van der Zee DC (2007) Duhamel procedure: a comparative retrospective study between an open and a laparoscopic technique. Surg Endosc 21:2163–2165
2. Mattioli G, Castagnetti M, Martucciello G, Jassoni V (2004) Results of a mechanical Duhamel pull-through for the treatment of Hirschsprung's disease and intestinal neuronal dysplasia. J Pediatr Surg 39:1349–1355
3. Minford JL, Ram A, Turnock RR, Lamont GL, Kenny SE, Rintala RJ, Lloyd DA, Baillie CT (2004) Comparison of functional outcomes of Duhamel and transanal endorectal coloanal anastomosis for Hirschsprung's disease. J Pediatr Surg 39:161–165

Finally, the rectal stump can be closed using one or two running sutures. If necessary, the stump can be trimmed to an appropriate size before closure

40 Pull-Through for High Imperforate Anus

M ARIO L IMA AND S TEFANO T URSINI

40.1 Operation Room Setup

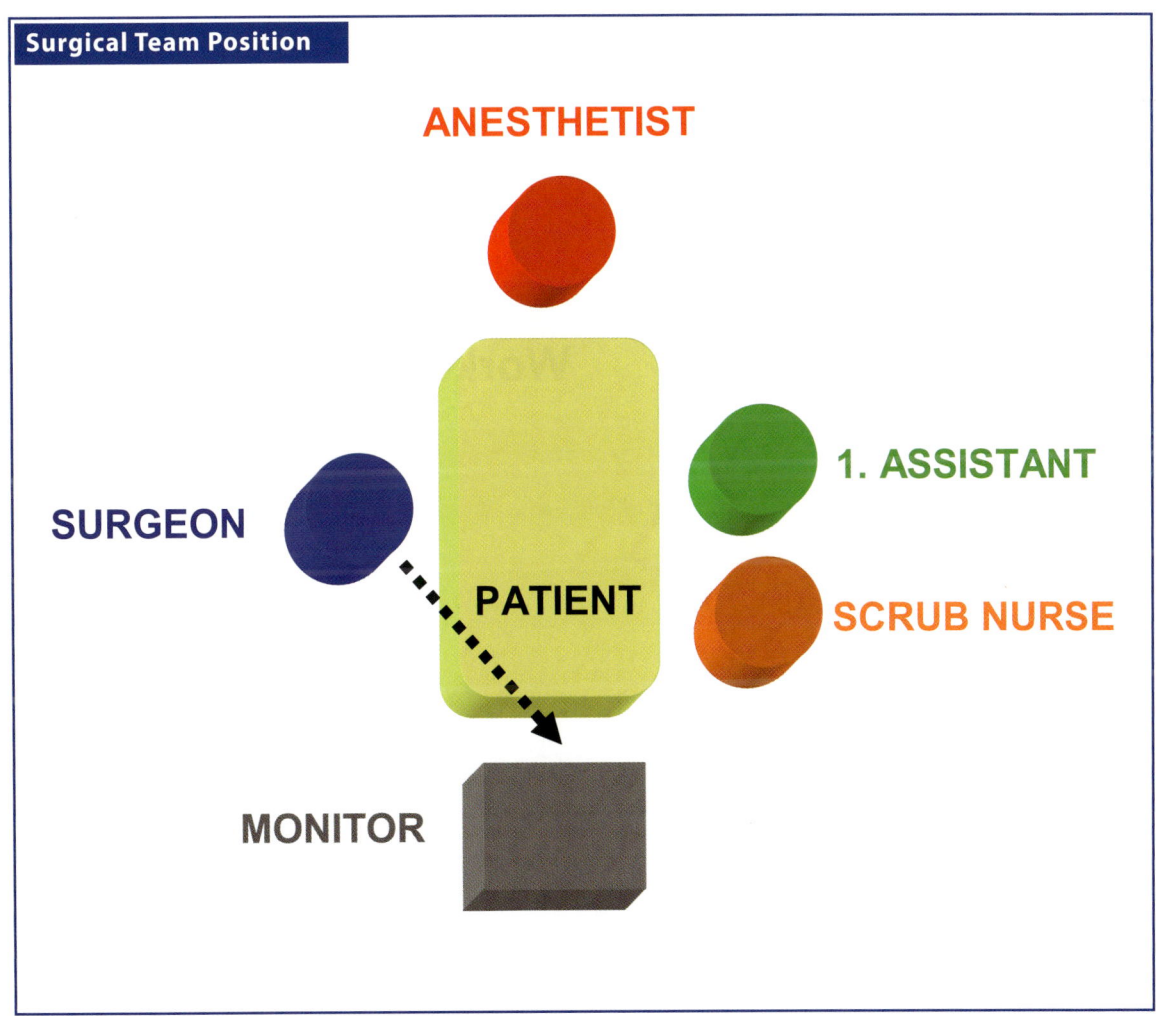

40.2   Patient Positioning

Supine, 30° Trendelenburg with a slight rotation of the table to the right. The patient is prepared and draped from chest to toes with legs in a light gynecological position; the buttocks are free for the secondary perineal approach.

40.3   Special Instruments

Transcutaneous muscle electrostimulator.

40.4   Location of Access Points

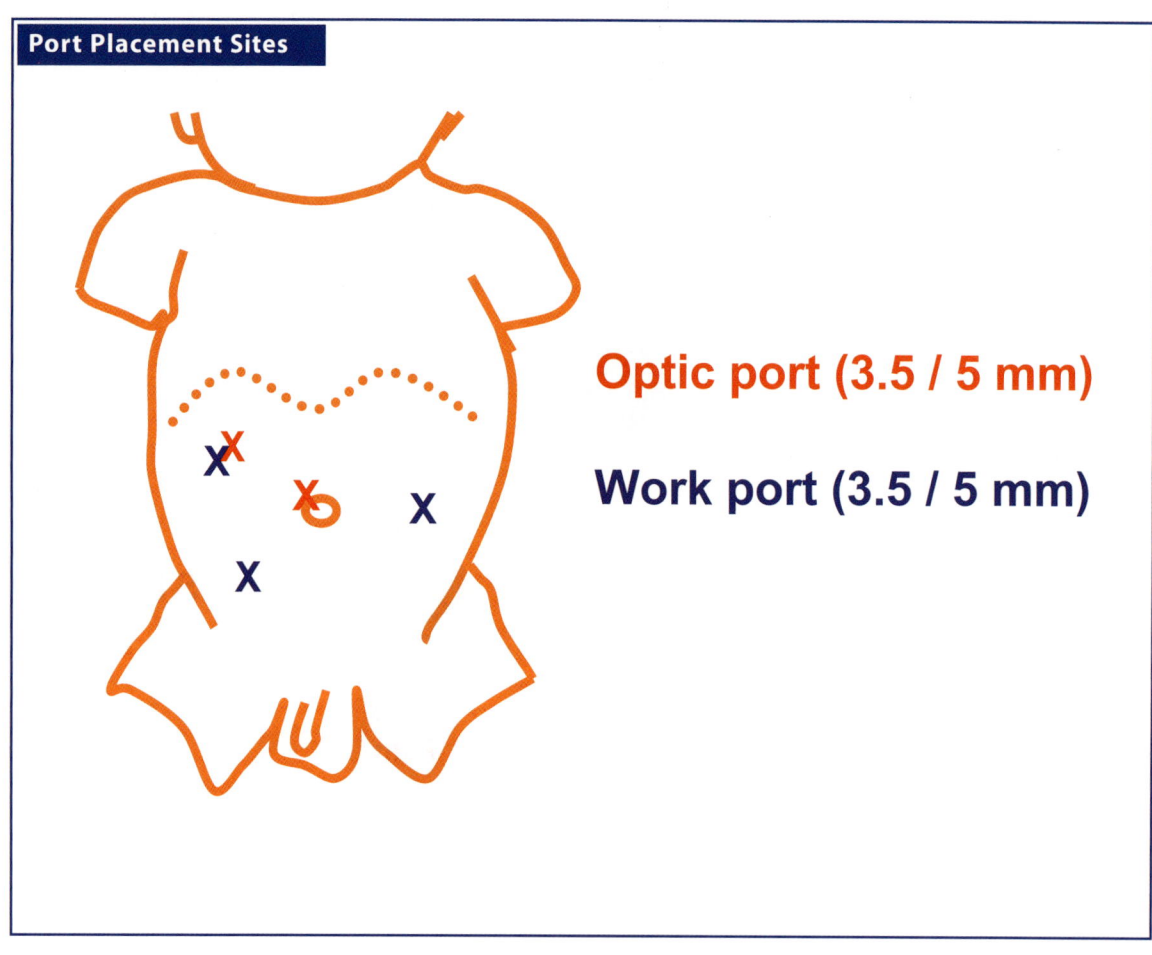

Port Placement Sites

Optic port (3.5 / 5 mm)

Work port (3.5 / 5 mm)

40.5   Indications

High imperforate anus in males or females either with fistula or without fistula.

40.6   Contraindications

General contraindications to laparoscopic surgery.

40.7   Technical Notes

1. The (3-mm) optic is positioned in the umbilicus. After the operative ports are inserted, the (5-mm) optic is moved to the right.
2. Precaution should be taken with colostomy positioning. A short distal pouch is difficult to pull through.
3. The fistula should be dissected and sectioned as distally as possible. It is preferably closed with a transfix suture. It is also recommended to leave a urethral tutor in place.
4. Mapping of the perineal area with a transcutaneous muscle electrostimulator is mandatory.
5. The laparoscopic view confirms the passage of the pull-through between the bellies of the pubococcygeus muscles.

40.8   Preoperative Considerations

1. A left-loop colostomy is performed at birth.
2. Decompression of the sigmoid tract is an advantage; it can allow an accurate evaluation of the fistula.
3. Associated malformations should be studied accurately.
4. The bladder should be empty (catheterization or Credé's maneuver).

40.9   Procedure Variations

1. Single-stage procedure without a diverting colostomy.
2. Veress needle is an option for pneumoperitoneum.
3. The bladder can be elevated using a transfix suture to the anterior abdominal plane.
4. A clip can be used to close the fistula distally.
5. Alternatively, the distal fistula can be left open with a urethral tutor.

40.10   Laparoscopic Step – Anorectal Pullthrough

Please see Figs. 1–6.

Figure 40.1

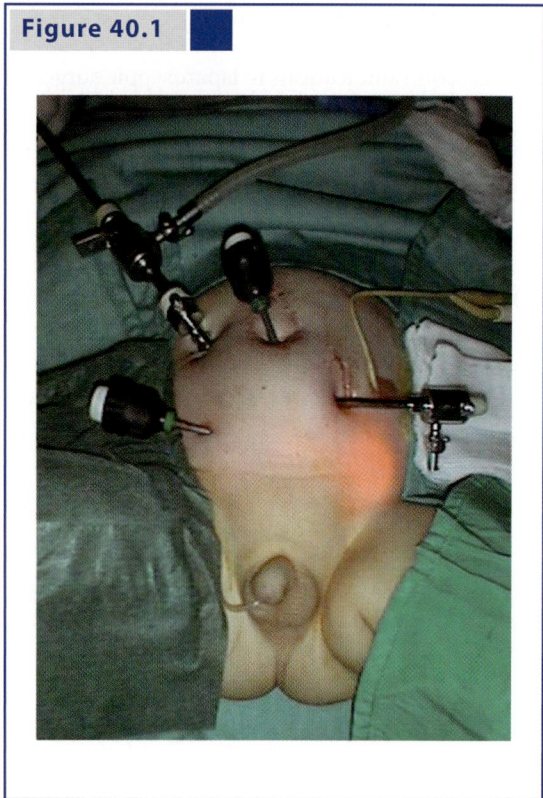

The patient in positioned in a 30° supine position. The optic is moved from the umbilicus to the right

Figure 40.2

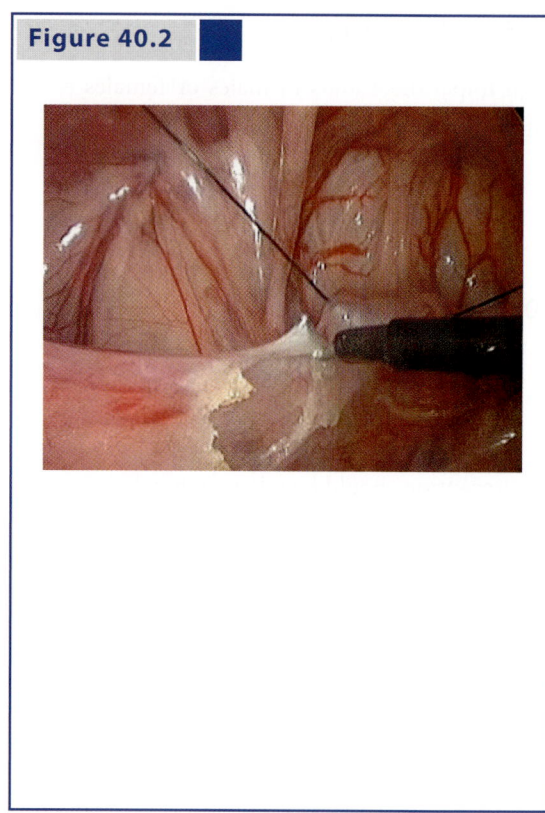

The peritoneum is opened and dissected to reach the fistula

Figure 40.3

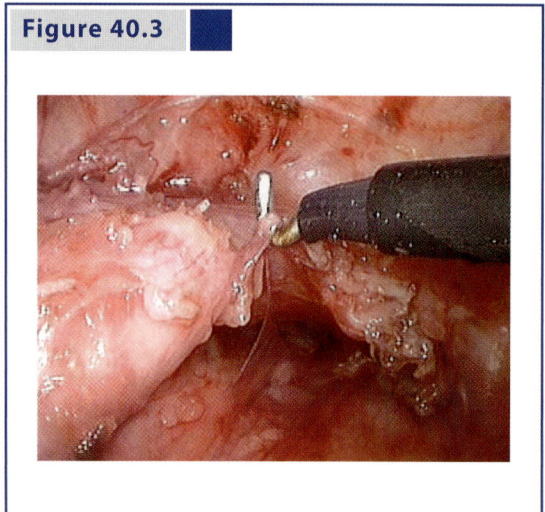

The fistula is located and grasped and the vessels are exposed and dissected with a monopolar hook

Figure 40.4

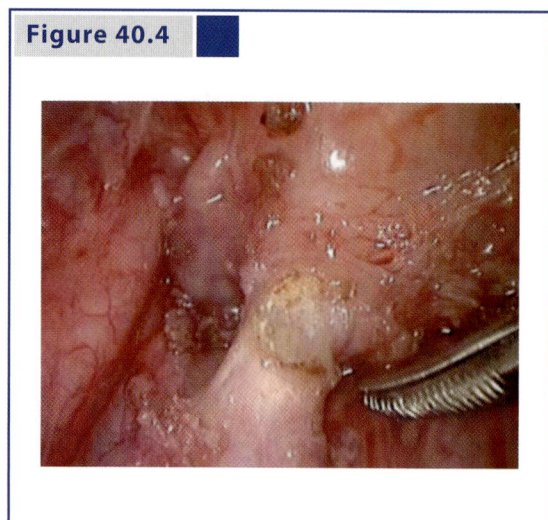

After careful dissection, the fistula is clearly exposed

Figure 40.5

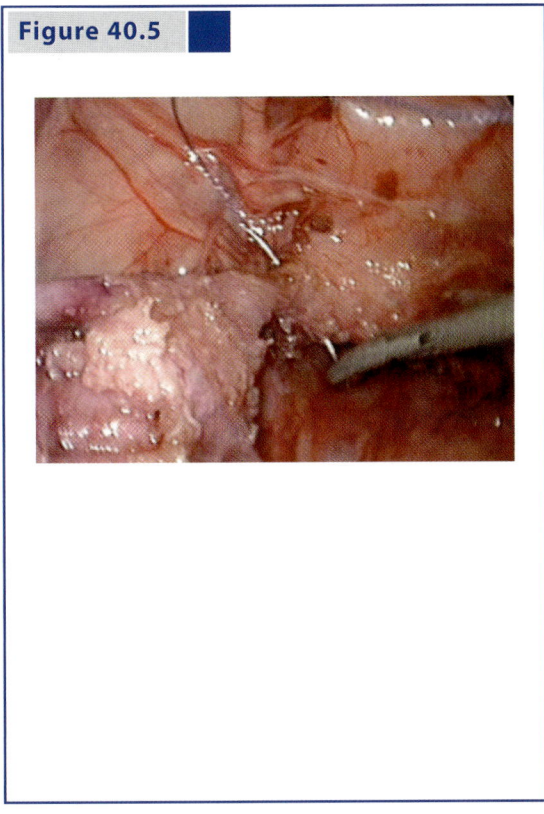

Figure 40.6

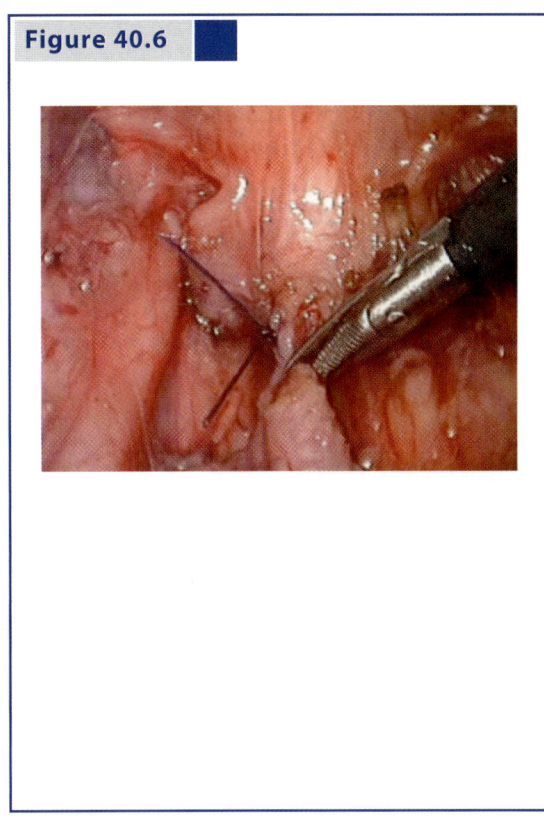

Ligation of the fistula is performed as distally as possible with a transfix absorbable suture

Scissors are used to section the ligated fistula

40.11   Perineal Step – Anorectal Pullthrough

40.11.1   Patient Position

Supine with legs in a light gynecological position to expose the perineal plane. The surgeon moves to the perineal plane.

Please see Figs. 7–13.

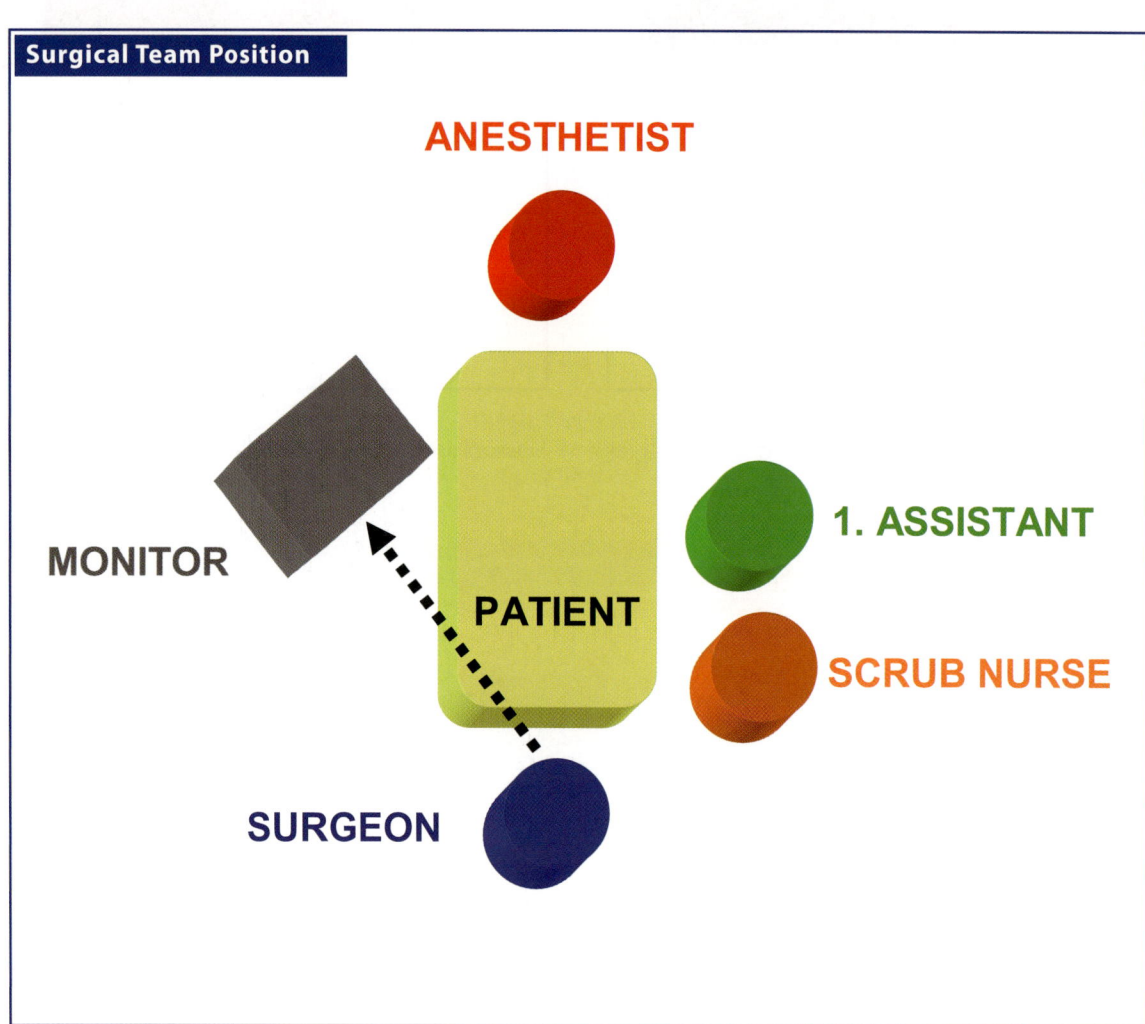

Figure 40.7

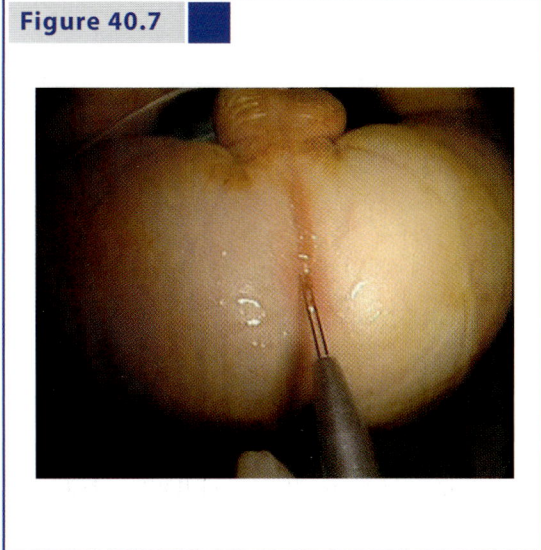

Mapping of the perineal area is performed with an transcutaneous muscle electrostimulator. The center of maximum contraction and cephalad elevation is identified as the location of the new-anus

Figure 40.8

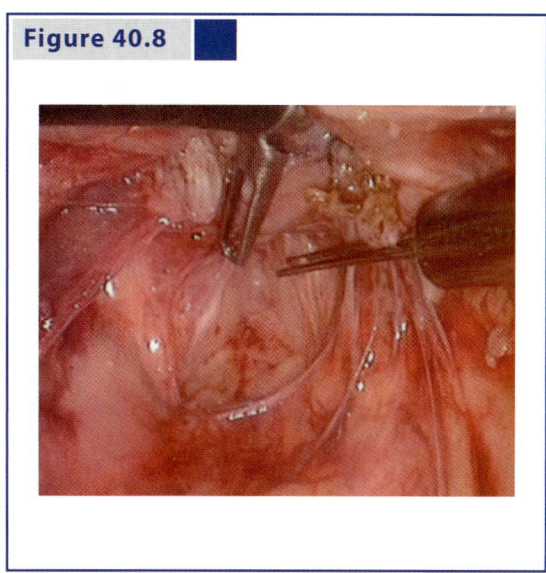

The pubococcygeus bellies are identified using a laparoscopic muscle electrostimulator with the current at an intensity of 60 mA

Figure 40.9

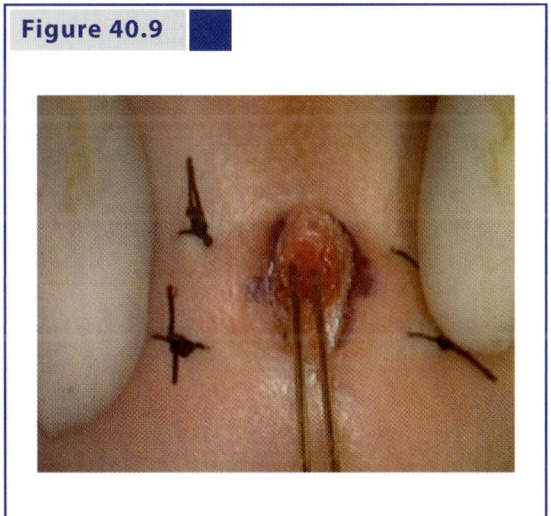

A vertical incision is made in the perineal area and a trocar is passed through the defined plane in the external sphincter muscle complex

Figure 40.10

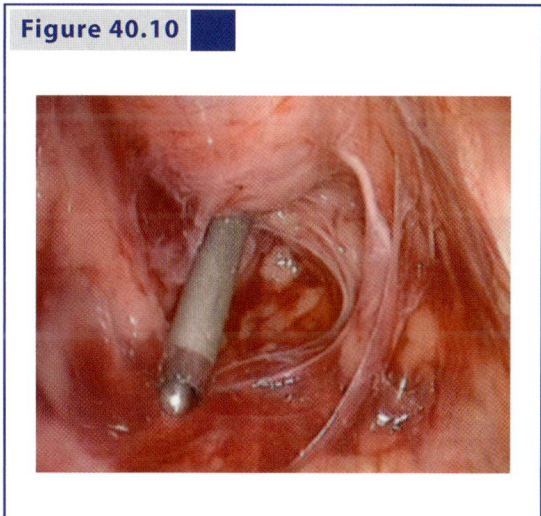

The trocar is advanced into the pelvis between the bellies of the pubococcygeus muscles

Figure 40.11

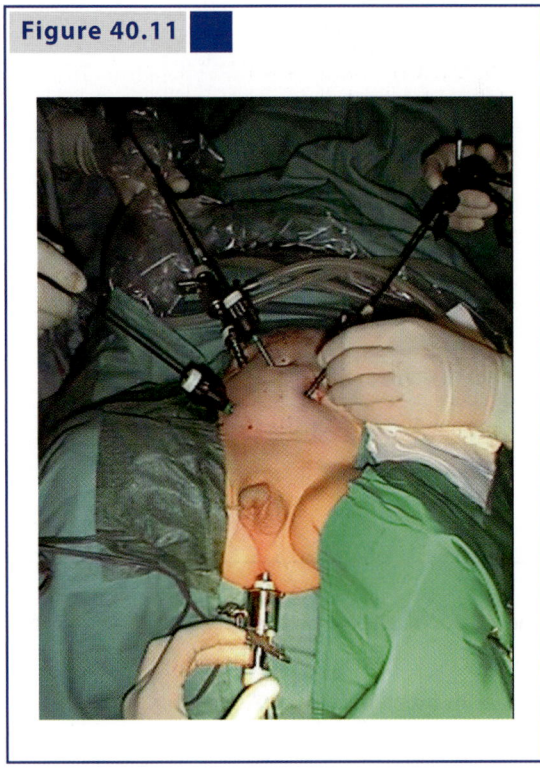

View of the "perineal" trocar at the point of insertion

Figure 40.12

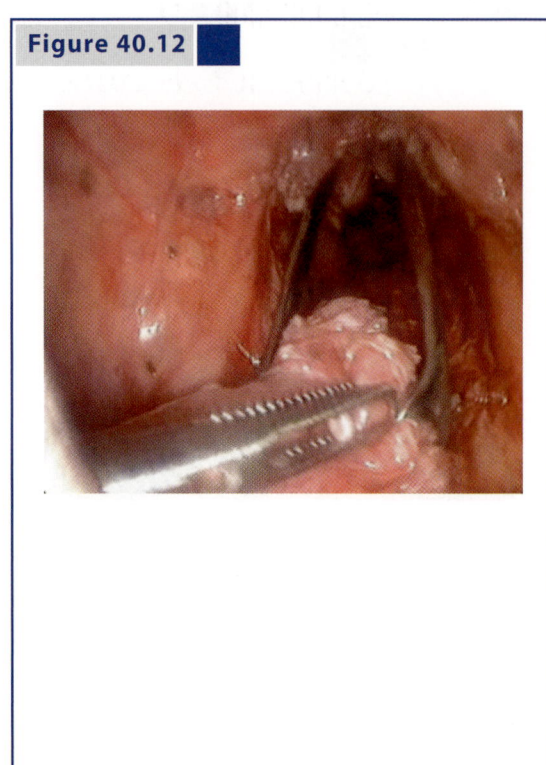

The rectal fistula is grasped and pulled through the incision to be exteriorized to the perineum

Figure 40.13

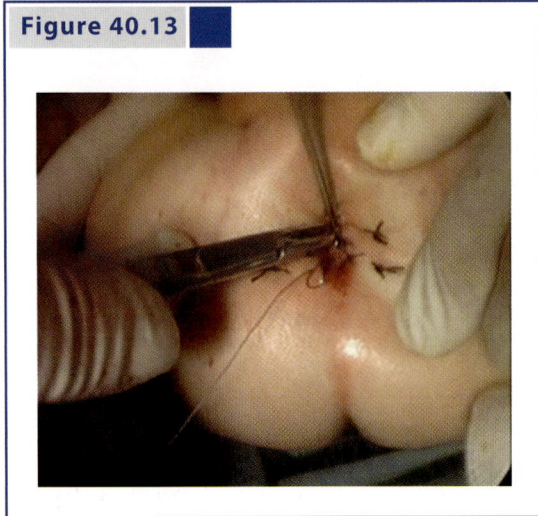

The rectum is sutured to the anus with interrupted 4-0 absorbable suture (Vicryl™; Ethicon, Somerville, NJ, USA)

Recommended Literature

1. Georgeson KE, Inge TH, Albanese CT (2000) Laparoscopically assisted anorectal pull-through for high imperforate anus – a new technique. J Pediatr Surg 35:927–930
2. Iwanaka T, Arai M, Kawashima H, Kudou S, Fujishiro J, Matsui A, Imaizumi S (2003) Findings of pelvic musculature and efficacy of laparoscopic muscle stimulator in laparoscopy-assisted anorectal pull-through for high imperforate anus. Surg Endosc 17:278–281
3. Lima M, Tursini S, Ruggeri G, Aquino A, Gargano T, De Biagi L, Ahmed A, Gentili A (2006) Laparoscopically assisted anorectal pull-through for high imperforate anus: three years experience. J Laparoendosc Adv Surg Tech A 16:63–66

41 Rectopexy

MUNTHER J. HADDAD AND AMULYA K. SAXENA

41.1   Operation Room Setup

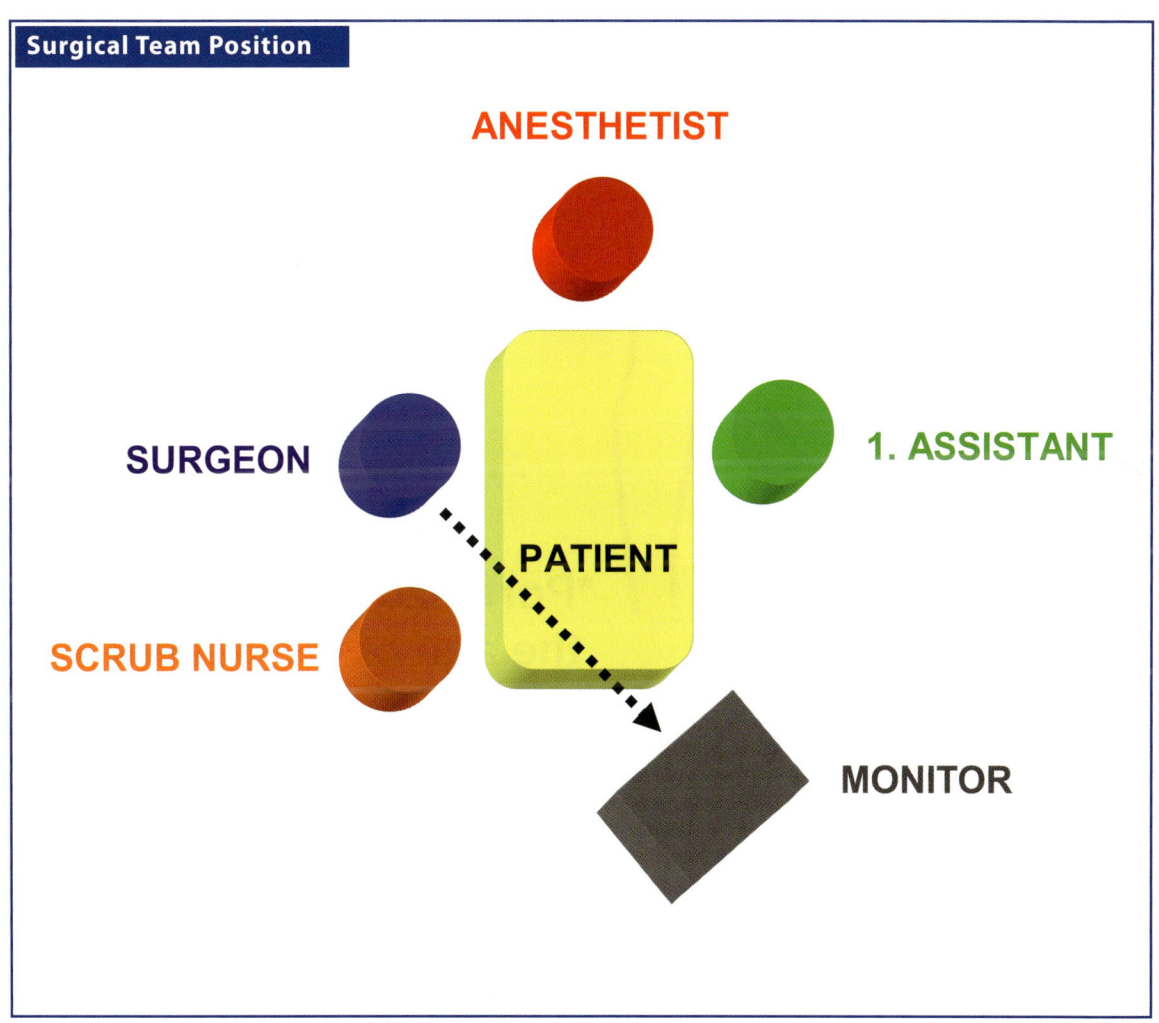

41.2   Patient Positioning

Supine position with arms tucked to the side.

41.3   Special Instruments

Polypropylene mesh.

41.4   Location of Access Points

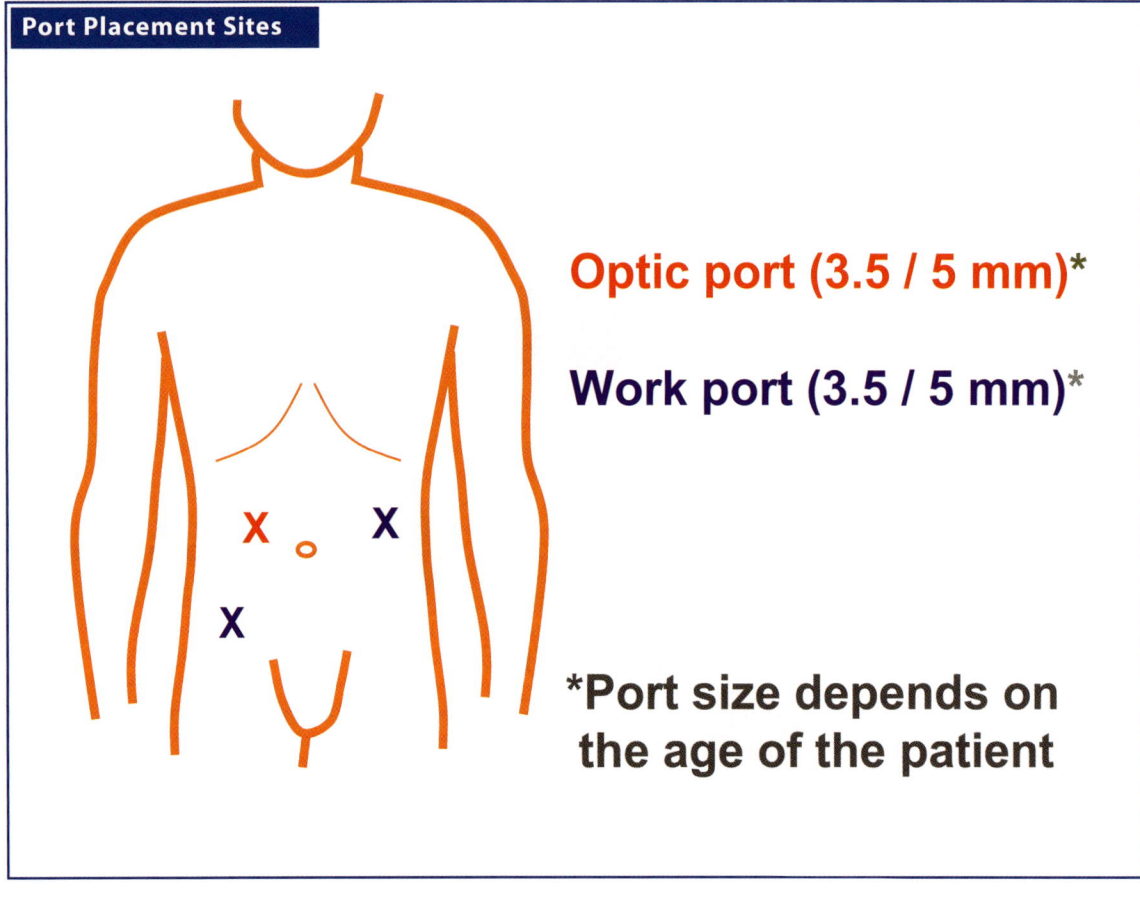

Port Placement Sites

Optic port (3.5 / 5 mm)*

Work port (3.5 / 5 mm)*

*Port size depends on the age of the patient

41.5 Indications

Severe rectal prolapse after failure of conservative management in:

1. Cystic fibrosis.
2. Chronic constipation.
3. Juvenile polyp (rare).

41.6 Contraindications

No absolute contraindication; however, only after failure of conservative therapy.

41.7 Preoperative Considerations

1. Bowel preparation is important to debulk the colon prior to surgery.
2. Preoperative antibiotics are administered: cefuroxime (30 mg/kg).
3. A nasogastric tube is placed to allow gastric decompensation.
4. A Foley catheter is placed for bladder drainage.

41.8 Technical Notes

1. Precaution must be taken when dissecting through the mesentery.
2. Care should be taken not to injure the ureters or the iliac vessels.
3. The sacral promontory, which is covered by a fascia, can be palpated as a hard, bone-like structure through which the sutures are placed.
4. Two sutures placed on either side of the colon must be placed at a distance of at least 2 cm from each other.

41.9 Procedure Variations

1. A polypropylene mesh is tacked to the presacral fascia under the colon with the aid of a hernia stapler. Care must be taken that the staples do not penetrate into the lumen of the bowel.
2. The retracted sigma colon is sutured to the left psoas muscle using nonabsorbable suture materials.
3. Perform a simple suture rectopexy with nonabsorbable sutures to secure the colon to the presacral fascia.

41.10 Laparoscopic Rectopexy Using Polypropylene Mesh

Please see Figs. 1–6.

Figure 41.1

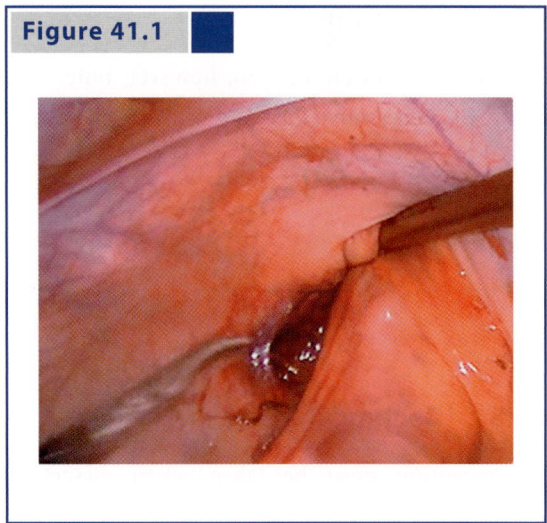

The rectosigmoid colon is retracted and the peritoneum is opened to facilitate sacral exposure

Figure 41.2

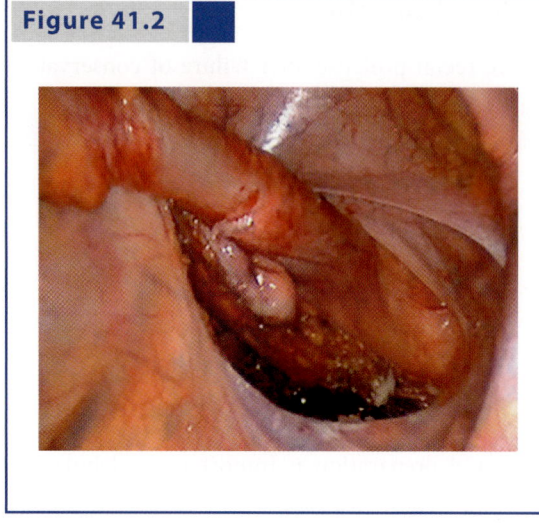

The peritoneum is incised circumferentially and care is take to avoid injury to the rectal vessels

Figure 41.3

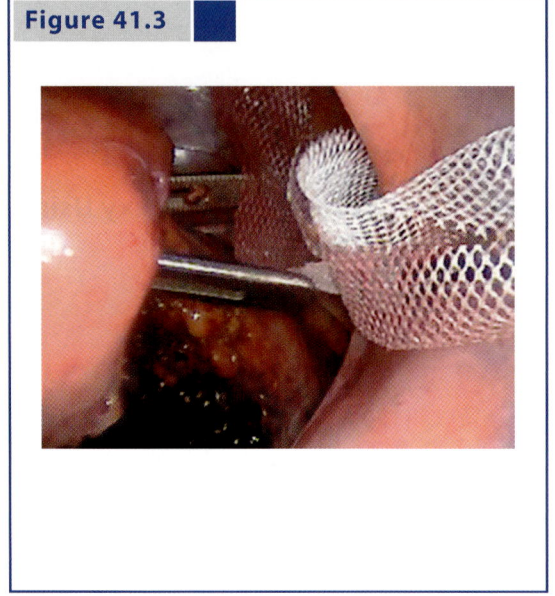

A grasper is passed behind the colon and a strip of polypropylene mesh is grasped and retrieved

Figure 41.4

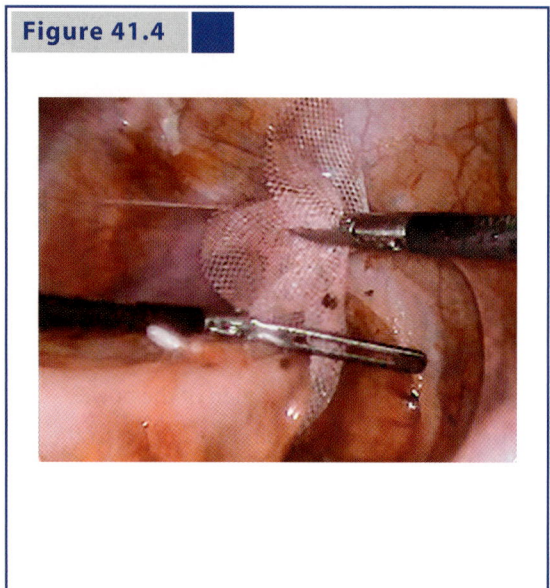

The polypropylene mesh is then wrapped around the rectum with the free end held upward

Figure 41.5

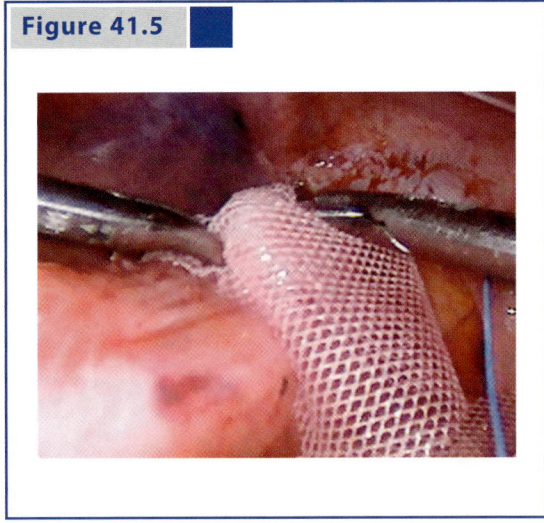

Figure 41.6

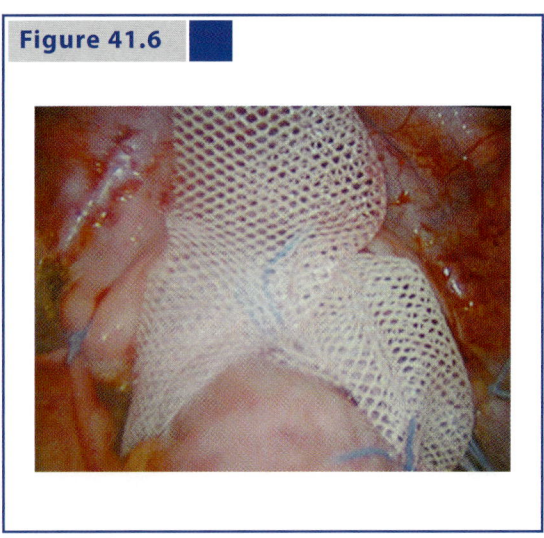

The bowel is held taut and the mesh is secured with sutures to the seromuscular bowel wall

Two sutures are placed on either side to secure the mesh to the sacral promontory fascia

41.11   Laparoscopic Suture Rectopexy

Please see Figs. 7–12.

Figure 41.7

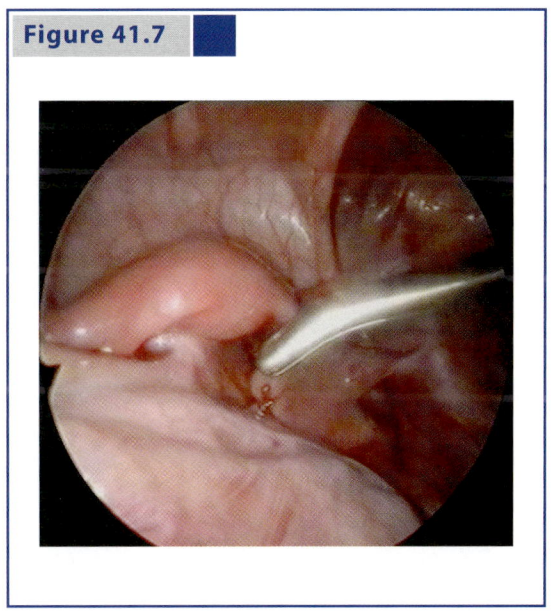

The rectosigmoid colon is retracted and the peritoneum lying over the sacrum is exposed

Figure 41.8

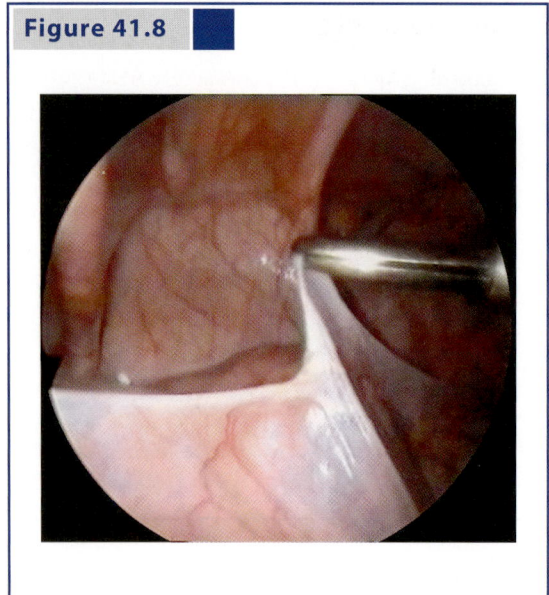

The peritoneum is raised and incised. This can be done using Metzenbaum scissors; electrocautery is not required

Figure 41.9

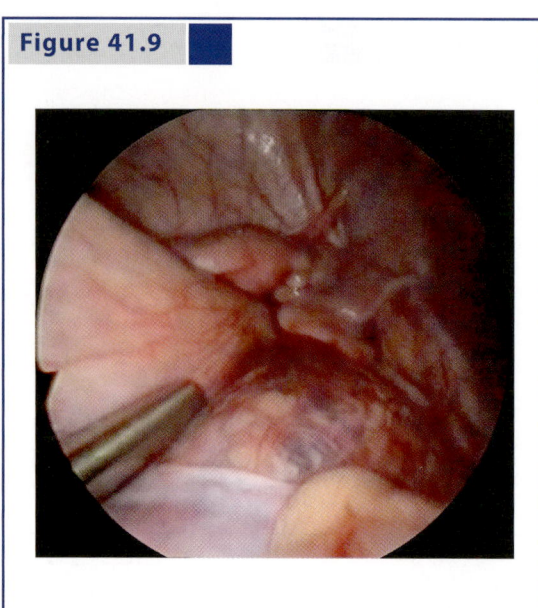

While the presacral facia is being exposed, care should be taken to identify the iliac vessels and the ureter

Figure 41.10

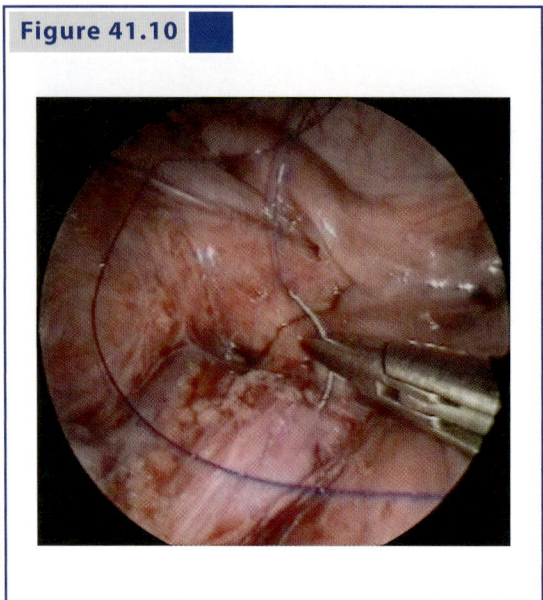

A nonabsorbable suture is passed through the presacral promontory fascia

Figure 41.11

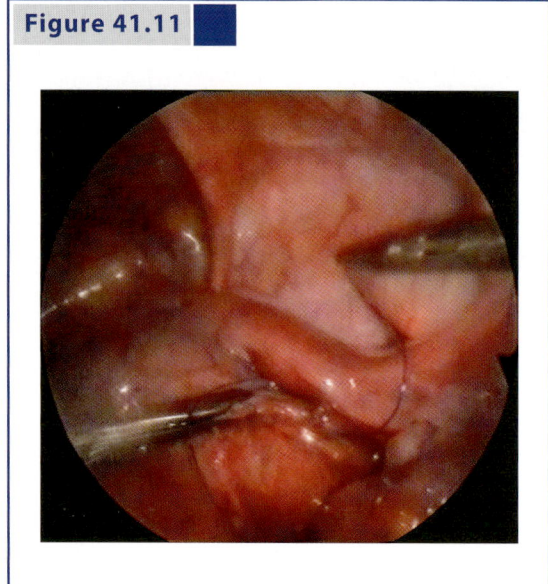

The bowel is held taut and the same suture is passed through the seromuscular layer of the rectosigmoid colon and the knot is tied

Figure 41.12

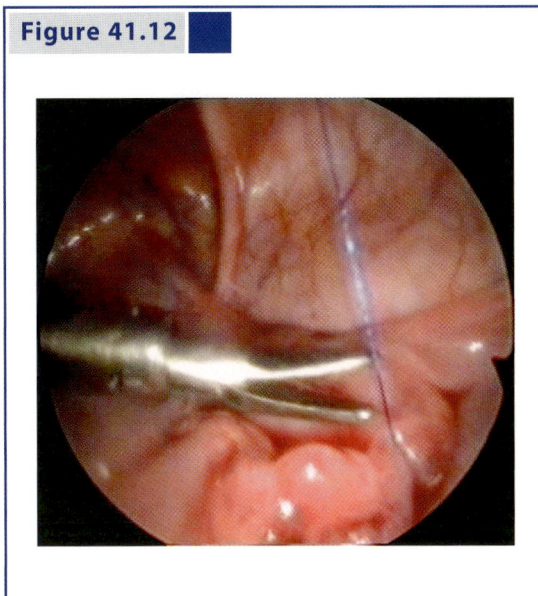

Two sutures are placed on either side to secure the rectosigmoid colon to the sacral promontory fascia

Recommended Literature

1. Bonnard A, Mougenot JP, Ferkdadji L, Huot O, Aigrain Y, De Lagausie P (2003) Laparoscopic rectopexy for solitary ulcer of rectum syndrome in a child. Surg Endosc 17:1156–1157

2. Koivusalo A, Pakarinen M, Rintala R (2006) Laparoscopic suture rectopexy in the treatment of persisting rectal prolapse in children: a preliminary report. Surg Endosc 20:960–963

3. Saxena AK, Metzelder ML, Willital GH (2004) Laparoscopic suture rectopexy for rectal prolapse in a 22-month-old child. Surg Laparosc Endosc Percutan Tech 14:33–34

42 Ventriculoperitoneal Shunt Implantation

Amulya K. Saxena and Hans G. Eder

42.1   Operation Room Setup

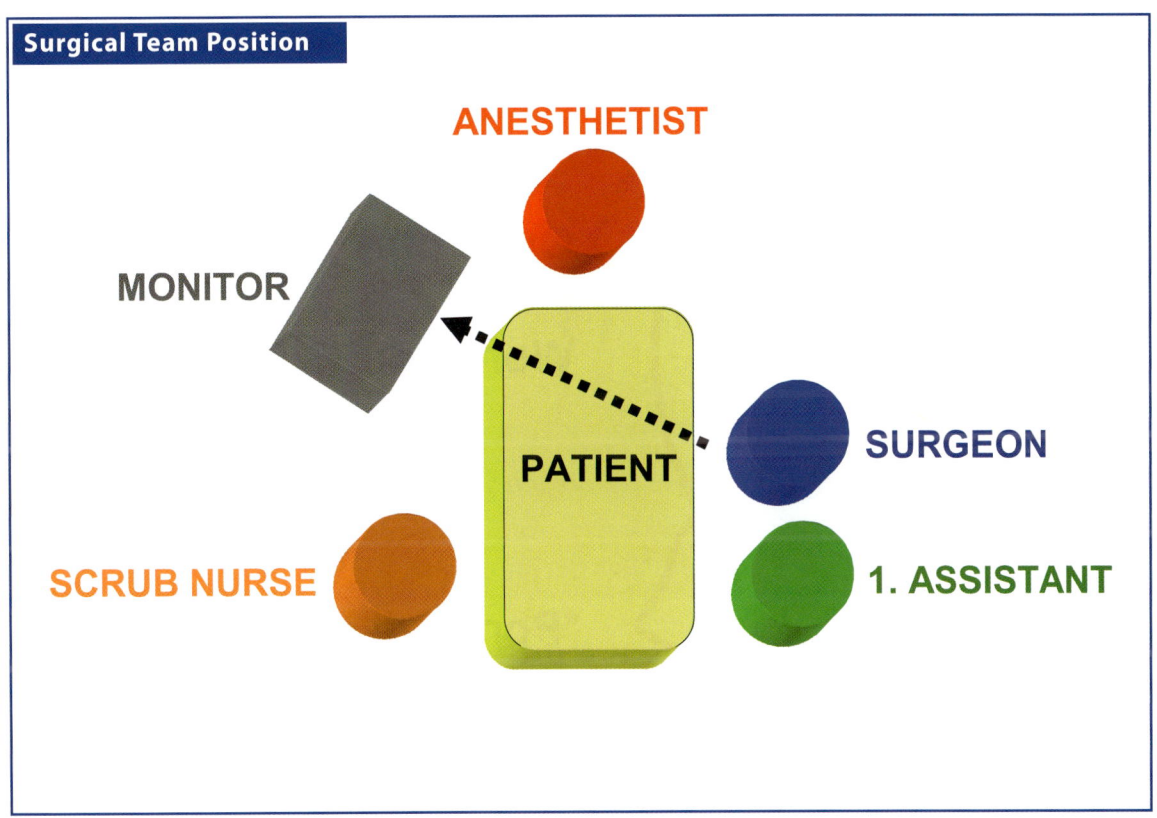

42.2   Patient Positioning

Supine position with arms tucked to the side.

42.3   Special Instruments

Ventriculoperitoneal shunt system.

42.4   Location of Access Points

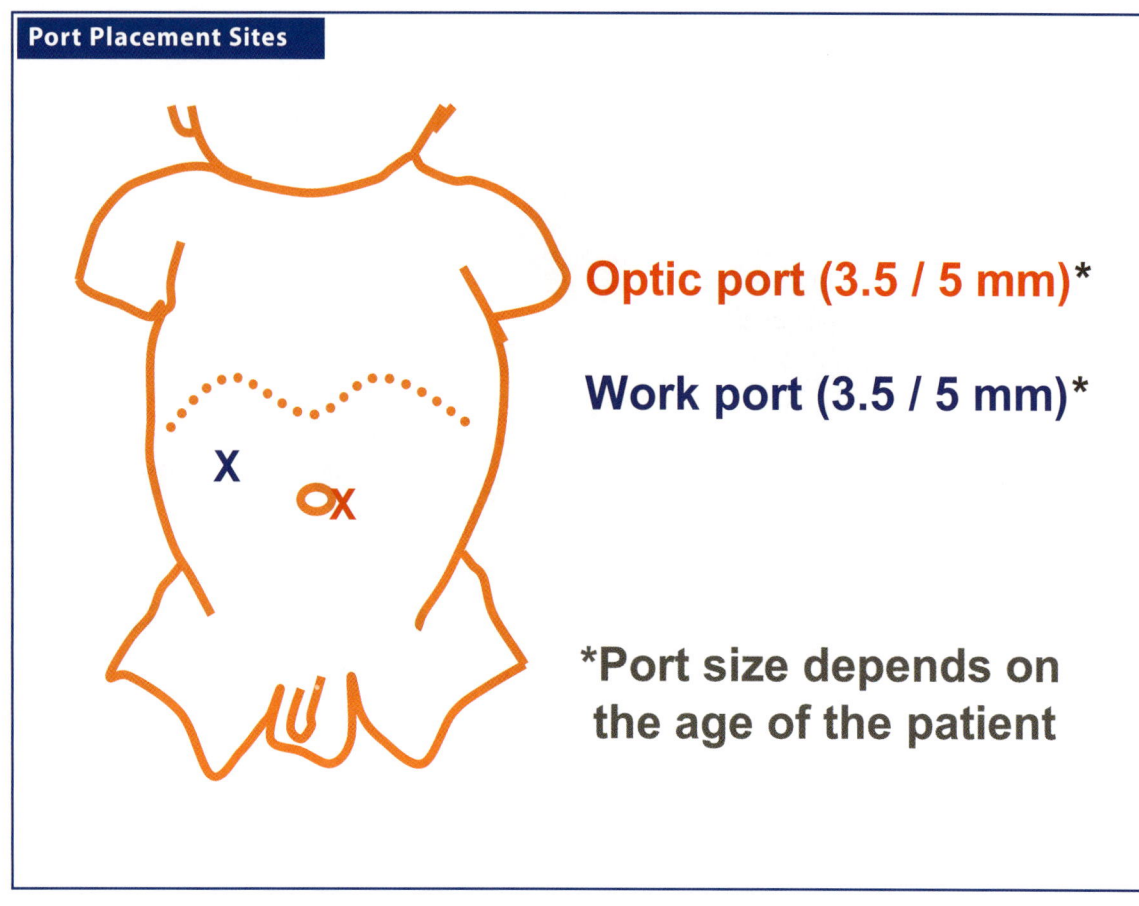

Port Placement Sites

Optic port (3.5 / 5 mm)*

Work port (3.5 / 5 mm)*

*Port size depends on the age of the patient

42.5   Indications

Communicating and noncommunicating forms of hydrocephalus in:

1. Intraventricular hemorrhage.
2. Inflammation.
3. Neoplastic diseases.
4. Congenital malformations.
5. Trauma-associated conditions.
6. Special indication is severe adhesions after prior abdominal surgery.

42.6   Relative Contraindications

Severe central nervous system malformations.

42.7   Preoperative Considerations

1. The patient is draped with the head and neck exposed on the side that the shunt is to be placed. The abdomen, however, is draped in a fashion suitable for abdominal procedures.
2. Consider rifampicin- or clindamycin-impregnated silicone shunts in complicated cases.
3. Antibiotics may be administered preoperatively.
4. Efforts should be taken to avoid hypothermia during surgery in infants.
5. The scalp is shaved at the site of intended catheter placement.

42.8   Technical Notes

1. Care is taken to minimize handling of the shunt throughout the entire surgical procedure.
2. In the case of abdominal adhesions, two ports are introduced and the adhesions are removed using conventional laparoscopic methods.
3. Using a port (peel-away sheath) to insert the shunt in the abdomen prevents direct contact of the shunt with the abdominal skin. Use of skin foil is also recommended.
4. The scope should control the placement and flow of the shunt before closure.

42.9   Procedure Variations

1. The abdominal portion of the procedure can be performed using a 5-mm trocar and a 10-Fr introducer for camera and catheter insertion.
2. Under laparoscopic control, a needle is introduced through a 5-mm incision in the right upper quadrant and the shunt tubing is tunneled to that site. A J-tipped guide wire is introduced, and the needle is exchanged for a dilator and peel-away sheath. The shunt is delivered through the sheath, which is sectioned and removed.

42.10   Laparoscopic-Assisted Ventriculoperitoneal Shunt Implantation

Please see Figs. 1–3.

Figure 42.1

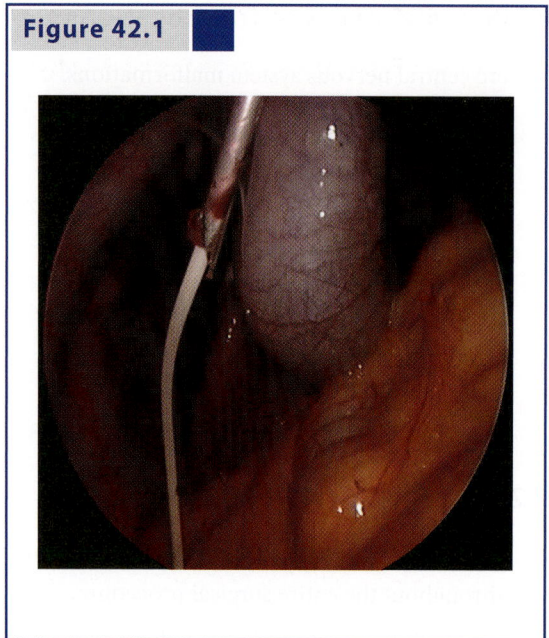

Figure 42.2

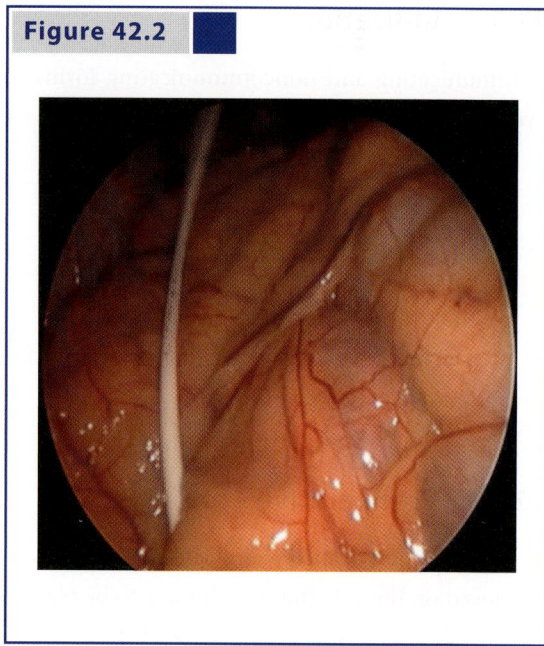

After insertion of the optic port, the shunt peel-away sheath is inserted directly through the abdominal wall under visual guidance

The final location of the shunt is controlled after the shunt peel-away sheath is removed

Figure 42.3

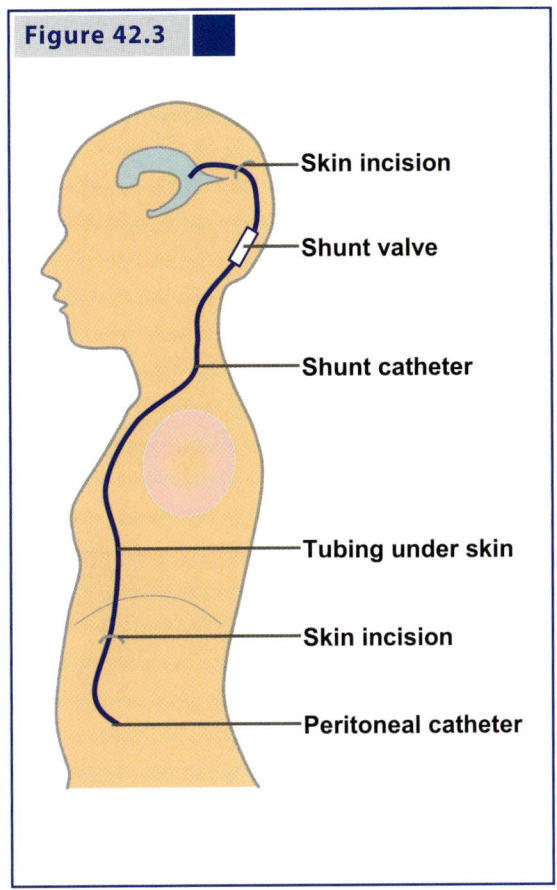

- Skin incision
- Shunt valve
- Shunt catheter
- Tubing under skin
- Skin incision
- Peritoneal catheter

Overview of shunt placement. Using a tunneler, the shunt is placed subcutaneously from the postauricular region, (where it is connected to the valve) to the abdominal insertion point. The other end of the valve is connected to the ventricular portion of the shunt through a small burr hole

Recommended Literature

1. Goitein D, Papasavas P, Gagne D, Ferraro D, Wilder B, Caushaj P (2006) Single trocar laparoscopically assisted placement of central nervous system – peritoneal shunts. J Laparoendosc Adv Surg Tech A 16:1–4
2. Konstantinidis H, Balogiannis I, Foroglu N, Spiliotopoulos A, Magras I, Kesisoglou I, Selviaridis P (2007) Laparoscopic placement of ventriculoperitoneal shunts: an innovative simplification of the existing techniques. Minim Invasive Neurosurg 50:62–64
3. Kurschel S, Eder HG, Schleef J (2005) CSF shunts in children: endoscopically-assisted placement of the distal catheter. Childs Nerv Syst 21:52–55

Section 4

Hepatobiliary, Splenic and Pancreatic Procedures

43 Cholecystectomy

Michael E. Höllwarth

43.1   Operation Room Setup

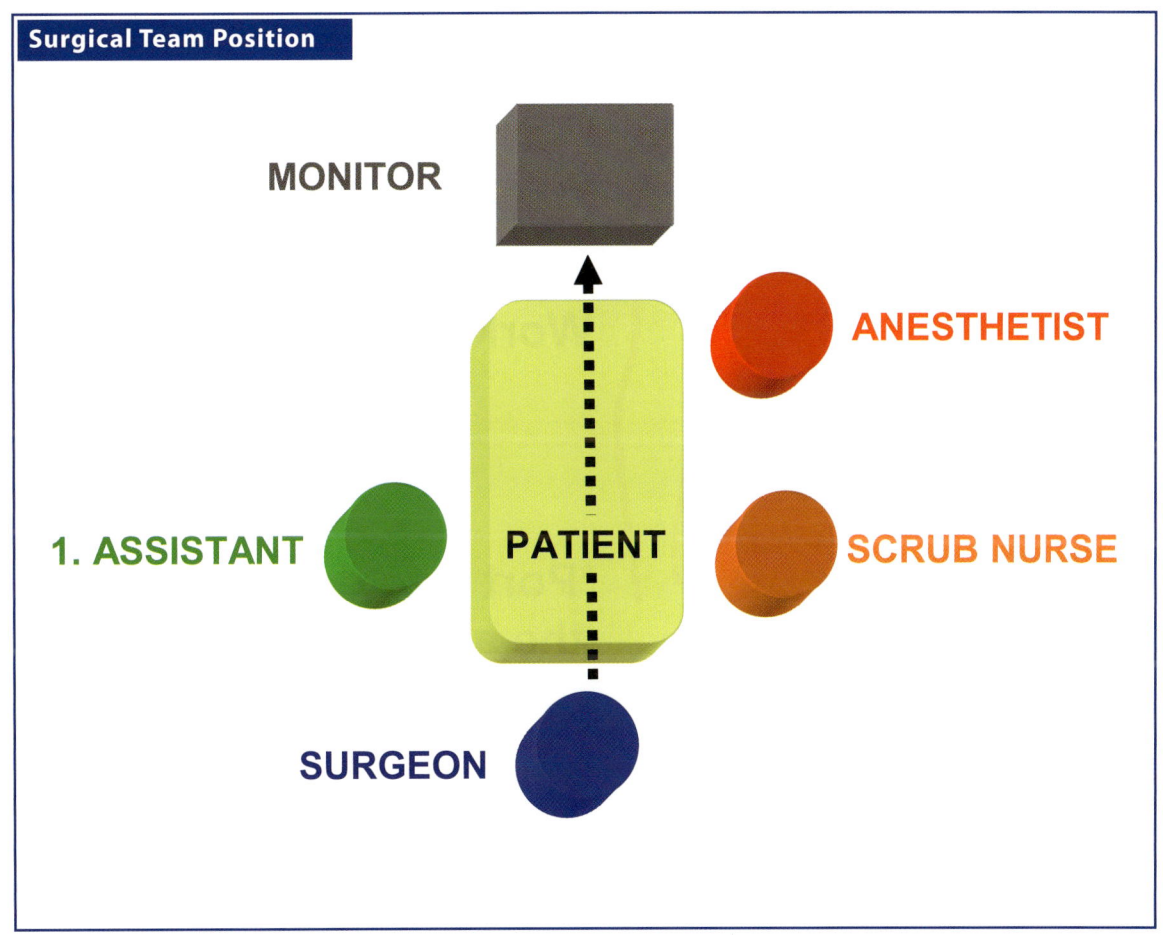

43.2   Patient Positioning

Supine position with the surgeon standing either on the left side or between the patient's legs.

43.3   Special Instruments

- Specimen retrieval bag
- Endoscopic clip applicator
- Ultracision® harmonic scalpel (Johnson & Johnson Medical Products, Ethicon Endo-Surgery, Cincinnati, OH, USA)

43.4   Location of Access Points

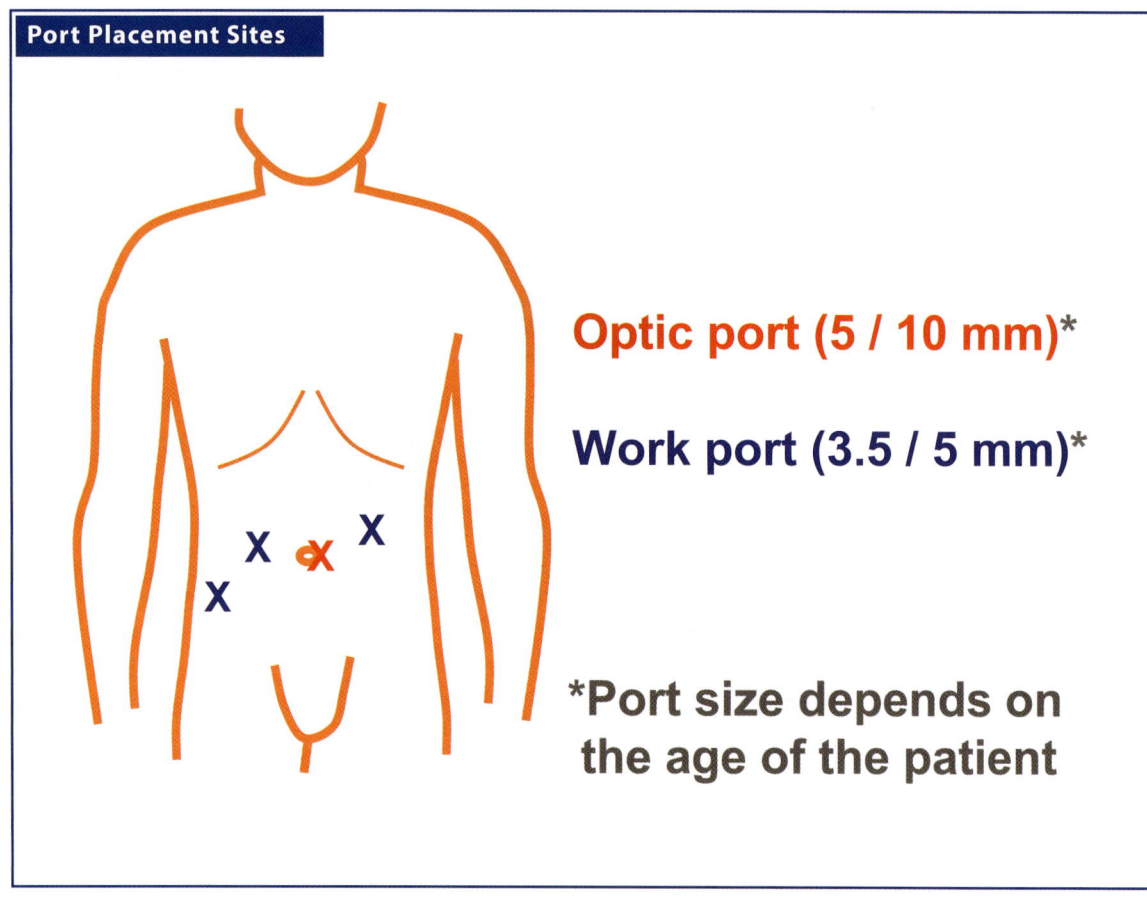

Port Placement Sites

Optic port (5 / 10 mm)*

Work port (3.5 / 5 mm)*

*Port size depends on the age of the patient

43.5   Indications

1. Cholelithiasis.
2. Cholecystitis.
3. Gallstone pancreatitis.
4. Cholangitis.

43.6   Relative Contraindications

1. Acute cholecystitis.
2. Choledocholithiasis.
3. Bowel obstruction.
4. Hepatic cirrhosis.

43.7   Preoperative Considerations

1. Patients are administered antibiotics (cefuroxime 30 mg/kg) at the time of induction of anesthesia
2. A nasogastric tube is placed for gastric decompression.
3. If intraoperative cholangiography is part of the procedure, the patient should be placed accordingly on the table and the entire staff be protected with appropriate vests, observing hospital radiation guidelines.

43.8   Technical Notes

1. The first grasper holds the gallbladder fundus and raises it toward the thorax to expose Calot's triangle.
2. Calot's triangle, which is bound by the cystic artery, cystic duct, and hepatic duct, should be dissected to safeguard essential structures. Anatomic variations from the norm should be considered.
3. Intraoperative cholangiography is not routinely used. Common bile duct stones are removed using endoscopic retrograde cholangiopancreatography (ERCP) either before or after cholecystectomy.

43.9   Procedure Variations

1. Use of laparoscopic ultrasound intraoperatively for imaging of the common bile duct.
2. Intraoperative cholangiography for exploration of the bile ducts.
3. Utilization of three ports for the procedure.
4. Application of the harmonic scalpel to dissect the gallbladder from the liver.
5. The gallbladder can be suspended using a snare loop to entrap and hold the fundus.

43.10   Laparoscopic Cholecystectomy

Please see Figs. 1–6.

Figure 43.1

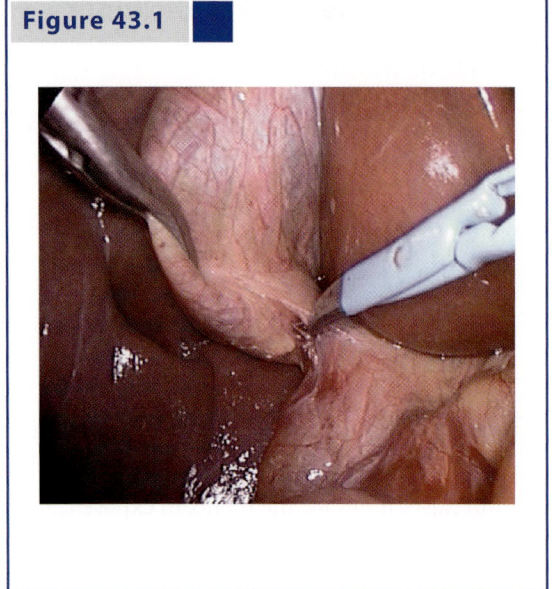

The gallbladder is retracted using graspers and Calot's triangle is cleared

Figure 43.2

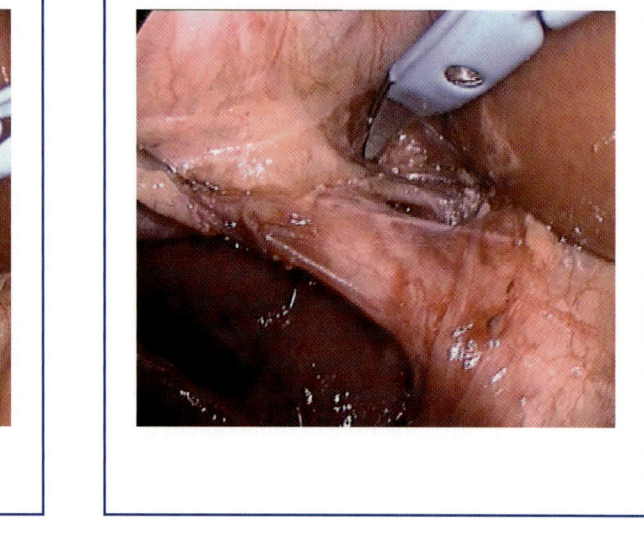

Adhesions are dissected free to allow clear visualization of the cystic duct and the cystic artery

Figure 43.3

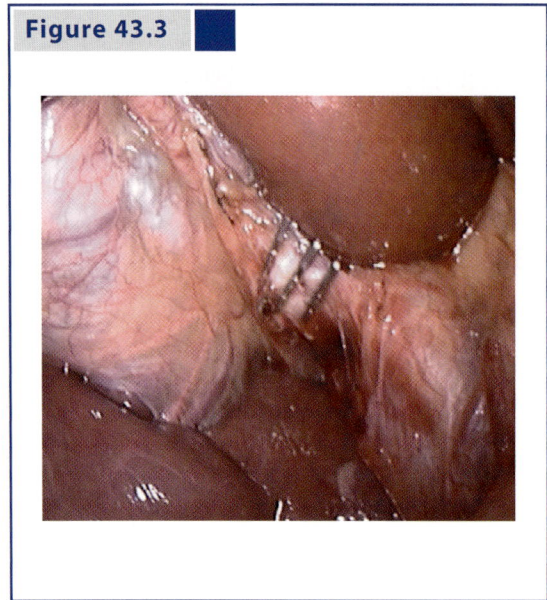

The endoscopic clip applicator is used to apply titanium clips in a dumbell formation separately on the cystic duct and the cystic artery

Figure 43.4

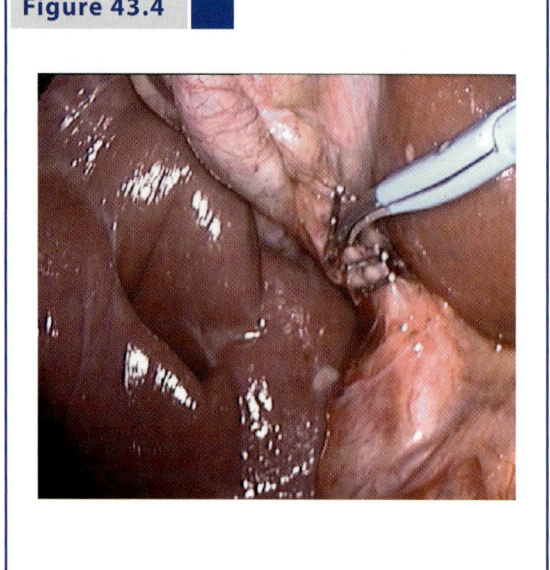

Using scissors, both the tissues are individually divided and checked for leaks

Figure 43.5

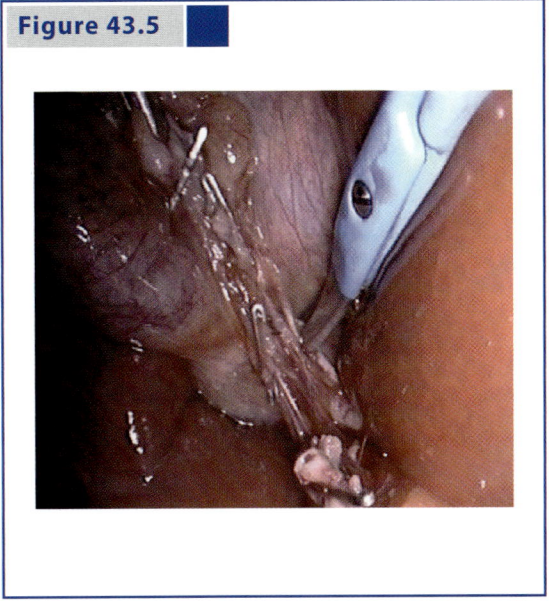

Figure 43.6

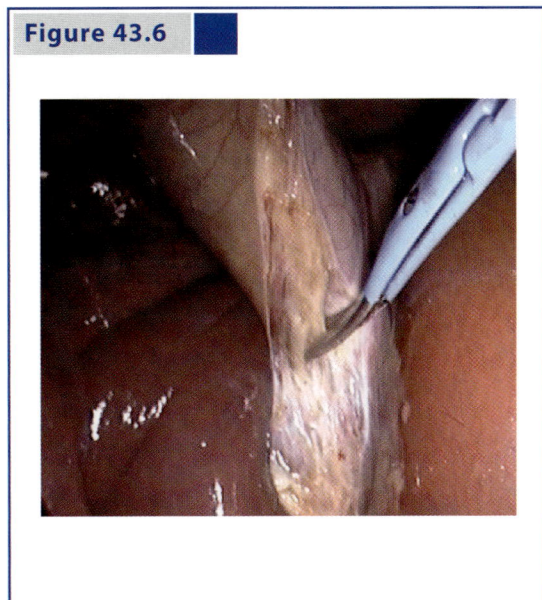

The gallbladder is dissected using electrosurgical bipolar scissors from the cystic duct end

After the gallbladder is dissected free, it is either extracted through a 10-mm port or placed into a specimen retrieval bag and removed

Recommended Literature

1. Bonnard A, Seguier-Lipszyc E, Liguory C, Benkerrou M, Garel C, Malbezin S, Aigrain Y, de Lagausie P (2005) Laparoscopic approach as primary treatment of common bile duct stones in children. J Pediatr Surg 40:1459–1463

2. Callery MP (2006) Avoiding biliary injury during laparoscopic cholecystectomy: technical considerations. Surg Endosc 20:1654–1658

3. Zacharakis E, Angelopoulos S, Kanellos D, Prameteftakis MG, Sapidis N, Stamatopolous H, Kanellos I, Tsalis K, Betsis D (2007) Laparoscopic cholecystectomy without intraoperative cholangiography. J Laparoendosc Adv Surg Tech A 17:620–625

44 Liver Biopsy

Kiyokazu Nakajima, Hideki Soh
and Toshirou Nishida

44.1 Operation Room Setup

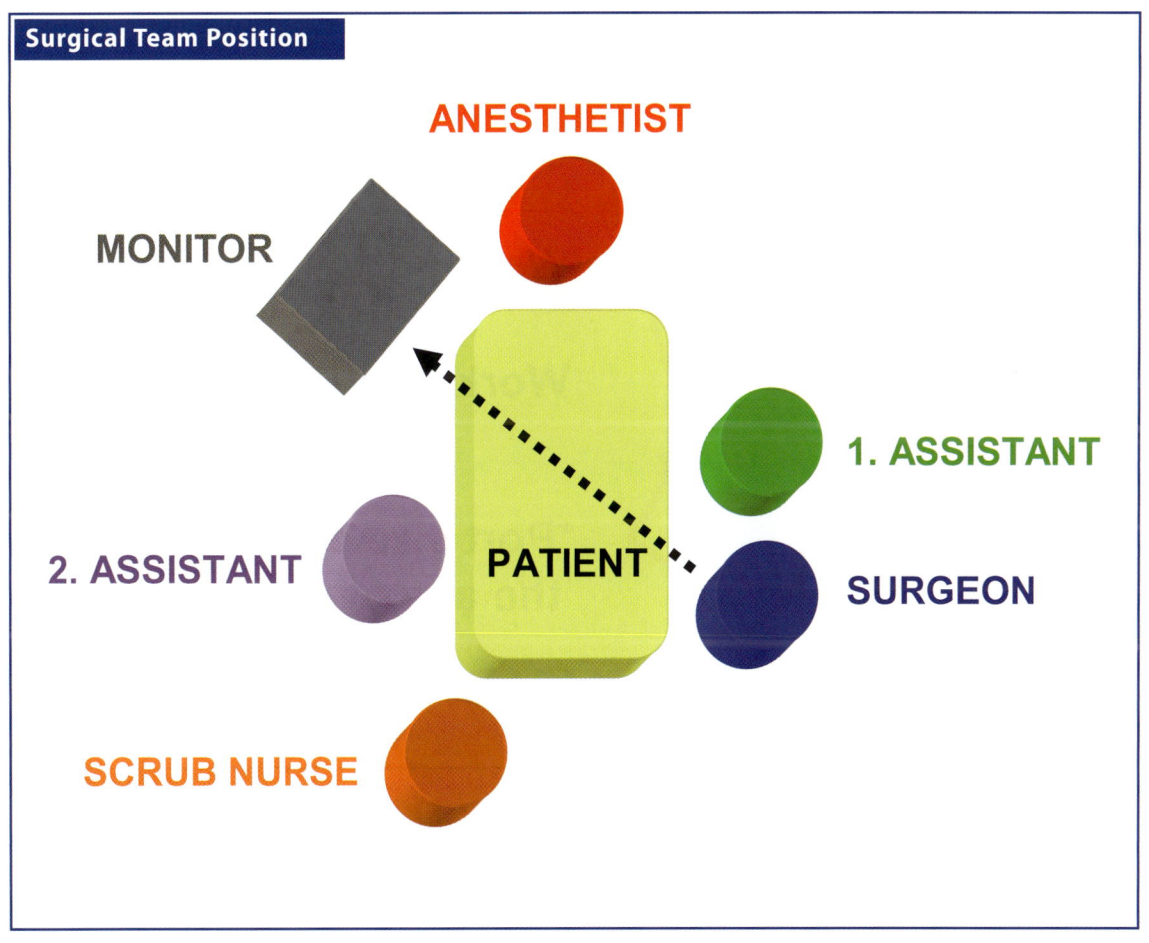

Surgical Team Position

ANESTHETIST

MONITOR

1. ASSISTANT

2. ASSISTANT   PATIENT

SURGEON

SCRUB NURSE

44.2   Patient Positioning

Supine position with arms tucked to the side. Right side up with mild reverse Trendelenburg position if needed.

44.3   Special Instruments

None.

44.4   Location of Access Points

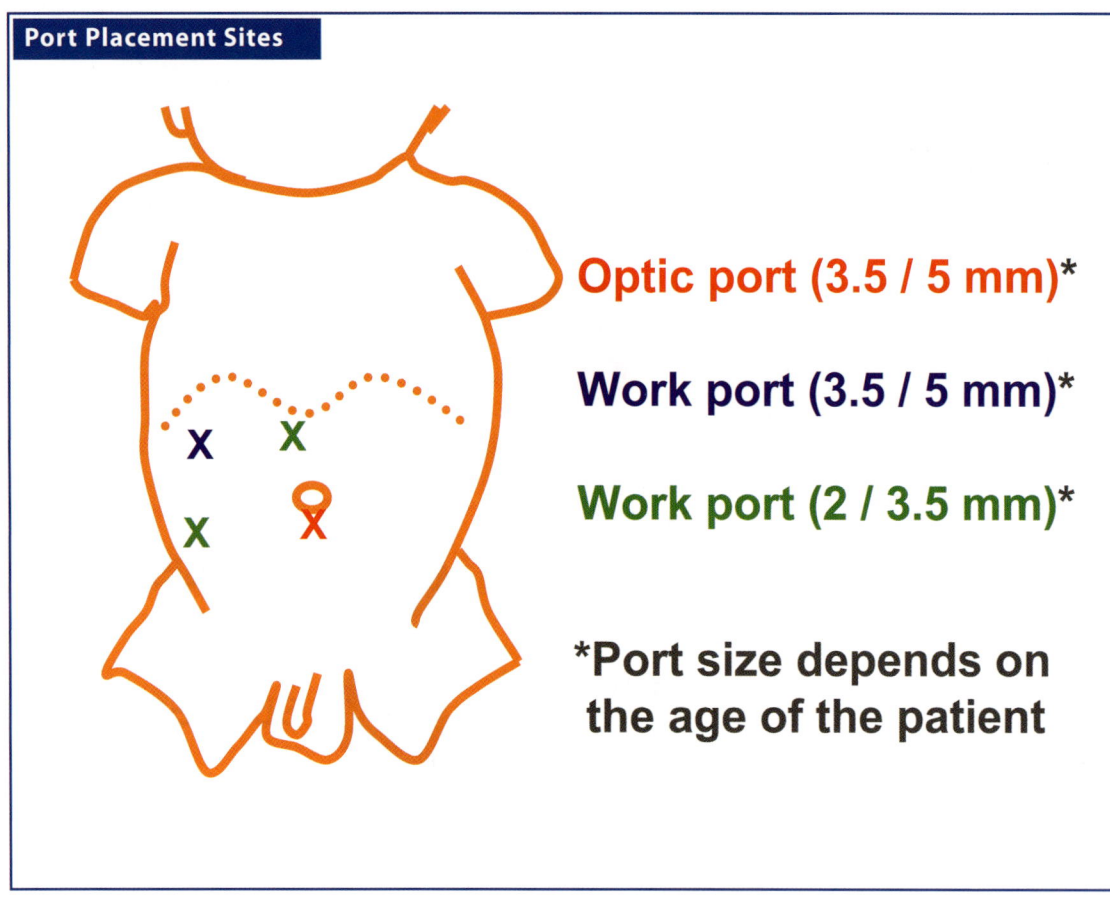

Port Placement Sites

Optic port (3.5 / 5 mm)*

Work port (3.5 / 5 mm)*

Work port (2 / 3.5 mm)*

*Port size depends on the age of the patient

44.5 Indications

1. Liver disorders of unknown origin, especially cases with failed diagnosis by percutaneous core-needle biopsy.
2. Staging of chronic hepatitis following serologic diagnosis.

44.6 Contraindications

1. Severe bleeding diathesis.
2. Severe liver cirrhosis.

44.7 Preoperative Considerations

1. The severity of hepatic damage should be evaluated fully prior to surgery.
2. Standard preoperative management should be carried out (e.g., draping, bladder emptying, antibiotics prophylaxis).
3. When concomitant abdominal surgery is planned, consideration of the accompanying procedure must also be taken into account.

44.8 Technical Notes

1. Evaluate the feasibility of hepatic clamping before starting the excision.
2. If the tissue is too cirrhotic to clamp, consider a core-needle biopsy procedure carried out under laparoscopic guidance.
3. A suction/irrigation line should be kept operational during the procedure.
4. Insertion of surgical gauze or sponge can be performed if a full-size laparoscopic port is available. Use of these materials greatly facilitates the procedure.

44.9 Procedure Variations

1. In adolescent patients, laparoscopic "stapled" wedge biopsy using Endo GIA™ stapler (Auto Suture, Norwalk, CT, USA) is optional. Use vascular cartridges to secure hemostasis.
2. A core-needle biopsy can be performed under laparoscopic guidance. Hemostasis is easily obtained at the biopsy site with the aid of electrocoagulation.
3. Laparoscopic ultrasound is optional to minimize perforation injury to major intrahepatic structures.

44.10 Laparoscopic Liver Wedge Biopsy

Please see Figs. 1–6.

Figure 44.1

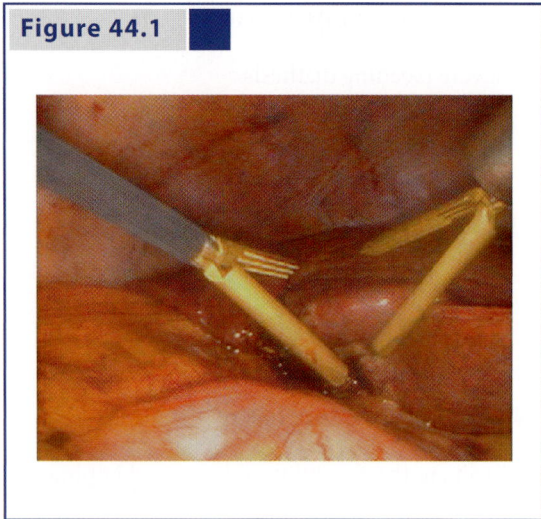

Two atraumatic bowel graspers are placed on the liver edge at a 90° angle

Figure 44.2

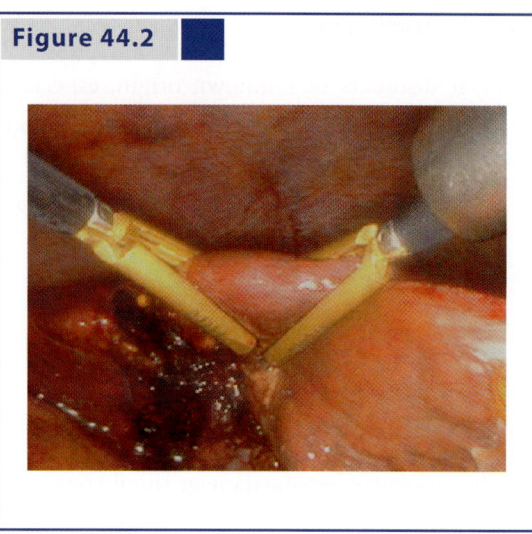

The hepatic tissue is tentatively clamped. Note the ischemic wedge between the two graspers, indicating effective clamping

Figure 44.3

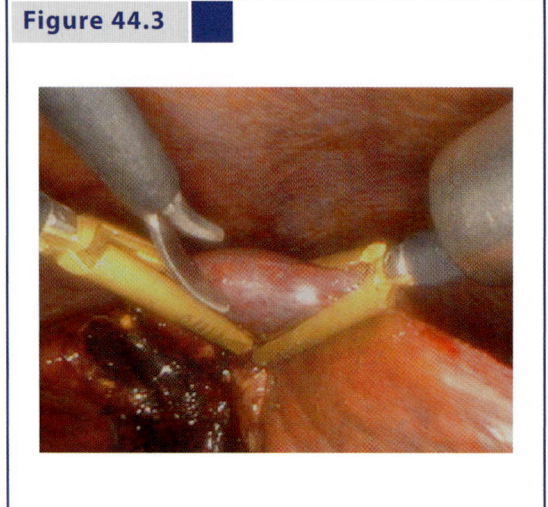

A curved endoscopic scissors is introduced while the graspers are held in situ by the assistant

Figure 44.4

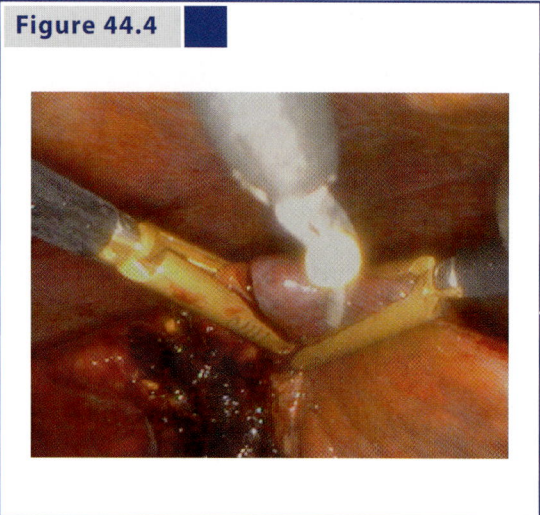

The tissue is excised between the two graspers. Bleeding is minimal when clamping is successful

Figure 44.5

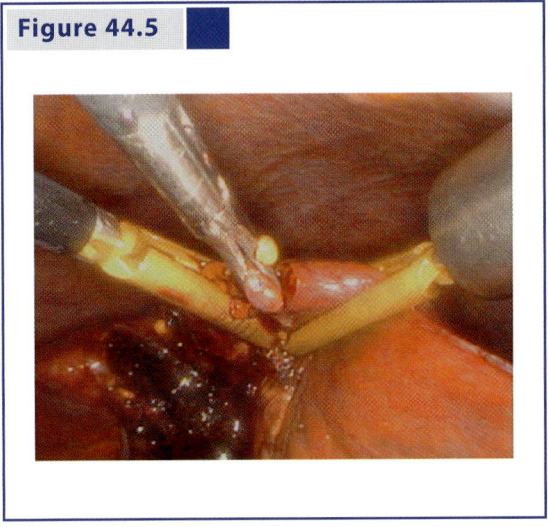

Figure 44.6

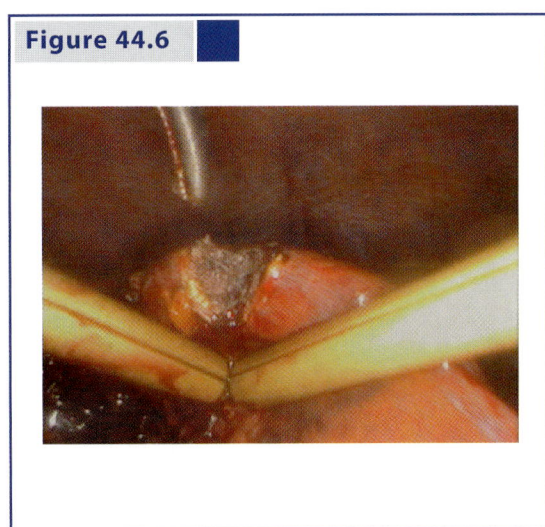

The specimen is retrieved using tissue-extracting forceps

The cut surfaces are coagulated with monopolar forceps. Additional coagulation is performed if any bleeding is noted after partial declamping

Recommended Literature

1. Lefor AT, Flowers JL (1994) Laparoscopic wedge biopsy of the liver. J Am Coll Surg 178:307–308

2. Nakajima K, Neze R, Sakamoto T, Suguira F, Yamamura N, Ito T, Nishida T (2007) A simple technique for wedge biopsy of the liver during laparoscopic surgery. J Laparoendosc Adv Surg Tech A 17:470–472

3. Sheela H, Seela S, Caldwell C, Boyer JL, Jain D (2005) Liver biopsy: evolving role in the new millennium. J Clin Gastroenterol 39:603–610

45 Choledochal Cyst Resection

Ramin Jamshidi and Hanmin Lee

45.1   Operation Room Setup

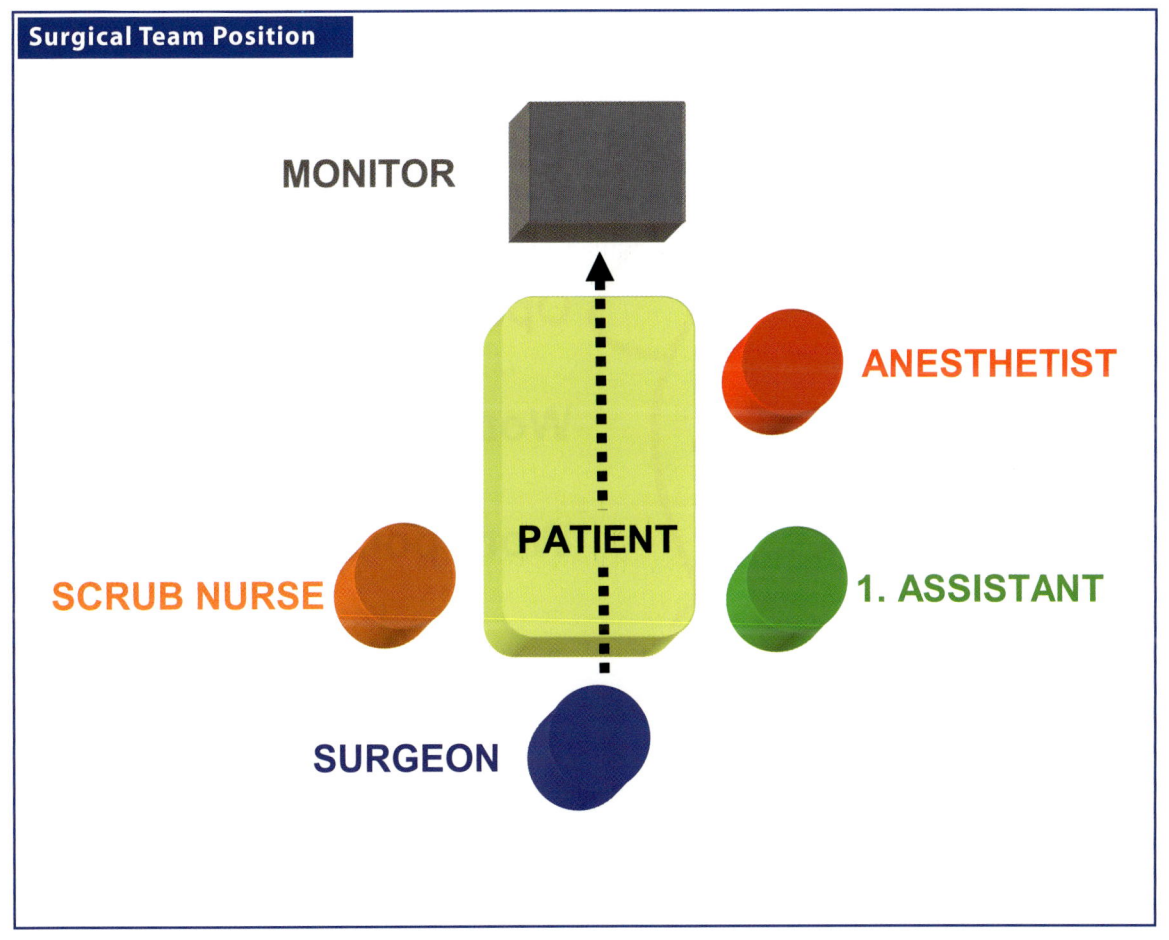

Surgical Team Position

MONITOR

ANESTHETIST

SCRUB NURSE

PATIENT

1. ASSISTANT

SURGEON

45.2   Patient Positioning

The patient is positioned supine at the foot end of the operating table with the arms extended. The legs should be in stirrups (older children) or "frog-legged" (infants).

45.3   Special Instruments

None.

45.4   Location of Access Points

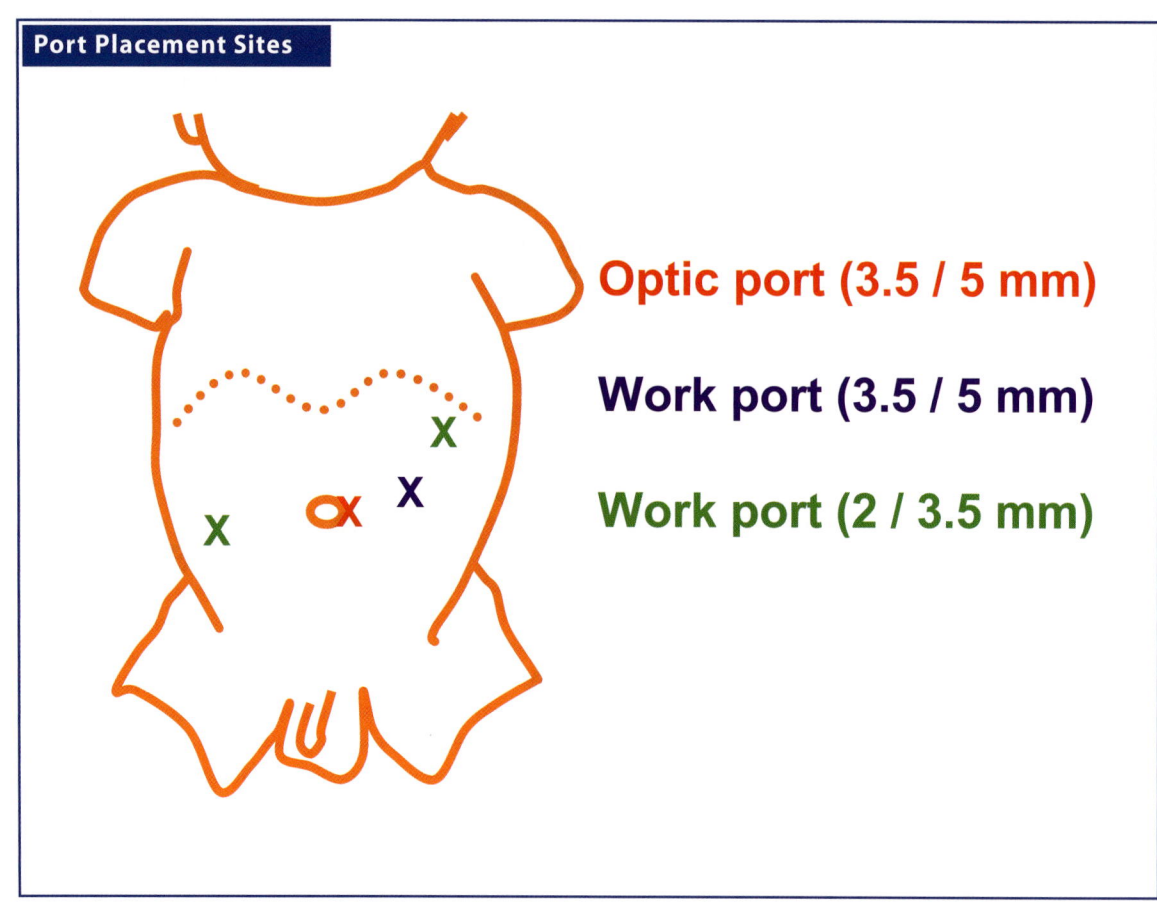

Port Placement Sites

Optic port (3.5 / 5 mm)

Work port (3.5 / 5 mm)

Work port (2 / 3.5 mm)

45.5   Indications

1. All choledochal cysts are resected due to the potential for cholangitis and malignant degeneration. Approximately 90% of choledochal cysts are Type I and Type II.
2. Type I cyst: fusiform extrahepatic biliary dilation.
3. Type II cyst: common bile duct diverticulum.
4. Type IVB cyst: primarily extrahepatic dilation with a limited intrahepatic component.

45.6   Contraindications

1. Type III cyst: "choledochocele" or intraduodenal dilation.
2. Type IVA cyst: extrahepatic as well as diffuse intrahepatic dilation.
3. Type V cyst: dilated intrahepatic biliary radicals.
4. Prior cholangitis or cholecystectomy are relative contraindications because adhesions may increase the technical complexity.

45.7   Preoperative Considerations

1. With entry into the enteric and biliary tracts, the operation is clean contaminated at best. A second-generation cephalosporin should be administered for perioperative antibiosis.
2. The average operating time is 4–7 h, so a urinary catheter should be placed at the start and antibiotics redosed if necessary.

45.8   Technical Notes

1. The gallbladder provides effective liver retraction and is less cumbersome than fan-type retractors.
2. A subxiphoid percutaneous suture can lasso the falciform ligament to further elevate the liver and obviate the need for another port.
3. If extreme inflammation causes common bile duct adherence to the portal vein, remove all internal components of the cyst and leave the posterior wall behind to avoid morbidity.

45.9   Procedure Variations

1. The completely laparoscopic method involves intracorporeal suturing for the jejunojejunostomy.
2. Alternately, the jejunum can be externalized and the Roux-en-Y constructed extracorporeally.
3. Cyst involvement of the confluence of right and left hepatic ducts requires reconstruction by either two separate hepaticojejunostomies or a "double-barrel hepaticojejunostomy."

45.10   Laparoscopic Choledochal Cyst Resection

Please see Figs. 1–8.

Figure 45.1

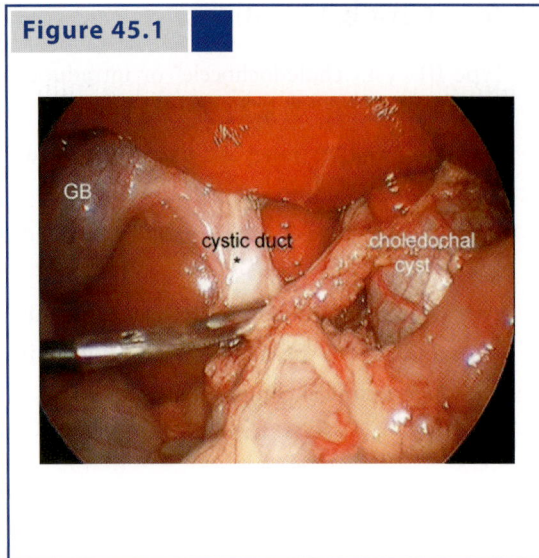

The gallbladder and choledochal cyst are dissected free and the anatomy confirmed; a cholangiogram is performed through the gallbladder if required. The cystic duct and artery are clipped and divided

Figure 45.2

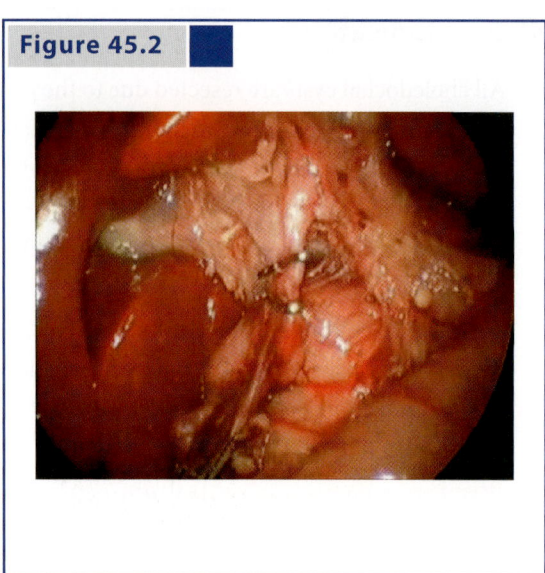

The gallbladder is retracted via the left subcostal port in order to elevate the liver cephalad. The proximal extent of the cyst is identified and the normal common hepatic duct clipped and divided

Figure 45.3

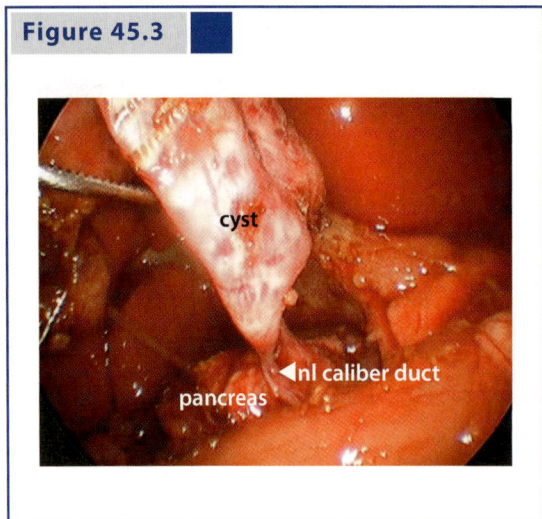

The distal extent of the cyst is dissected free to where it enters the pancreas. The normal common bile duct is clipped and divided. *nl* normal

Figure 45.4

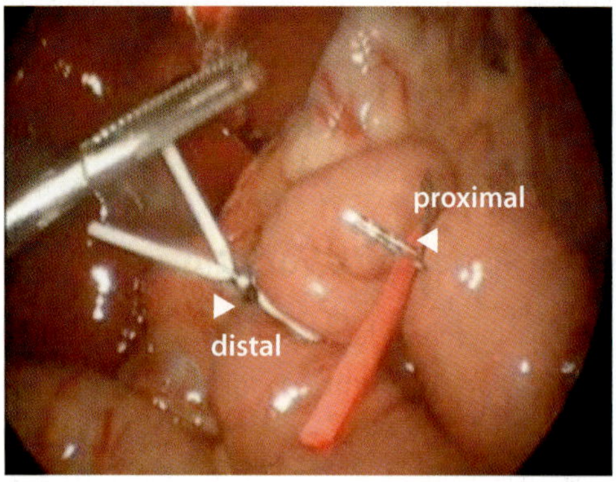

The jejunum is traced for 15 cm from the ligament of Treitz and the proximal and distal ends are labeled with colored vessel loops

Figure 45.5

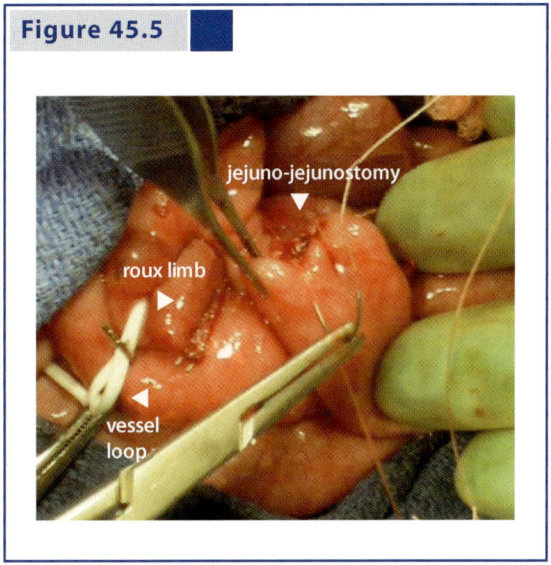

The umbilical port is lengthened to 1.5 cm and the labeled jejunum is externalized to allow construction of the Roux-en-Y jejunojejunostomy with a 20- to 30-cm Roux limb

Figure 45.6

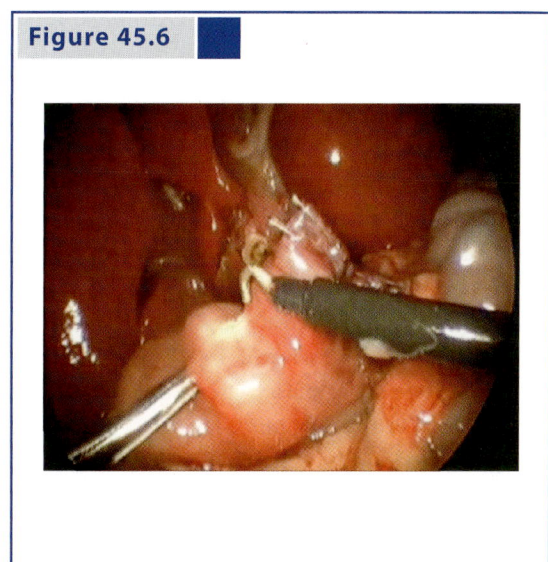

The bowel is internalized and pneumoperitoneum re-established. The Roux limb is passed through the transverse mesocolon and approximated to the common hepatic duct with stay sutures; a size-matched enterotomy is made

Figure 45.7

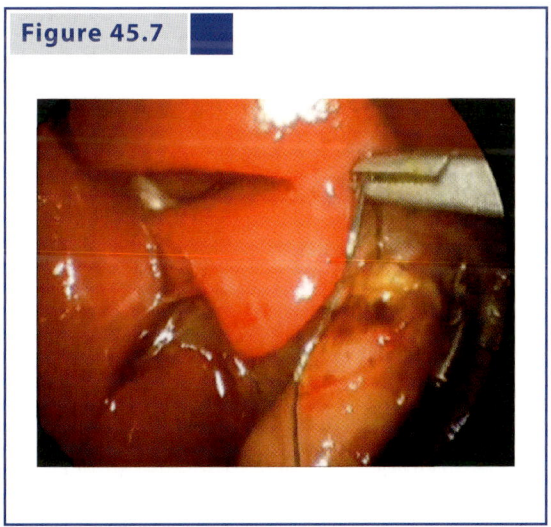

An end-to-side duct to mucosa anastomosis is fashioned, running along the posterior wall and interrupting the anterior wall

Figure 45.8

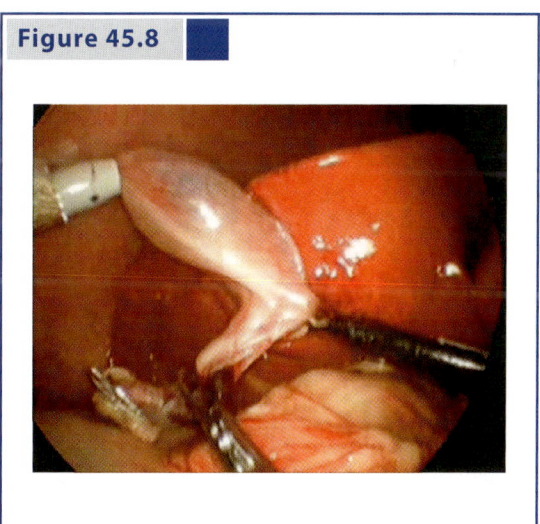

The cholecystectomy is completed, the cyst and gallbladder removed, and the operation terminated

Recommended Literature

1. Lee H, Hirose S, Bratton B, Farmer D (2004) Initial experience with complex laparoscopic biliary surgery in children: biliary atresia and choledochal cyst. J Pediatr Surg 39:804–807
2. Li L, Feng W, Jing-Bo F, Qi-Zhi Y, Gang L, Liu-Ming H, Yu L, Jun J, Ping W (2004) Laparoscopic-assisted total cyst excision of choledochal cyst and Roux-en-Y hepatoenterostomy. J Pediatr Surg 39:1663–1666
3. Martinez-Ferro M, Esteves E, Laje P (2005) Laparoscopic treatment of biliary atresia and choledochal cyst. Semin Pediatr Surg 14:206–215

46 Portoenterostomy (Kasai Procedure)

Marcelo H. Martinez-Ferro

46.1 Operation Room Setup

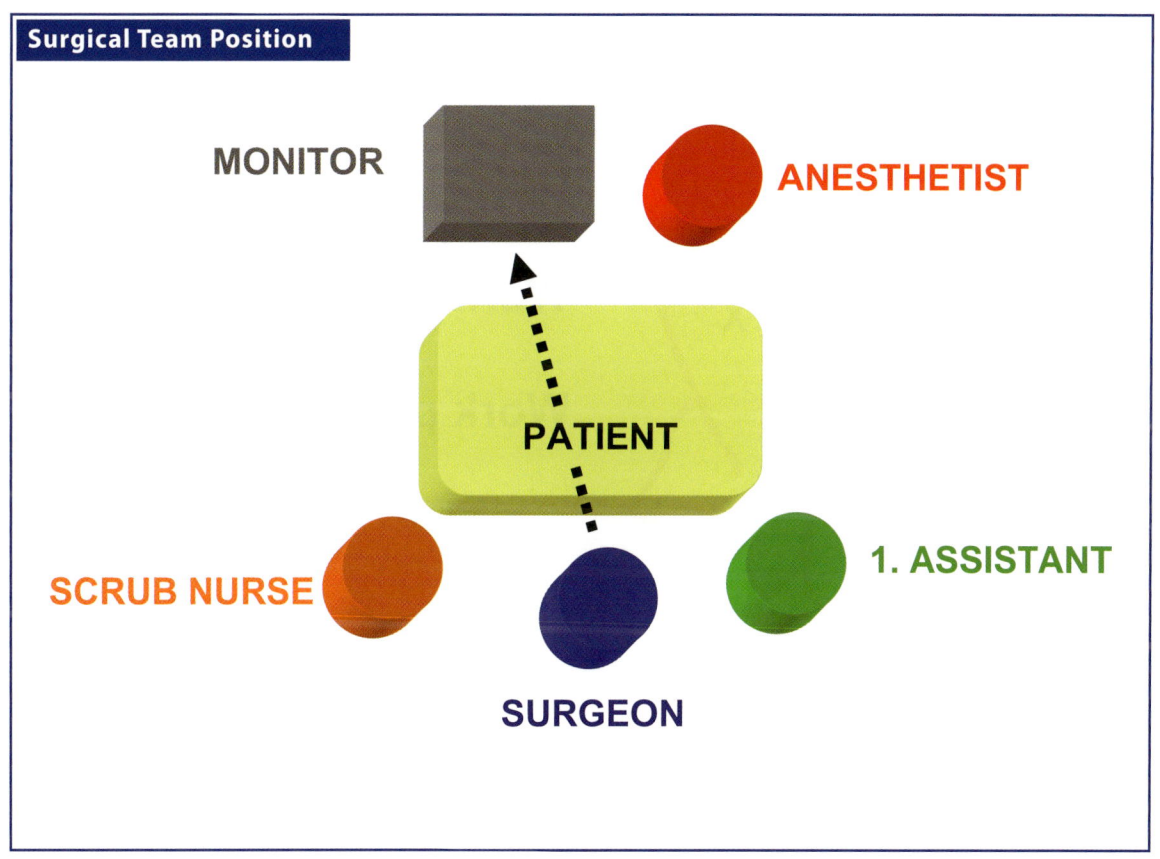

46.2   Patient Positioning

The patient is placed across the table and positioned over an elevated platform in order to achieve maximum instrument mobility.

46.3   Special Instruments

None.

46.4   Location of Access Points

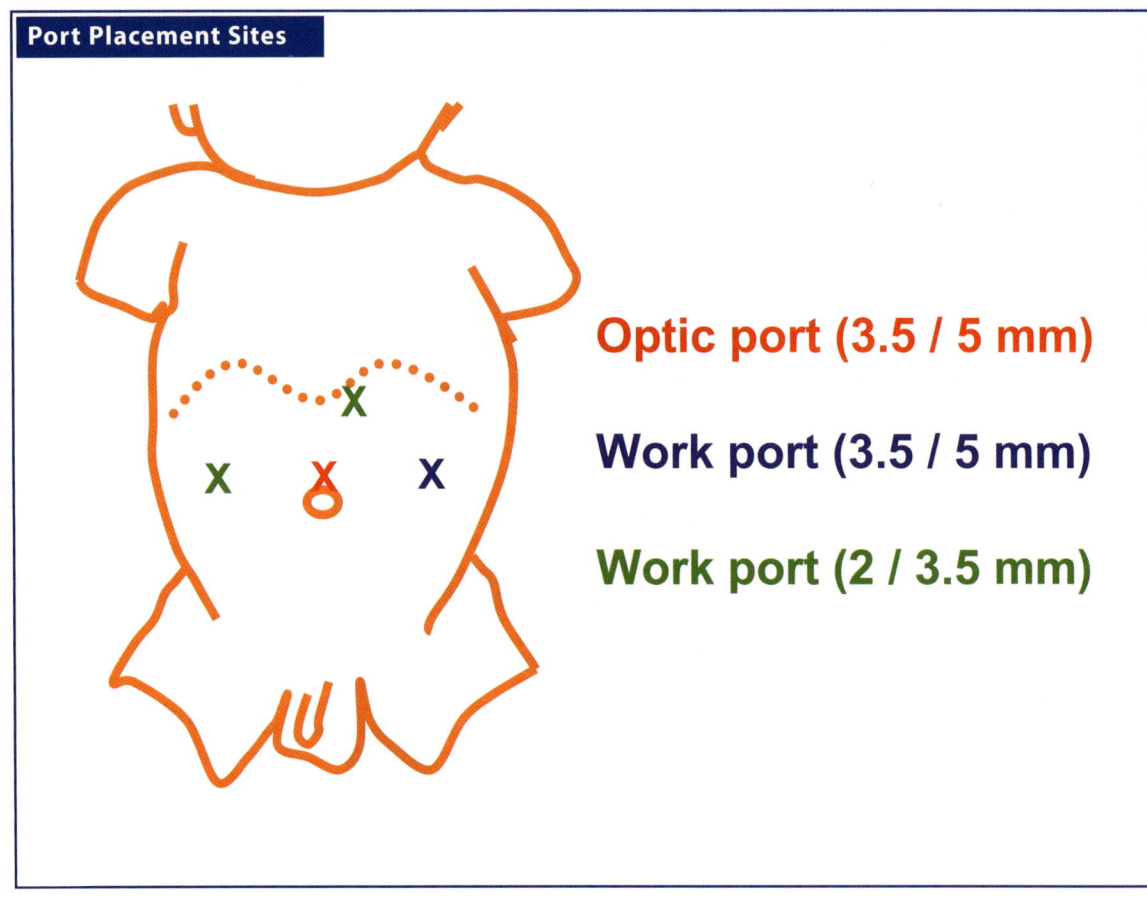

Port Placement Sites

Optic port (3.5 / 5 mm)

Work port (3.5 / 5 mm)

Work port (2 / 3.5 mm)

46.5 Preoperative Considerations

1. Bowel cleansing with 100 ml/kg polyethylene glycol 3350 (GoLYTELY®, BAREX®) solution is preferred.
2. Otherwise, three or four saline enemas (30 ml/kg each) are indicated at 6, 3, and 1 h prior to surgery.
3. After induction of anesthesia, a soft rubber catheter is inserted through the anus and advanced to the sigma colon to evacuate residual air or intestinal contents.

46.6 Technical Notes: Access Related

1. The use of a wide-angle scope provides an optimal vision in a limited working field.
2. Liver stay sutures are very convenient for an adequate exposure of the biliary tree.
3. For additional retraction, a percutaneous stitch from just below the xiphoid can be used to snare the round ligament and retract the liver superiorly.
4. If cholangiography is needed, a 22-gauge angiocath is used to access the gallbladder percutaneously.

46.7 Technical Notes: Procedure Related

1. The main hepatic arteries (left and right) and the portal vein are the anatomical landmarks that establish the boundaries of the portal plate.
2. After cutting the plate, profuse bleeding will occur. Avoid using monopolar cautery as it can destroy the still-patent microscopic bile ducts. Instead, apply gentle irrigation with saline and pack the plate with absorbable hemostat such as Surgicel® (Ethicon, Somerville, NJ, USA) while the Roux-en-Y is performed.
3. Placement of two initial percutaneous stay sutures at both posterior corners of the anastomosis will facilitate the precise placement of the posterior central stitches.

46.8 Procedure Variations

1. An extra fifth port can be placed at the right lower quadrant for the introduction of the aspiration device as well as for duodenal and colonic retraction.
2. The Roux-en-Y limb can be passed either antecolic or retrocolic up to the porta hepatis.
3. Intestinal anastomosis to the portal plate can be performed with posterior and anterior running sutures.

46.9 Laparoscopic Portoenterostomy (Kasai Procedure)

Please see Figs. 1–12.

Figure 46.1

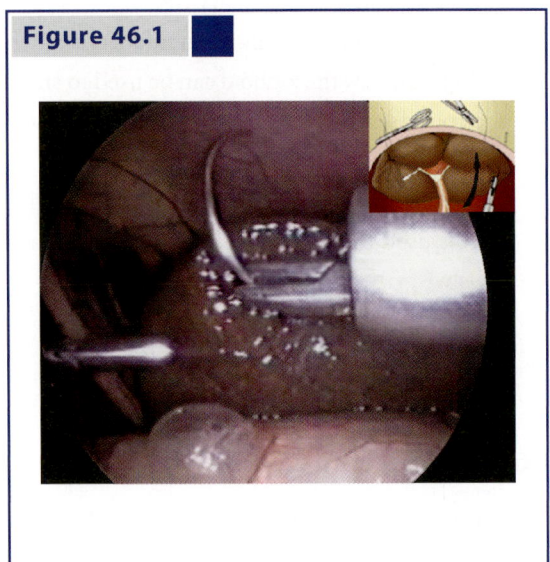

Figure 46.2

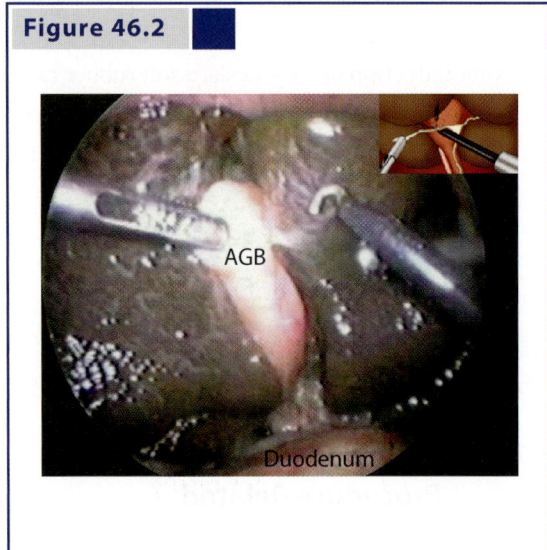

Two percutaneous transhepatic stitches are placed entering the abdominal cavity near the border of the left and right costal margins, passing through the liver parenchyma and exiting the abdominal cavity 1 cm away from its entrance point

The atretic gallbladder and cystic duct are dissected free from the liver and the dissection carried towards the fibrous remnant of the common bile duct and hepatic duct. *AGB* Atretic gallbladder

Figure 46.3

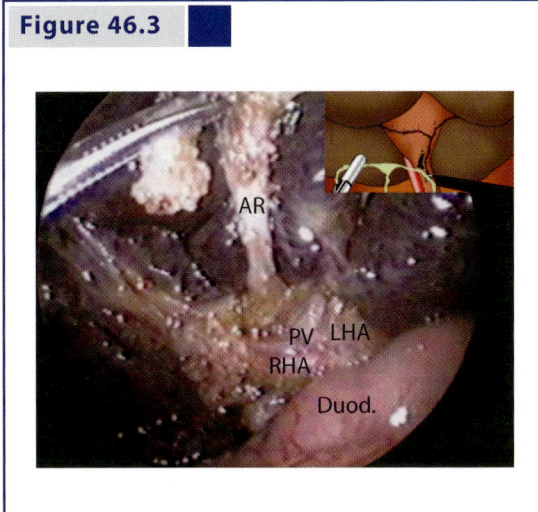

The dissection is then progressed to the duodenum and pancreas distally following the choledochal remnants, which are transected using the monopolar hook. Proximally, the atretic biliary tree leads directly to the portal plate. **AR** Atretic remnants, **PV** portal vein, **LHA** left hepatic artery, **RHA** right hepatic artery, **Duod** duodenum

Figure 46.4

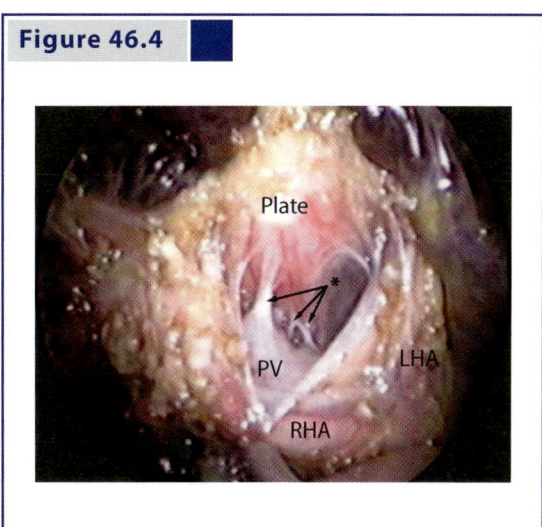

Main hepatic arteries (left and right) and the portal vein are the anatomical landmarks that establish the boundaries of the portal plate. Special attention must be given to the small portal vessels (***asterisk and arrows***) that emerge vertically from the portal plate to the portal vein

Figure 46.5

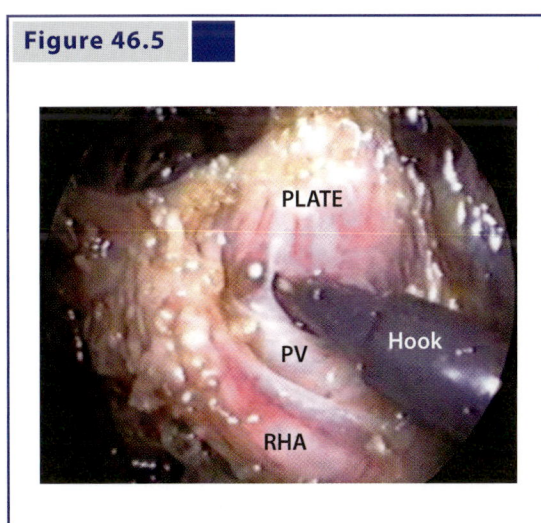

Small portal vein branches bridging the portal vein to the portal bile duct remnants are divided with monopolar hook electrocautery

Figure 46.6

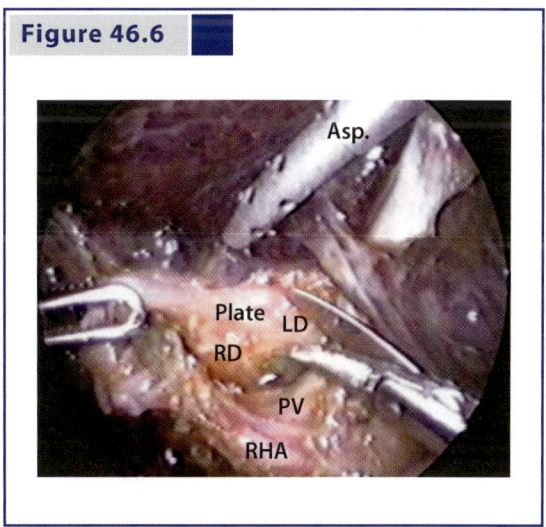

The fibrous remnant of the portal plate is excised sharply with 3-mm curved endoscopic scissors. **RD** Right duct, **LD** left duct, **Asp** aspirator

Figure 46.7

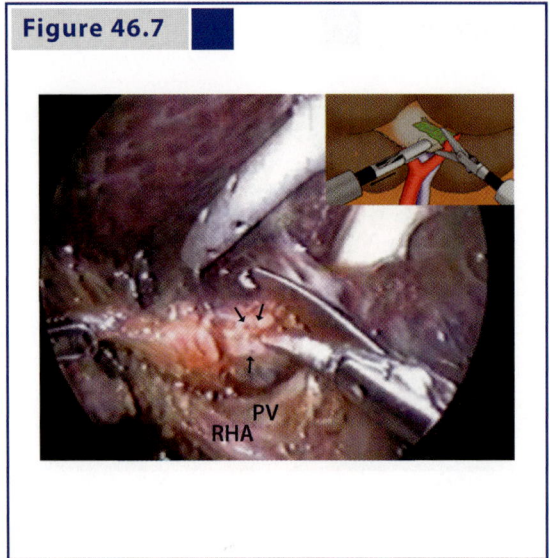

Figure 46.8

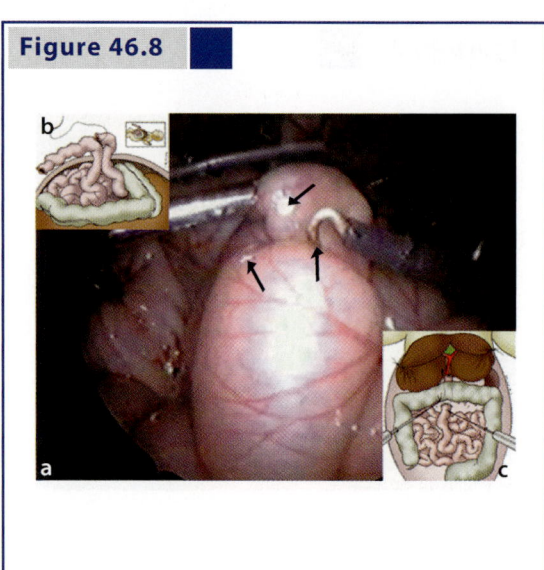

In the majority of cases, under magnification, bile can be observed flowing from the still-patent small bile ducts (***arrows***) at the portal plate

(a) Using a monopolar hook, the proximal jejunum (20- 40-cm distal to the Treitz ligament) is marked with one dot and the distal end with two dots. (b) The marked jejunum is exteriorized through the umbilical port wound and divided. (c) A 30-cm Roux-en-Y limb is created. Finally, the Roux-en-Y limb is passed either antecolic or retrocolic up to the porta hepatis

Figure 46.9

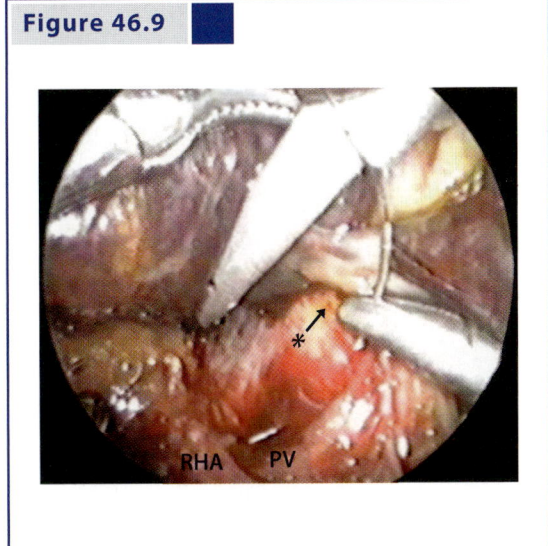

Figure 46.10

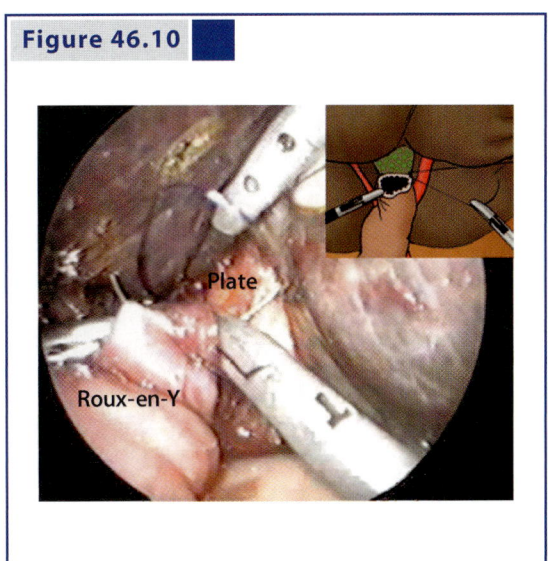

The anastomosis to the portal plate is performed with 5/0 absorbable monofilament suture (PDS™; Ethicon, Somerville, NJ, USA) with a C1 needle. Posterior central stitches must enter the portal plate near its posterior border and exit very close to the portal vein. Note the bile draining from the still-patent bile duct (*)

For the anastomosis, extracorporeal Roeder knot-tying is recommended. The anterior face of the portojejunostomy can be performed either by interrupted stitches or by running suture

Figure 46.11

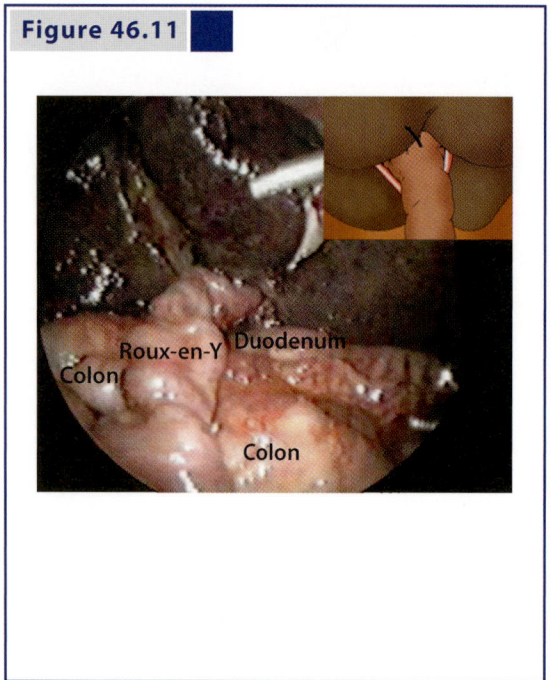

Figure 46.12

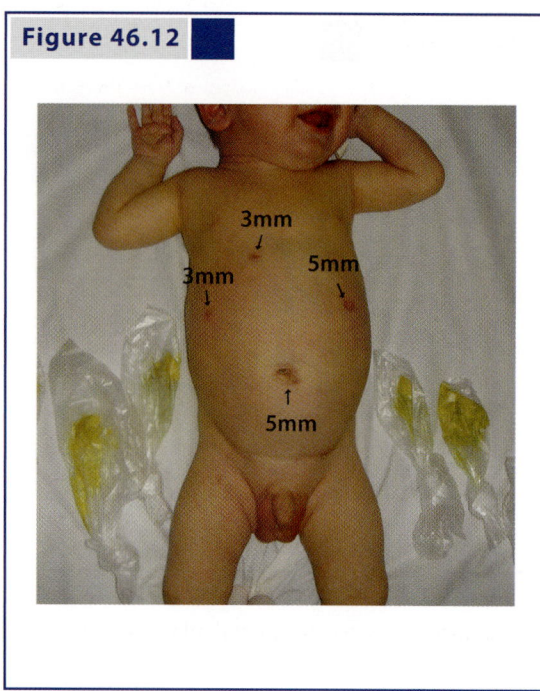

Final view of the completed anastomosis. Note that in this case, the Roux-en-Y limb has been passed in an antecolic fashion

Postoperative results demonstrating the healed port site incisions 1 week after laparoscopic portoenterostomy for biliary atresia. Note the colored stools

Recommended Literature

1. Aspelund G, Ling SC, Ng V, Kim PC (2007) A role for laparoscopic approach in the treatment of biliary atresia and choledochal cysts. J Pediatr Surg 42:869–872
2. Esteves E, Neto EC, Neto MO, Devanir J, Pereira RE (2002) Laparoscopic Kasai portoenterostomy for biliary atresia. Pediatr Surg Int 18:737–740
3. Martinez-Ferro M, Esteves E, Laje P (2005) Laparoscopic atresia and choledochal cyst. Semin Pediatr Surg 14:206–215

47 Liver Resection

Chung N. Tang and Michael K. Li

47.1 Operation Room Setup

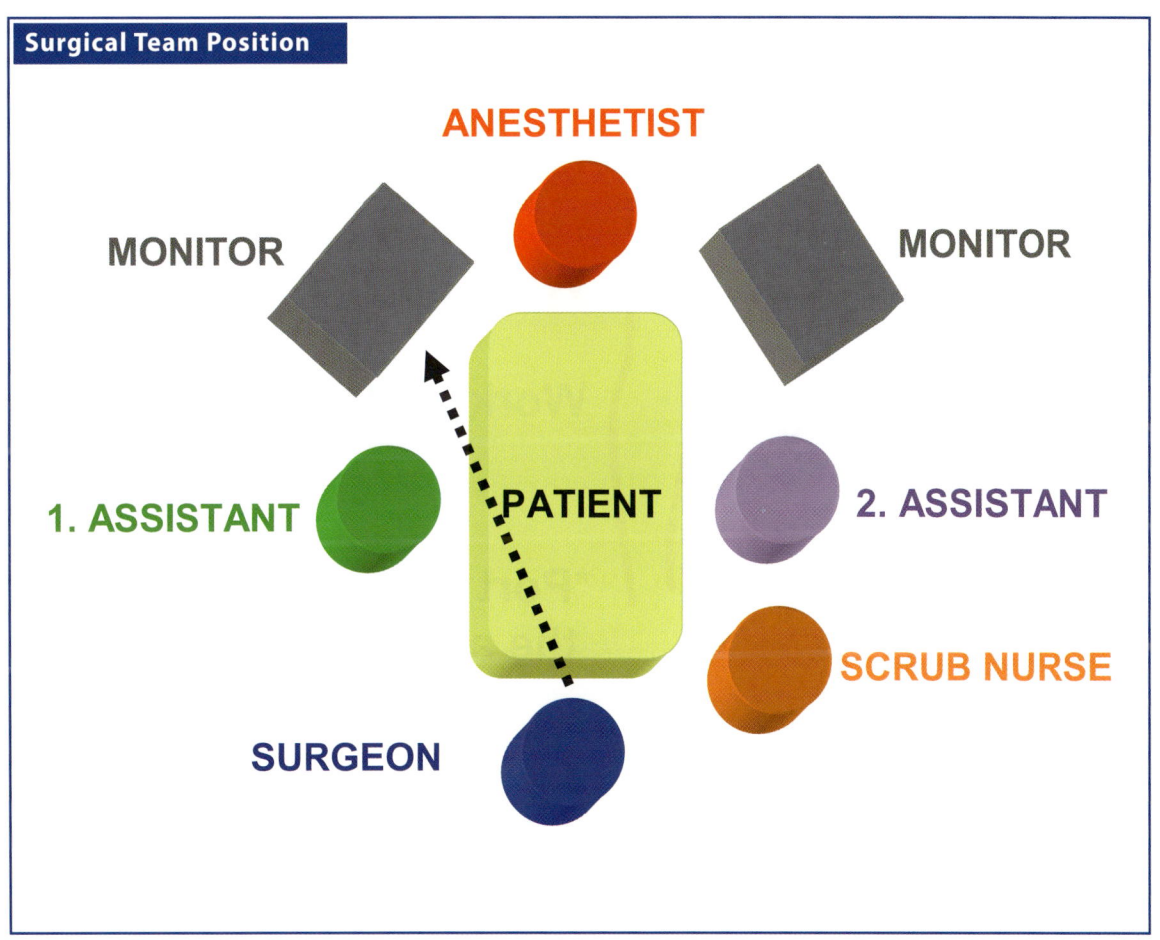

47.2 Patient Positioning

Lloyd-Davis position. The surgeon stands in between the legs of the patient with assistants on either side.

47.3 Special Instruments

- Ultracision® harmonic scalpel (Johnson & Johnson Medical Products, Ethicon Endo-Surgery, Cincinnati, OH, USA)
- Laparoscopic ultrasound probe
- Specimen retrieval bag

47.4 Location of Access Points

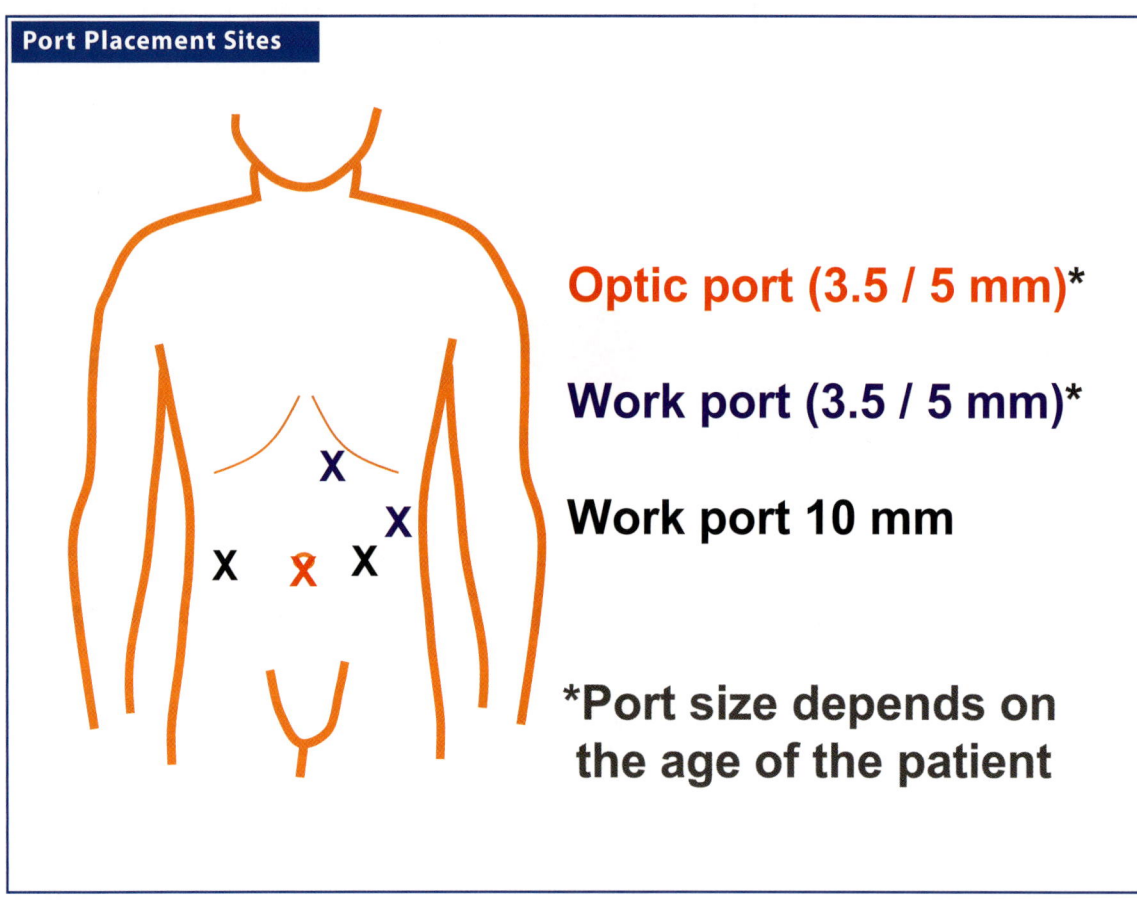

Port Placement Sites

Optic port (3.5 / 5 mm)*

Work port (3.5 / 5 mm)*

Work port 10 mm

*Port size depends on the age of the patient

47.5   Indications

Benign liver tumor (solitary lesion in the antero-lateral segments of the liver); this procedure is still under investigation for pediatric patients.

47.6   Contraindications

1. Insufficient liver function.
2. Severe portal hypertension.
3. Cardiorespiratory dysfunction.
4. Coagulopathies.
5. Previous surgeries (relative contraindication).

47.7   Preoperative Considerations

1. Ensure there is enough blood available together with fresh frozen plasma and platelets (depending on conditions).
2. Have an intensive care unit bed available for the patient should it be needed postoperatively.
3. Insert a urinary catheter.
4. Place a central venous line and/or an arterial catheter.
5. Prophylactic antibiotics are administered and light bowel preparation is beneficial.

47.8   Technical Notes

1. The use of a 30° laparoscope is recommended as it can provide a wider range of view.
2. For a patient with good liver reserves, the Pringle maneuver is recommended, which can significantly decrease operative blood loss.
3. Lowering the central venous pressure to $<5\,cmH_2O$ (i.e., $<3.7\,mmHg$) is an effective means of reducing operative blood loss.

47.9   Procedure Variations

1. Total laparoscopic liver resections.
2. Hand-assisted laparoscopic resections.

47.10   Laparoscopic Liver Resection

Please see Figs. 1–8.

Figure 47.1

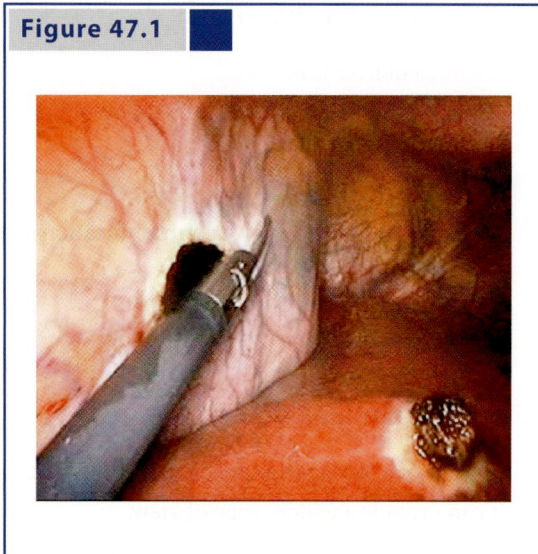

The liver is mobilized to expose the surface on either sides of the falciform ligament.

Figure 47.2

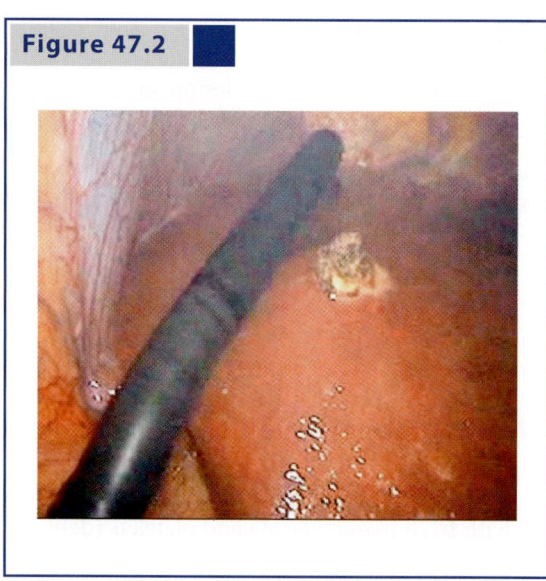

Laparoscopic ultrasonography is used to confirm the number and size of the lesions, and to define their relationship with the intrahepatic vascular structures

Figure 47.3

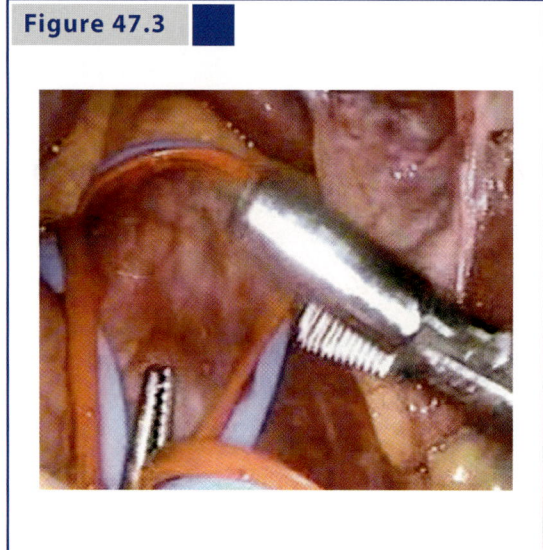

The avascular lesser omentum is divided and a vascular sling is passed around the hepatoduodenal ligament. If portal control is required, the tension can be tightened and retained by artery forceps

Figure 47.4

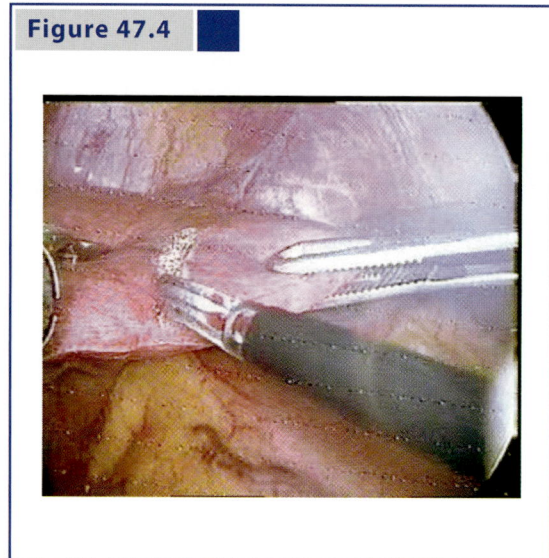

The desired plane of transection is marked on the liver surface with diathermy

Figure 47.5

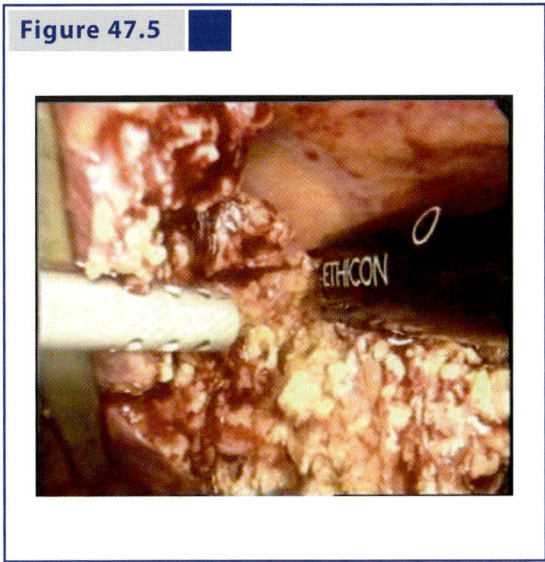

Hepatic transection is performed with a harmonic scalpel

Figure 47.6

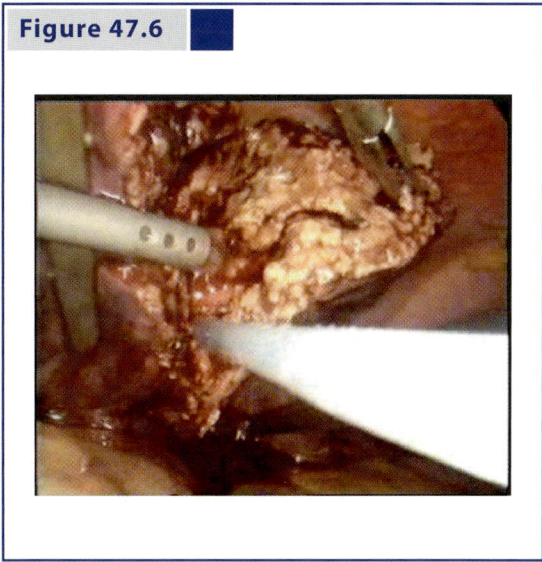

Transection is performed cautiously to circumvent the lesion

Figure 47.7

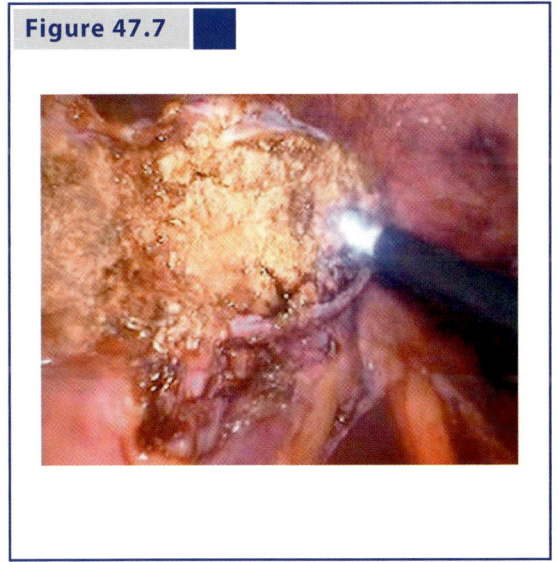

Bipolar electrocoagulation or an argon-beam coagulator is used for minor bleeding, and larger structures are secured with clips. Portal pedicles and major hepatic veins are divided by application of an endoscopic stapler

Figure 47.8

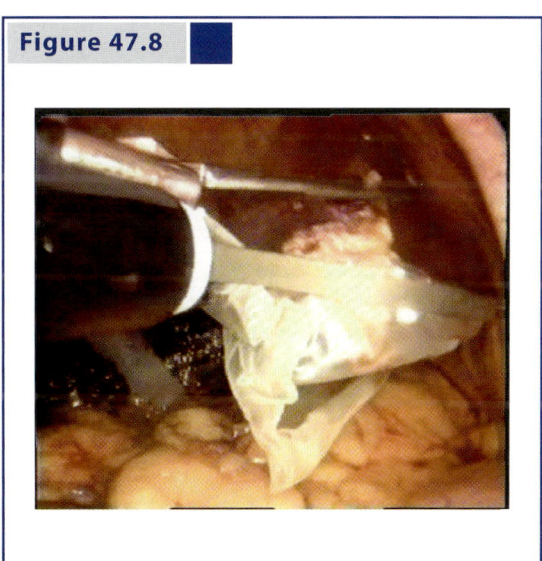

The resected specimen is placed in a specimen retrieval bag and then extracted

Recommended Literature

1. Dutta S, Nehra D, Woo R, Cohen I (2007) Laparoscopic resection of a benign liver tumor in a child. J Pediatr Surg. 42:1141–1145
2. Tang CN, Tsui KK, Ha JP, Yang GP, Li MK (2006) A single-centre experience of 40 laparoscopic liver resections. Hong Kong Med J 12:419–425
3. Yoon YS, Han HS, Choi YS, Lee SI, Jang JY, Suh KS, Kim SW, Lee KU, Park YH (2006) Total laparoscopic left lateral sectionectomy performed in a child with benign liver mass. J Pediatr Surg 41:25–28

48 Management of Hydatid Cysts

Francisco J. Berchi

48.1 Operation Room Setup

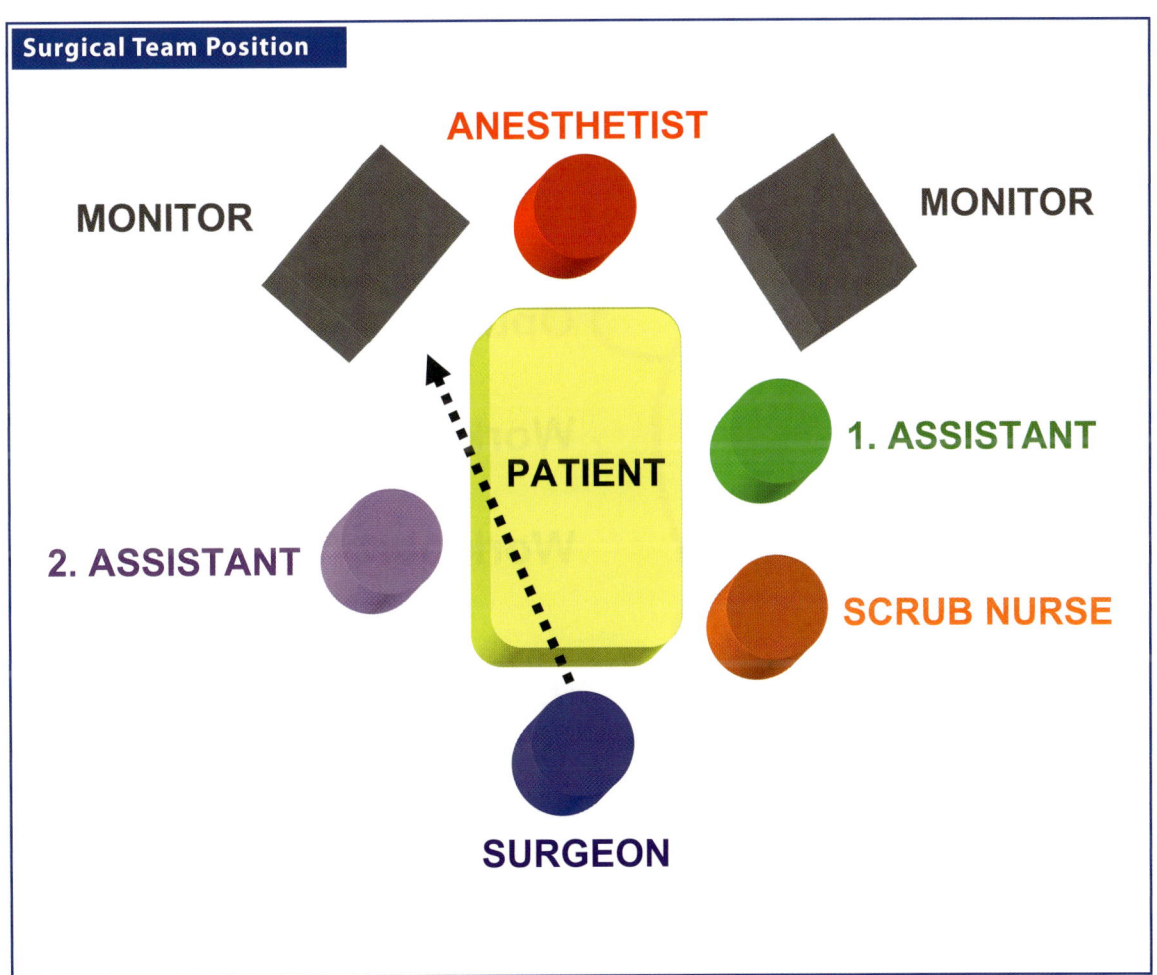

Surgical Team Position

ANESTHETIST

MONITOR

MONITOR

PATIENT

1. ASSISTANT

2. ASSISTANT

SCRUB NURSE

SURGEON

48.2   Patient Positioning

The patient is positioned "supine" at the end of the operating table with arms tucked to the side. The surgeon stands between the patient's legs.

48.3   Special Instruments

- LigaSure™ (Valleylab, Boulder, CO, USA) or Ultracision® harmonic scalpel (Johnson & Johnson Medical Products, Ethicon Endo-Surgery, Cincinnati, OH, USA)
- Tru-cut needle (Tru-cut®; Allegiance Healthcare Corp., McGraw Park, IL, USA)
- Five culture test tubes
- Specimen retrieval bag

48.4   Location of Access Points

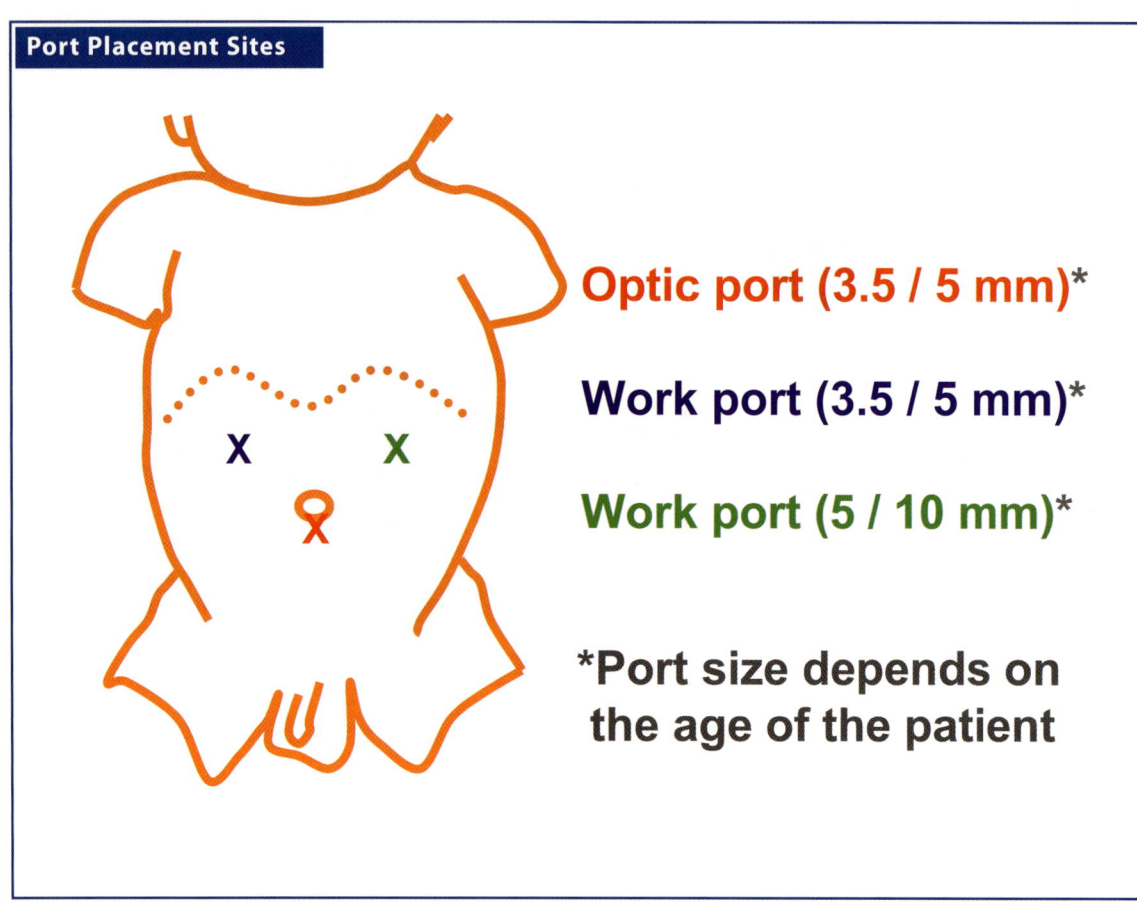

Port Placement Sites

Optic port (3.5 / 5 mm)*

Work port (3.5 / 5 mm)*

Work port (5 / 10 mm)*

*Port size depends on the age of the patient

48.5   Indications

1. *Echinococcus* cysts (single and multiple).
2. Small multivesicular cysts with calcification and located near the liver surface.

48.6   Contraindications

1. Infected cysts (sepsis).
2. Peritonitis.
3. Anaphylactic reaction or dissemination of disease.

48.7   Preoperative Considerations

1. The medical treatment is albendazole 15 mg/kg/day for 4 weeks with cessation for 2 weeks. This is repeated for three or more cycles: Hepatic function is monitored during the entire course of this therapy.
2. It is important to inform the family about the complications of surgery; particularly that of perioperative intra-abdominal dissemination of hydatids (scolices and anaphylactic reaction).
3. Nasogastric tube, urinary bladder catheter, and broad-spectrum antibiotics.

48.8   Technical Notes

1. A 14-gauge, conventional, intravenous catheter or a Veress needle is introduced into the abdominal cavity for continuous irrigation of the surface of the liver and the cyst with 10% saline.
2. A percutaneous transhepatic (never directly in to the cyst) Tru-Cut-type needle or Advocat-cannula that is connected to a suction/irrigation device is inserted into the cyst.
3. Inject 20 ml hypertonic 20% or 10% saline into the cyst and leave it for 5–10 min.
4. Suction is performed at the base of the cyst.

48.9   Procedure Variations

1. Multivesicular cysts, which are usually small with calcifications and located near the liver surface can be treated by complete laparoscopic resection using electrocautery, ultrasonic cavitron device, laser, or LigaSure™.
2. Hemostasis is essential and bile leakage may be stopped by directly suturing; with or without fibrin glue.
3. An omental patch may be used to obliterate the cavity left by the cyst.

48.10   Laparoscopic Management of Hydatid Cysts

Please see Figs. 1–6.

Figure 48.1

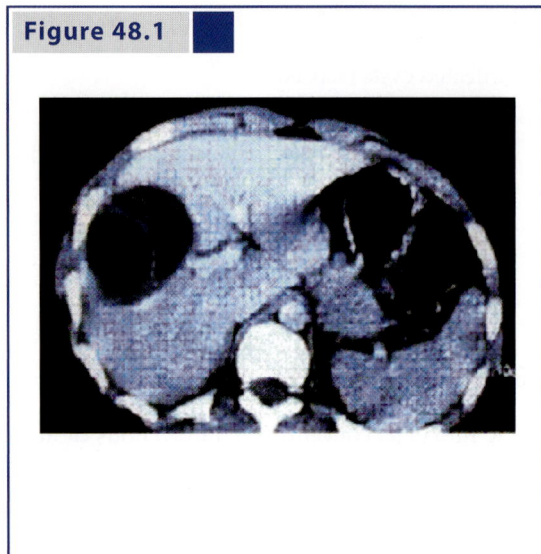

Axial computed tomography is obtained to assist in the planning of the laparoscopic procedure

Figure 48.2

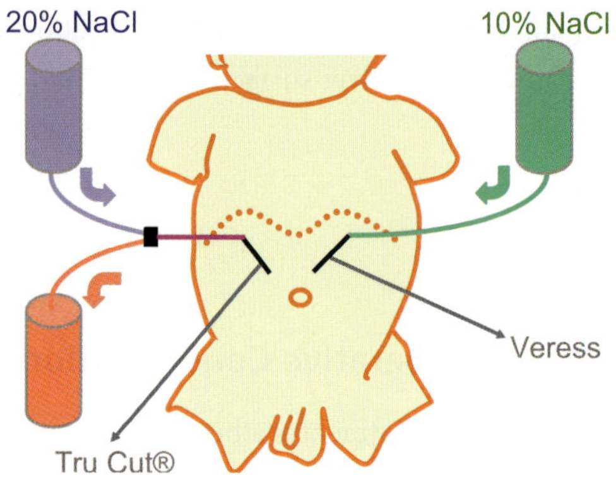

20% NaCl

10% NaCl

Veress

Tru Cut®

Setup overview: a Veress needle is used for continuous liver surface irrigation with 10% NaCl. The Tru-Cut® needle is placed in the cyst to allow the application of 20% NaCl application and aspiration of the cyst contents

Figure 48.3

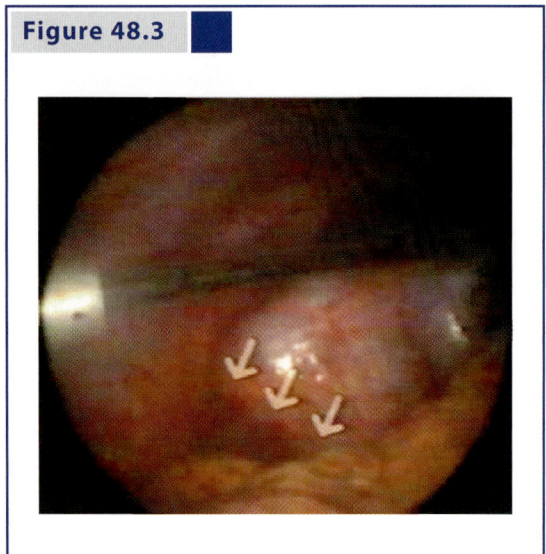

Exploration of the entire abdomen is performed. The liver surface is carefully examined to identify the cyst

Figure 48.4

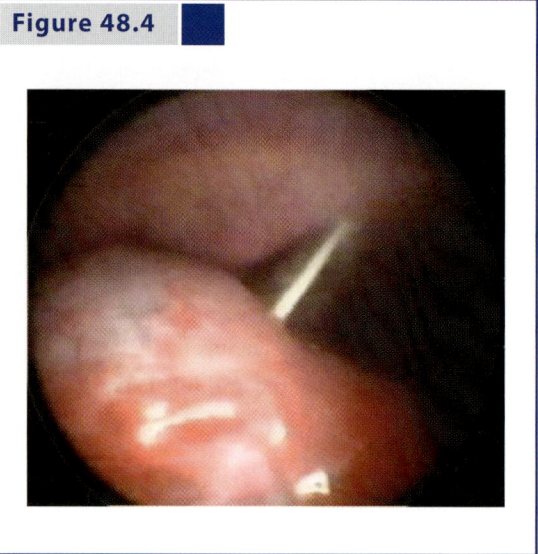

A percutaneous transhepatic Tru-Cut® needle is inserted into the cyst and suction and irrigation is carried out a minimum of five times

Figure 48.5

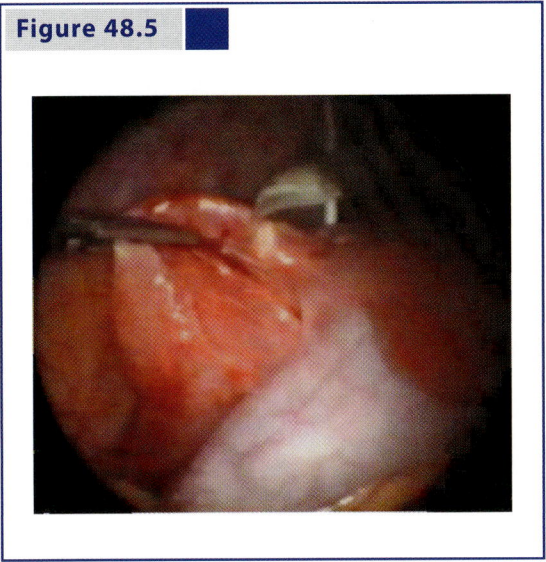

Figure 48.6

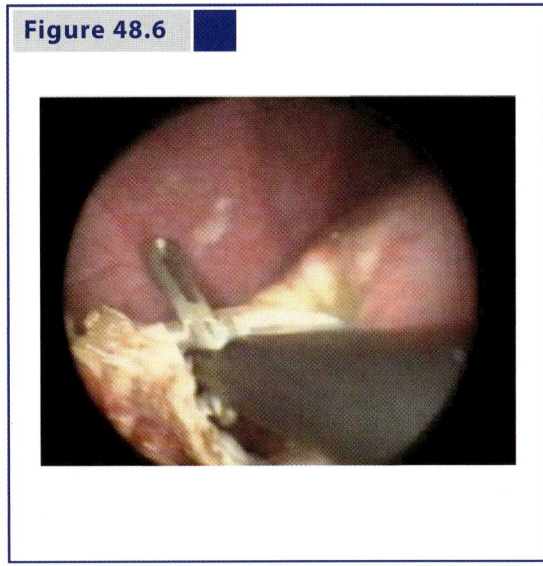

Once the cavity is completely cleared, the cyst is incised directly with electrosurgical scissors and the germinal layer is removed

The cyst wall is resected with a harmonic device and retrieved using a specimen retrieval bag. A Jackson-Pratt drain is placed before closure

Recommended Literature

1. Berchi FJ (1981) Tratamiento Endoquirurgico de la Hidatidosis Heptica en la Infancia. Premio Video-Med, Badajoz/España
2. Chen W, Xusheng L (2007) Laparoscopic surgical techniques in patients with hepatic hydatid cyst. Am J Surg 194:243–247
3. Maazoun K, Mekki M, Chioukh F, Sahnoun L, Ksia A, Jouini R, Jallouli M, Krichene I, Belghith M, Nouri A (2007) Laparoscopic treatment of hydatid cyst of the liver in children. A report on 34 cases. J Pediatr Surg 42:1683–1686

49 Management of Pancreatic Pseudocysts

CHINNUSAMY PALANIVELU
AND MUTHUKUMARAN RANGARAJAN

49.1 Operation Room Setup

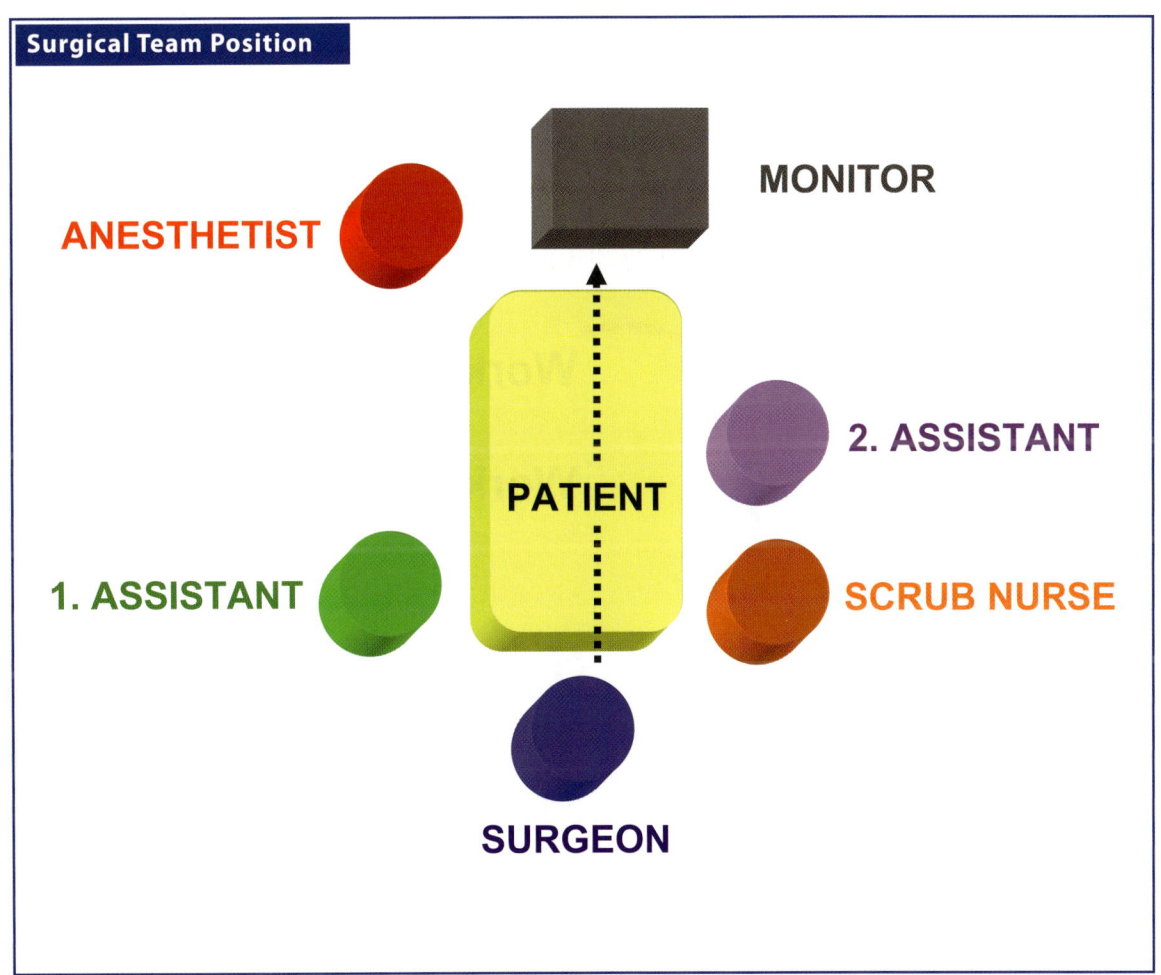

49.2   Patient Positioning

Supine position with the patient's arms outstretched.

49.3   Special Instruments

- Ultracision® shears (Johnson&Johnson Medical Products, Ethicon Endo-Surgery, Cincinnati, OH, USA)
- EndoGIA™ stapler (Auto Suture, Norwalk, CT, USA)

49.4   Location of Access Points

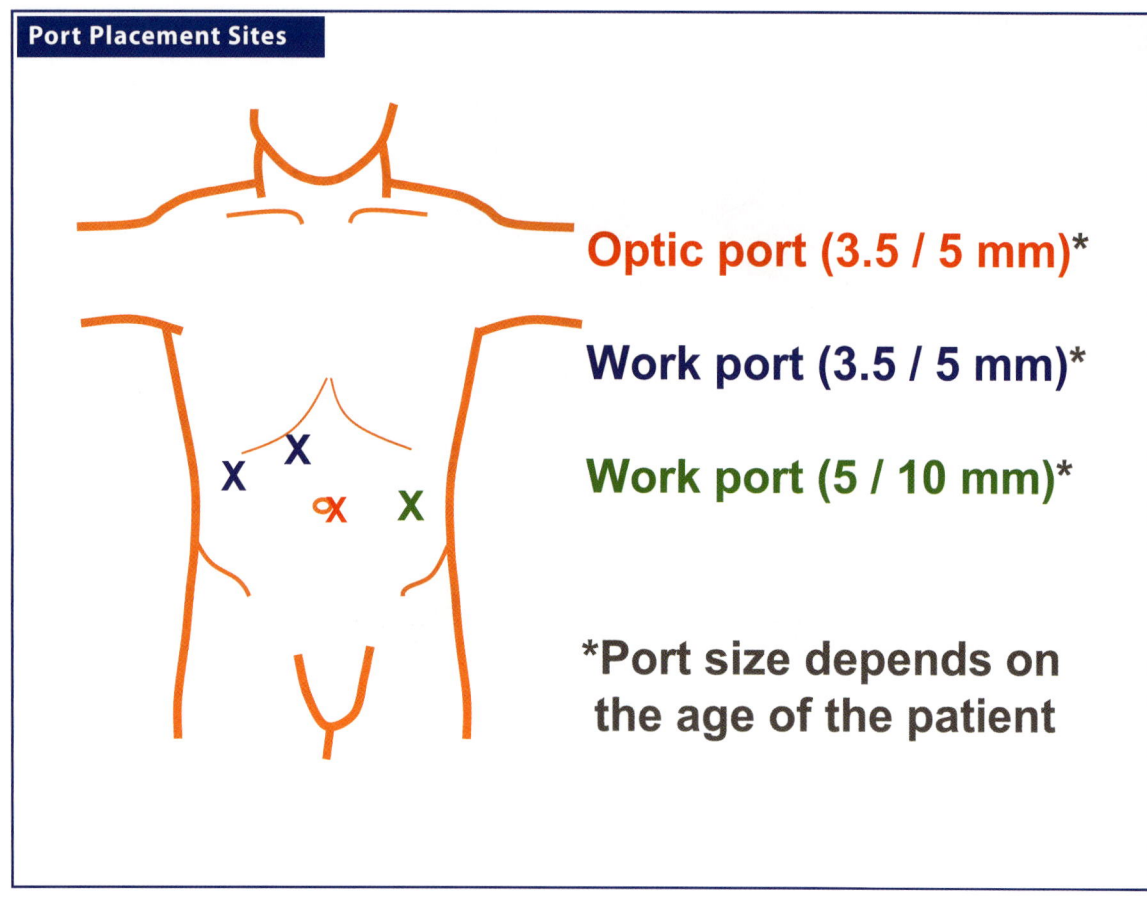

49.5   Indications

1. Symptomatic cysts
2. Rapidly enlarging cysts.
3. Cyst with diameter > 6 cm.
4. Surgery is performed 6 weeks after the development of the cyst.
5. Presence of pancreatic necrosis.
6. Development of complications like rupture, infection, and obstruction of the bile duct, duodenum, and other adjacent organs.

49.6   Contraindications

1. Extensive contamination or peritonitis.
2. Four weeks or less from the onset of the pancreatitis.

49.7   Preoperative Considerations

1. Complete blood count, renal profile, liver-function tests, coagulation profile, serum amylase and lipase, ultrasonography, and dual-phase computed tomography with a specific pancreatic-imaging protocol are mandatory.
2. Magnetic resonance cholangiopancreatography may be used selectively.
3. Team set up depends on the location of the pseudocyst.
4. Adequate resuscitation if needed preoperatively.

49.8   Technical Notes

1. Anterior gastrotomy at the summit of the cyst is the first step.
2. Diagnostic aspiration should be done under direct vision using a spinal needle attached to a 10-ml syringe.
3. A stoma of approximately 4 cm diameter should be created using ultrasonic shears between the cyst and posterior wall of the stomach.
4. The cyst cavity is best examined using a 30° telescope.

49.9   Procedure Variations

1. Cystojejunostomy is a suitable technique for pseudocysts of the gastrocolic omentum or those present in the paracolic gutter at the left iliac fossa.
2. In the cystojejunostomy procedure, a Roux-en-Y jejunal loop is created using an EndoGIA™ stapler.
3. Furthermore, after debridement, a 4-cm, handsewn, pseudocystojejunal anastomosis is performed with continuous sutures.

49.10   Laparoscopic Cystogastrostomy for Pancreas Pseudocyst

Please see Figs. 1–6.

Figure 49.1

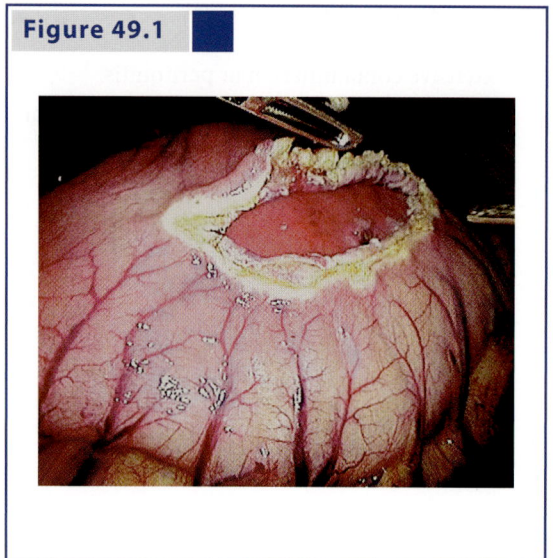

An anterior gastrotomy is performed with Ultracision® shears. The pseudocyst can be seen bulging through the posterior wall of the stomach

Figure 49.2

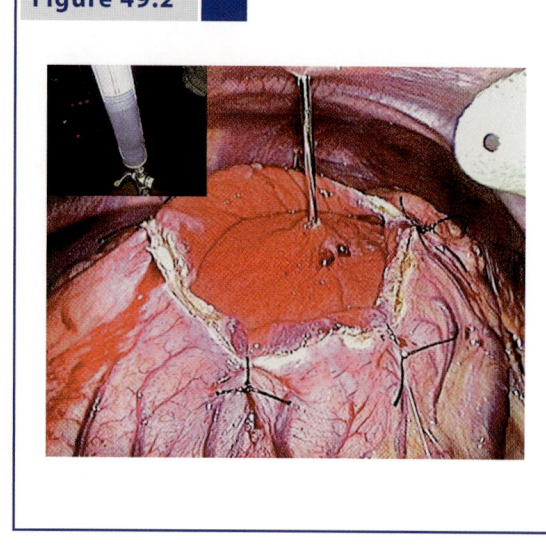

Diagnostic percutaneous aspiration of fluid from the cyst is performed

Figure 49.3

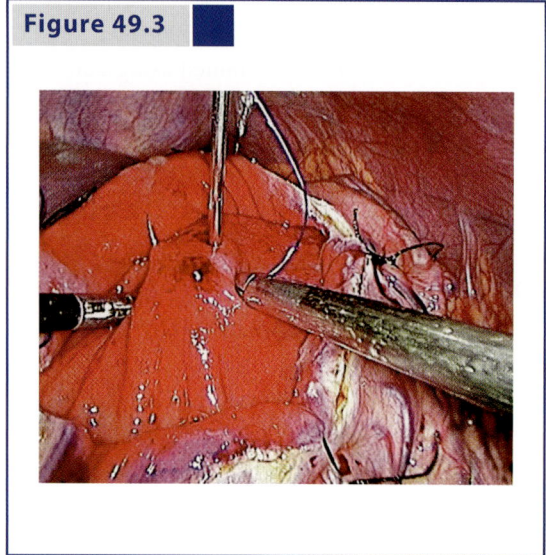

A summit stitch is placed on the posterior wall of the stomach

Figure 49.4

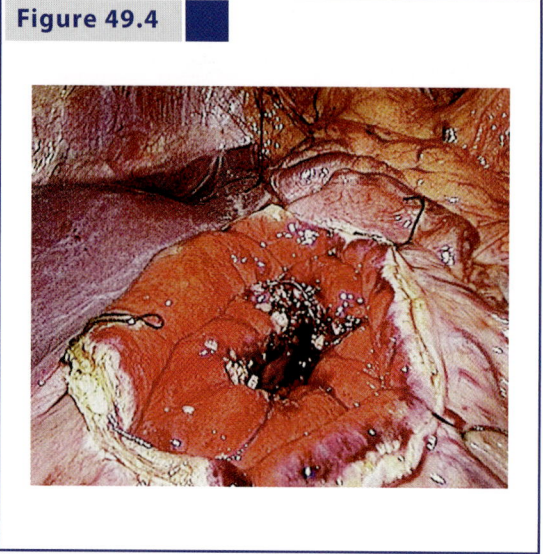

A cystostomy is performed through the posterior gastric wall using Ultracision® shears

Figure 49.5

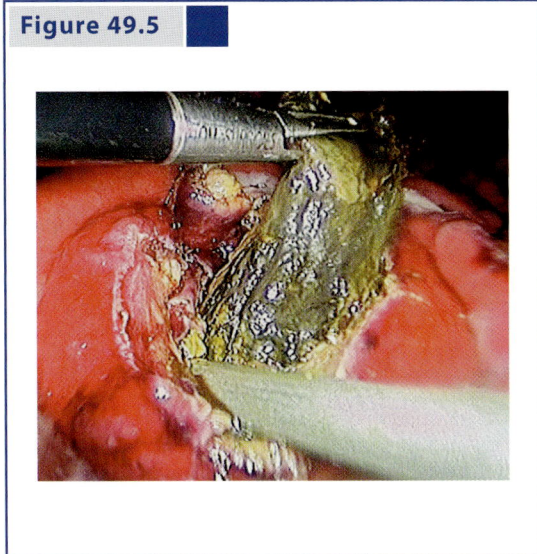

Figure 49.6

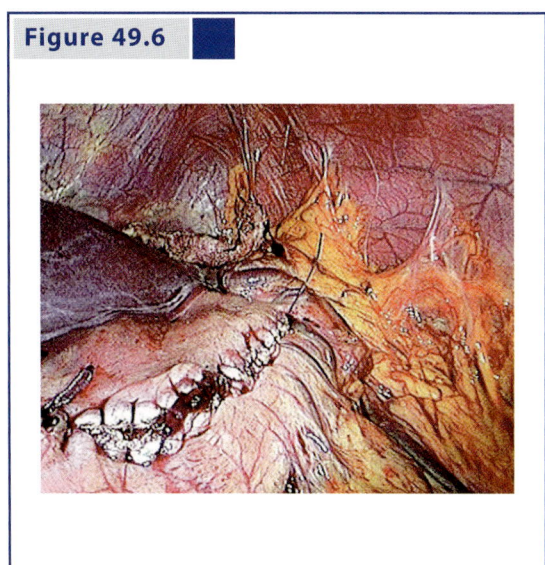

A necrosectomy is performed and the debris attached to the wall of the cyst is removed

The anterior gastrotomy is closed with continuous intracorporeal sutures

Recommended Literature

1. Bufo AJ (2004) Endolaparoscopic cystogastrostomy: pushing the envelope of minimally invasive surgery in children. Pediatr Endosurg Inn Tech 8:344–347
2. Saad DF, Gow KW, Cabbabe S, Heiss KF, Wulkan ML (2005) Laparoscopic cystogastrostomy for the treatment of pancreatic pseudocysts in children. J Pediatr Surg 40:e13–17
3. Seitz G, Warmann SW, Kirschner HJ, Haber HP, Schaefer JW, Fuchs J (2006) Laparoscopic cystojejunostomy as a treatment option for pancreatic pseudocysts in children – a case report. J Pediatr Surg 41:e33–35

50 Pancreatectomy

Mark L. Wulkan

50.1 Operation Room Setup

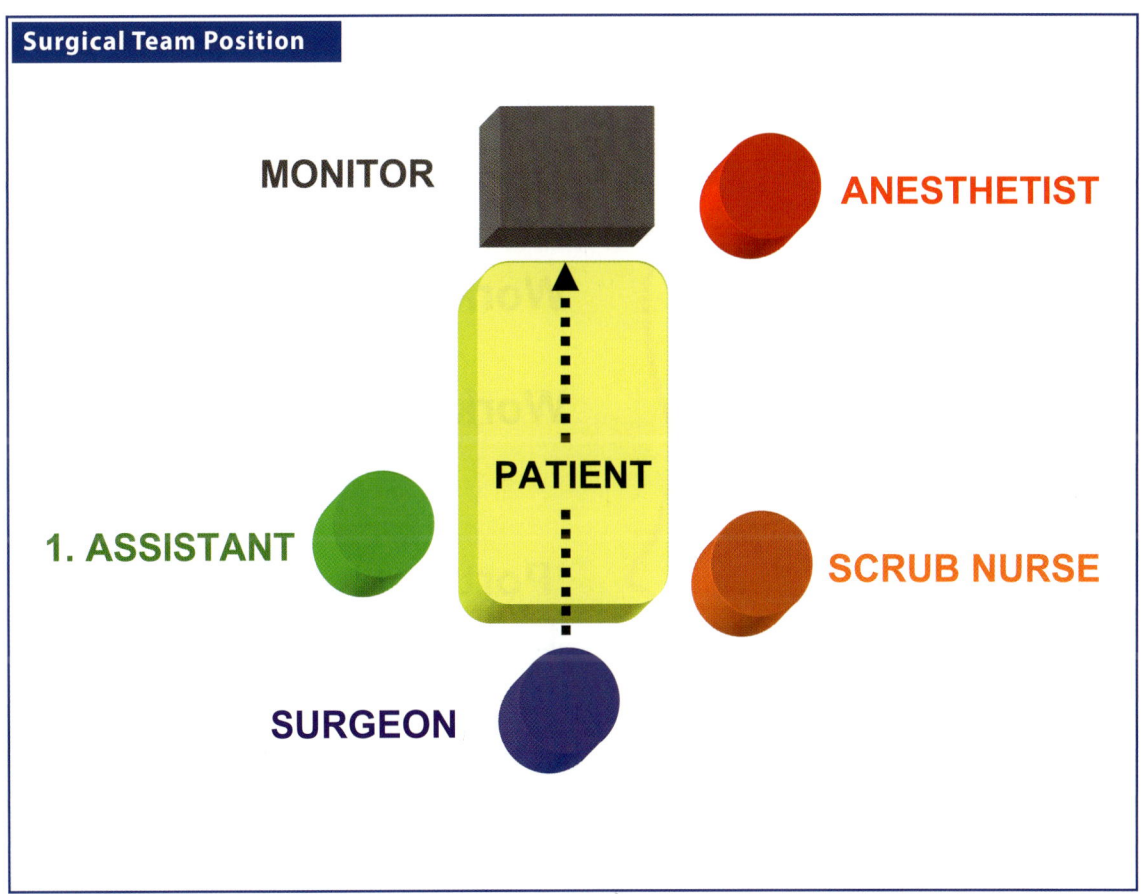

Surgical Team Position

MONITOR

ANESTHETIST

1. ASSISTANT

PATIENT

SCRUB NURSE

SURGEON

50.2   Patient Positioning

Young patients are placed in the frog-leg position. Older patients are placed in the lithotomy position. The surgeon stands in the "French" position, between the patient's legs or at the foot of the bed.

50.3   Special Instruments

- Ultracision® shears (Johnson & Johnson Medical Products, Ethicon Endo-Surgery, Cincinnati, OH, USA)
- LigaSure™ (Valleylab, Boulder, CO, USA).
- Specimen retrieval bag

50.4   Location of Access Points

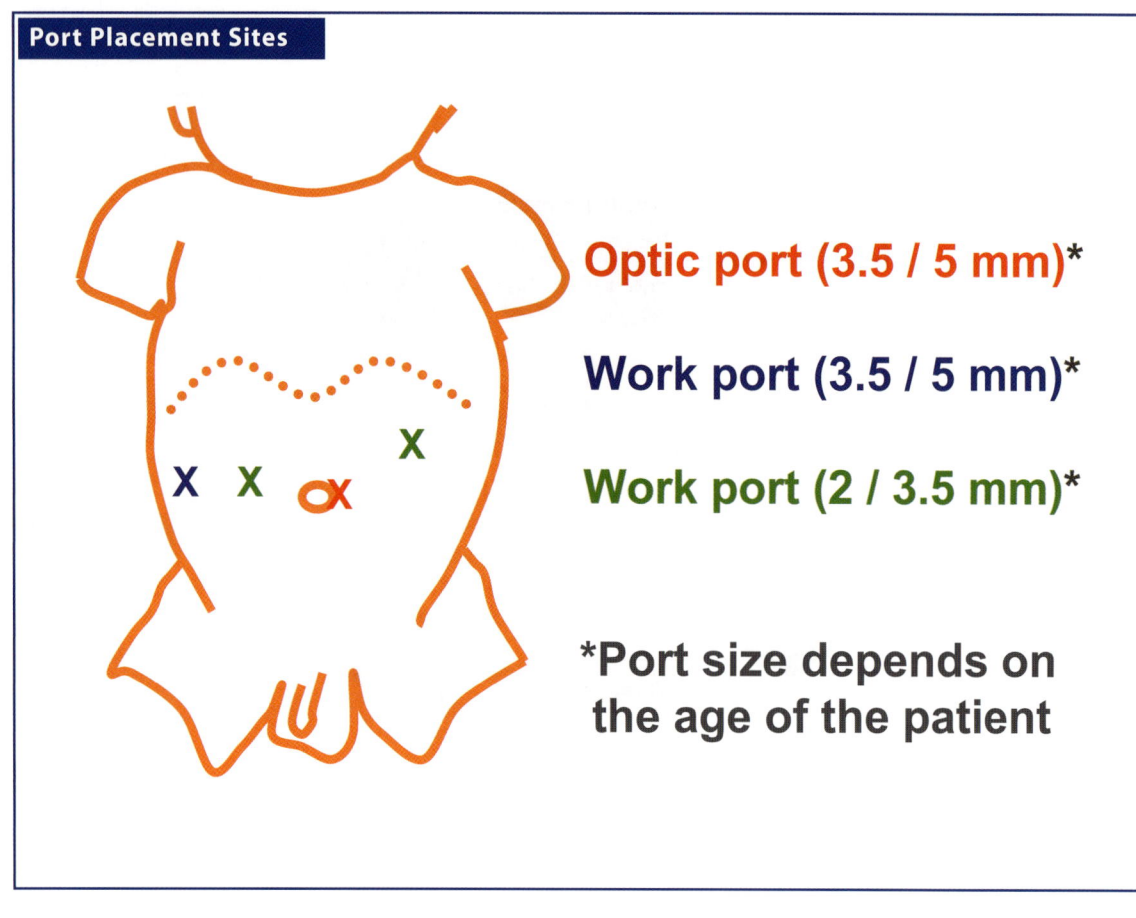

Port Placement Sites

Optic port (3.5 / 5 mm)*

Work port (3.5 / 5 mm)*

Work port (2 / 3.5 mm)*

*Port size depends on the age of the patient

50.5   Indications

1. Insulinoma.
2. Hyperinsulinism.
3. Trauma.
4. Other pancreatic tumors.

50.6   Contraindications

General contraindications to laparoscopic surgery.

50.7   Preoperative Considerations

1. Glucose levels should be controlled.
2. Preoperative work-up for hyperinsulinism may include magnetic resonance imaging, computed tomography, selective venous sampling, or a selective calcium stimulation test.
3. New nuclear medicine scans are being developed to help localize insulinoma.

50.8   Technical Notes

1. Suspend the stomach from the abdominal wall with a heavy suture.
2. Ultrasonic shears and the LigaSure™ bipolar device are effective at dividing the parenchyma.
3. Cholangiography may be necessary to identify the location of the common bile duct.

50.9   Procedure Variations

1. With the patient positioned on the right lateral side, the plane located between the left kidney and the posterior aspects of the spleen and pancreas can be dissected.
2. Application of tissue sealant to prevent fistula formation after pancreatectomy.
3. The Penrose drain "lasso" technique can be employed for atraumatic manipulation of the pancreas during the procedure.

50.10   Laparoscopic Pancreatectomy

Please see Figs. 1–9.

Figure 50.1

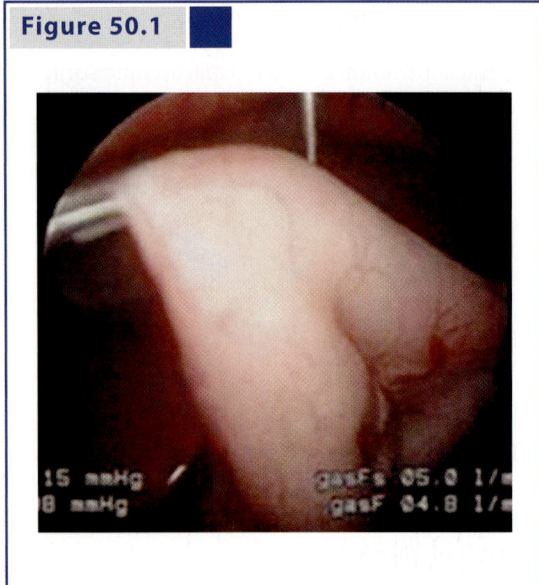

The stomach is suspended from the anterior wall using heavy suture material on a big needle through the abdominal wall

Figure 50.2

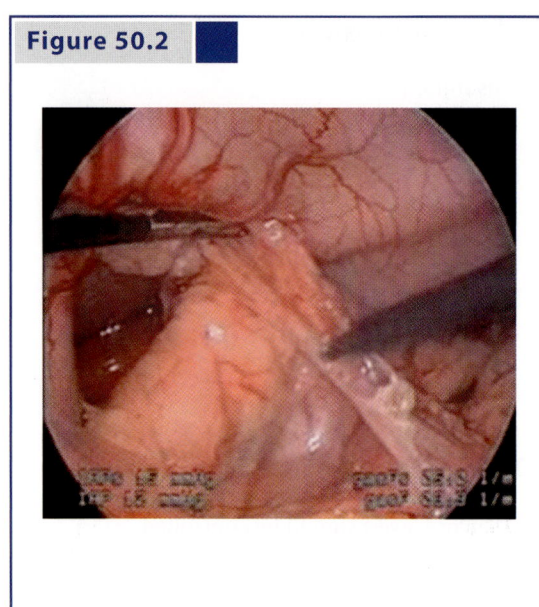

After the lesser sac is entered, the inferior margin of the pancreatic tail is dissected from the retroperitoneum

Figure 50.3

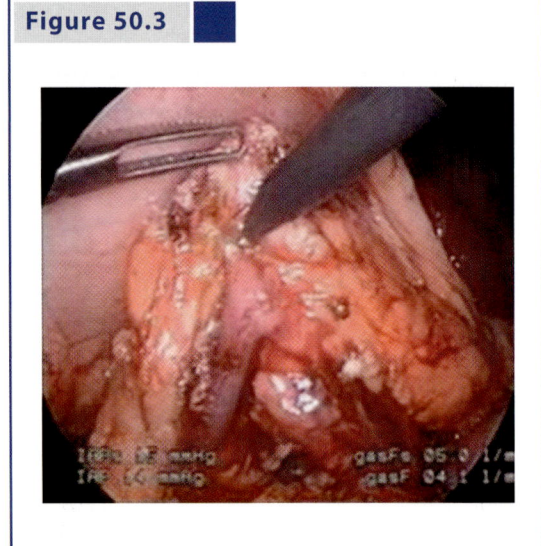

The small branches of the splenic vein are dissected and divided using hook electrocautery. Ultrasonic shears may also be used

Figure 50.4

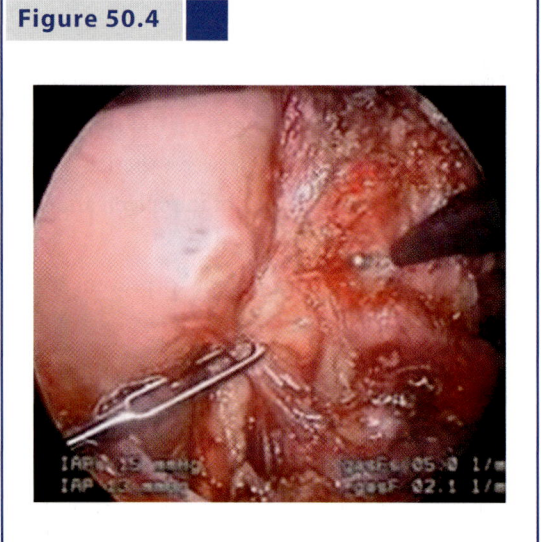

In a similar fashion, the splenic artery is dissected off the tail of the pancreas

Figure 50.5

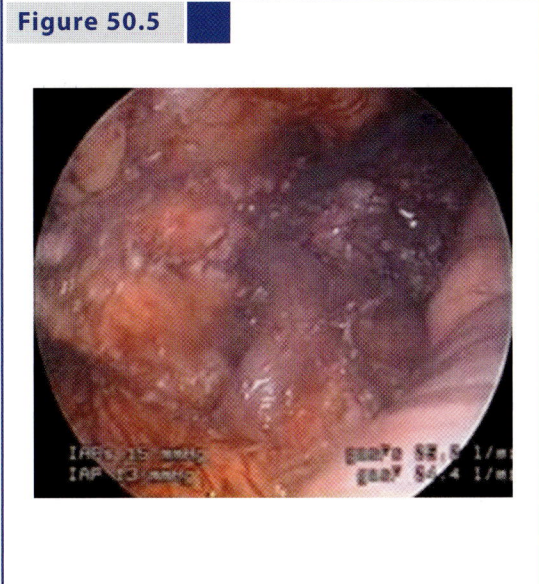

The tail is free and the uncinate process can be seen next to the confluence of the splenic and superior mesenteric arteries. The uncinate process is dissected off the superior mesenteric artery using hook electrocautery

Figure 50.6

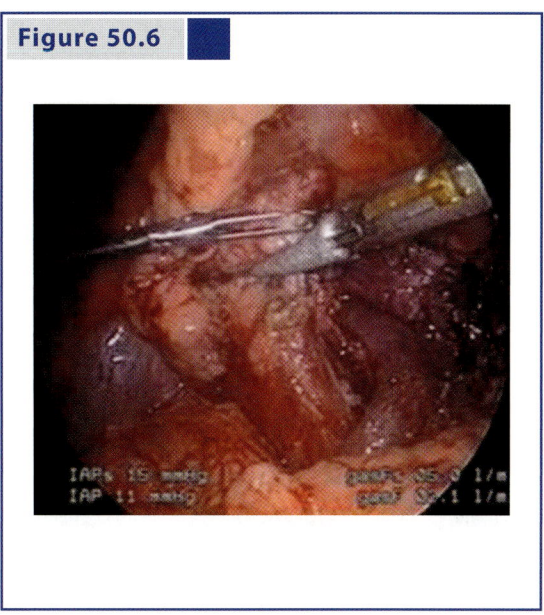

The transverse pancreatic arteries are controlled using the LigaSure™ device as the gland is divided

Figure 50.7

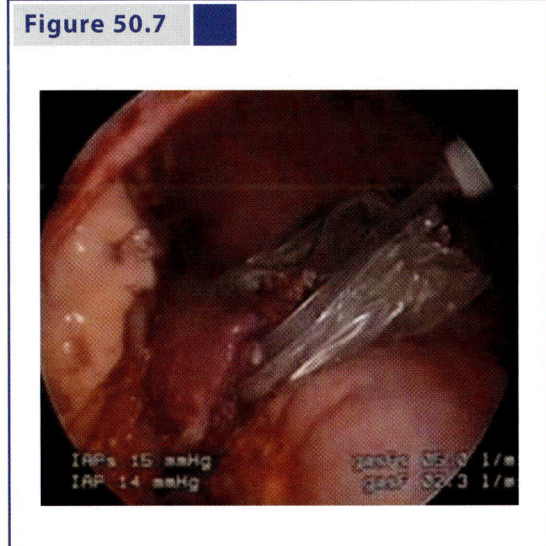
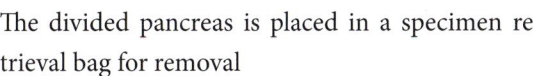

The divided pancreas is placed in a specimen retrieval bag for removal

Figure 50.8

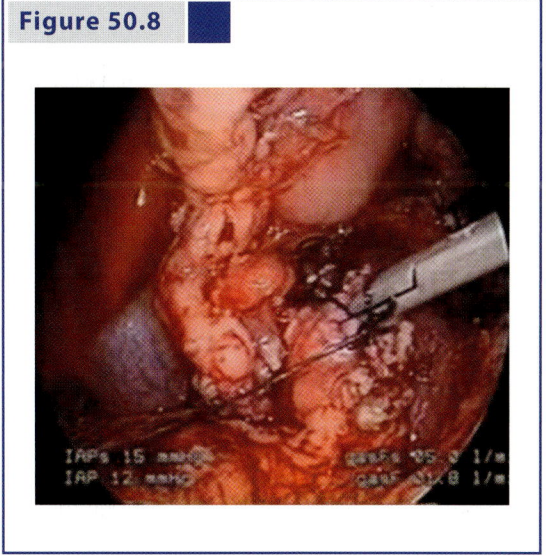

The pancreatic stump is over sewn

Figure 50.9

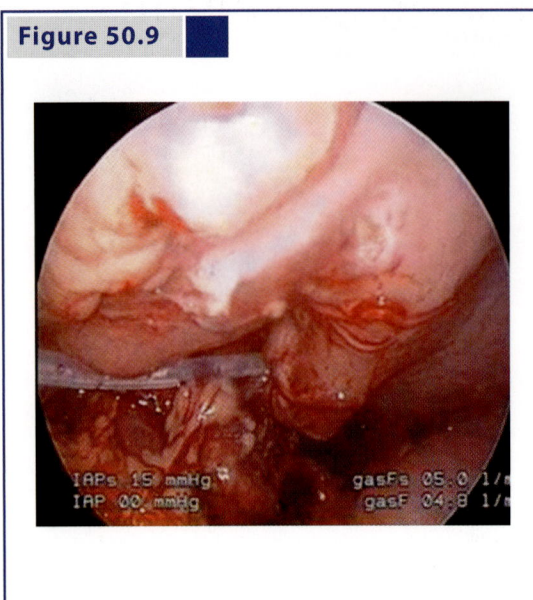

A drainage catheter is left in place

Recommended Literature

1. Bax KN, van der Zee DC (2007) The laparoscopic approach towards hyperinsulinism in children. Semin Pediatr Surg 16:245–251
2. Melotti G, Butturini G, Piccoli M, Casetti L, Bassi C, Mullineris B, Lazzaretti MG, Pederzolli P (2007) Laparoscopic distal pancreatectomy: results on a consecutive series of 58 patients. Ann Surg 246:77–82
3. Takaori K, Tanigawa N (2007) Laparoscopic pancreatic resection: the past, present and future. Surg Today 37:535–545

51 Splenectomy and Related Procedures

PAUL PHILIPPE

51.1 Operation Room Setup

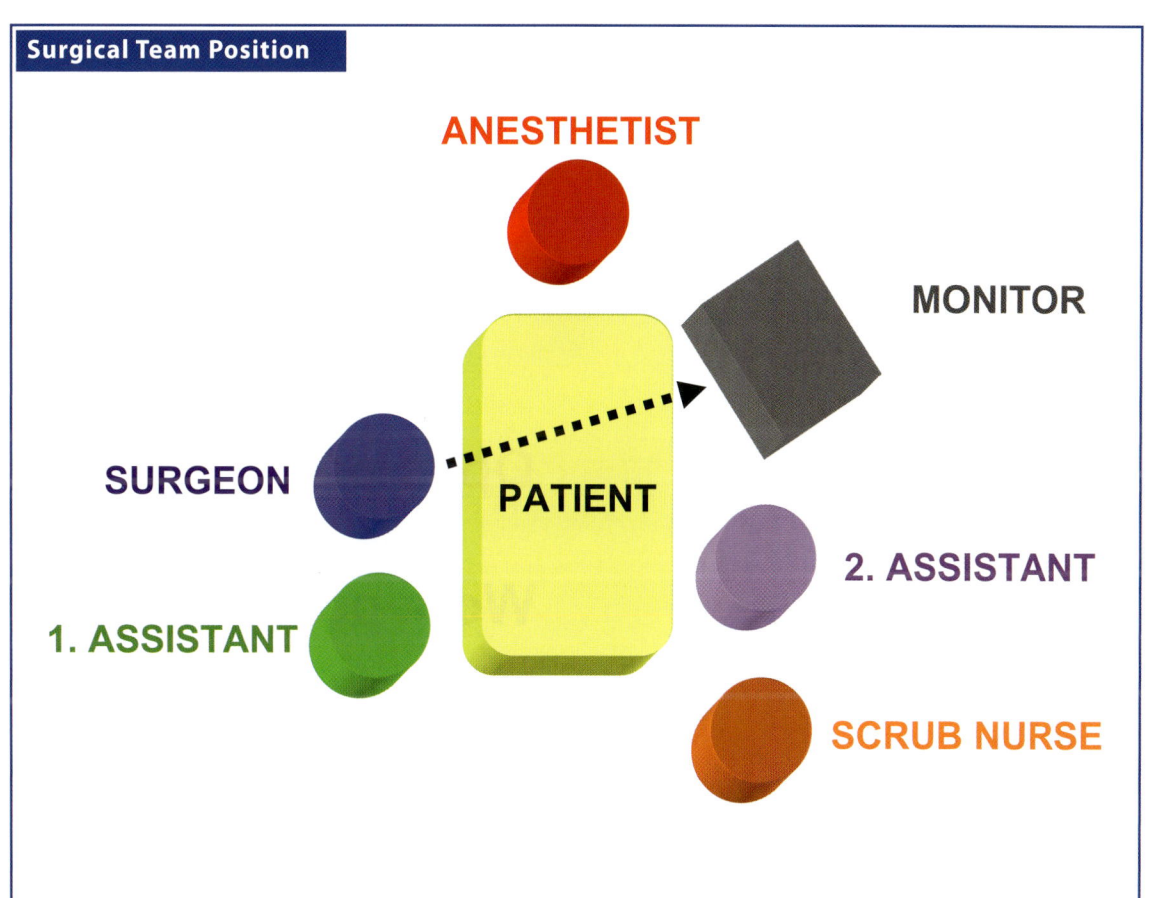

51.2   Patient Positioning

Right lateral decubitus with a roll under the right flank. If associated with cholecystectomy, a 45° lateral decubitus position is preferred (the table is tilted to the side for the splenic part and returned to neutral position for the biliary part of the procedure).

51.3   Special Instruments

- EnSeal® (SurgRx, Redwood City, CA, USA) Tissue Sealing Device (TSD) or
- Ultracision® harmonic scalpel (Johnson & Johnson Medical Products, Ethicon Endo-Surgery, Cincinnati, OH, USA) or
- 5-mm clip applicator
- Tachosil® (Nycomed GmbH, Zürich, Switzerland)

51.4   Location of Access Points

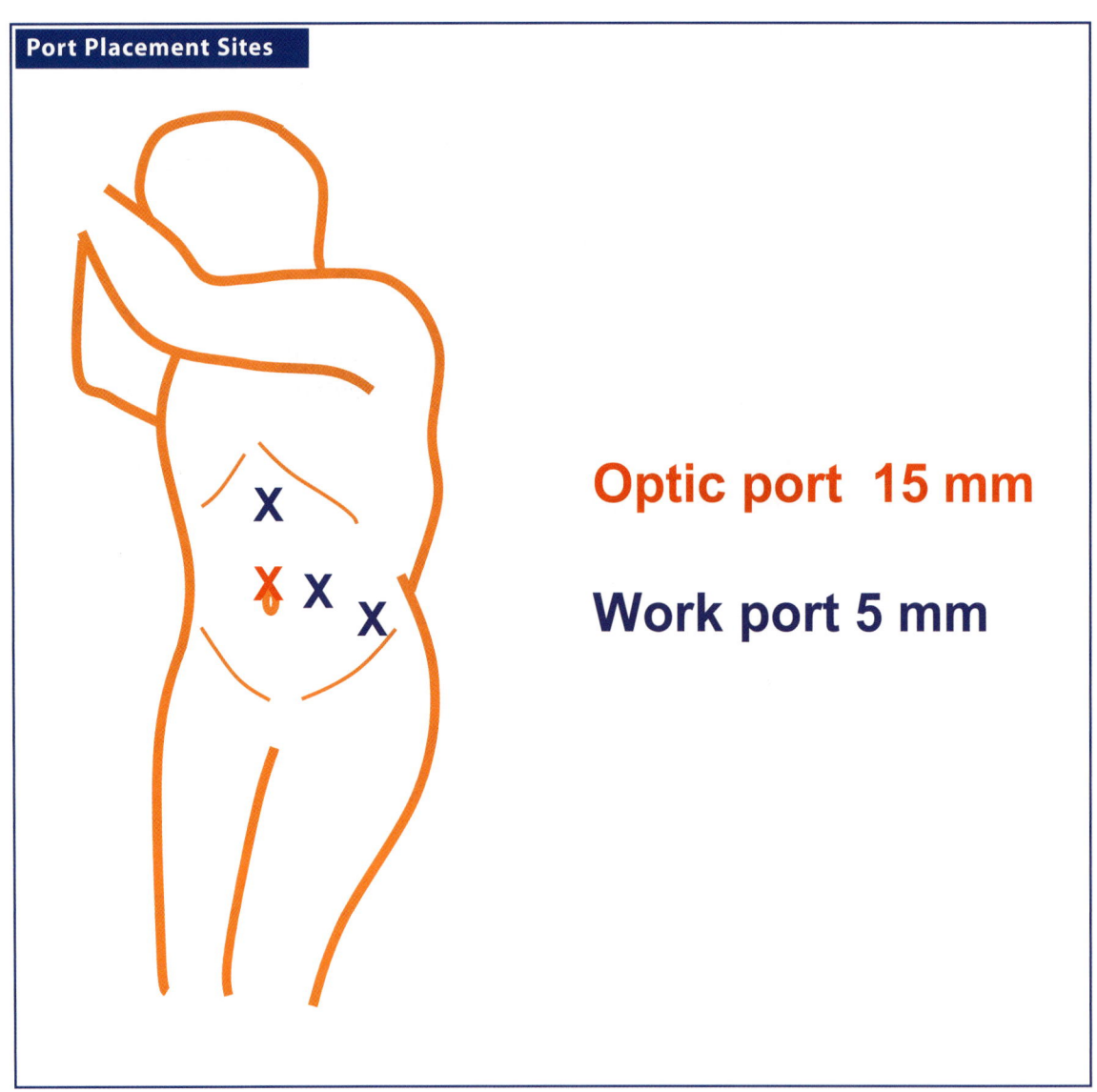

Port Placement Sites

Optic port 15 mm

Work port 5 mm

51.5 Total Splenectomy

51.5.1 Indications

1. Hematologic disorders including hereditary spherocytosis.
2. Immune thrombocytopenic purpura.
3. Sickle cell anemia.
4. Tumors.

51.5.2 Contraindications

1. Hemodynamic instability (trauma).
2. Splenic abscesses.
3. Massive splenomegaly requires advanced skills and experience. Consider preoperative embolization.

51.5.3 Preoperative Considerations

1. Consider pneumococcal vaccination and perioperative penicillin administration.
2. Consider partial splenectomy in hemolytic disorders. The extent of resection depends on the severity of hemolysis (resect the larger part of the spleen if hemolysis is severe).
3. Type- and cross-matching is prudent in partial splenectomies. Platelet transfusion may be necessary.

51.5.4 Technical Notes

1. Insert trocars under visual guidance to avoid splenic injury in cases of splenomegaly.
2. The artery and vein should be dissected and occluded separately.
3. Keep the spleen attached to the left upper quadrant and use gravity to retract the stomach and colon.
4. A large, spring-loaded specimen-retrieval bag allows the surgeon to "scoop" the spleen from its lower pole upward.
5. Retrieve the bag through an enlarged umbilical incision. Use fingers or atraumatic forceps to morcelate the spleen, since rupture of the specimen-retrieval bag carries the risk of splenosis.

51.5.5 Procedure Variations

1. Dorsal decubitus positioning of the patients can be done; however, this requires more ports for exposure.
2. Vascular control can be achieved safely with intracorporeal ligatures, but it is faster with a TSD.
3. The specimen can be extracted through a Pfannenstiel incision in the case of massive splenomegaly or if an intact specimen is required for pathological evaluation.

51.5.6 Laparoscopic Total Splenectomy

Please see Figs. 1–8.

Figure 51.1

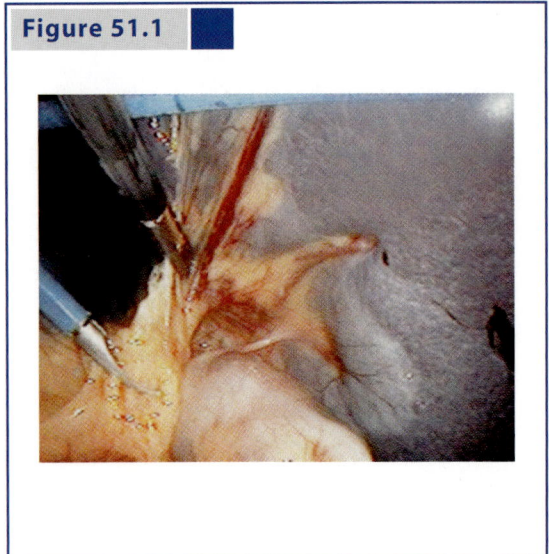

With the spleen lifted by the flank instrument, the colosplenic ligaments are taken down

Figure 51.2

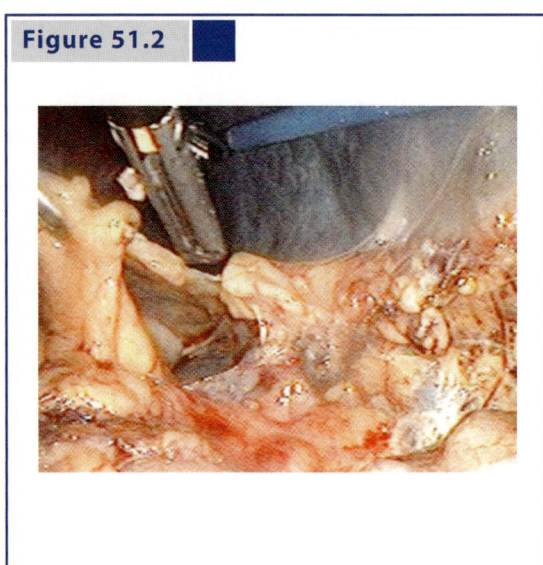

The gastrosplenic ligament (short gastric vessels) is opened with the LigaSure™ tissue-sealing device

Figure 51.3

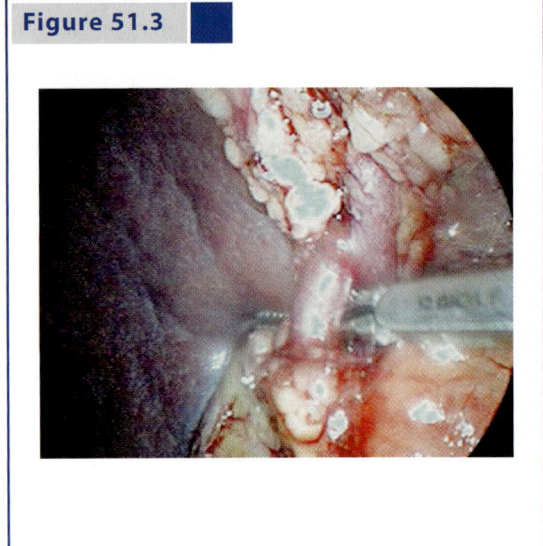

The dissection of the splenic hilus is performed with the intention of isolating the splenic artery from the vein

Figure 51.4

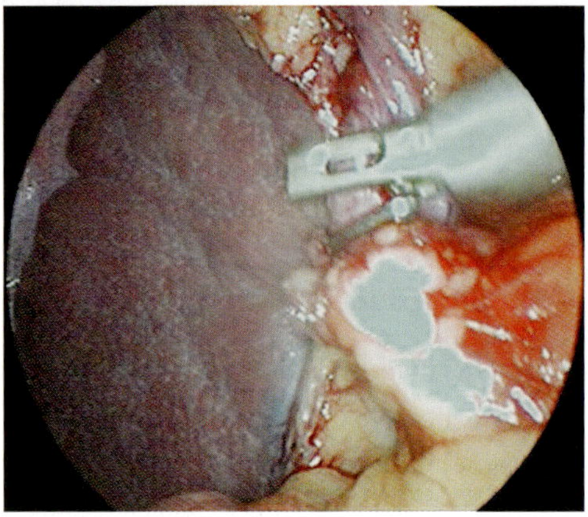

The artery can be ligated and divided using a variety of techniques. The most preferred devices for ligation are clips, hand ligatures, or tissue-sealing devices

Figure 51.5

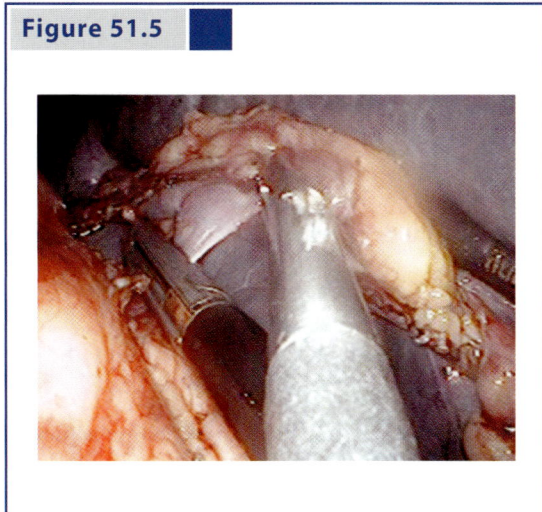

The vein is ligated and divided similarly. A tissue-sealing device as shown here is preferred for this purpose

Figure 51.6

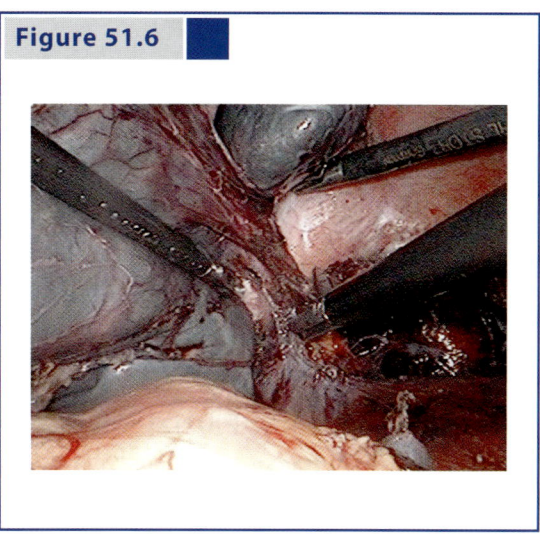

The posterior attachments are taken down, keeping the spleen "hung" to facilitate specimen retrieval bag insertion

Figure 51.7

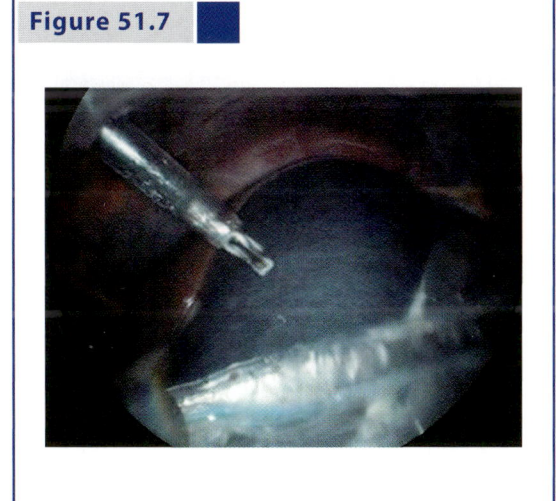

The spleen is "scooped" into a large specimen retrieval bag, with the lower pole being introduced into the bag first

Figure 51.8

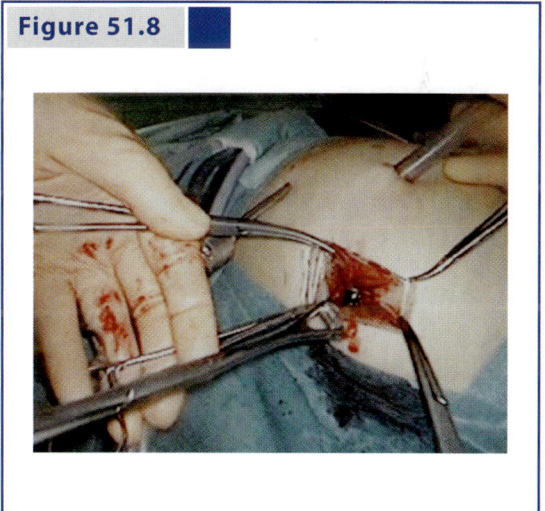

The specimen is fragmented in the bag using a finger or an atraumatic forceps, and then extracted

51.6   Partial Splenectomy

51.6.1   Indications

1. Cysts and tumors (hamartomas).
2. Hemolytic disorders with preservation of splenic function.
3. Gaucher's disease.

51.7   Laparoscopic Partial Splenectomy

Please see Figs. 9–12.

51.6.2   Technical Notes

1. Both upper and lower partial splenectomies are possible.
2. Divide the arterial branches to the part to be resected. Prior isolation of the main splenic artery is optional.
3. Parenchymal dissection is facilitated by the use of a TSD or harmonic scalpel.
4. If necessary, hemostasis can be further achieved with fibrin glue (spray) or fibrinogen/thrombin-coated collagen sponge (Tachosil®).

Figure 51.9

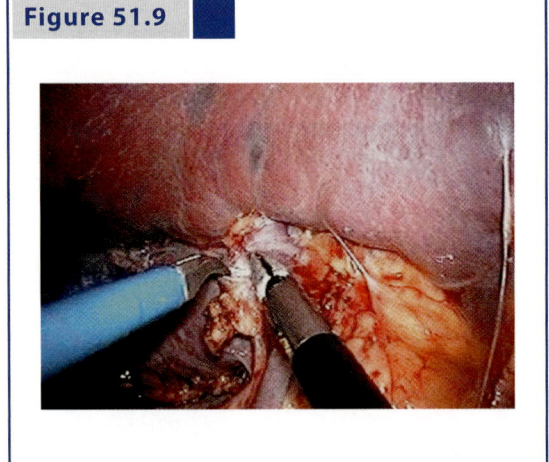

For partial splenectomy, the vessels supplying the part to be resected are selectively divided and dissected

Figure 51.10

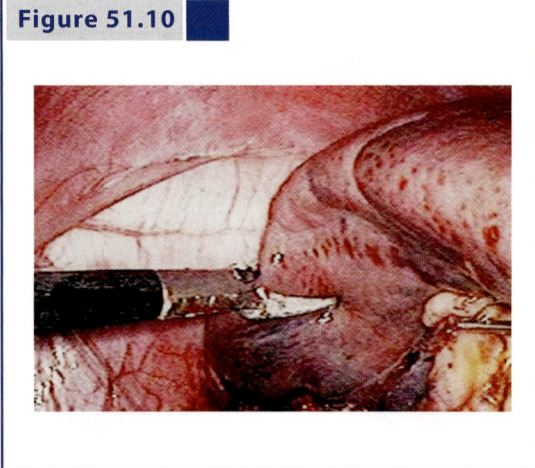

The parenchyma is divided with a tissue-sealing device along the demarcation line

Figure 51.11

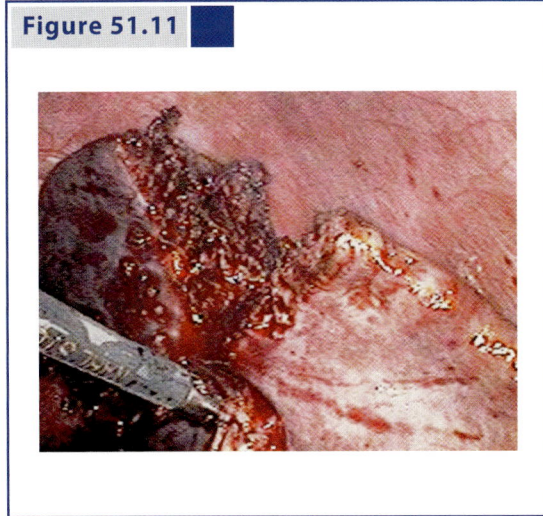

Figure 51.12

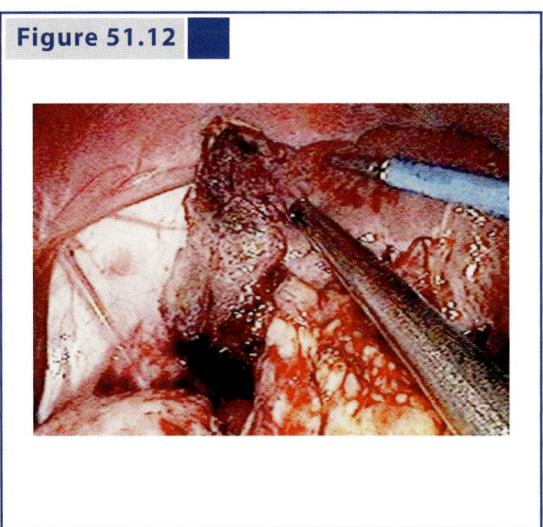

The parenchymal resection is completed with minimal bleeding

Hemostasis is further achieved with the placement of a fibrinogen/thrombin-coated collagen sponge (Tachosil®) on the resected parenchymal surface

Recommended Literature

1. Breitenstein S, Scholtz T, Schefer M, Decurtins M, Clavien PA (2007) Laparoscopic partial splenectomy. J Am Coll Surg 204:179–181
2. Rescorla FJ, West KW, Engum SA, Grosfeld JL (2007) Laparoscopic splenic procedures in children: experience in 231 children. Ann Surg 246:683–687
3. Sheshadri PA, Poulin EC, Mamazza J, Schlachta CM (2000) Technique for laparoscopic partial splenectomy. Surg Laparosc Endosc Percutan Tech 10:106–109

52 Mesh Splenopexy for Wandering Spleen

Chinnusamy Palanivelu
and Muthukumaran Rangarajan

52.1 Operation Room Setup

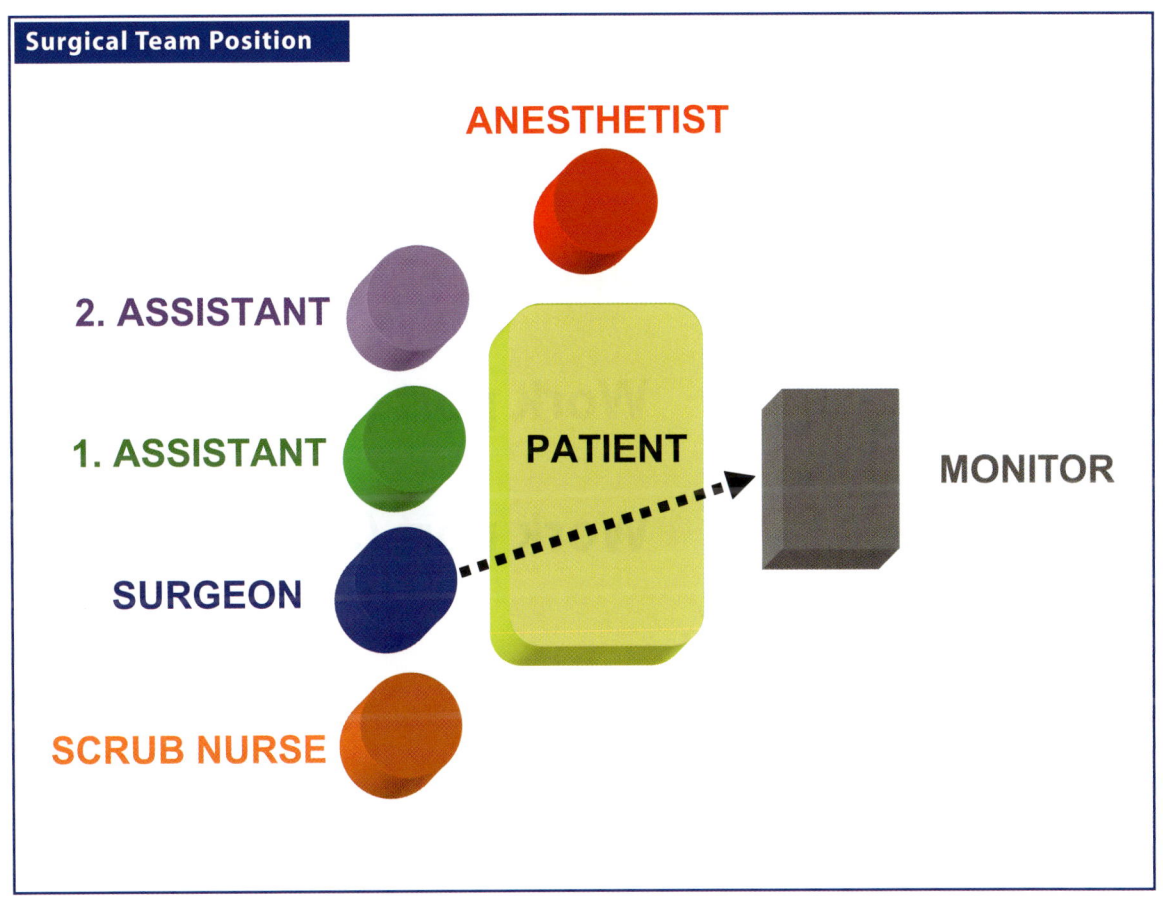

52.2   Patient Positioning

Right lateral decubitus position with a roll placed under the right flank.

52.3   Special Instruments

Polypropylene composite mesh.

52.4   Location of Access Points

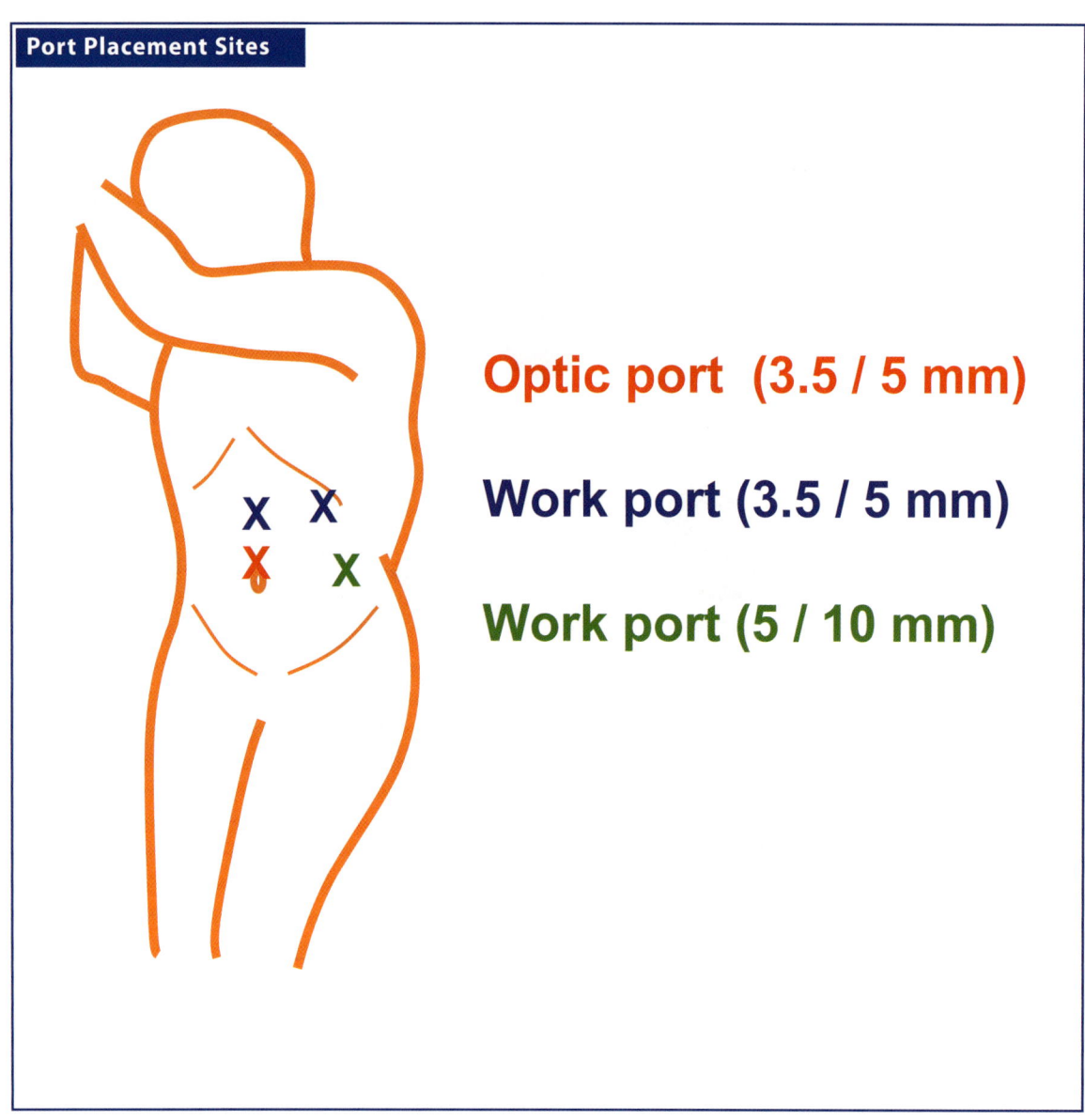

Port Placement Sites

Optic port (3.5 / 5 mm)

Work port (3.5 / 5 mm)

Work port (5 / 10 mm)

52.5   Indications

1. Wandering spleen.
2. Pelvic spleen.
3. Torsion of the spleen.
4. Large splenic cysts that require laparoscopic mobilization of the spleen and its reattachment in the left upper quadrant.

52.6   Contraindications

Asymptomatic splenic infarct requires no surgical intervention.

52.7   Preoperative Considerations

1. Ultrasonography and color Doppler study should confirm the diagnosis by revealing the exact location and the status of the spleen.
2. Vaccination (pneumococcal, *Haemophilus influenzae*, meningococcal) is mandatory.
3. The patient or the parents must be informed about the possibility of complete splenectomy if the viability of the spleen is found to be questionable during surgery.

52.8   Technical Notes

1. The spleen is generally found attached to an abnormally long tortuous vascular pedicle with no gastrosplenic or phrenicosplenic ligaments.
2. The posterior peritoneum over the left kidney is opened and a flap that includes the peritoneum over the anterior abdominal wall is lifted up to create a raw area.
3. A composite polypropylene mesh of 15 × 15 cm is sutured over the raw area with 3–0 nonabsorbable sutures and wrapped around the spleen.

52.9   Procedure Variations

1. Splenectomy is an option if vascular compromise is present.
2. Splenopexy without mesh is possible by creating an extraperitoneal pouch.
3. Splenopexy with double mesh ("sandwich techniques") is another alternative.

52.10   Laparoscopic Mesh Splenopexy for Wandering Spleen

Please see Figs. 1–6.

Figure 52.1

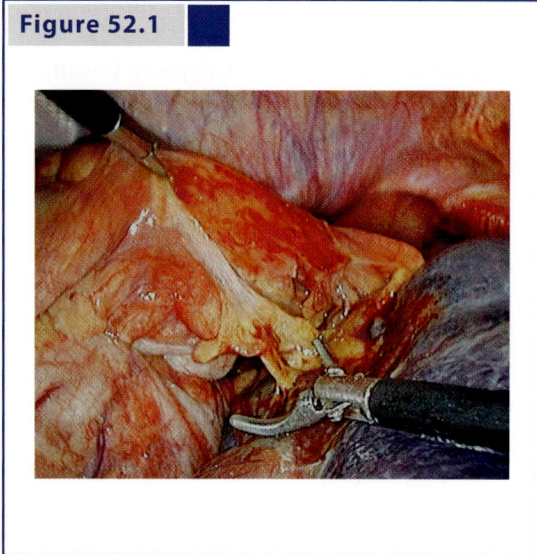

The wandering spleen is localized in the left iliac fossa

Figure 52.2

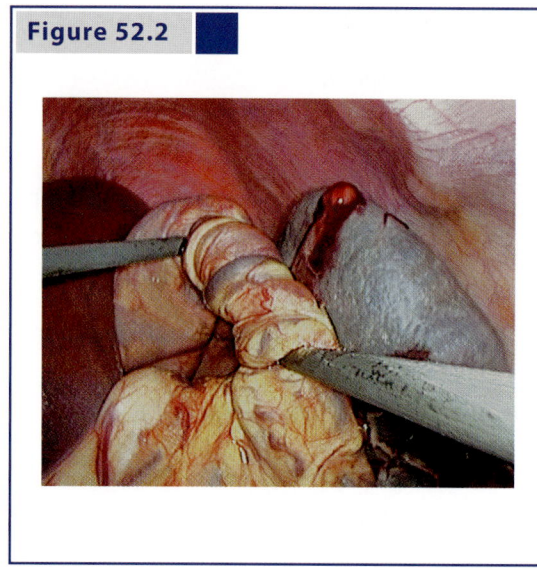

The spleen is positioned in the left hypochondrium. Torsion of the vascular pedicle is observed without evidence of vascular compromise to the spleen

Figure 52.3

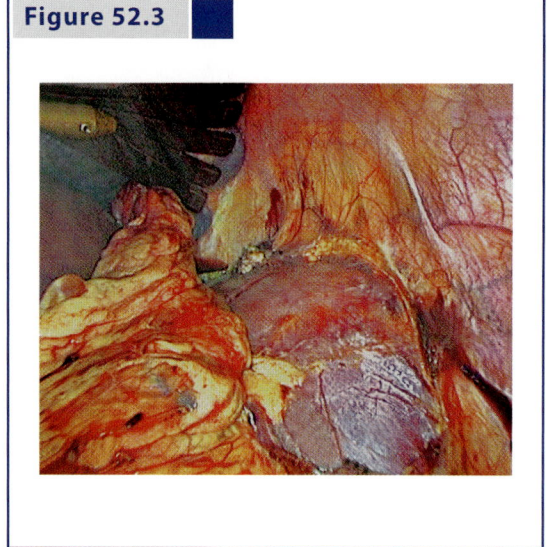

A raw area is created by raising the peritoneal flap around the area foreseen for the positioning of the spleen

Figure 52.4

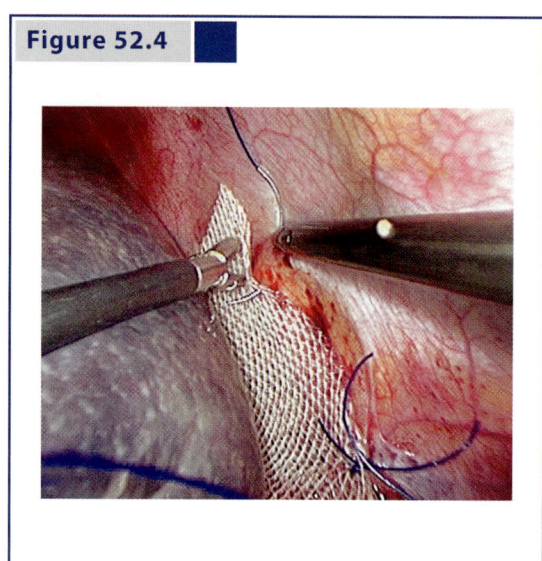

A 15×15-cm composite mesh is introduced in the abdomen and sutured over the raw peritoneal area

Figure 52.5

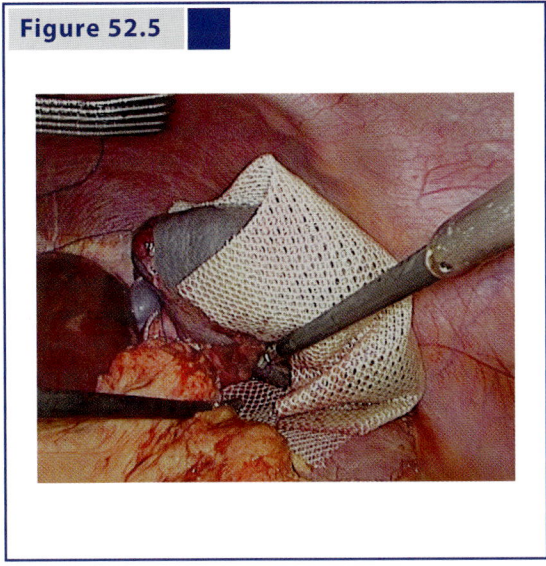

Figure 52.6

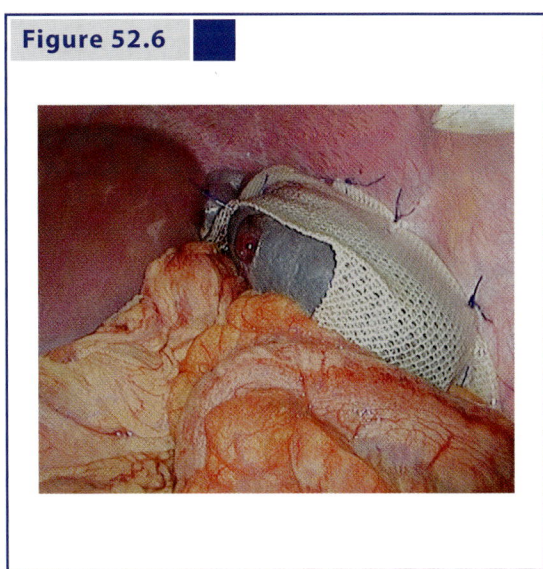

The mesh is wrapped around the spleen to secure it from both the sides. The edges of the mesh meet in the area around the vascular pedicle and are sutured

The spleen is "wrapped" between the two flanks of the mesh, along with reinforcement using omentum

Recommended Literature

1. Fukuzawa H, Urushihara N, Ogura K, Miyazaki E, Matsuoka T, Fukumoto K Kimura S, Mitsunaga M, Hasegawa S (2006) Laparoscopic splenopexy for wandering spleen: extraperitoneal pocket splenopexy. Pediatr Surg Int 22:931–934

2. Hedeshian MH, Hirsh MP, Danielson PD (2005) Laparoscopic splenopexy of a pediatric wandering spleen by creation of a retroperitoneal pocket. J Laparoendosc Adv Surg Tech A 15:670–672

3. Nomura H, Haji S, Kuroda D, Yasuda K, Ohyanagi H, Kudo M (2000) Laparoscopic splenopexy for adult wandering spleen: Sandwich method with two sheets of absorbable knitted mesh. Surg Laparosc Endosc Percutan Tech 10:332–334

Section 5

Genitourinary Procedures

53 Inguinal Hernia Repair

FRANÇOIS BECMEUR

53.1 Operation Room Setup

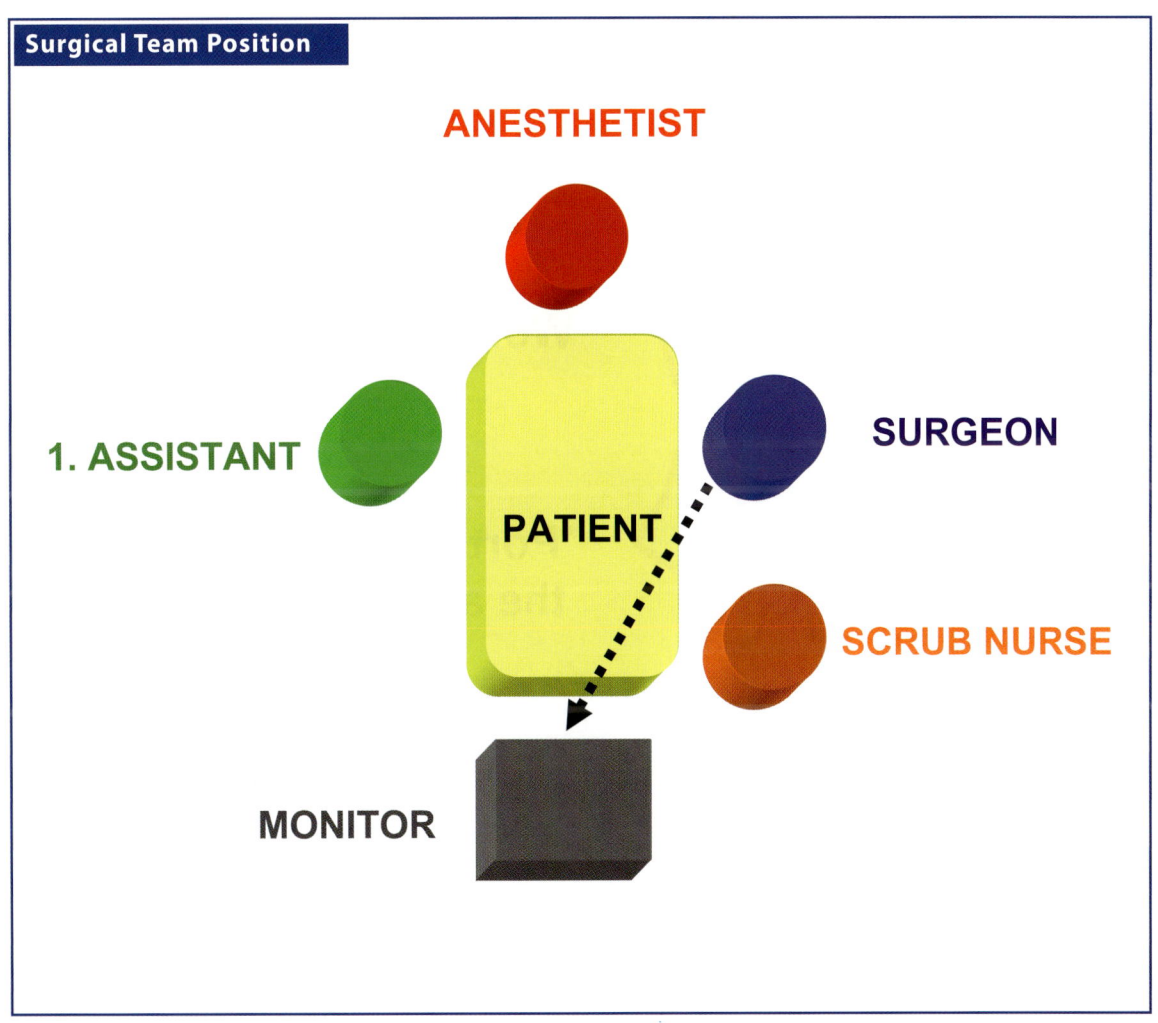

Surgical Team Position

ANESTHETIST

1. ASSISTANT

PATIENT

SURGEON

SCRUB NURSE

MONITOR

53.2   Patient Positioning

Supine position with arms tucked to side. Staff position for right hernia repair is shown (for the left side the surgeon and assistant switch places).

53.3   Special Instruments

- Atraumatic forceps
- Needle holders

53.4   Location of Access Points

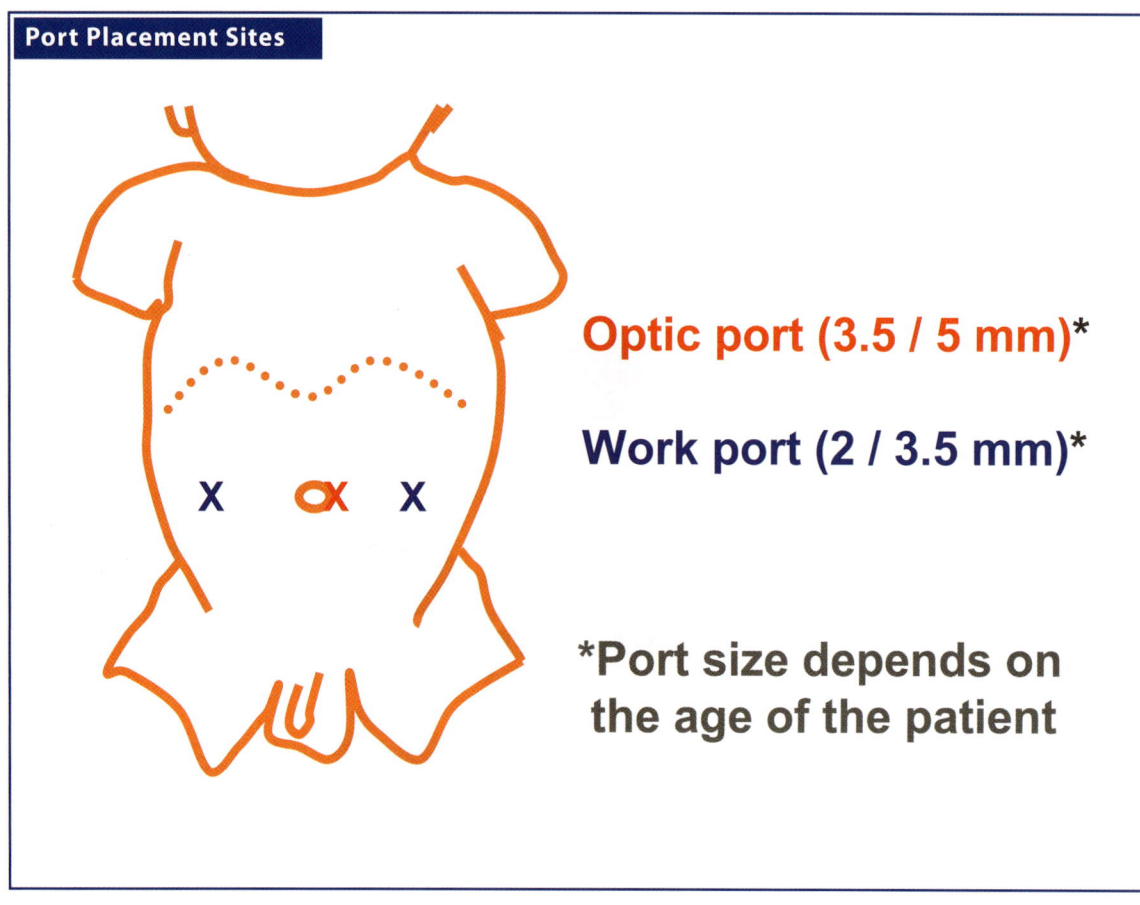

Port Placement Sites

Optic port (3.5 / 5 mm)*

Work port (2 / 3.5 mm)*

*Port size depends on the age of the patient

53.5 Indications

1. Patent processus vaginalis.
2. Inguinal hernia (in both sexes).
3. Incarcerated hernia.
4. Femoral hernia.
5. Direct hernia.
6. Recurrence of groin hernias.

53.6 Contraindications

1. Premature infants (relative contraindication).
2. Contraindications to general anesthesia.

53.7 Preoperative Considerations

1. Similar to day-care preparation procedures.
2. Empty the urinary bladder before the procedure.
3. A Foley catheter is not necessary for the procedure.

53.8 Technical Notes

1. Identify the type of hernia and evaluate the contralateral side.
2. Open the peritoneal fold at the outer circumference of the internal inguinal ring.
3. Hernia sac dissection is aided by insufflation. The sac must be divided and a peritoneal ring around the sac must be removed.
4. Ensure that there is no residual processus vaginalis. Nonabsorbable 3–0 sutures are used.

53.9 Procedure Variations

1. Laparoscopic inversion and ligation of inguinal hernia in girls. In this procedure the sac is grasped, inverted, and then ligated with an endoloop using 3-mm instruments without ports.
2. Subcutaneous endoscopically assisted ligation (SEAL): A stab incision is made on the skin above the internal inguinal ring and under endoscopic visualization the internal inguinal ring is encircled passing a nonabsorbable suture on a large needle (T12 or T20).

53.10 Laparoscopic Inguinal Hernia Repair

Please see Figs. 1–4.

Figure 53.1

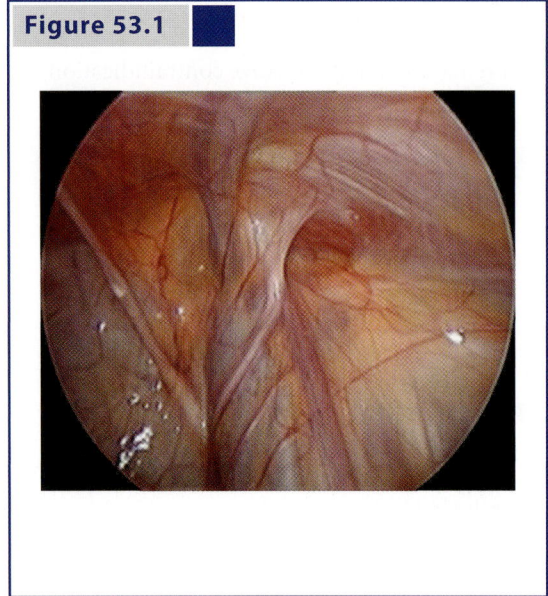

Laparoscopic view of a patent process vaginalis on the right side

Figure 53.2

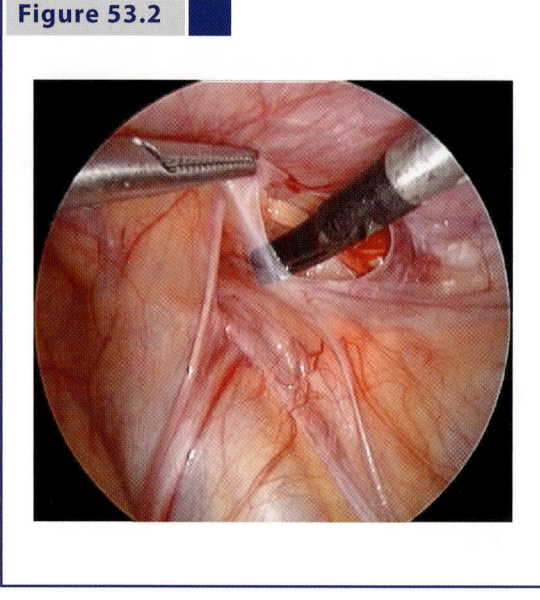

The edge of the inguinal sac is held with a grasper and the peritoneum is opened

Figure 53.3

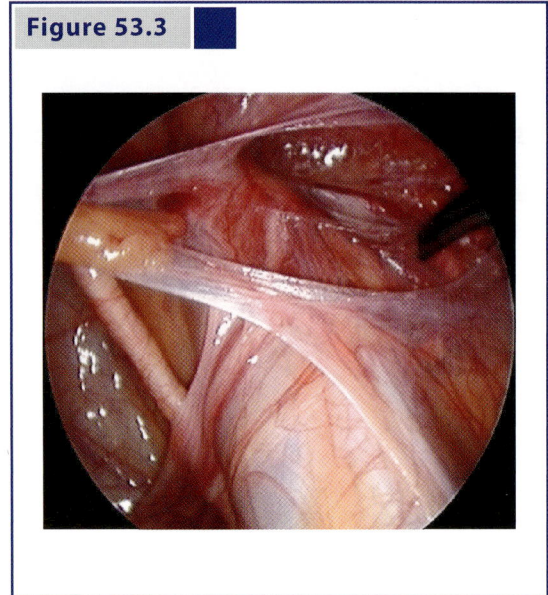

After circular preparation the peritoneum is divided from the inguinal sac

Figure 53.4

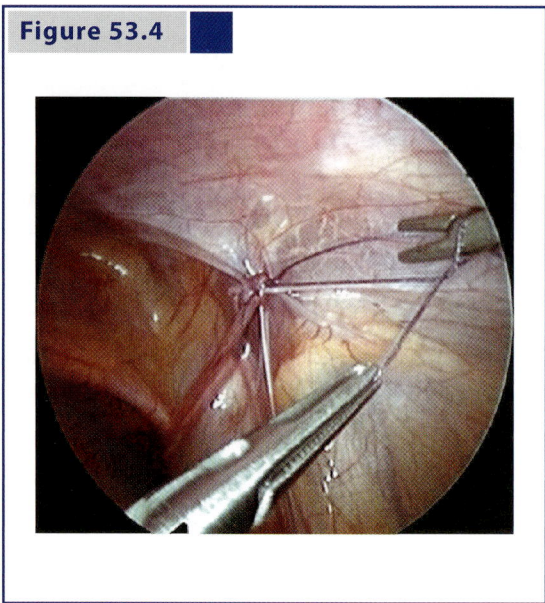

The suture needle is introduced through the abdominal wall and the sac sutured

Figure 53.5

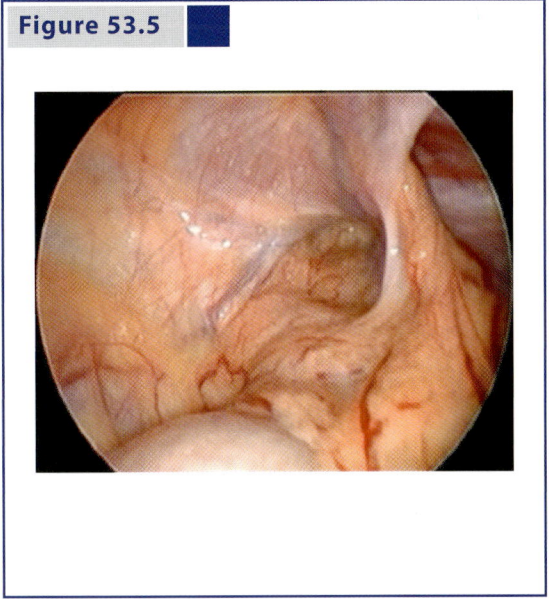

Figure 53.6

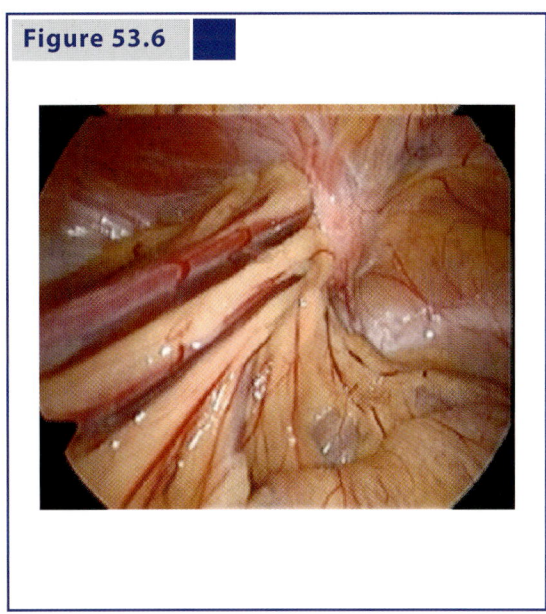

Example of right femoral hernia with a patent process vaginalis

Example of incarceration of the greater omentum in the left inguinal ring

Recommended Literature

1. Becmeur F, Philippe P, Lemandat-Schultz A, Moog R, Grandadam S, Lieber A, Toledano D (2004) A continuous series of 96 laparoscopic inguinal hernia repairs in children by a new technique. Surg Endosc 18:1738–1741
2. Montupet P, Esposito C (1999) Laparoscopic treatment of congenital inguinal hernia in children. J Pediatr Surg 34:420–423
3. Schier F, Klizaite J (2004) Rare inguinal hernias forms in children. Pediatr Surg Int 20:748–752

54 Procedure Options in Undescended Testis

OLIVER J. MUENSTERER AND HOLGER TILL

54.1 Operation Room Setup

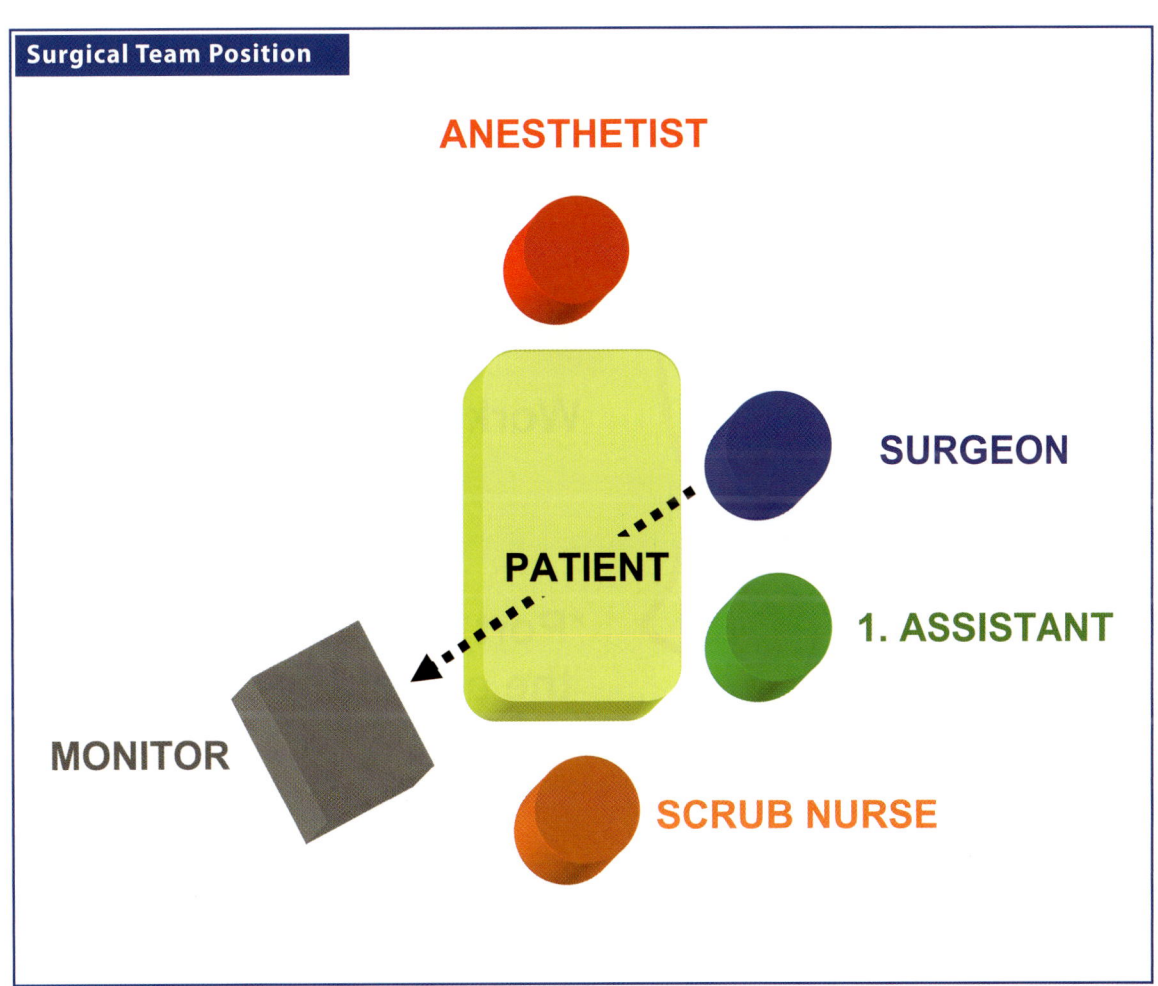

Surgical Team Position

ANESTHETIST

SURGEON

PATIENT

1. ASSISTANT

MONITOR

SCRUB NURSE

54.2   Patient Positioning

Supine position with arms tucked to the side. The ipsilateral side may be abducted if required. Staff position for right-side exploration is shown here.

54.3   Special Instruments

- Ultracision® shears (Johnson & Johnson Medical Products, Ethicon Endo-Surgery, Cincinnati, OH, USA) or
- Endoscopic clip applicator

54.4   Location of Access Points

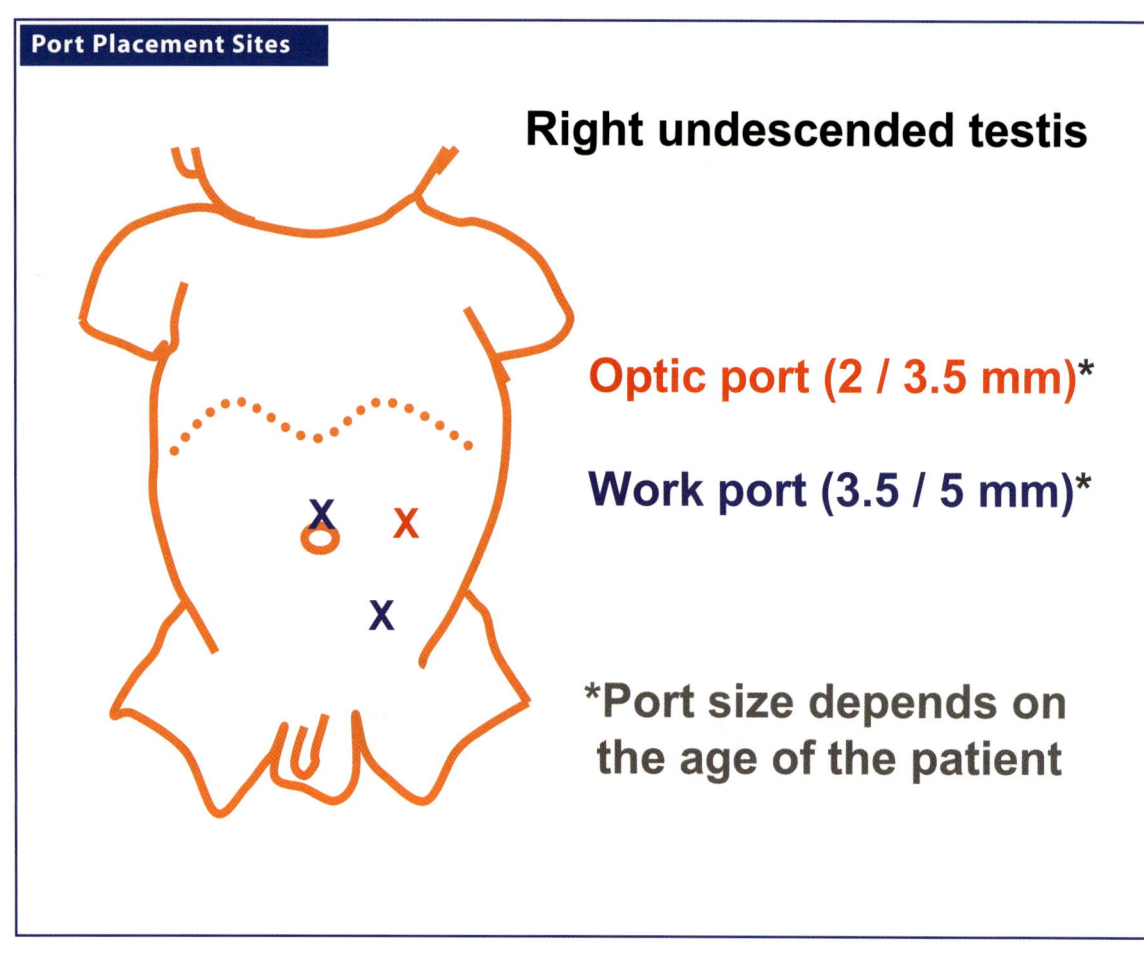

Port Placement Sites

Right undescended testis

Optic port (2 / 3.5 mm)*

Work port (3.5 / 5 mm)*

*Port size depends on the age of the patient

54.5 Indications

1. Nonpalpable unilateral testis.
2. Nonpalpable bilateral testis with male karyotype and positive human chorionic gonadotrophin (hCG) test.

54.6 Contraindications

Patients with nonpalpable bilateral testis and negative hCG test require a preoperative pediatric endocrine work-up.

54.7 Preoperative Considerations

1. Imaging studies cannot reliably rule out intra-abdominal testes.
2. Place a Foley catheter before the procedure to drain the bladder and maximize the operating space in the lower pelvis.
3. The Trendelenburg position aids in better visualization of the lower abdomen and pelvis.
4. The operating table should be tilted ipsilateral side up.

54.8 Technical Notes

1. Place the umbilical port and perform a diagnostic laparoscopy to identify the position and morphology of the affected testis, vas, and vessels.
2. In order to mobilize the testicle, the gubernaculum is transected.
3. Grasp the testis only by the remaining gubernacular attachments to avoid tissue trauma.
4. Deflating the pneumoperitoneum may add length to the spermatic cord for orchidopexy.

54.9 Procedure Variations

1. Finding a testis with normal vessels and a blind-ending or absent vas may indicate cystic fibrosis. If possible, an orchidopexy should be performed in these patients.
2. In case of dysplastic or malformed testes, orchiectomy or biopsy should be performed.

54.10 Laparoscopic Approach to Undescended Testis

Please see Figs. 1–6.

Figure 54.1

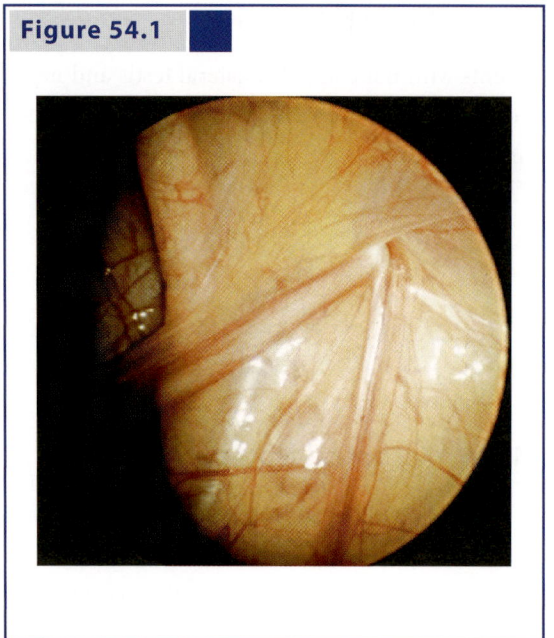

Figure 54.2

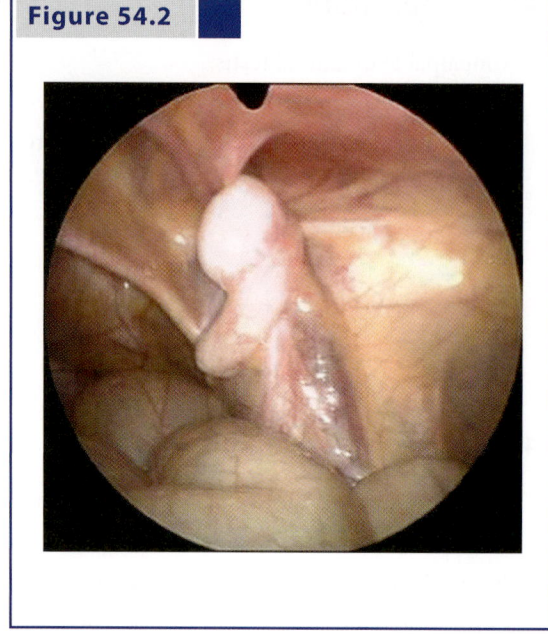

If both the vas deferens and vessels enter the inguinal canal, laparoscopy is terminated and open standard inguinal exploration is performed

If the vas and vessels lead to a normal intra-abdominal testis, determine if the testis is low (< 3 cm from the inguinal ring or below the iliac vessels) or high. Low testes are treated by conventional or laparoscopic orchidopexy

Figure 54.3

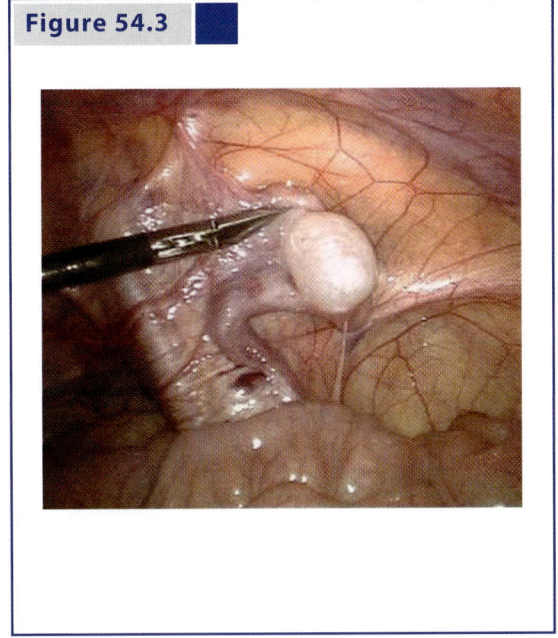

Figure 54.4

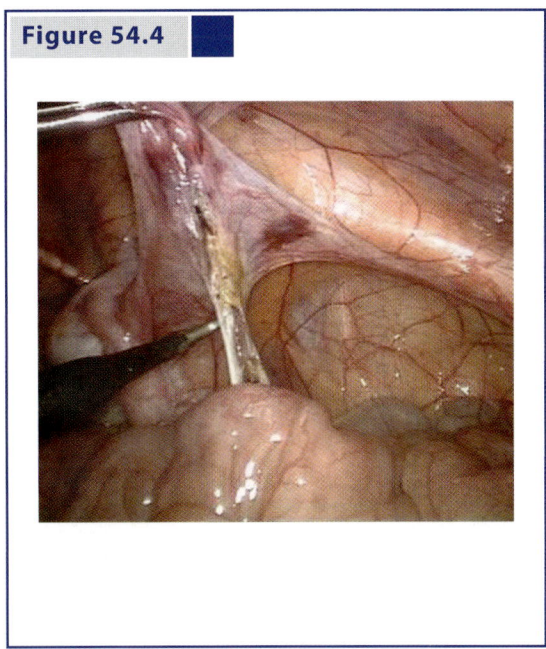

High-lying intra-abdominal testes may require a two-stage Fowler-Stephens procedure

The first stage comprises transection of the testicular vessels and placing the testicle near the internal inguinal ring. After a 6-month interval, orchidopexy is performed (at this time a strip of the peritoneum around the testicle is preserved and mobilized along with the testis)

Figure 54.5.1

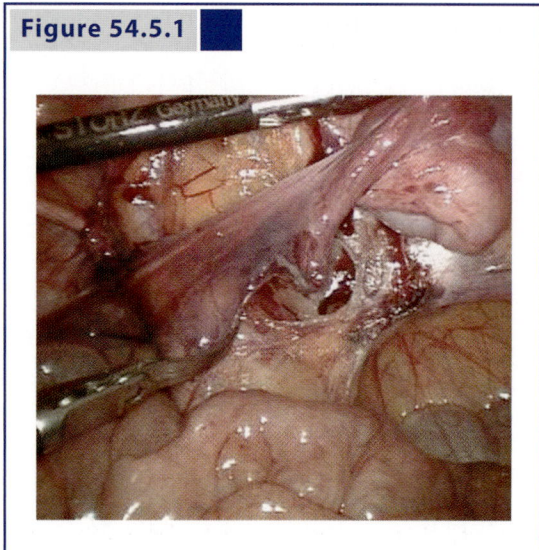

In the second stage, the testis is mobilized along with a generous flap of peritoneum, which assures adequate blood supply

Figure 54.5.2

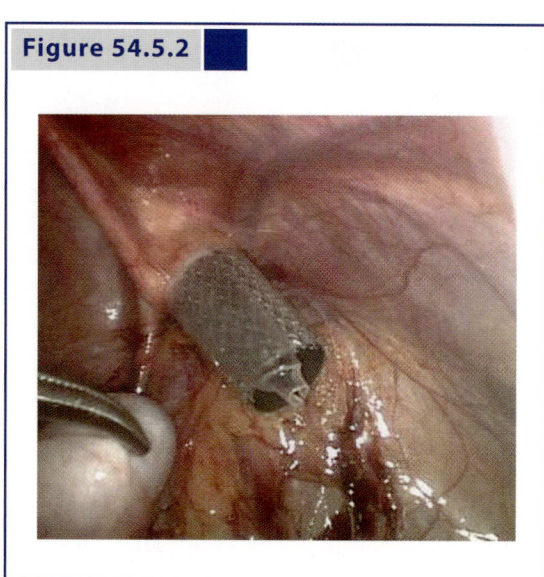

Using a 12 mm expandable port (STEP trocar) introduced through the base of the scrotum, a neo-ring medial to the epigastric vessels is created (Prentiss maneuver)

Figure 54.5.3

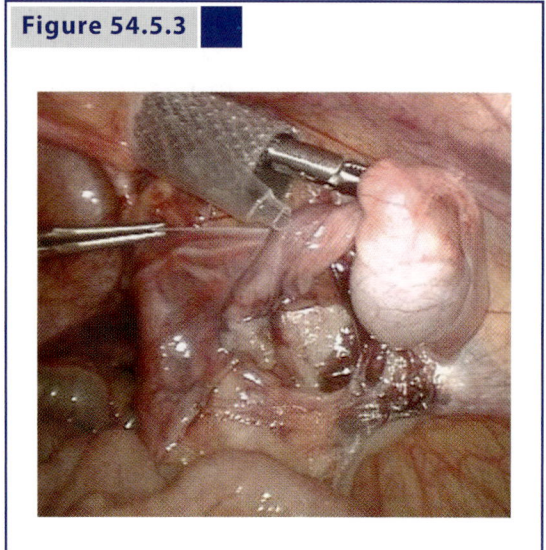

The testis is then grasped by a forceps (introduced through the scrotal expandable port) and pulled down into the scrotum. The port is removed, and the testis is secured in the scrotum in the conventional way

Figure 54.5.4

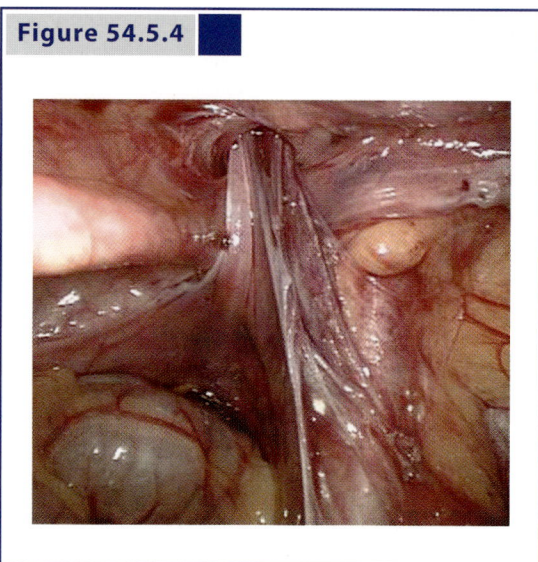

Torsion-free passage and location of the vas and peritoneal flap are endoscopically verified

Figure 54.6

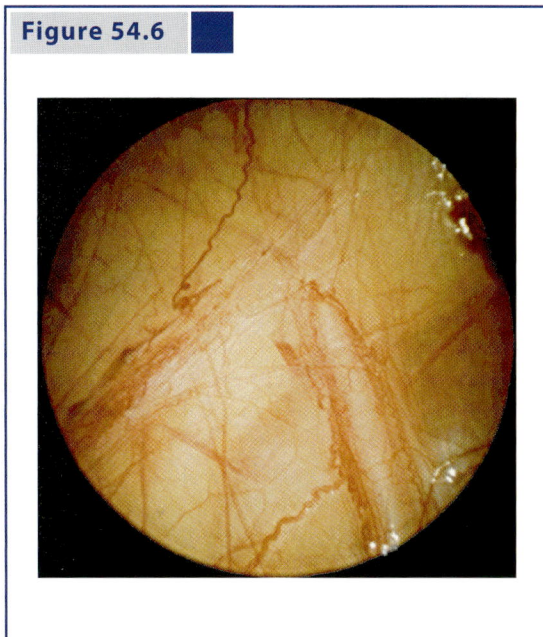

If the vas and vessels end blindly before the inguinal ring and no testes are identified despite a thorough search (intrauterine torsion, atrophy, or aplasia), the operation is terminated (Courtesy of Prof Jürgen Waldschmidt)

Recommended Literature

1. Patil KK, Green JS, Duffy PG (2005) Laparoscopy for impalpable testes. BJU Int 95:704–708
2. Peters CA (2004) Laparoscopy in pediatric urology. Curr Opin Urol 14:67–73
3. Schleef J, von Bismark S, Burmucic K, Gutmann A, Mayr J (2002) Groin exploration for nonpalpable testes: laparoscopic approach. J Pediatr Surg 37:1552–1555

55 First Step Fowler-Stephens in Prune-Belly Syndrome

Amulya K. Saxena

55.1 Operation Room Setup

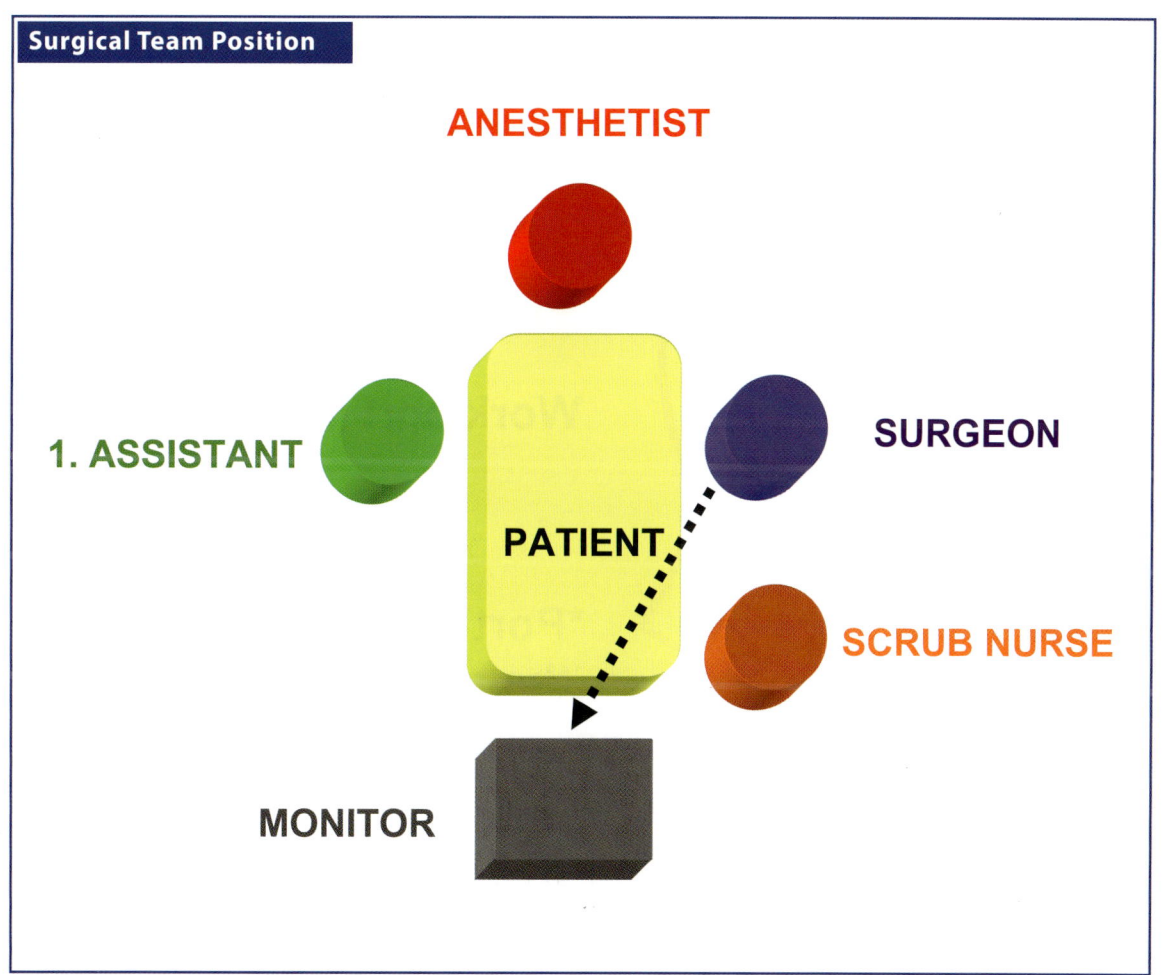

55.2   Patient Positioning

Supine position with arms tucked to the side.

55.3   Special Instruments

- Bipolar electrocautery forceps or
- Endoscopic clip applicator or
- LigaSure™ (Valleylab, Boulder, CO, USA) or
- Ultracision® shears (Johnson & Johnson Medical Products, Ethicon Endo-Surgery, Cincinnati, OH, USA).

55.4   Location of Access Points

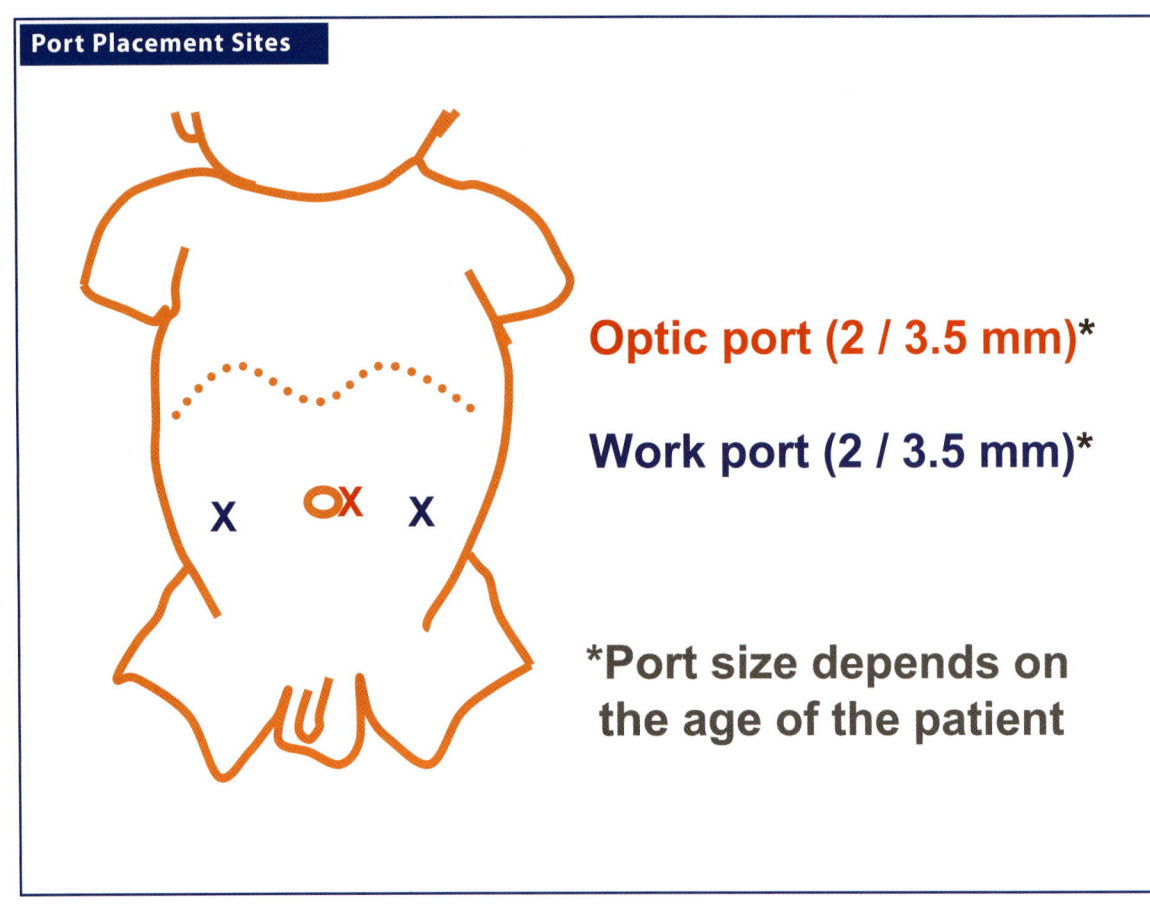

Port Placement Sites

Optic port (2 / 3.5 mm)*

Work port (2 / 3.5 mm)*

*Port size depends on the age of the patient

55.5   Considerations in Laparoscopy

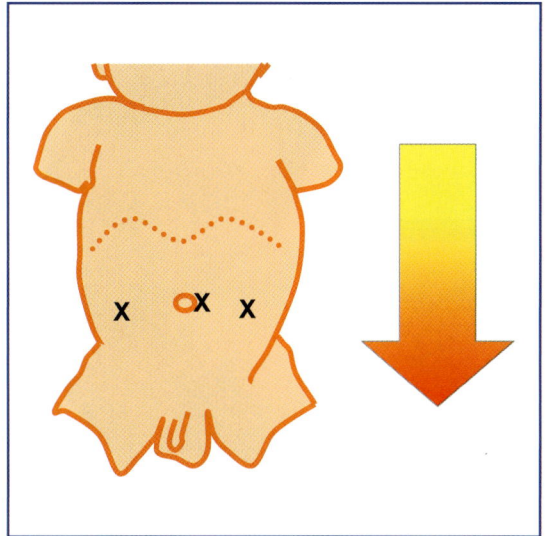

The bold arrow showing gradual increases in the scarcity and weakness of the abdominal muscles toward the pelvis, where port placement is desired.

55.6   Preoperative Considerations

1. The upper abdominal and diaphragm muscles are not or less involved, and normal ventilation pressures can be used during anesthesia.
2. Single-dose antibiotics are administered, since prune-belly patients have problems with respiratory toilet (that are the sequelae to an impaired cough mechanism), which is difficult without the assistance of abdominal musculature and hence could lead to increased postoperative pulmonary problems after general anesthesia.

55.7   Technical Notes

1. Abdominal access must be gained using the open-access technique due to the lack of abdominal wall resistance.
2. A purse-string suture is tied to secure the ports at the point of insertion as well as to seal the point of entry from escape of insufflated gas.
3. Longer laparoscopic instruments 310–430 mm are recommended, since abdominal insufflation causes a marked increase in the abdominal diameter.

55.8   Procedure Variations

1. Ligation of vessels can be done by: clips, LigaSure™ tissue-sealing device, Ultracision® shears, or suture ligation.
2. Threaded port sleeves provide better gripping of the abdominal wall than smooth port sleeves.

55.9   Laparoscopic First Step Fowler-Stephens Procedure in Prune-Belly Syndrome

Please see Figs. 1–6.

Figure 55.1

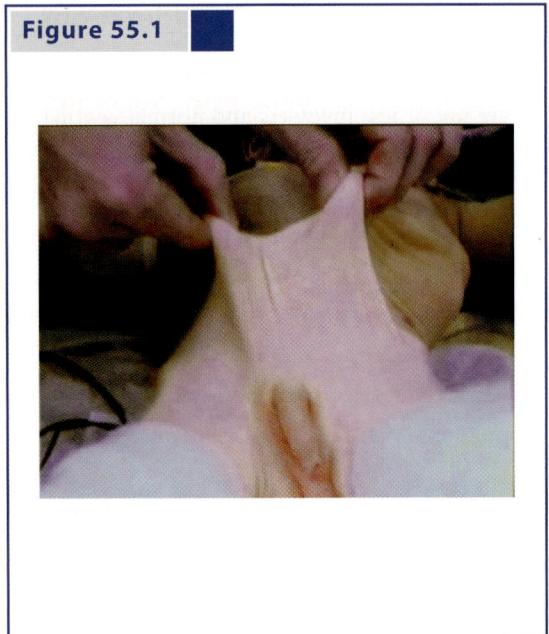

The lax abdomen of a patient with prune-belly syndrome can pose challenges in endoscopic surgery with regard to insufflation and port placement

Figure 55.2

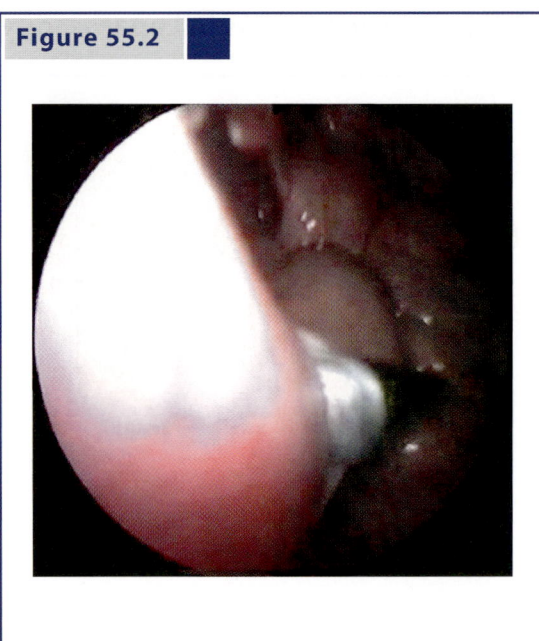

Trocars cross the midline with conventional insertion methods due to lack of abdominal resistance and hence open insertion is the preferred option

Figure 55.3

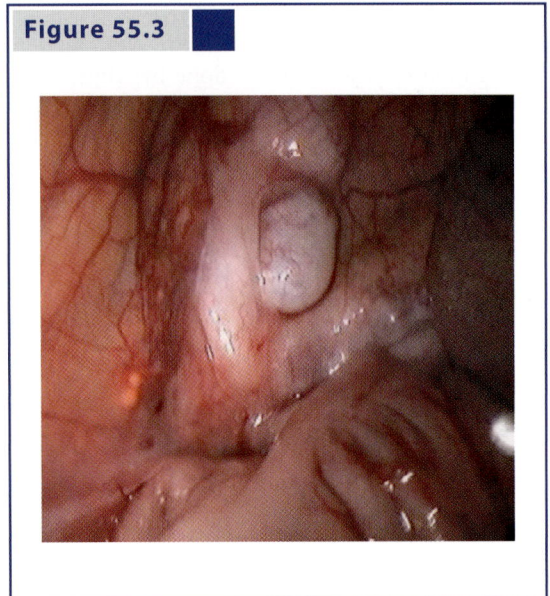

The weak internal spermatic vessels are visualized cranial to the high-lying abdominal testis

Figure 55.4

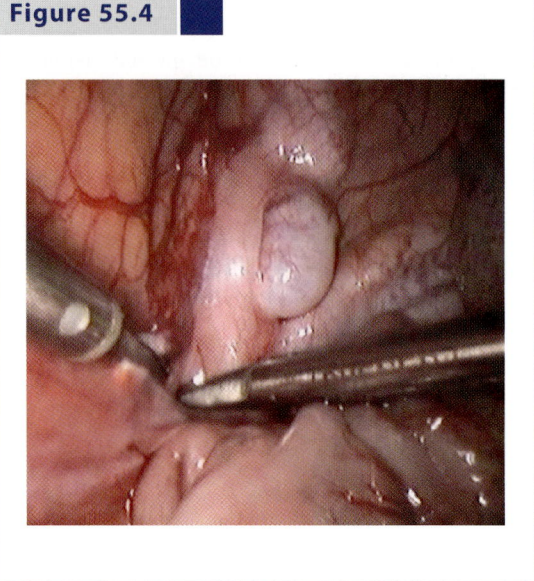

Using bipolar electrocautery forceps, the vessels are cauterized and care is taken not to cause thermal injury to the testicle

Figure 55.5

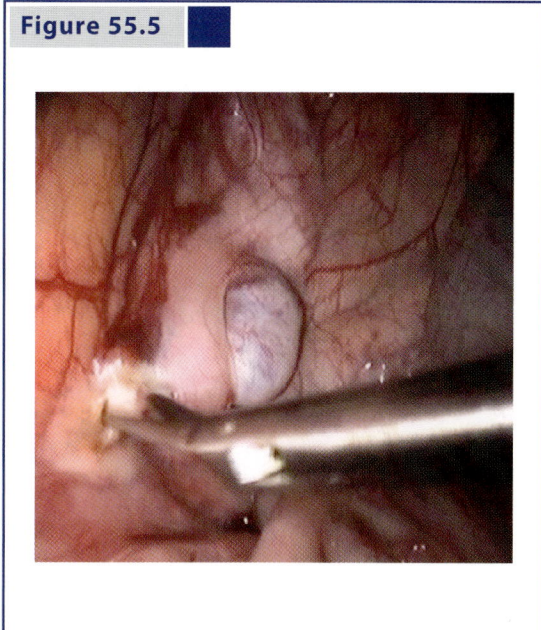

Figure 55.6

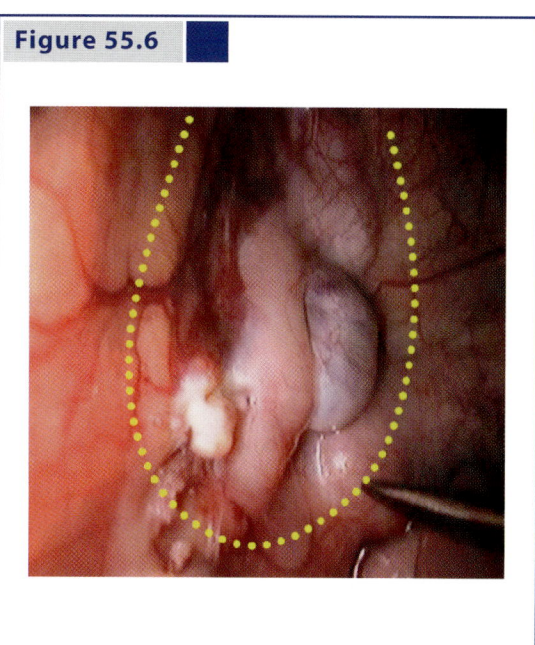

The vessels are divided using scissors, and the testis is lodged close to the inguinal ring. The collateral vas deferens vessels maintain the testicular vascular supply

The second step of the Fowler-Stephens procedure is performed after 6 months; the strip of peritoneum (***dotted lines***) overlying the vas and testis is preserved and mobilized with the testis

Recommended Literature

1. Docimo SG, Moore R, Kavoussi L (1995) Laparoscopic orchidopexy in the prune belly syndrome: a case report and review of the literature. Urology 45:679–681
2. Saxena AK, Brinkmann OA (2007) Unique features of prune belly syndrome in laparoscopic surgery. J Am Coll Surg 205:217–221
3. Yu TJ, Lai MK, Chen WF, Wan YL (1995) Two-stage orchiopexy with laparoscopic clip ligation of the spermatic vessels in prune-belly syndrome. J Pediatr Surg 30:870–872

56 Management of Ovarian Cysts

LUTZ STROEDTER

56.1 Operation Room Setup

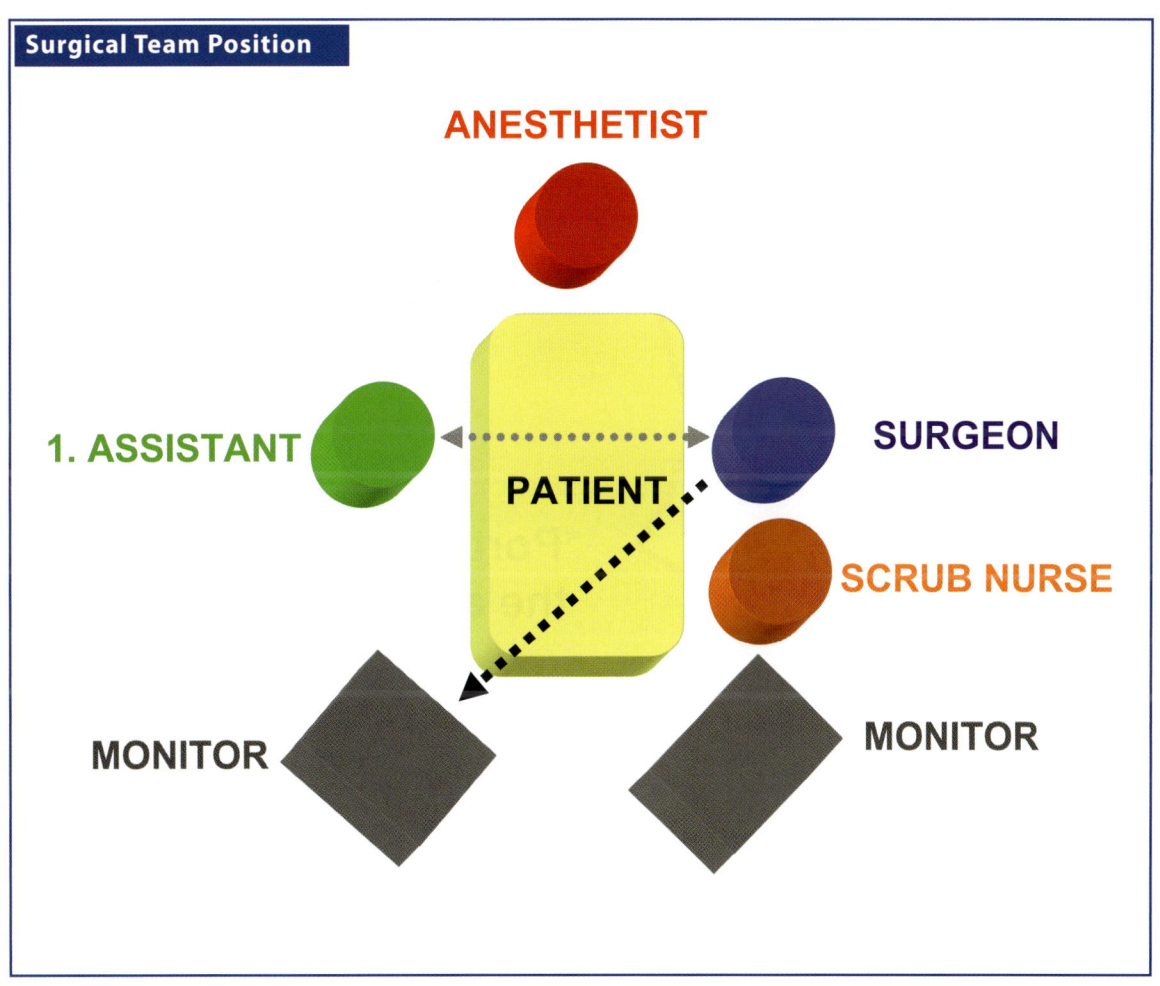

56.2   Patient Positioning

Supine Trendelenburg position with arms tucked to the side. Operation room position shown for a right-side cyst. The team switches for the left side.

56.3   Special Instruments

None.

56.4   Location of Access Points

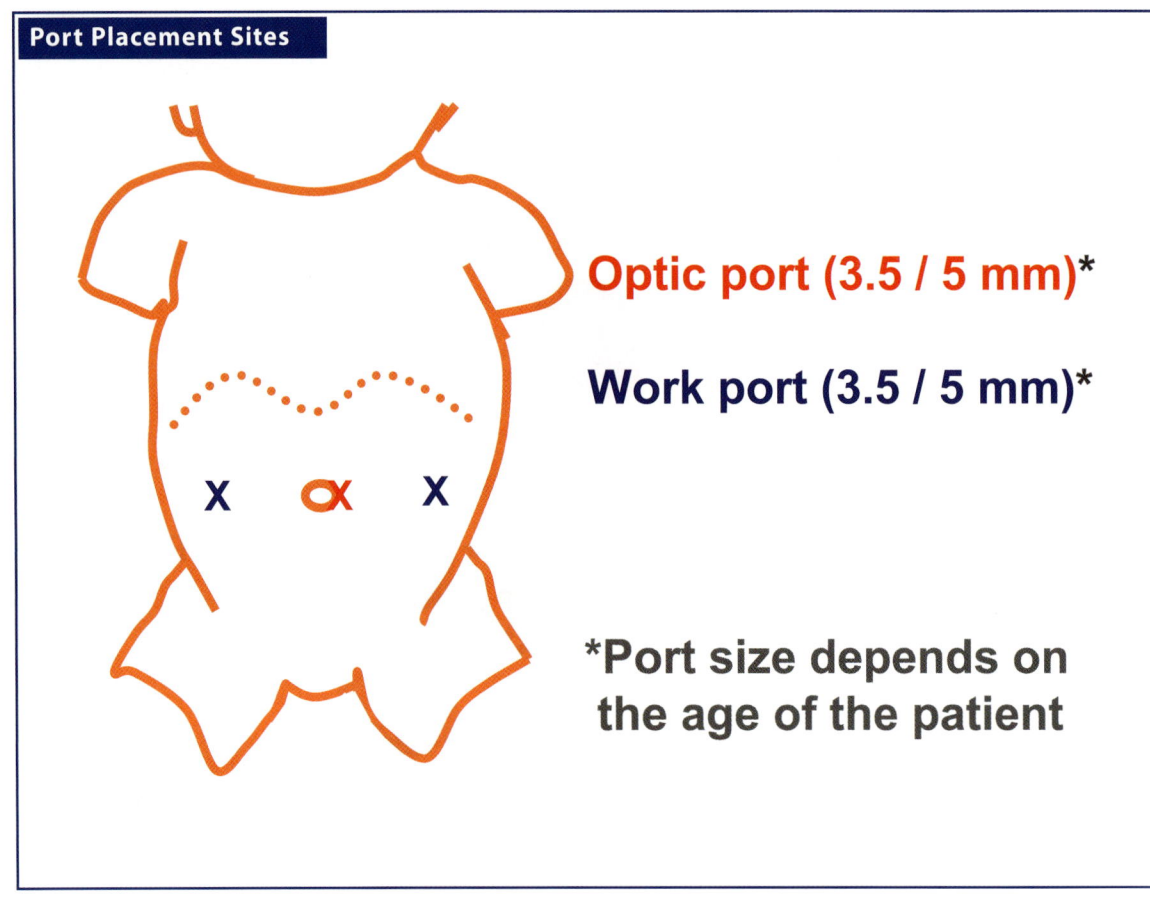

Port Placement Sites

Optic port (3.5 / 5 mm)*

Work port (3.5 / 5 mm)*

*Port size depends on the age of the patient

56.5   Indications

1. Ovarian cysts (larger than 5 cm in diameter) associated with abdominal pain.
2. Ovarian-cyst-associated torsion.
3. Suspected ovarian abscess.

56.6   Relative Contraindications

1. Multiple previous upper abdominal procedures.
2. Suspicion of ovarian malignancy.
3. General contraindications to laparoscopy.

56.7   Preoperative Considerations

1. Ovarian enlargement secondary to impaired venous and lymphatic drainage is the most common sonographic finding in ovarian torsion.
2. Combination of Doppler flow imaging with the morphologic assessment of the ovary may improve diagnostic accuracy. However, the interpretation of Doppler sonography is inconsistent due to the dual ovarian blood supply from the uterine artery and the ovarian artery.

56.8   Technical Notes

1. Puncture the ovarian cyst with a transcutaneous laparoscopically guided needle and send the contents for examination.
2. In cases of torsion, wait for 10 min after relieving the torsion to access ovarian vascular recirculation.
3. During oophoropexy, caution should be taken not to injure the ureter and the vessels close to the site of suture.

56.9   Procedure Variations

1. Laparoscopically assisted extracorporeal ovarian cystectomy.
2. Laparoscopically assisted transumbilical ovarian cystectomy in neonates.

56.10   Laparoscopic Approach to Ovarian Cysts

Please see Figs. 1–6.

Figure 56.1

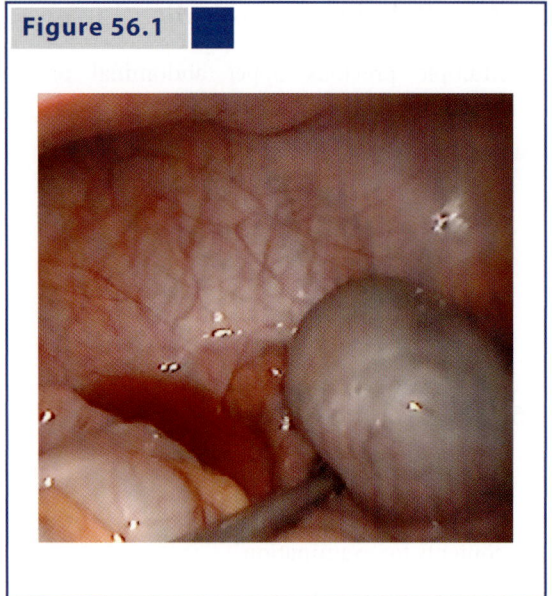

Laparoscopic view of a hemorrhagic right ovarian cyst leading to ovarian torsion

Figure 56.2

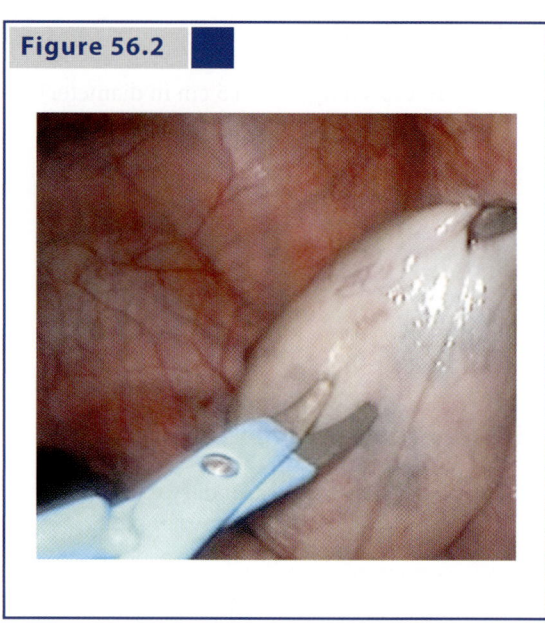

The ovary is twisted appropriately to reduce the torsion. An area for cyst decompression is marked using electrocautery scissors

Figure 56.3

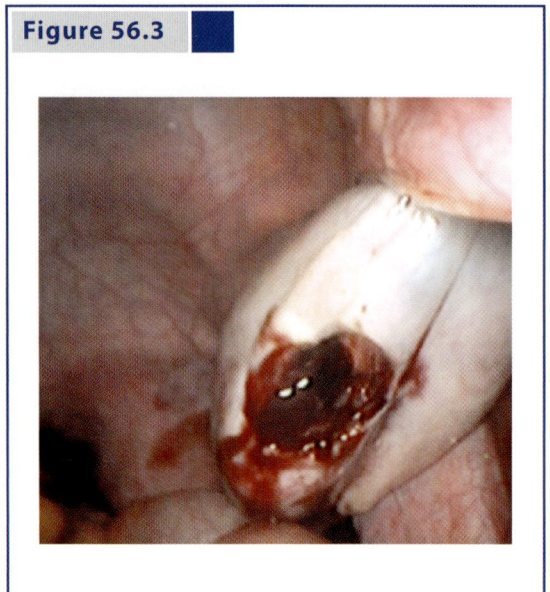

The cap of the hemorrhagic cyst is then dissected to release the accumulated blood

Figure 56.4

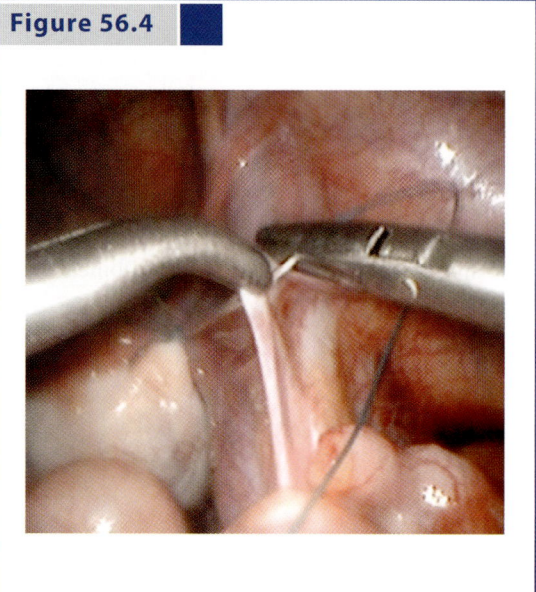

Using two nonabsorbable sutures the affected ovary is sutured to the pelvic peritoneum

Figure 56.5

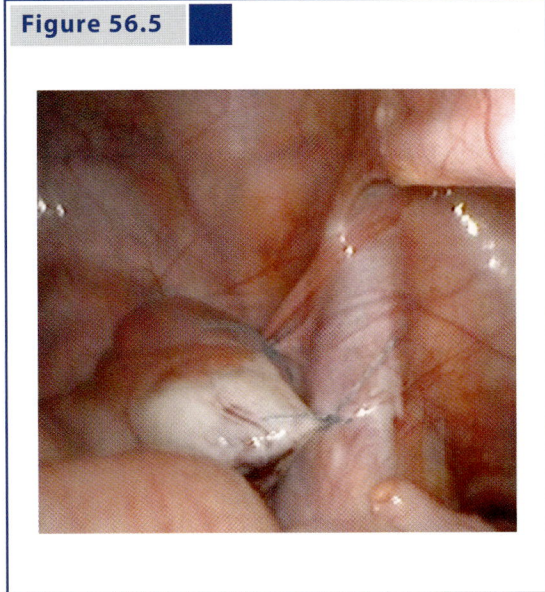

Figure 56.6

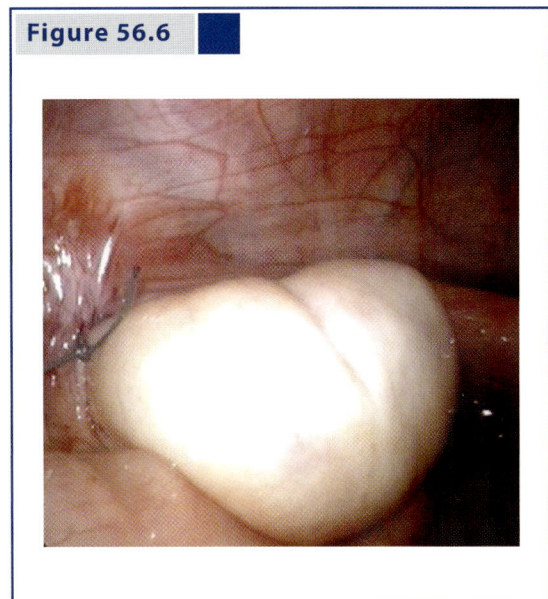

Postoperative view of the right ovary on completion of the procedure

A contralateral oophoropexy of the normal unaffected ovary is performed only in cases of ovarian torsion with severe ischemia and necrosis

Recommended Literature

1. Oelsner G, Cohen SB, Soriano D, Admon D, Mashiach S, Carp H (2003) Minimal surgery for the twisted ischaemic adnexa can preserve ovarian function. Hum Reprod 18:2599–2602
2. Steyaert H, Meynol F, Valla JS (1998) Torsion of the adnexa in children: the value of laparoscopy. Pediatr Surg Int 13:384–387
3. White M, Stella J (2005) Ovarian torsion: 10-year perspective. Emerg Med Australas 17:231–237

57 Adrenalectomy

STEVEN Z. RUBIN AND MARCOS BETTOLLI

57.1 Operation Room Setup

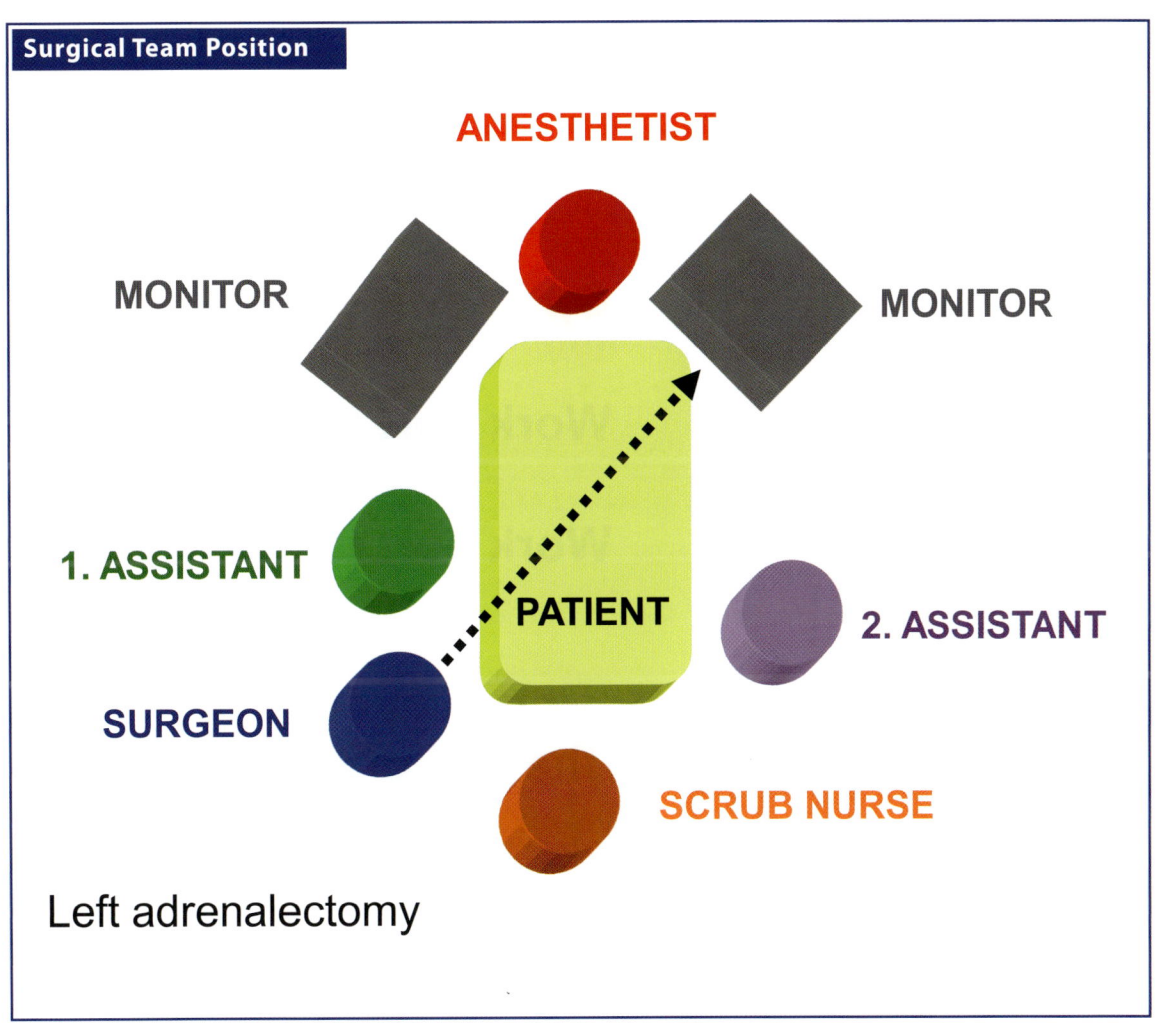

57.2   Patient Positioning

Right lateral decubitus for left adrenalectomy (shown). Mirror image for staff positions in right adrenalectomy.

57.3   Special Instruments

- Liver retractor
- Specimen retrieval bag
- LigaSure™ (Valleylab, Boulder, CO, USA) or
- Ultracision® harmonic scalpel (Johnson & Johnson Medical Products, Ethicon Endo-Surgery, Cincinnati, OH, USA)

57.4   Location of Access Points

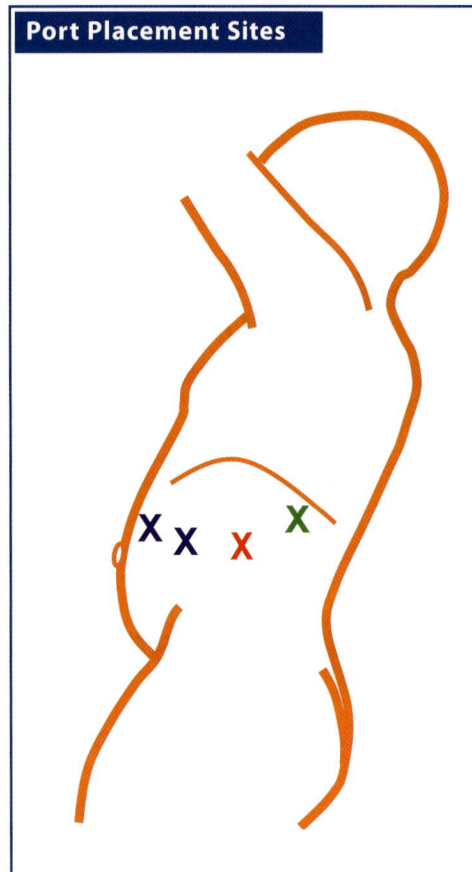

Port Placement Sites

Left adrenalectomy

Optic port (3.5 / 5 mm)*

Work port (3.5 / 5 mm)*

Work port (5 / 10 mm)*

***Port size depends on the age of the patient**

57.5   Indications

1. Tumor biopsy.
2. Adrenal tumors up to 6 cm.
3. Resection of adrenal metastasis.
4. Nonfunctioning adrenal incidentaloma > 4 cm.

57.6   Contraindications

1. Large (> 6 cm) or irresectable mass-laparoscopic biopsies only.
2. Mass not localized to adrenal-laparoscopic biopsies only
3. Preoperatively diagnosed adrenal cancer.
4. Noncorrectable coagulopathy.

57.7   Preoperative Considerations

1. Ensure accurate anatomical delineation and radiological staging.
2. Endocrinological management (e.g., pheochromocytoma) is essential.
3. Foley catheter and naso-(oro-)gastric tube are inserted.
4. Bilateral antisepsis of the skin of the abdomen and lower chest is required.

57.8   Technical Notes

1. Avoid grasping the adrenal gland, especially for pheochromocytoma.
2. LigaSure™/Ultracision® harmonic scalpel is utilized for dissection and hemostasis.
3. Initial isolation and division of adrenal vessels is ideal (left adrenal vein; right adrenal vessels are multiple and short).
4. The specimen is extracted in a specimen-retrieval bag.
5. In the face of uncontrolled complications, conversion to an open procedure is recommended.

57.9   Procedure Variations

1. Retroperitoneal approach.
2. Bilateral adrenalectomy.

57.10   Laparoscopic Transabdominal Adrenalectomy

Please see Figs. 1–6.

Figure 57.1

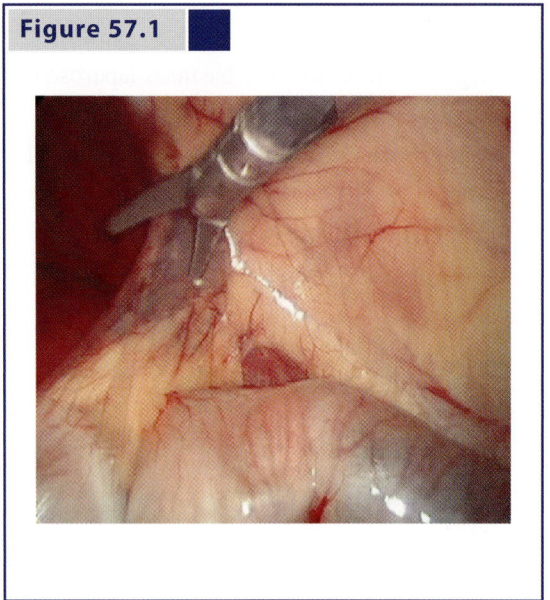

Left-side adrenalectomy; the dissection is started by mobilizing the splenic flexure of the colon

Figure 57.2

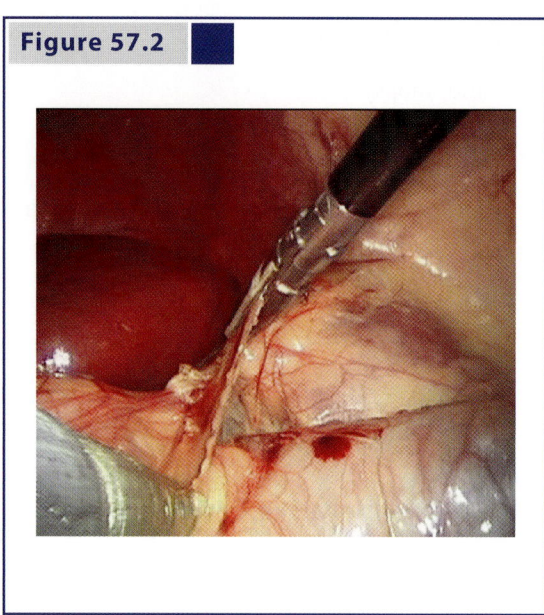

The lienophrenic ligament is divided and Gerota's fascia is opened

Figure 57.3

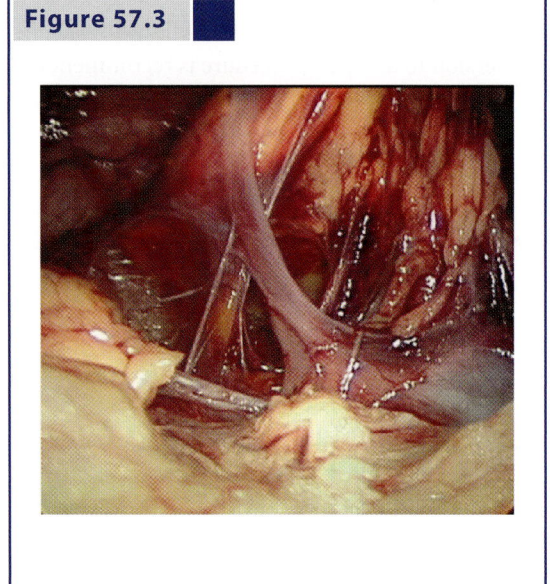

The left renal vein is dissected allowing exposure of the left adrenal vein

Figure 57.4

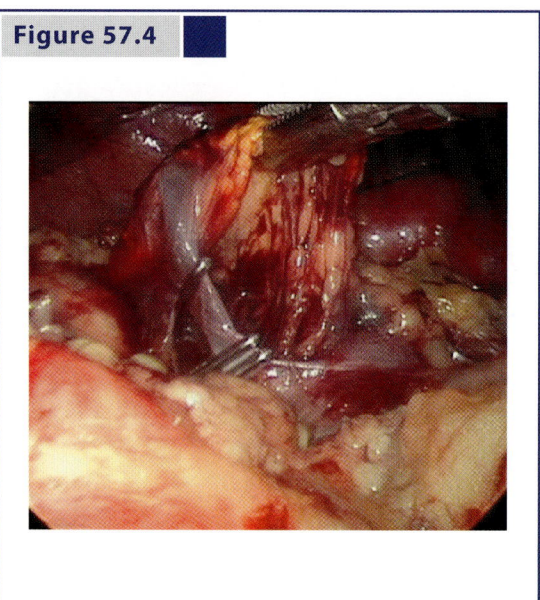

The left adrenal vein is ligated with clips and divided

Figure 57.5

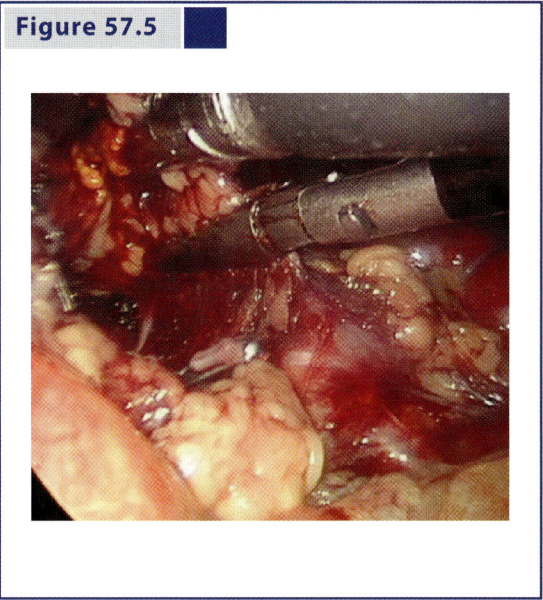

Figure 57.6

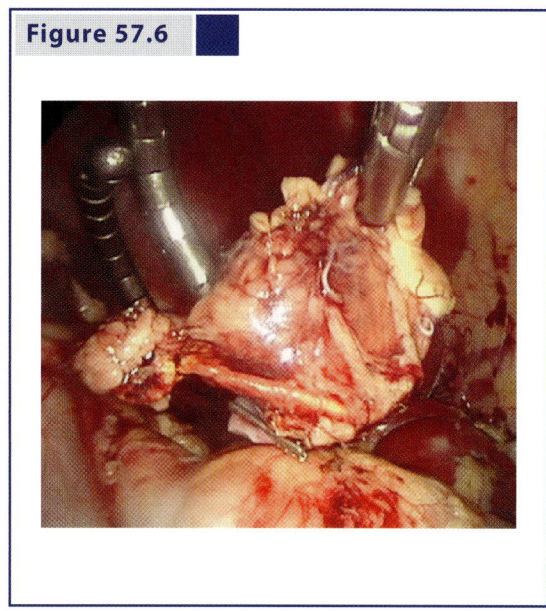

The gland is freed of its attachments using LigaSure™-aided dissection

The isolated gland is placed in a specimen retrieval bag and extracted through the 10-mm port

Recommended Literature

1. Assalia A, Gagner M (2004) Laparoscopic adrenalectomy. Br J Surg 91:1259–1274
2. Lal G, Clark OH (2003) Laparoscopic adrenalectomy – indications and technique. Surg Oncol 12:105–123
3. Miller KA, Albanese C, Harrison M, Farmer D, Ostlie DJ, Gittes G, Holcomb GW 3rd (2002) Experience with laparoscopic adrenalectomy in pediatric patients. J Pediatr Surg 37:979–982

58 Nephroureterectomy

Benno M. Ure and Martin L. Metzelder

58.1 Operation Room Setup

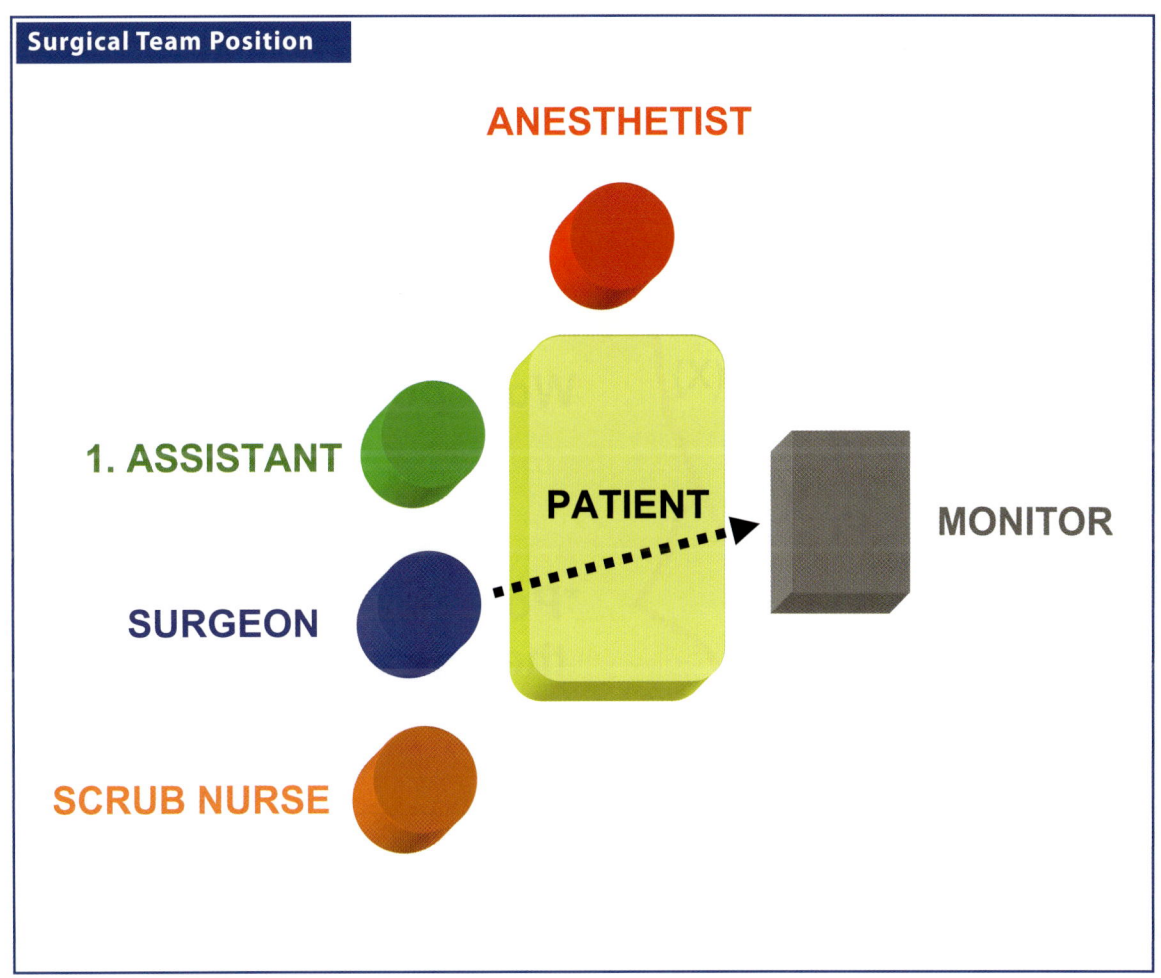

58.2   Patient Positioning

Semilateral position with 45° elevation on the contralateral side and fixation of the unilateral arm above the head. Staff positions for left nephroureterectomy is shown.

58.3   Special Instruments

- 5-mm LigaSure™ (Valleylab, Boulder, CO, USA) or
- Endoscopic clip applicator
- Specimen retrieval bag
- 10-mm scope

58.4   Location of Access Points

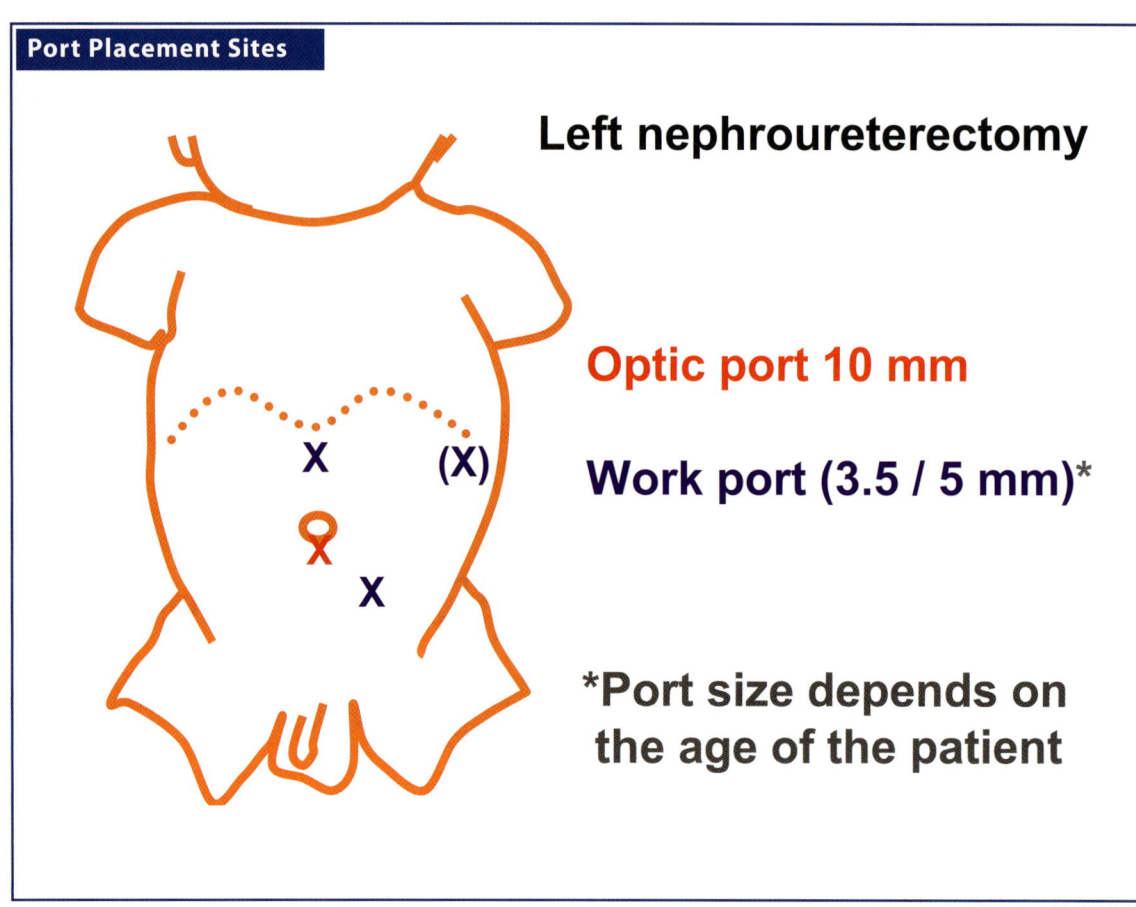

Port Placement Sites

Left nephroureterectomy

Optic port 10 mm

Work port (3.5 / 5 mm)*

***Port size depends on the age of the patient**

58.5   Indications

1. Nonfunctional refluxive kidney.
2. Nonfunctional kidney after obstruction of the vesicoureteral junction.
3. Multicystic renal dysplasia.

58.6   Contraindications

1. Urinary tract infection or sepsis.
2. Renal transplantation of the ipsilateral side.
3. Liver cirrhosis with portal hypertension.
4. Severe coagulation disorders.

58.7   Preoperative Considerations

1. Bladder emptying is not necessary for this procedure.
2. Antibiotics are generally not administered.
3. Bowel preparation is also not obligatory.

58.8   Technical Notes

1. The peritoneum is opened over the kidney and medial reflection of the bowel and colon.
2. In cases with difficulty in orientation, the ureter may be used for mobilization.
3. A careful approach to the renal vessels must be taken regardless of the ligation technique.
4. The specimen can be removed via an enlarged incision at the infraumbilical access point. If necessary, the renal tissue may be morcellated in the specimen retrieval bag.

58.9   Procedure Variations

1. The kidney can be secured by a suture passed through the abdominal wall. This facilitates easier mobilization of the kidney.
2. In case of multicystic kidney, the large cysts should be punctured to reduce the volume of the kidney. This facilitates both easier dissection of the perirenal tissue as well as aids in the easier extraction and retrieval of the specimen.

58.10   Laparoscopic Transabdominal Nephrectomy

Please see Figs. 1–6.

Figure 58.1

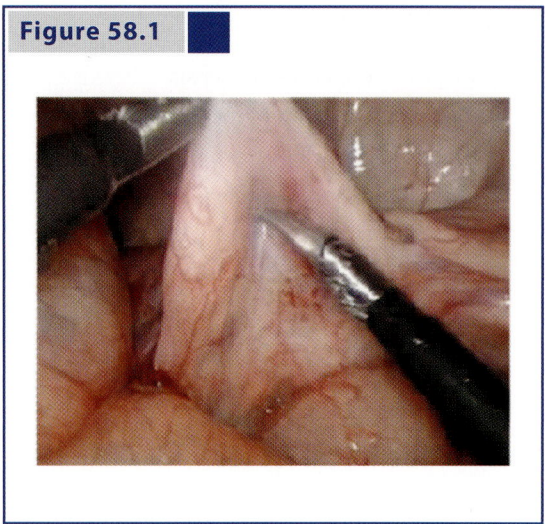

The ureter is mobilized first in small dysplastic kidneys to facilitate the identification of the structures

Figure 58.2

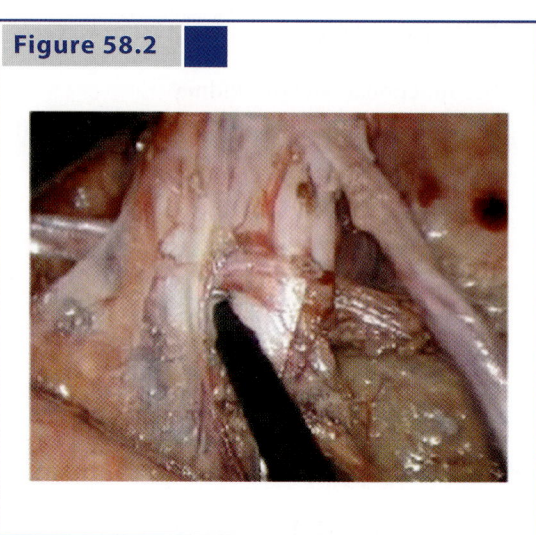

The kidney and the pelvis are mobilized using a monopolar hook cautery

Figure 58.3

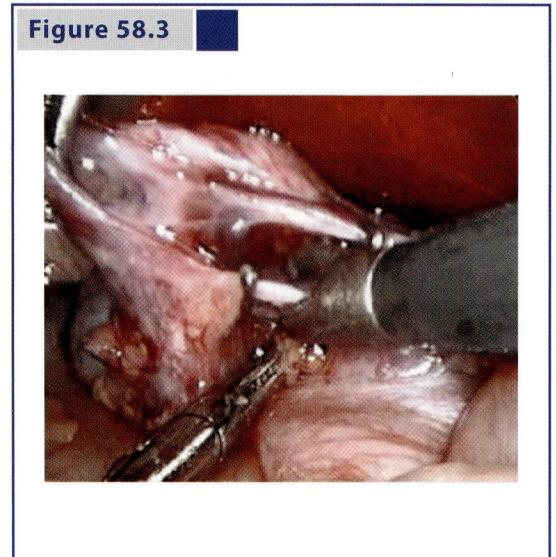

The renal vessels can be ligated and divided using clips or sutures

Figure 58.4

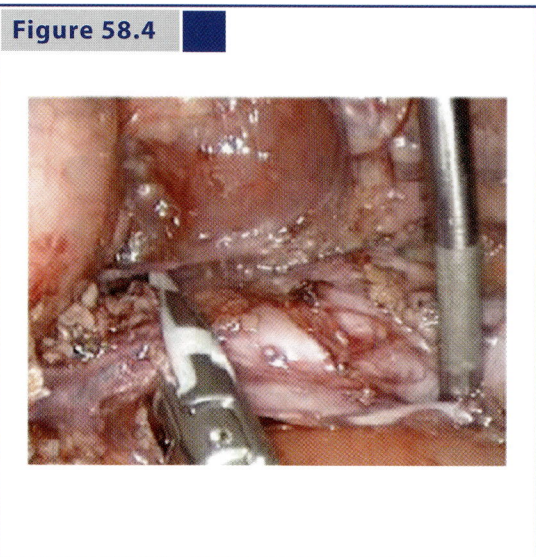

Alternatively, vessels can be divided and ligated using the LigaSure™ device

Figure 58.5

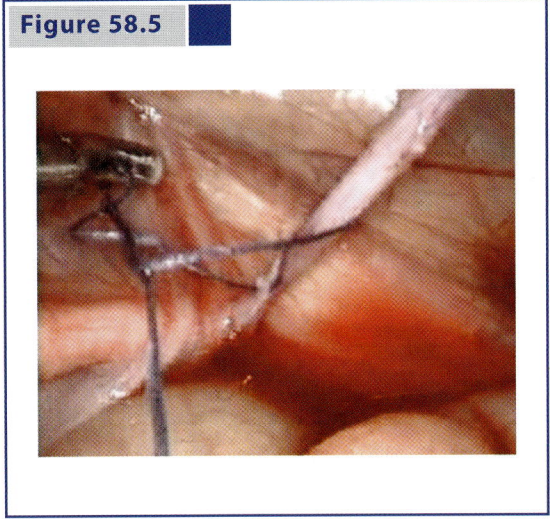

The distal ureter is ligated using a suture close to its point of entry in the urinary bladder

Figure 58.6

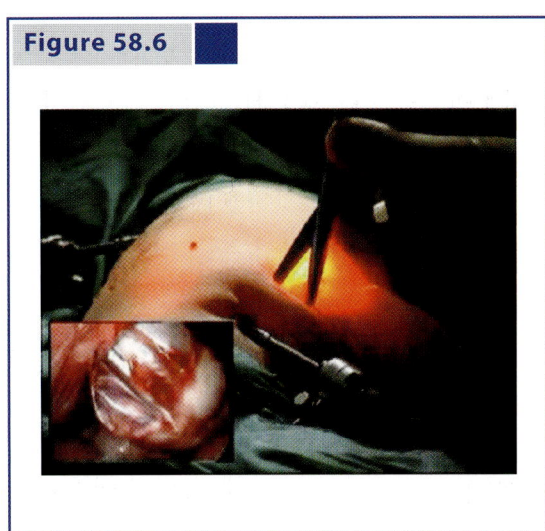

The kidney is removed in a specimen retrieval bag (*inset*) via the enlarged infraumbilical port incision

Recommended Literature

1. Jesch NK, Metzelder ML, Kuebler JF, Ure BM (2006) Laparoscopic transperitoneal nephrectomy is feasible in the first year of life and not affected by kidney size. J Urol 176:1177–1179

2. Metzelder ML, Kuebler J, Petersen C, Gluer S, Nustede R, Ure BM (2006) Laparoscopic nephroureterectomy in children: a prospective study on Ligasure™ versus clip/ligation. Eur J Pediatr Surg 16:241–244

3. Najmaldin AS (1999) Transperitoneal laparoscopic nephrectomy. In: Bax NMA, Georgeson KE, Najmaldin AS, Valla J-S (eds) Endoscopic Surgery in Children. Spinger, New York, pp 371–378

59 Transabdominal Pyeloplasty

JAMES G. YOUNG AND FRANCIS X. KEELEY

59.1   Operation Room Setup

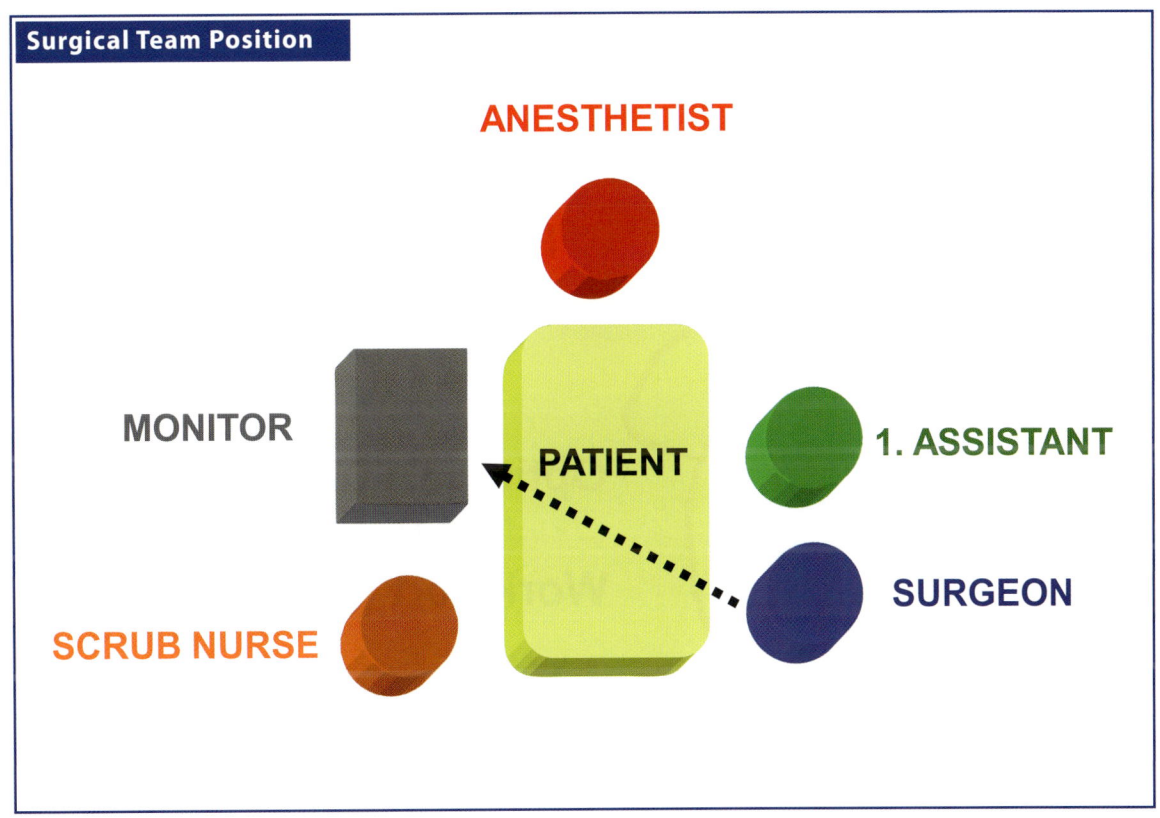

59.2   Patient Positioning

For right transperitoneal pyeloplasty (reverse positions for left) position the patient on left lateral side leaning back at an angle approximately 30° perpendicular to table. Support position with strap around table and patient's lower buttocks. Wedge supports are applied to upper buttock. The patient's right hand is supported on a padded board. Right knee is straightened; left knee flexed and pillow placed between legs. Positions for right side pyeloplasty shown.

59.3   Special Instruments

- Gyrus bipolar Trisector® (ACMI-Gyrus, Maple Grove, MN, USA)
- Needle holder

59.4   Location of Access Points

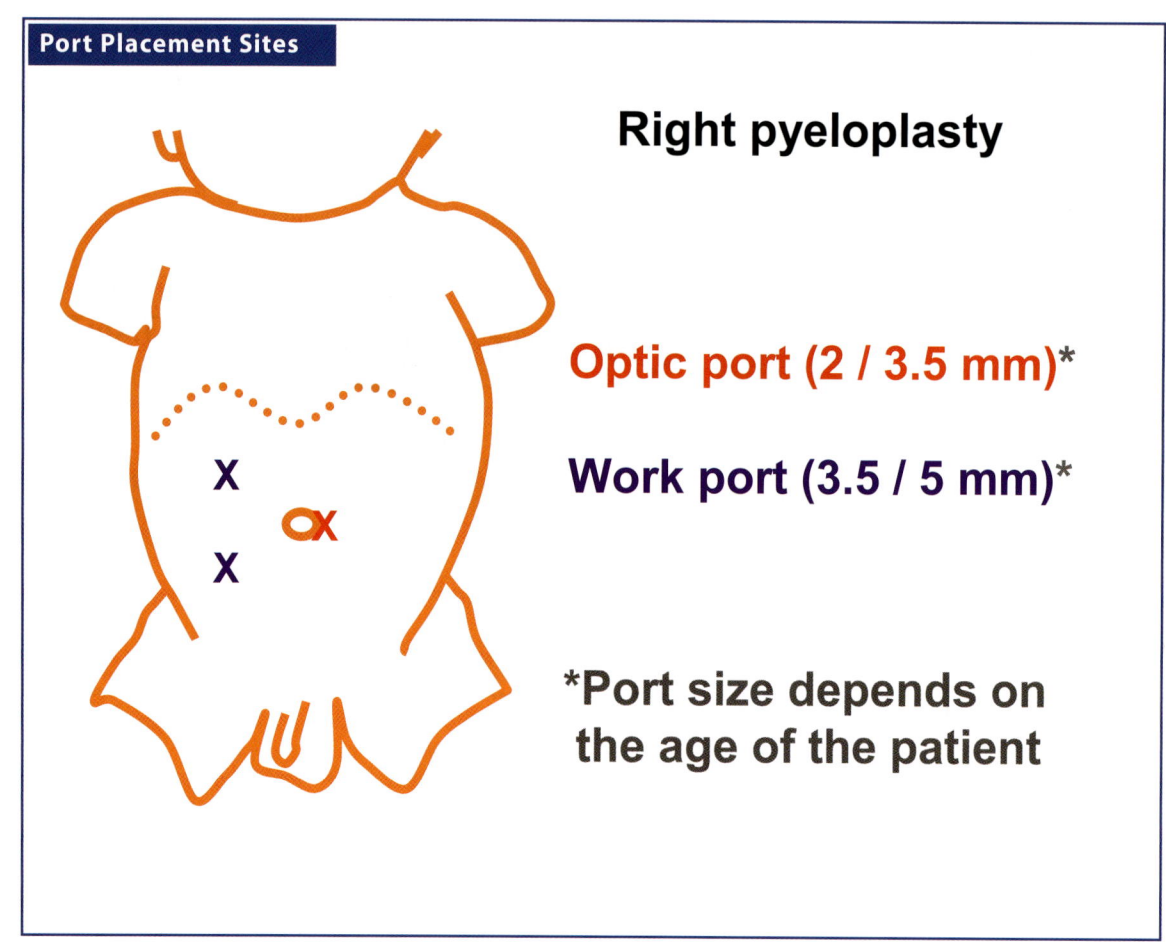

Port Placement Sites

Right pyeloplasty

Optic port (2 / 3.5 mm)*

Work port (3.5 / 5 mm)*

***Port size depends on the age of the patient**

59.5   Indications

1. Primary pelviureteric junction obstruction (PUJO).
2. Secondary PUJO if due to a crossing vessel.
3. Treatment is particularly indicated if the patient is symptomatic or if there is impairment of renal function.

59.6   Contraindications

1. Nonfunctioning kidney.
2. Active urological sepsis in the affected kidney.
3. Coagulopathy.

59.7   Preoperative Considerations

1. PUJO should be demonstrated clinically and radiologically with ultrasound and diuretic MAG3 (Mercapto Acetyl Tri Glycine) renography.
2. The Whitaker test may be considered if renography is indeterminate.
3. Secondary causes should be excluded and on-table retrograde pyelography considered.
4. Give gentamicin prophylaxis on induction of anesthesia.

59.8   Technical Notes

1. Freeing up a reasonable area of the renal pelvis is crucial to a tension-free anastomosis.
2. Resist the urge to place a stent in a retrograde fashion before starting the laparoscopy; instead, place the stent in an antegrade fashion after completing the posterior wall of the anastomosis. The stent is placed over a guidewire introduced through a large-caliber needle. Use a longer stent than usual so that the proximal curl does not interfere with the anastomosis.
3. Suturing the anastomosis can be taxing. Adjust the height of the table to ensure that your shoulders are relaxed.

59.9   Procedure Variations

Retroperitoneal approach: the dissection is more direct, but the anastomosis can be much more challenging (see Chap. 60).

59.10   Laparoscopic Transabdominal Pyeloplasty

Please see Figs. 1–4.

Figure 59.1

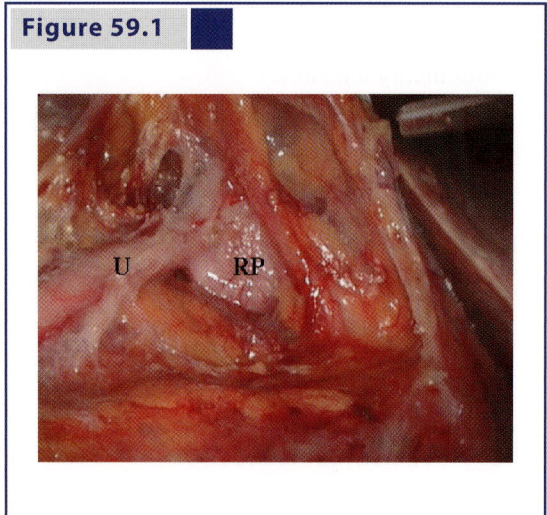

The right kidney is exposed by mobilizing colon. The lower pole is identified and is retracted laterally to expose the renal pelvis (**RP**). The renal pelvis is dissected circumferentially and traced to the ureter (**U**)

Figure 59.2

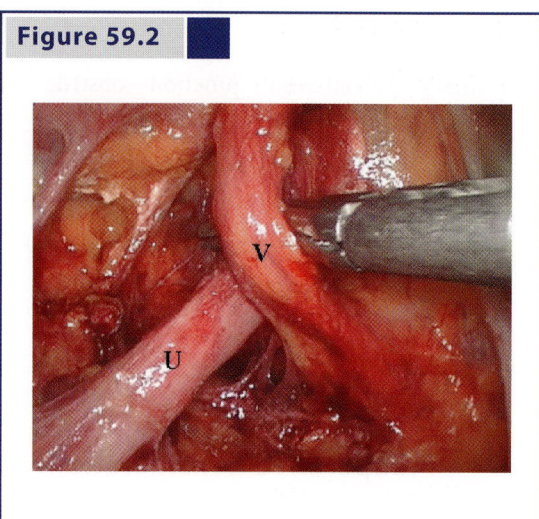

If the renal pelvis is collapsed or there is little hydronephrosis, the ureter can be located and dissected up to the renal pelvis. Not infrequently, a lower pole vessel (**V**) is seen crossing the ureter

Figure 59.3

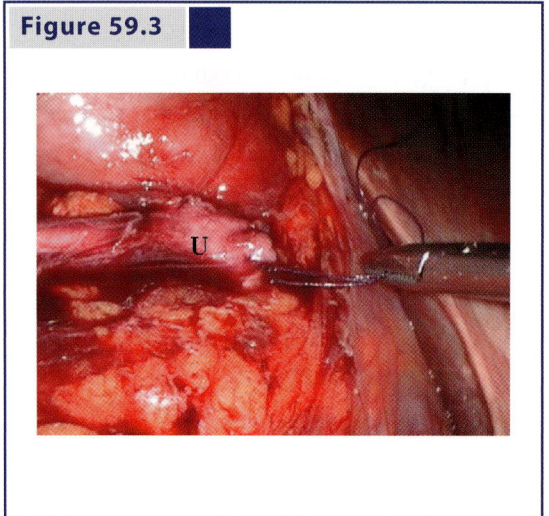

Dismembered pyeloplasty is performed with a stay suture in place to prevent the ureter retracting. The ureter is widely spatulated

Figure 59.4

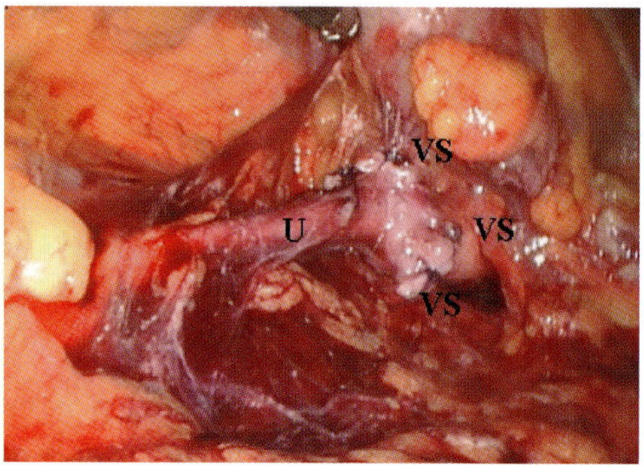

Ureteropelvic anastomosis is performed with three interrupted absorbable sutures at the apex of the spatulation followed by a continuous running suture. A Robinson drain is inserted at the end of the procedure. **VS** Absorbable suture (Vicryl™; Ethicon, Somerville, NJ, USA)

Recommended Literature

1. Davenport K, Minervini A, Timoney AG, Keeley FX Jr (2005) Our experience with retroperitoneal and transperitoneal laparoscopic pyeloplasty for pelviureteric junction obstruction. Eur Urol 48:973–977

2. Piaggio LA, Franc-Guimond J, Noh P, Wehry M, Figueroa T, Barthold J, González R (2007) Transperitoneal laparoscopic pyeloplasty for primary repair of ureteropelvic junction obstruction in infants and children: comparison with open surgery. J Urol 178:1579–1583

3. Smaldone MC, Sweeney DD, Ost MC, Docimo SG (2007) Laparoscopy in paediatric urology: present status. BJU Int 100:143–150

60 Retroperitoneal Robot-Assisted Pyeloplasty

Lars H. Olsen and Troels M. Jørgensen

60.1   Operation Room Setup

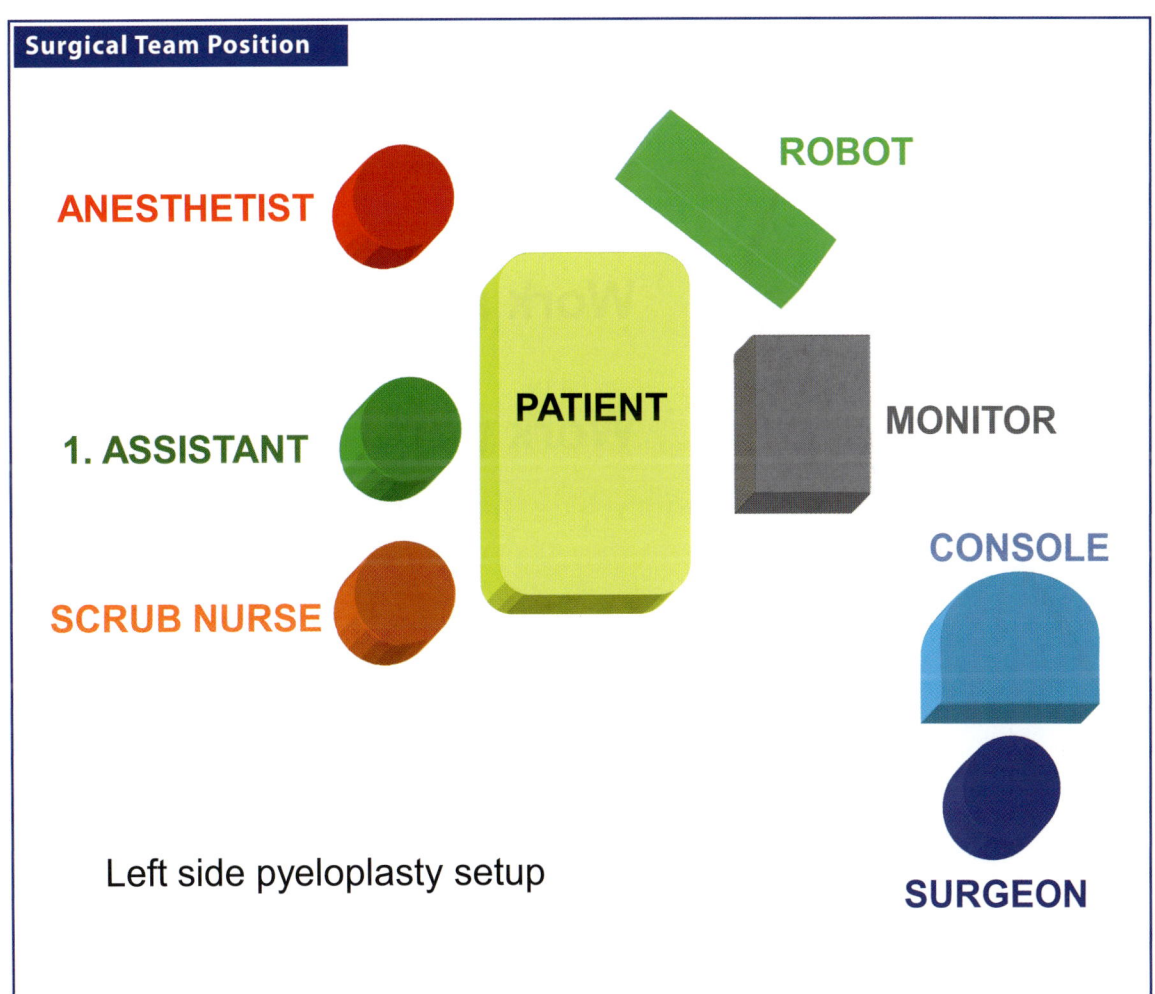

Surgical Team Position

ANESTHETIST

ROBOT

PATIENT

1. ASSISTANT

MONITOR

SCRUB NURSE

CONSOLE

SURGEON

Left side pyeloplasty setup

60.2   Patient Positioning

For left retroperitoneal pyeloplasty (reverse positions for right pyeloplasty) the patient is placed in the right lateral recumbent position.

60.3   Special Instruments

Balloon catheter (for creation of a retroperitoneal space).

60.4   Location of Access Points

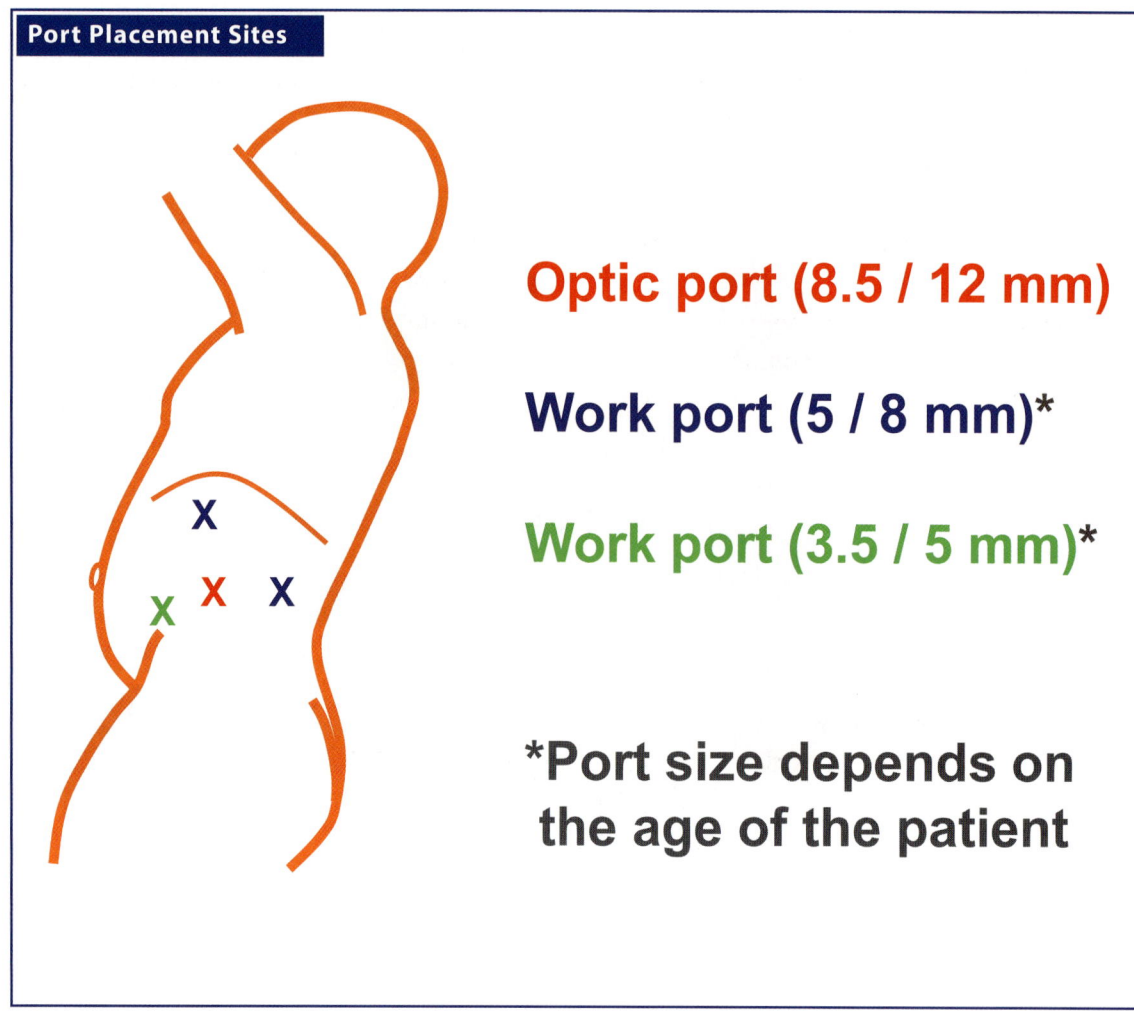

Port Placement Sites

Optic port (8.5 / 12 mm)

Work port (5 / 8 mm)*

Work port (3.5 / 5 mm)*

***Port size depends on the age of the patient**

60.5 Indications

1. Pelviureteric junction obstruction (PUJO).
2. Treatment is particularly indicated if the patient is symptomatic or there is impairment of renal function.
3. Kidney stones in addition to PUJO.

60.6 Relative Contraindications

1. Re-do procedures.
2. Infants below 6 months–1 year.

60.7 Preoperative Considerations

1. A single dose of antibiotics is administered if the placement of a double-J ureteral stent is planned or indwelling catheters are expected to be removed after 24 h.
2. Epidural catheter placement should be considered.
3. Patients are placed with the upper leg stretched and the lower leg flexed. A small gel cushion or roll should be placed under the contralateral iliac crest. Internal rotation of the upper hip joint should be avoided in older children.

60.8 Technical Notes

1. The DeBakey grasper is manipulated by the surgeon's left hand.
2. The surgeon's right hand manipulates the monopolar hook or scissors and the large needle holder.
3. The assistant assists with other 3.5/5-mm instruments (scissors, grasper, and suction/irrigation) as required.
4. Suturing of the anastomosis is performed using absorbable 5–0 or 6–0 suture material.

60.9 Procedure Variations

1. Transabdominal pyeloplasty.
2. Nondismembered pyeloplasty should be done only if surgery on the lower ureter is anticipated.

60.10 Robot-Assisted Laparoscopic Retroperitoneal Pyeloplasty

Please see Figs. 1–10.

Figure 60.1

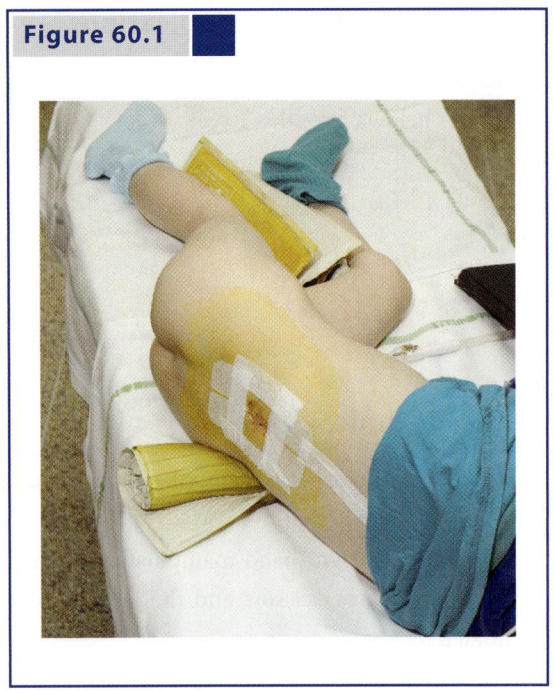

The patient is positioned with the upper leg stretched and the lower leg flexed. Position shown for left side pyeloplasty

Figure 60.2

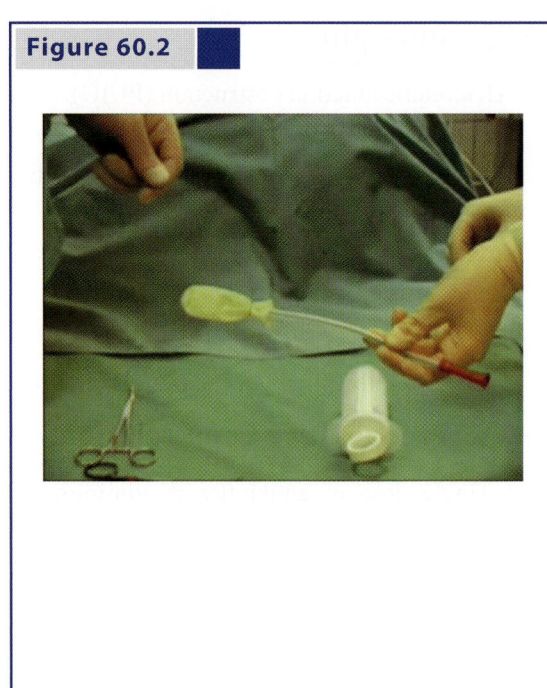

The retroperitoneal space is developed with a simple surgical-glove-finger-catheter balloon. Do not inflate more than 200–300 ml of air/saline (to avoid tearing of the peritoneum). In adolescents, commercially available balloon dilatators can be used

Figure 60.3

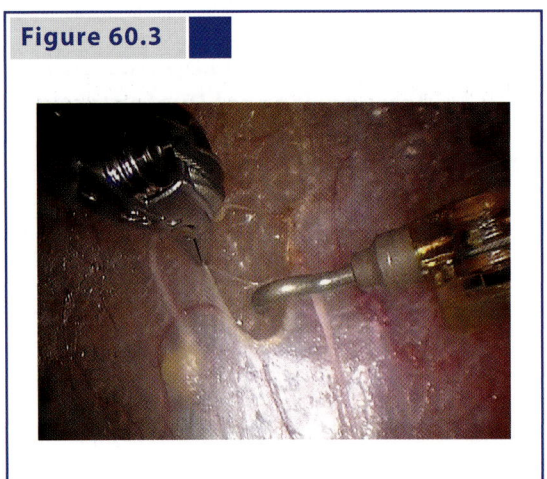
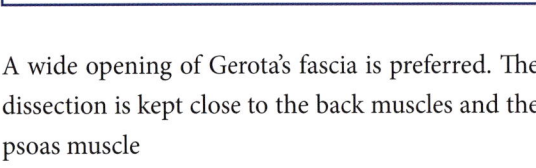

A wide opening of Gerota's fascia is preferred. The dissection is kept close to the back muscles and the psoas muscle

Figure 60.4

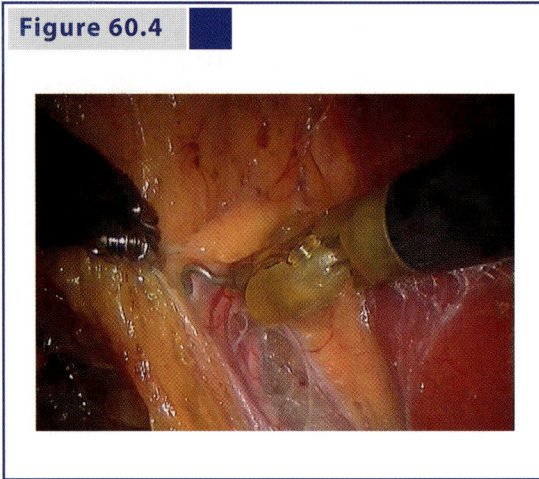

Dissection is carried out cranially to caudally, from the pelvis down to the ureter, in the lesser-vascularized areas

Figure 60.5

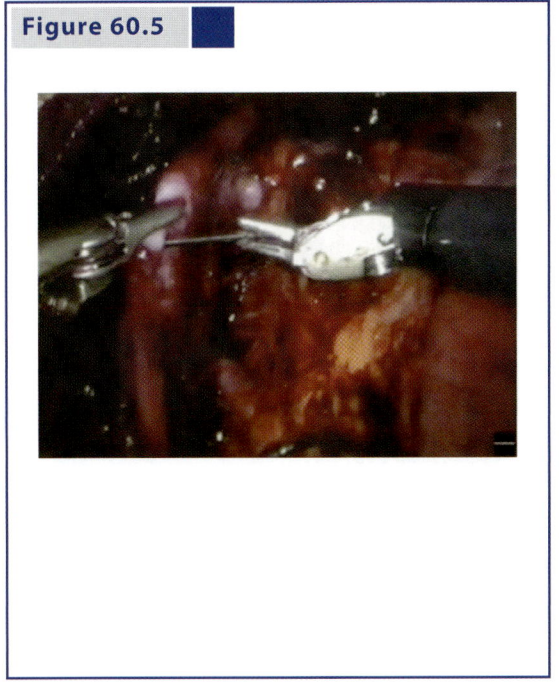

Stay sutures are placed on both ends of the pelvis and the upper end of the ureter. This helps to keep blood and urine out of the operating field. The stay sutures further align the ureter and the pelvis and facilitate suturing of the anastomosis

Figure 60.6

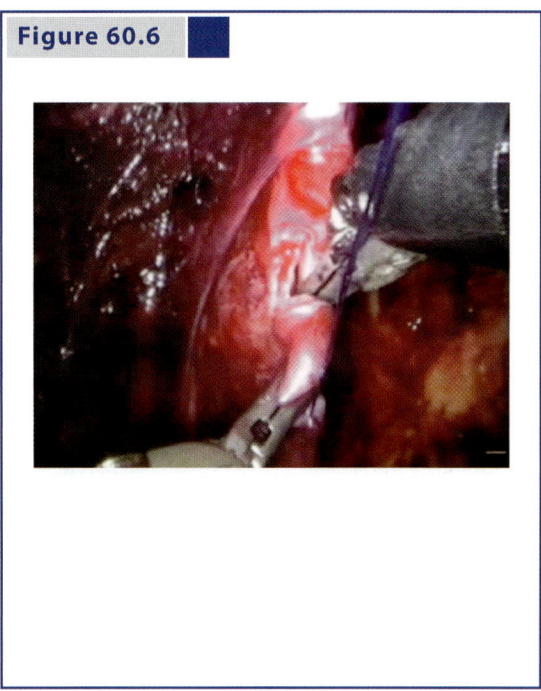

The pelvis and ureter are dismembered. The stenotic area of the ureter is preserved and is used as a handle during suturing. If an aberrant vessel is present, the ureter is transposed before the stay suture is placed

Figure 60.7

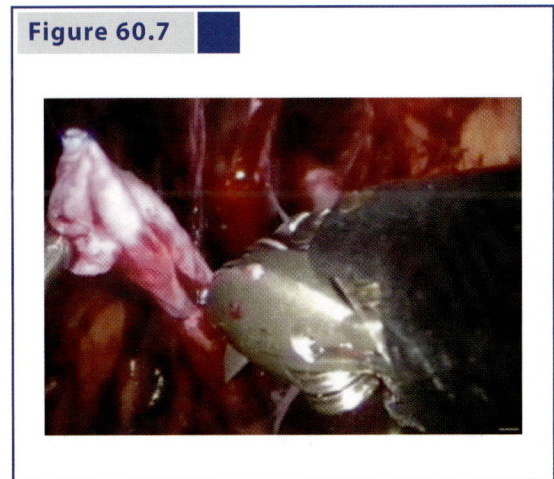

The ureter is spatulated for a length of approximately 2 cm

Figure 60.8

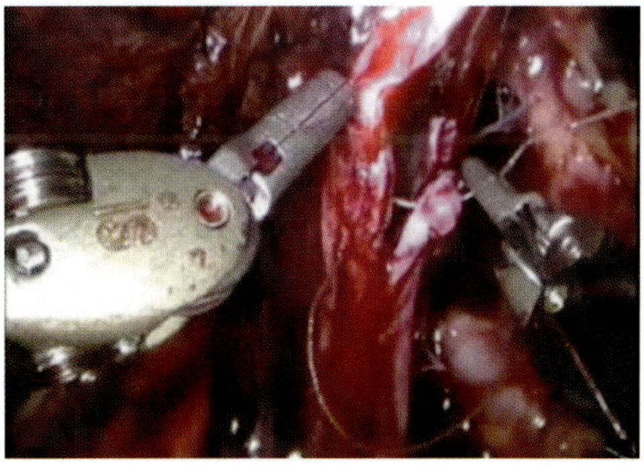

One half, either anterior or posterior (as preferred), of the anastomosis is closed with 5-0 or 6-0 running sutures

Figure 60.9

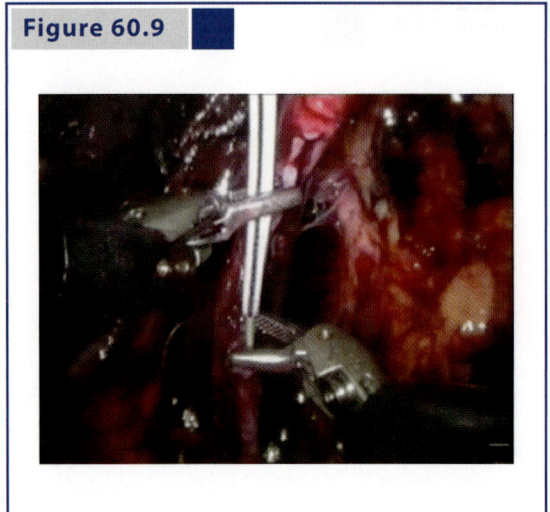

Figure 60.10

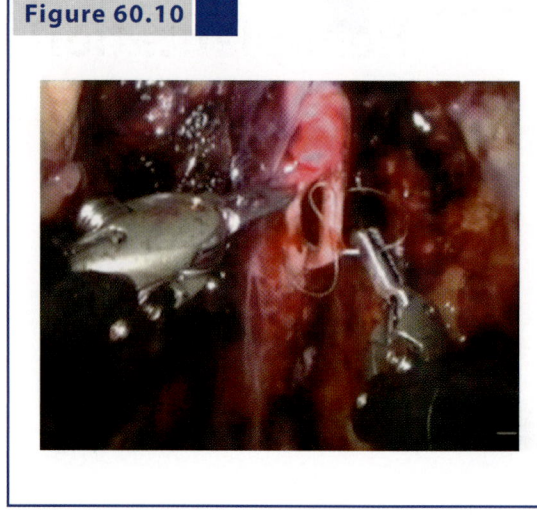

A guidewire is inserted through the 5-mm assistant port. A desired-size double-J stent is pushed down the guidewire to the bladder until the upper end is visible. The guidewire is removed and the upper coil of the stent is placed in the pelvis

The second half of the anastomosis is then completed. A drain is not necessary when opting for retroperitoneal access. The fascia of the camera port and the medial assistant port are closed before skin closure

Recommended Literature

1. Kutikov A, Nguyen M, Guzzo T, Cantar D, Casale P (2006) Robot assisted pyeloplasty in the infant – lessons learned. J Urol 176:2237–2239
2. Lee RS, Retik AB, Borer JG, Peters CA (2006) Pediatric robot assisted laparoscopic dismembered pyeloplasty: comparison with a cohort of open surgery. J Urol 175:683–687
3. Olsen LH, Rawashdeh YF, Jorgensen TM (2007) Pediatric robot assisted retroperitoneoscopic pyeloplasty: a 5-year experience. J Urol 178:2137–2141

61 Transvesicoscopic Ureteric Reimplantation

Jean-Stéphane Valla

61.1 Operation Room Setup

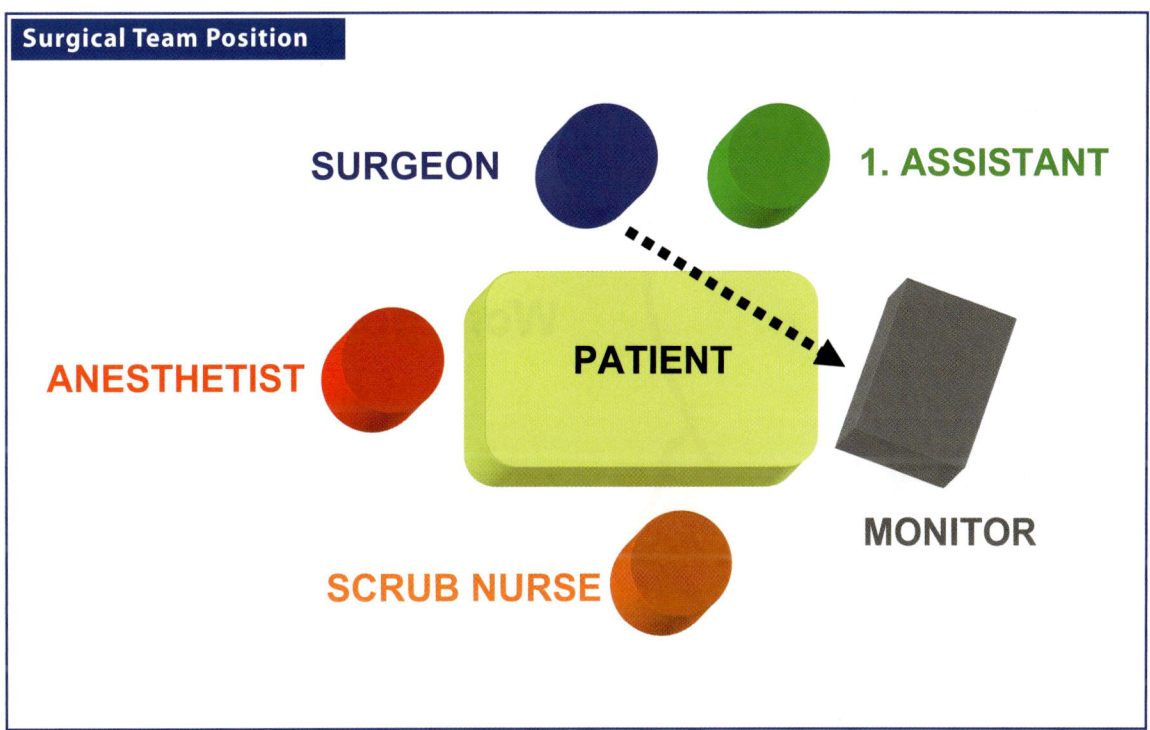

Surgical Team Position

SURGEON

1. ASSISTANT

ANESTHETIST

PATIENT

MONITOR

SCRUB NURSE

61.2   Patient Positionings

Supine in the modified lithotomy position with abducted thighs. The lower part of the abdomen and genitalia are draped in a sterile fashion.

61.3   Special Instruments

- Cystoscopy set
- 3-mm instruments
- 3-mm ports

61.4   Location of Access Points

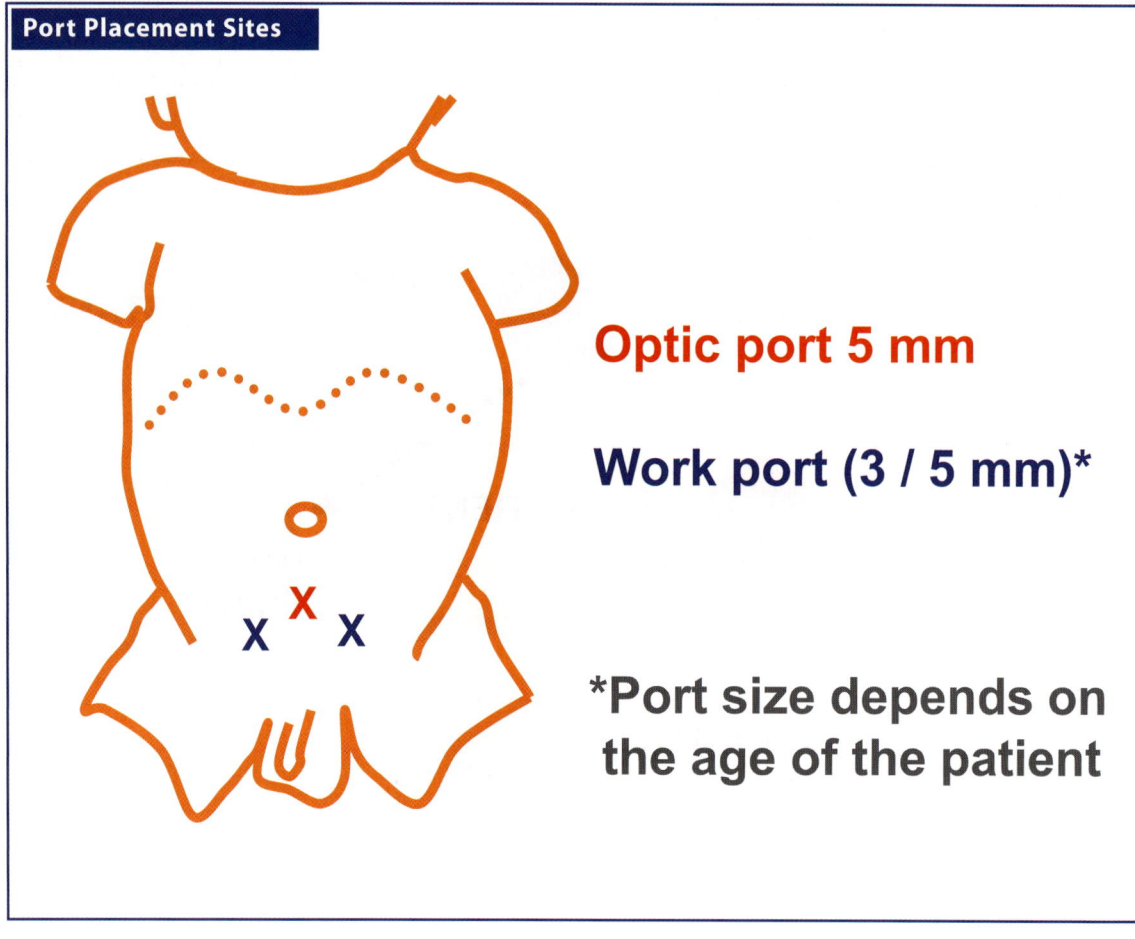

Port Placement Sites

Optic port 5 mm

Work port (3 / 5 mm)*

*Port size depends on the age of the patient

61.5   Indications

1. Persistent high-grade reflux.
2. Failure of endoscopic submucosal injection.
3. Major anatomical anomalies: duplex system, reflux of ureterocele incision, reflux-associated with large diverticulum.

61.6   Contraindications

1. Children under 6 months of age (the working space is too small).
2. Huge megaureter.

61.7   Preoperative Considerations

1. Verify the sterility of the patient's urine.
2. Complete a preoperative assessment of urinary tract to exclude any bladder obstruction or dysfunction.
3. Obtain informed consent from the parents since this is a new technique that is not yet considered as the gold-standard in the management of vesicoureteral reflux.

61.8   Technical Notes

1. First step: the bladder is distended with saline instilled using transureteral cystococopy. The three ports are placed under cystoscopic guidance. The bladder wall must be approximated to the abdominal wall to avoid trocar dislodgement during the procedure by the use of special ports (self-retaining ports with balloon or umbrella tips) or a suture passed percutaneously.
2. Second step: the bladder is insufflated with carbon dioxide using pressures of 8–10 mmHg. The ureteral reimplantation is performed in a manner similar to that followed in the open procedure.
3. Leave a bladder catheter (transurethral or suprapubic) for 2 days postoperatively.
4. Try to close the bladder wall port incisions.

61.9   Procedure Variations

1. The urethra could be used to pass a 3-mm instrument and could be used as the third operating access.
2. The urethra could also be used to place a catheter that can be utilized to aspirate smoke and urine during the procedure.
3. A mechanical camera holder is useful to obtain stable vision at the time of suturing.
4. There is no need to occlude the urethra, even in female patients, as the gas leak through the urethra is minimal.

61.10   Transvesicoscopic Cohen's Right-Side Ureteric Reimplantation

Please see Figs. 1–11.

Figure 61.1

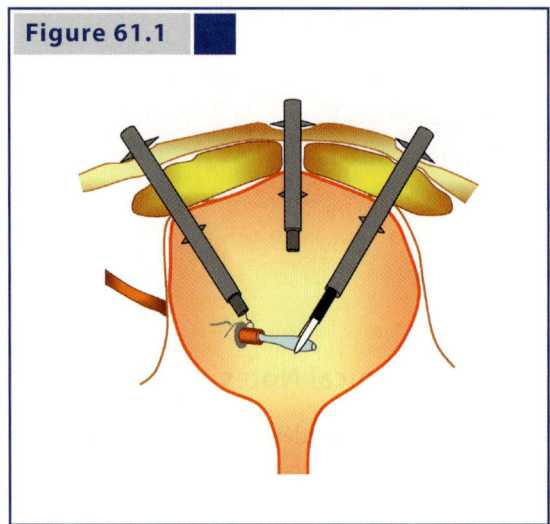

Schematic representation of the transvesicoscopic ureteric reimplantation procedure showing the points of port placement and intervention

Figure 61.2

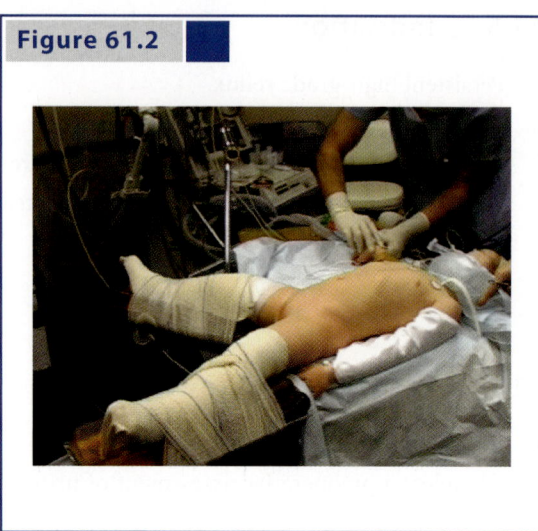

The patient is positioned toward the end of the operating table since this procedure involves the simultaneous implementation of cystoscopy

Figure 61.3

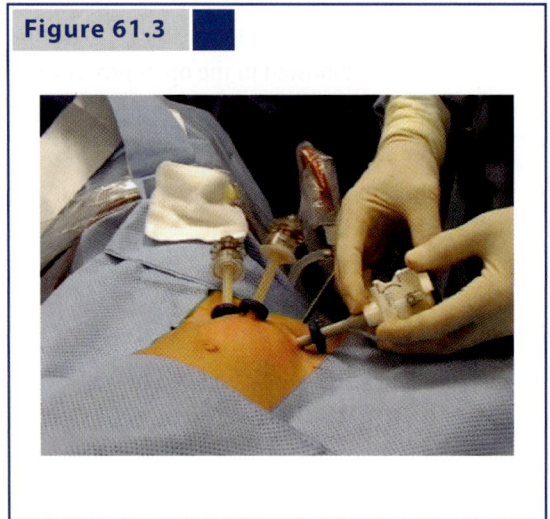

The ports are inserted under cystoscopic visualization. The ports are placed closer to the umbilicus in small children (bladder = abdominal organ) and closer to the pubis in older children (bladder=pelvic organ)

Figure 61.4

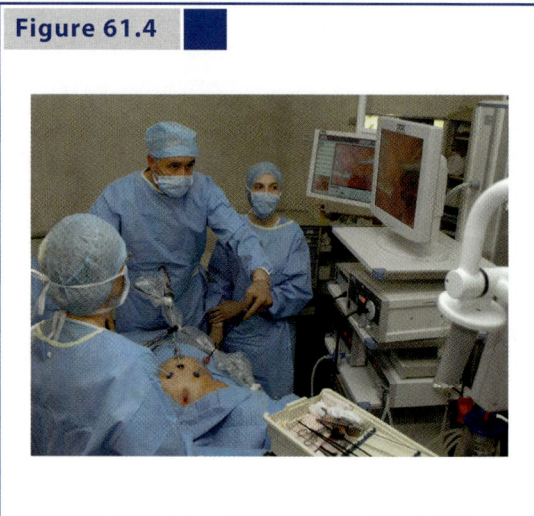

The surgeon stands toward the head of the patient in children under the age of 5 years and on the left side of the patient in older children

Figure 61.5

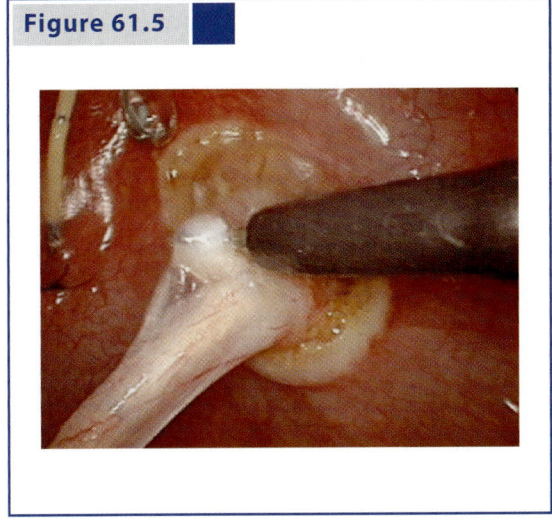

The right ureter is dissected circumferentially from the urinary bladder with a 3-mm hooked monopolar cautery

Figure 61.6

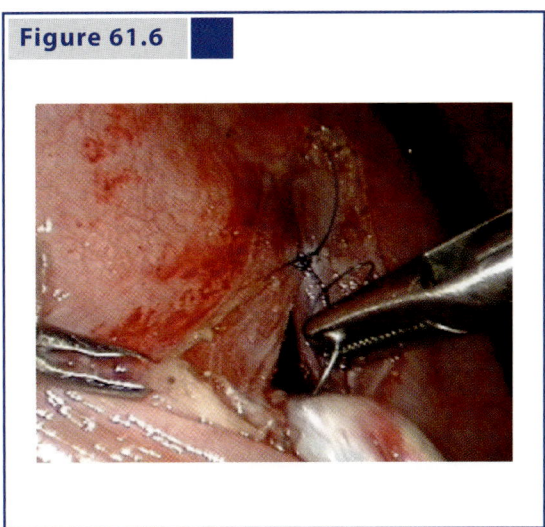

The muscular defect or the ureteric hiatus created during the ureter dissection is sutured

Figure 61.7

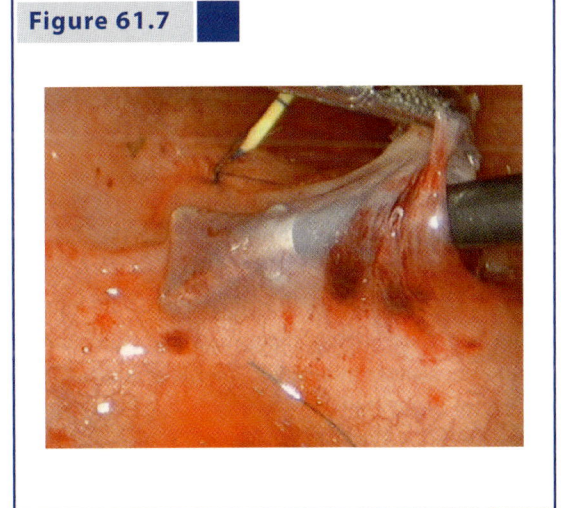

A submucosal tunnel is created with blunt dissection to the desired position of ureter reimplantation

Figure 61.8

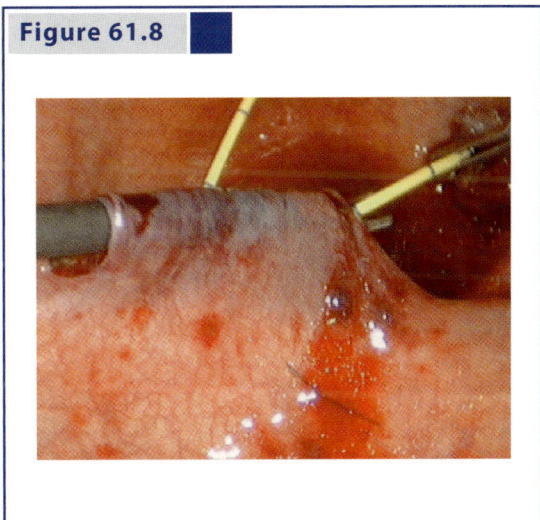

After the tunnel is created, a grasper is passed through it to grasp the ureteric stent

Figure 61.9

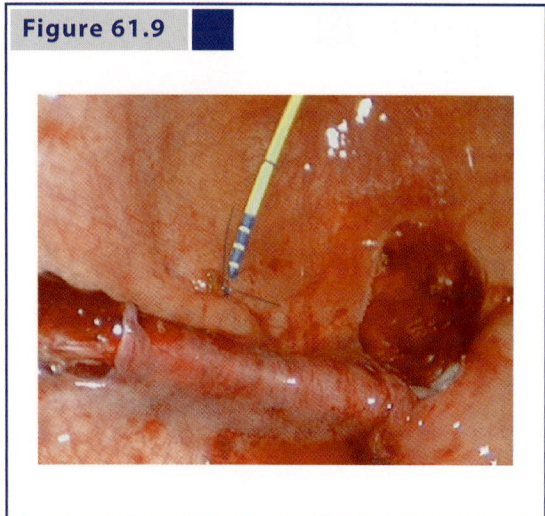

Figure 61.10

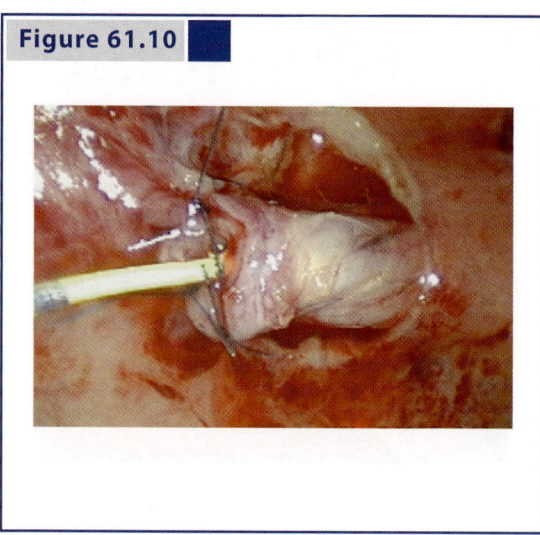

The ureter is then passed through the tunnel and sufficiently exposed on the other side

After resection of the distal part of the ureter a ureteroneocystostomy is performed with interrupted sutures

Figure 61.11

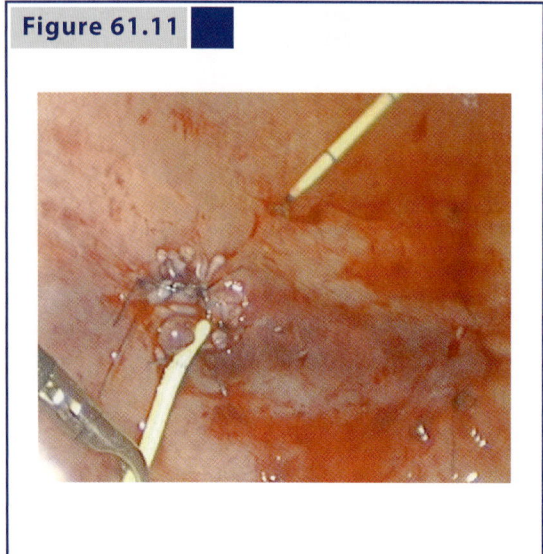

The procedure is completed with circumferential interrupted sutures to secure the ureter to its new position

Recommended Literature

1. Kutikov A, Guzzo TJ, Canter DJ, Casale P (2006) Initial experience with laparoscopic transvesical ureteral reimplantation at the Children's Hospital of Philadelphia. J Urol 176:2222–2225
2. Ogan K, Pohl HG, Carlson D, Belaman AB, Rushton HG (2001) Parental preferences in the management of vesicoureteral reflux. J Urol 166:240–243
3. Yeung CK, Sihoe JD, Borzi PA (2005) Endoscopic cross-trigonal ureteral reimplantation under carbon dioxide bladder insufflation: a novel technique. J Endourol 19:295–299

62 STING Procedure for Vesicoureteral Reflux

PREM PURI

62.1 Operation Room Setup

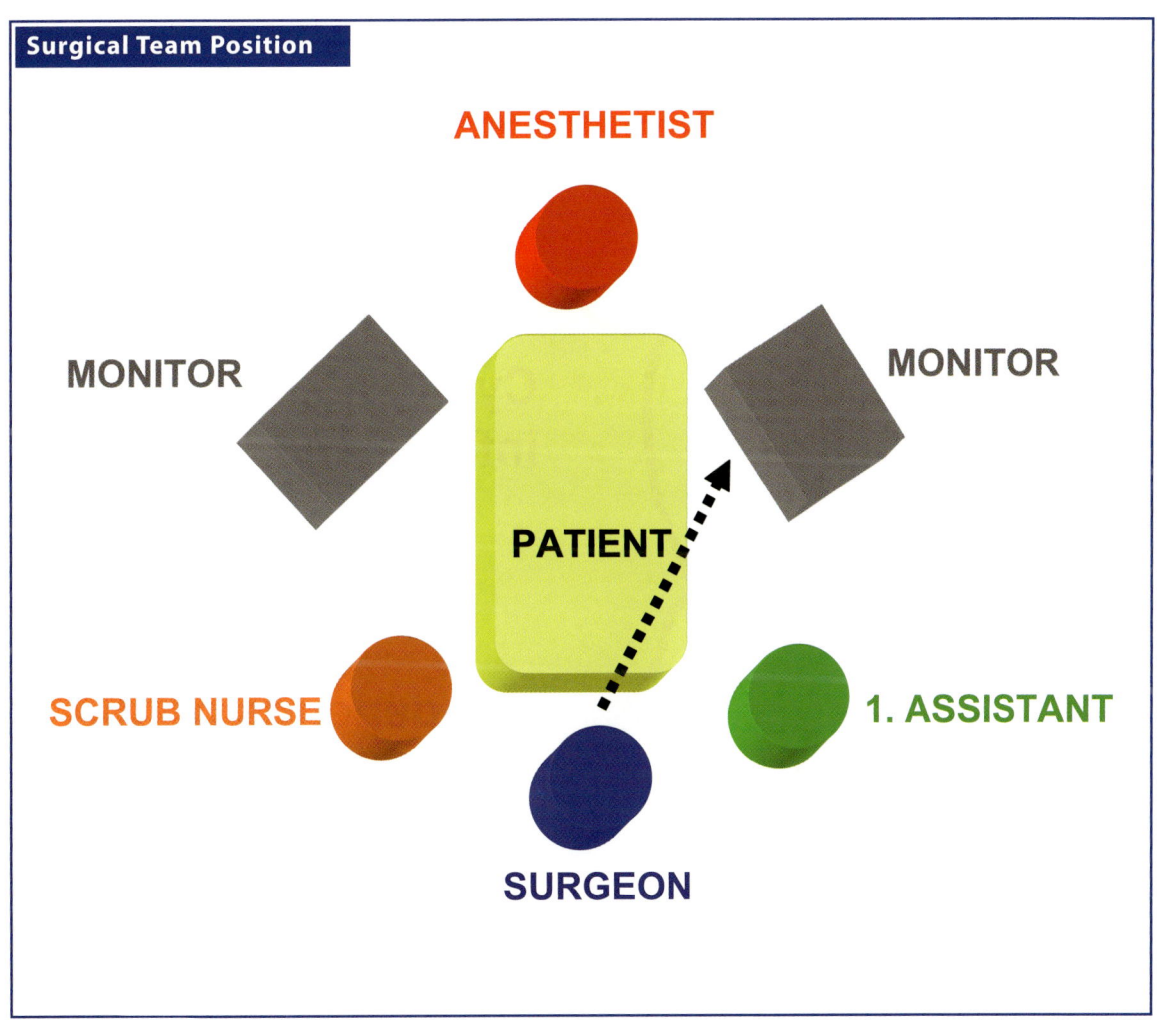

Surgical Team Position

ANESTHETIST

MONITOR

MONITOR

PATIENT

SCRUB NURSE

1. ASSISTANT

SURGEON

62.2   Patient Positioning

Toward the end of the table in a supine position with arms tucked to the side.

62.3   Special Instruments

- Cystoscope
- Puri flexible catheter (Karl Storz, Tuttlingen, Germany)
- Deflux™ (Q-Med Scandinavia, Uppsala, Sweden)

62.4   Location of Access Points

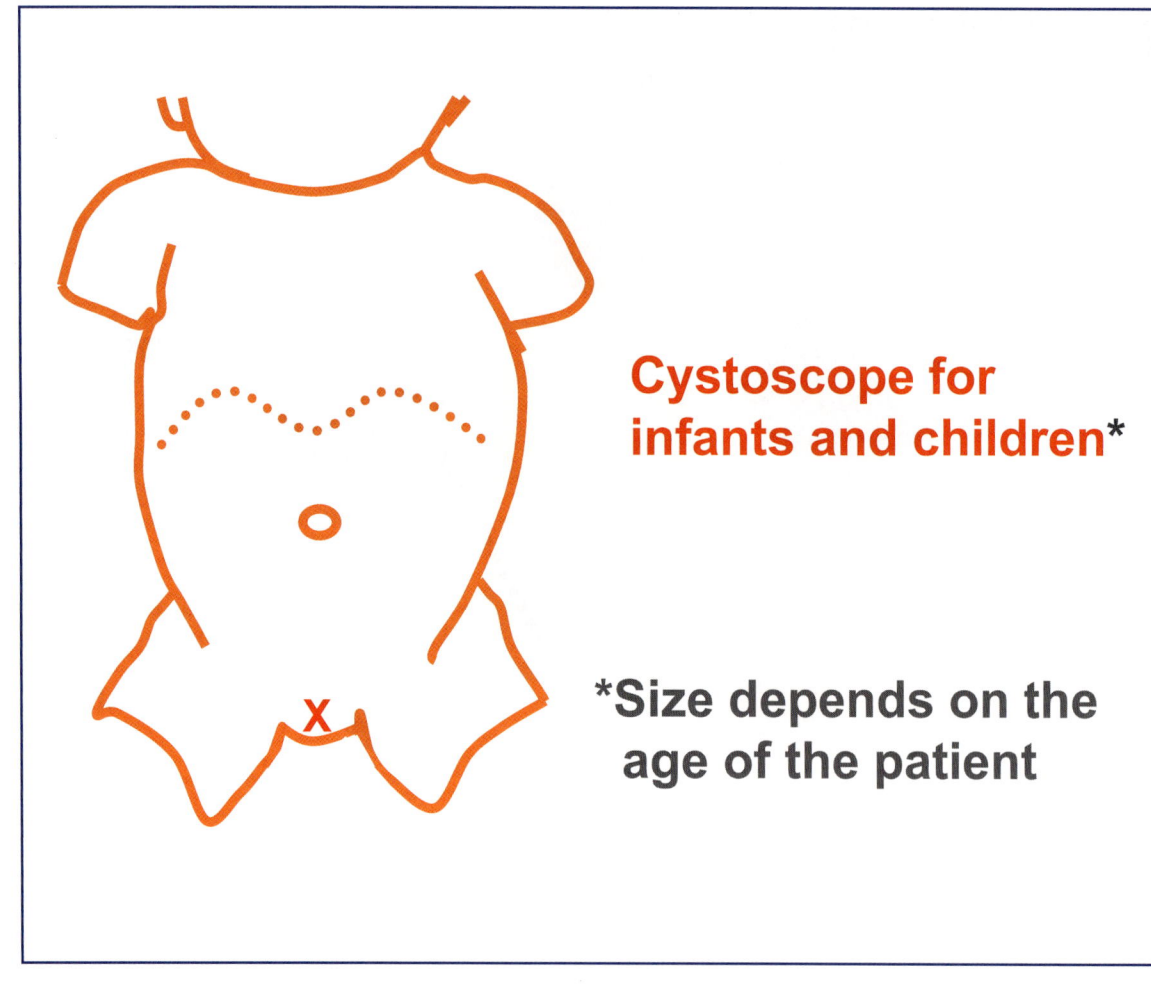

Cystoscope for infants and children*

*****Size depends on the age of the patient**

62.5   Indications

1. High-grade primary vesicoureteral reflux (VUR; grade III–V).
2. VUR in duplex renal systems.
3. VUR secondary to neuropathic bladder and posterior urethral valves.
4. VUR in failed reimplanted ureters.
5. VUR into refluxing ureteral stumps.

62.6   Preoperative Considerations

62.6.1   Tissue-Augmenting Substances

The tissue-augmenting substance most commonly used for subureteral injection is dextranomer/hyaluronic acid copolymer (Deflux™). It consists of microspheres in 1% high-molecular-weight sodium hyaluronan solution. Each milliliter of Deflux contains 0.5 ml sodium hyaluronan and 0.5 ml dextranomer.

62.7   Technical Notes I

1. All cystoscopes available for infants and children can be used for this procedure.
2. The disposable Puri flexible catheter or a rigid metallic catheter can be used for injection.
3. A 1-ml syringe filled with Deflux™ is attached to the injection catheter.
4. Under direct vision through the cystoscope, the needle is introduced under the bladder mucosa 2–3 mm below the affected ureteral orifice at the 6 o'clock position.

62.8   Technical Notes II

1. In grades IV and V reflux with wide ureteral orifices, the needle should be inserted not below, but directly into the affected ureteral orifice.
2. The needle is advanced about 4–5 mm under the mucosa and the injection started slowly.
3. As the Deflux™ is injected a bulge appears in the floor of the submucosal ureter. A correctly placed injection creates the appearance of a nipple on the top of which is a slit-like or inverted crescent orifice.
4. Patients are treated as day cases and a voiding cystourethrogram and ultrasound are performed 6–12 weeks after discharge.

62.9   STING Procedure for the Treatment of VUR

Please see Figs. 1–14.

Figure 62.1

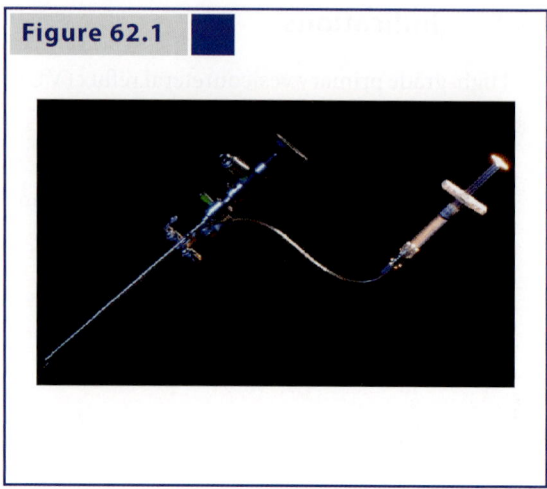

Equipment set-up for the STING procedure is shown here. A-1ml syringe prefilled with Deflux™ is attached to the Puri flexible catheter for injection and introduced through a cystoscope

Figure 62.2

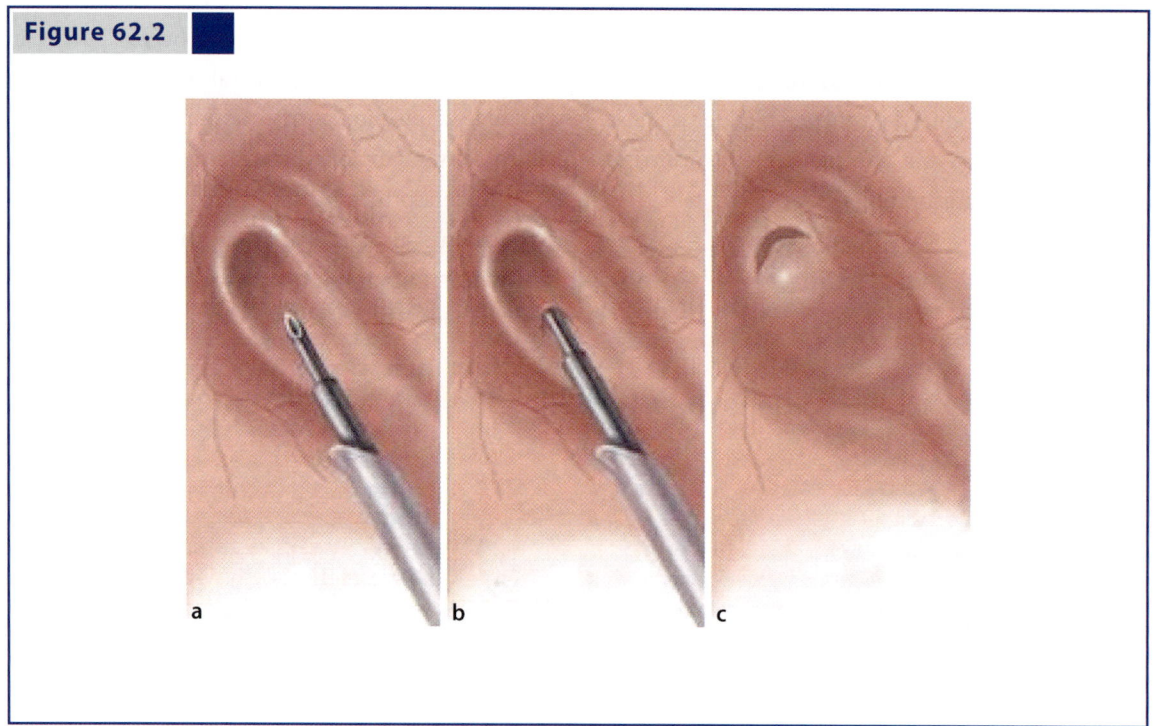

Schematic representation of the STING procedure. The needle is introduced under the mucosa of the affected ureteral orifice at the 6 o'clock position (a) and is advanced 4–5 mm before the injection is started (b). At the end of the injection the ureteral orifice is slit-like (c)

Figure 62.3

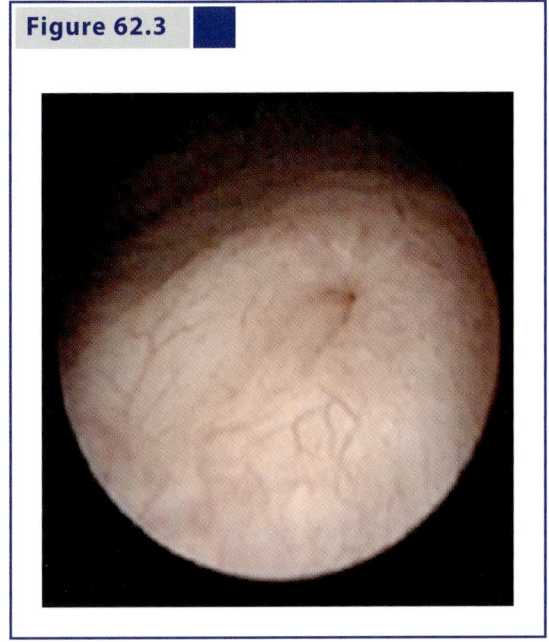

Endoscopic appearance of a grade III refluxing ureteral orifice

Figure 62.4

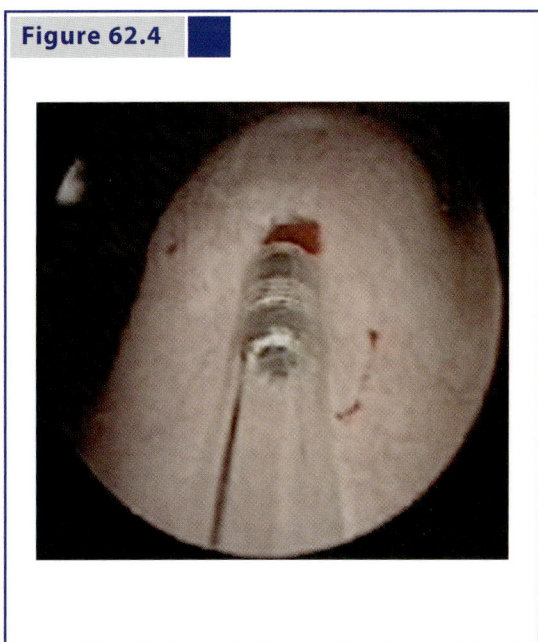

Endoscopic appearance of STING. A correctly placed Deflux™ implant gives the appearance of a nipple on top of which is a slit-like orifice

Figure 62.5

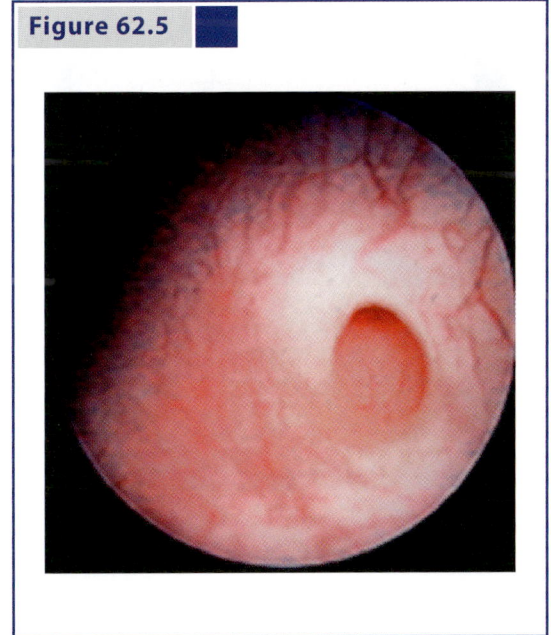

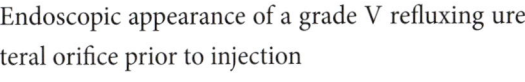

Endoscopic appearance of a grade V refluxing ureteral orifice prior to injection

Figure 62.6

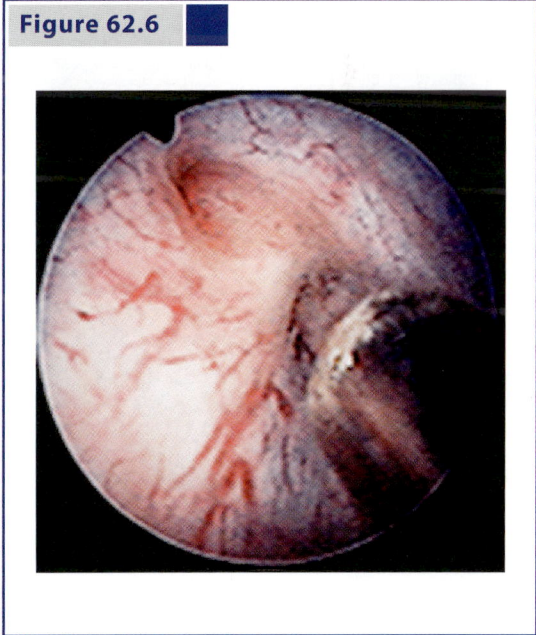

Endoscopic appearance of a grade V refluxing ureteral orifice with the injection in progress

Figure 62.7

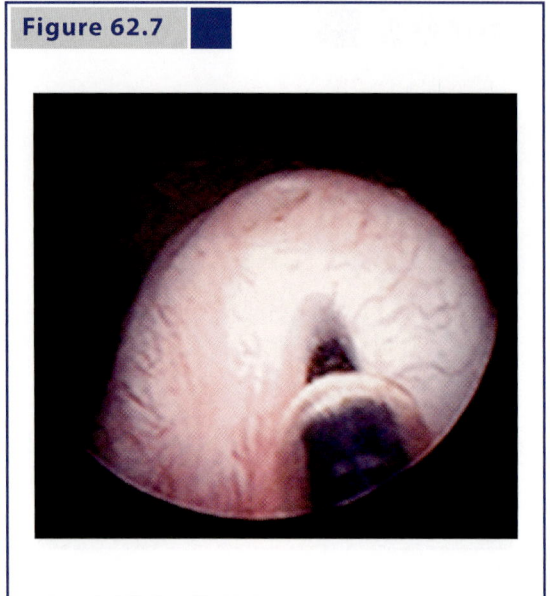

During the injection the needle is slowly withdrawn until a "volcanic" bulge of paste is seen

Figure 62.8

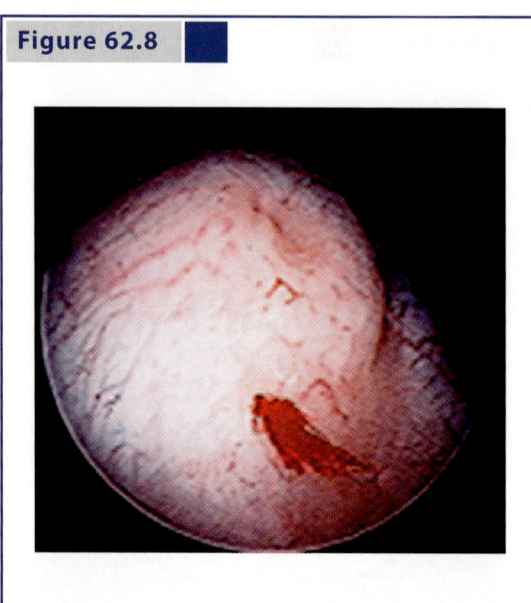

A correctly placed injection creates the appearance of a nipple with a slit like orifice on the top of it

Figure 62.9

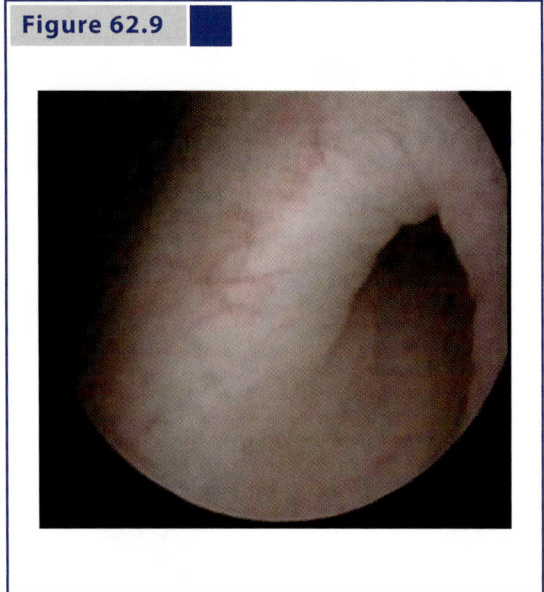

Endoscopic appearance of a grade V wide ureteral orifice in an infant

Figure 62.10

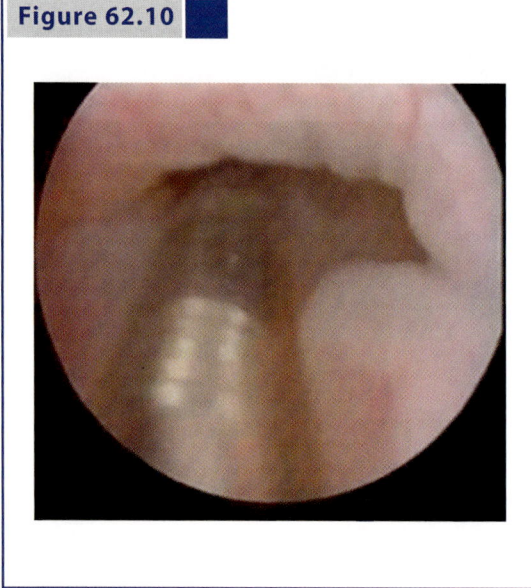

The needle for injection is inserted under the mucosa directly inside the affected ureteral orifice

Figure 62.11

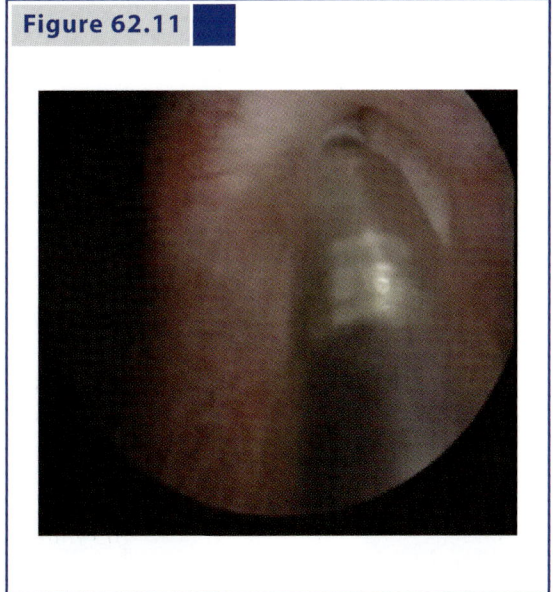

Figure 62.12

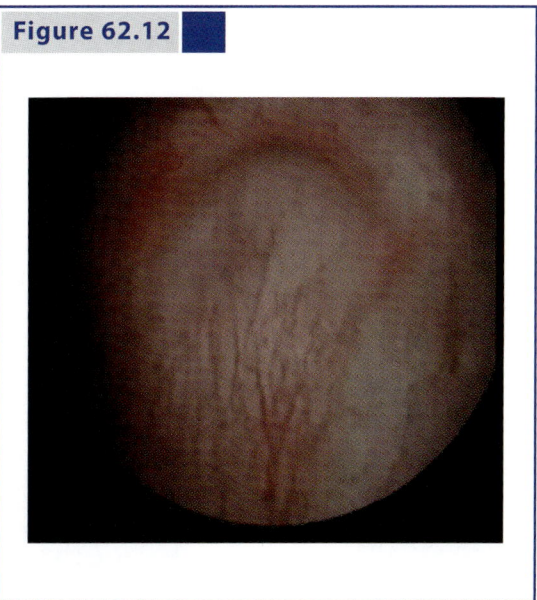

Injection in progress showing a bulge of paste appearing in the floor of the affected ureteral orifice

At the end of the injection the ureteral orifice has a slit-like appearance

Figure 62.13

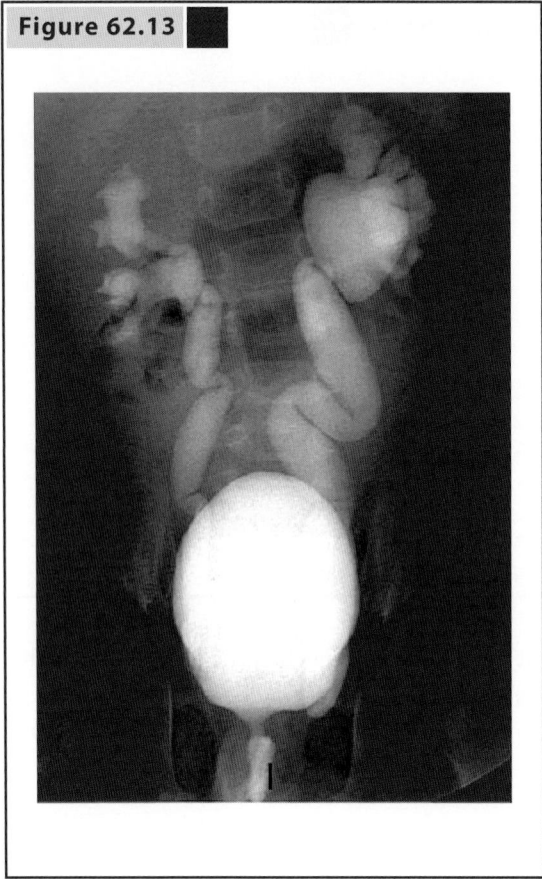

Figure 62.14

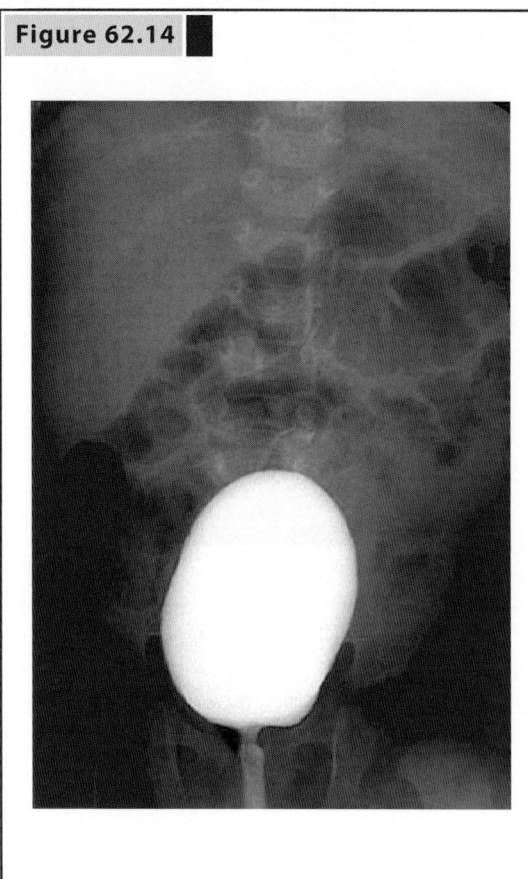

Voiding cystourethrogram showing bilateral grade V reflux

Voiding cystourethrography in the same child showing no evidence of reflux 3 months after the STING procedure

Recommended Literature

1. Menezes M, Puri P (2007) The role of endoscopic treatment in the management of grade 5 primary vesicoureteral reflux. Eur Urol 52:1505–1510

2. Puri P (2006) Endoscopic treatment of vesicoureteral reflux. In: Puri P, Höllwarth ME (eds) Pediatric Surgery (Springer Surgery Atlas Series). Springer Heidelberg, pp 493–498

3. Puri P, Pirker M, Mohanan M, Dawrant M, Dass L, Colhoun E (2006) Subureteral dexranomer\hyaluronic acid injection as first line treatment in the management of high grade vesicoureteral reflux. J Urol 176:1856–1860

63 Varicocele Ligation

Oliver J. Muensterer

63.1 Operation Room Setup

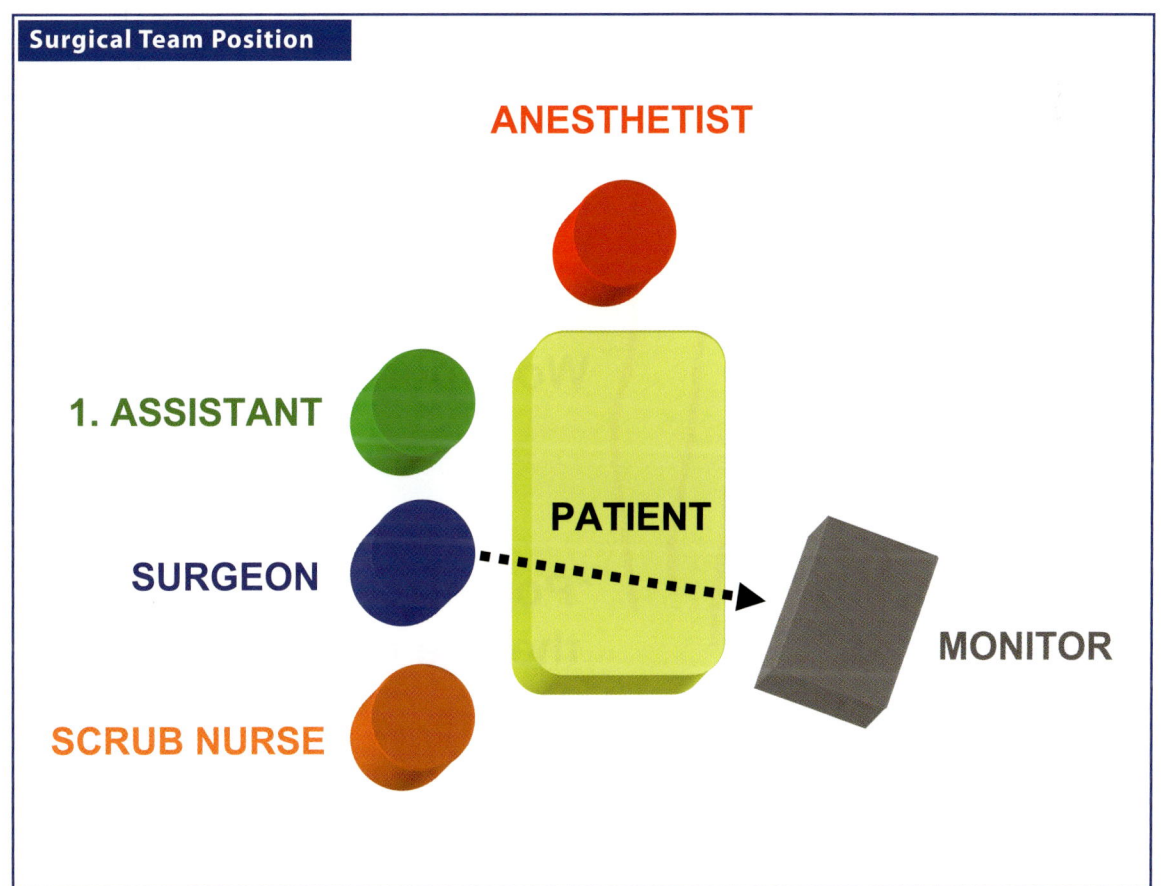

Surgical Team Position

ANESTHETIST

1. ASSISTANT

SURGEON

SCRUB NURSE

PATIENT

MONITOR

63.2   Patient Positioning

Supine position with arms tucked to the side; the ipsilateral side may be abducted. The positioning shown here is for left-side varicocele, which occurs more frequently.

63.3   Special Instruments

- Ultracision® shears (Johnson & Johnson Medical Products, Ethicon Endo-Surgery, Cincinnati, OH, USA)
- Endoscopic clip applicator

63.4   Location of Access Points

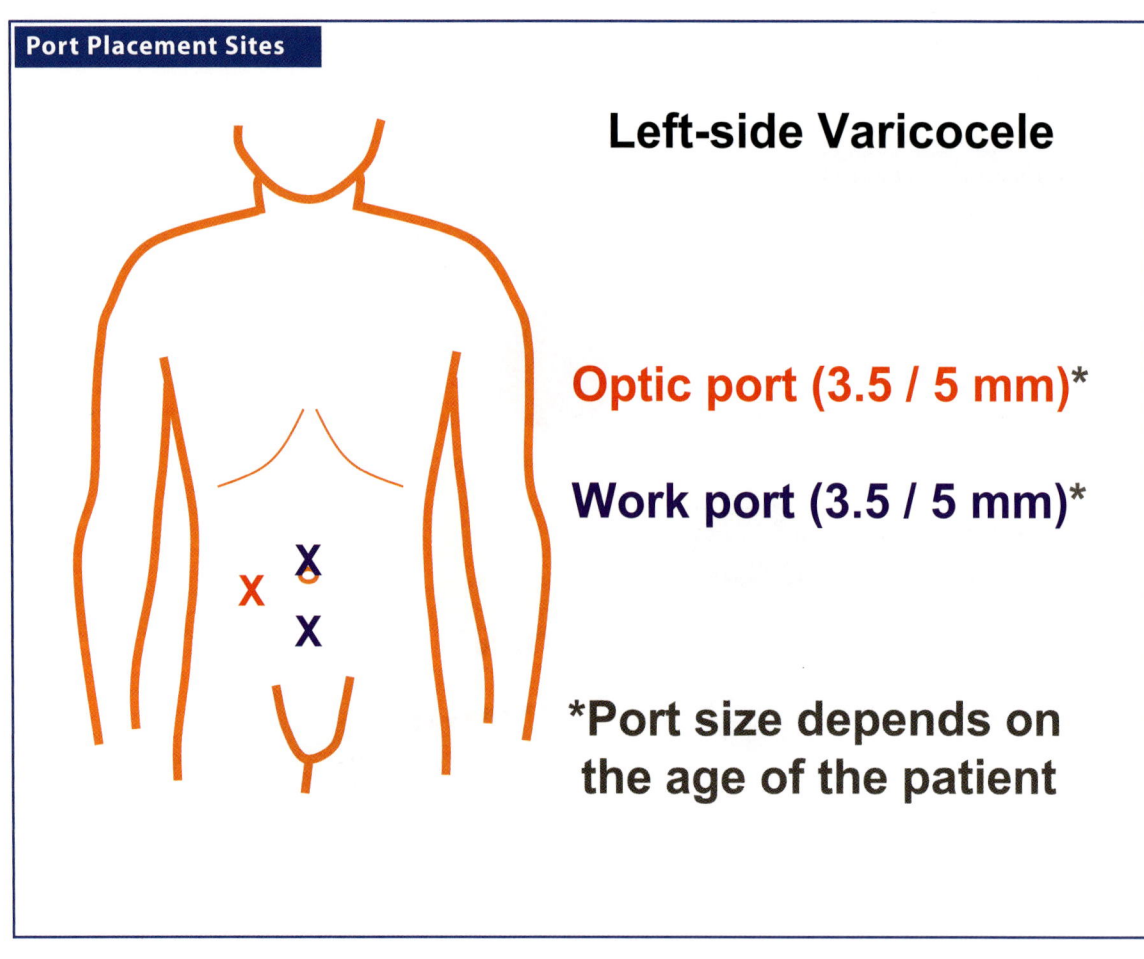

63.5   Indications

Symptomatic varicocele (low sperm count, scrotal pain, testicular atrophy compared to the contralateral side, severe cosmetic impairment).

63.6   Contraindications

1. Suspected malignancy of the ipsilateral kidney.
2. Other testicular or scrotal pathologies mimicking varicocele.
3. Previous surgery that may have compromised the blood supply to the affected testes (orchidopexy).

63.7   Preoperative Considerations

1. In children under 5 years or right-sided varicocele, use ultrasound to rule out renal tumor or hydronephrosis causing mechanical compression of the testicular vein.
2. Usually left-sided (90%); however 9% are bilateral and only 1% are right-sided.
3. The recurrence rate is under 4% for mass ligation (artery and vein), up to 20% with artery preservation, and 16% for the inguinal open approach.
4. The most common complications are hydrocele formation (7%) and sensory loss in the distribution of the cutaneous femoral lateral nerve.

63.8   Technical Notes

1. Tilting the table with the ipsilateral side up and head down may facilitate exposure of the spermatic vessels.
2. A large incision in the peritoneum should be made to grasp all identified vessels and to mobilize them well into the abdominal cavity. This helps to facilitate a complete and safe ligation.

63.9   Procedure Variations

1. Depending on personal preference and the equipment available, ligation of the spermatic vessels may be performed by electrocautery, ultrasound scissors, or clips.
2. Preoperative subdartos injection of isosulfan blue may help the surgeon to identify and preserve the lymphatic vessels during dissection and thereby reduce the risk of postoperative hydrocele formation.

63.10   Laparoscopic Palomo Varicocele Ligation

Please see Figs. 1–6.

Figure 63.1

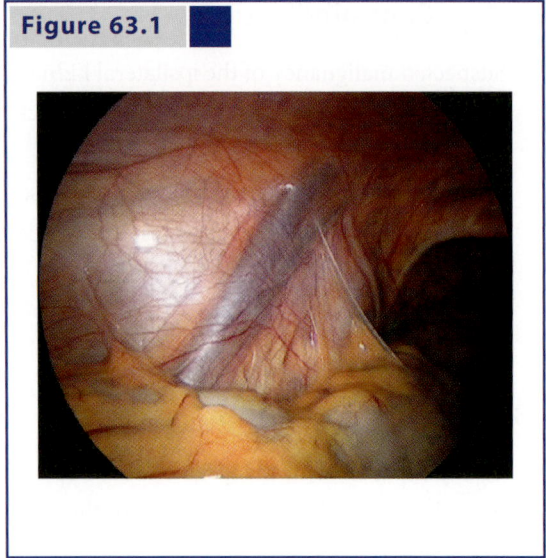

The spermatic vessels leading to the internal inguinal ring are identified

Figure 63.2

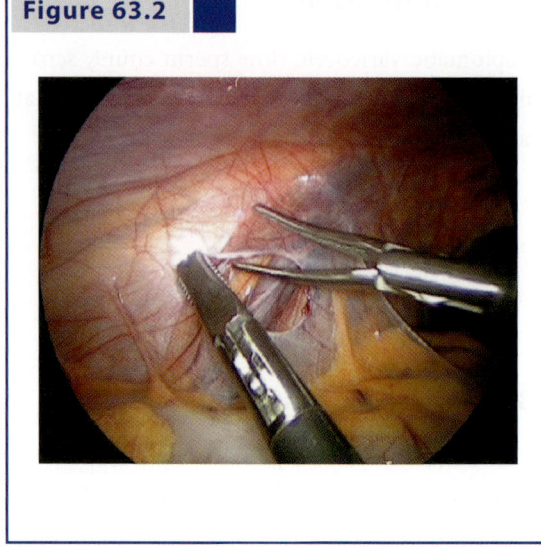

The peritoneum overlying the vessels is incised

Figure 63.3

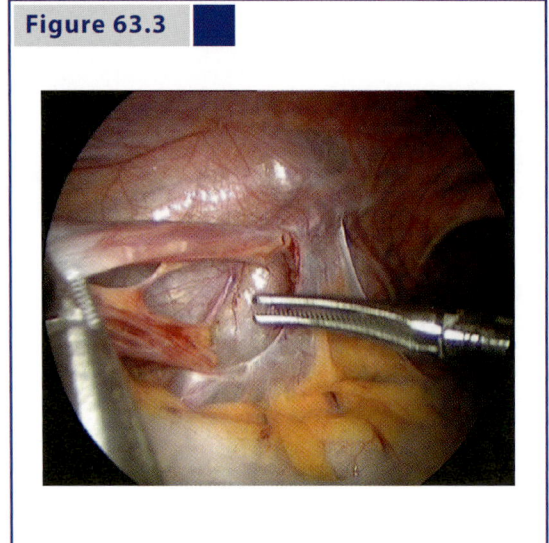

The vessels are prepared and mobilized into the abdominal cavity

Figure 63.4

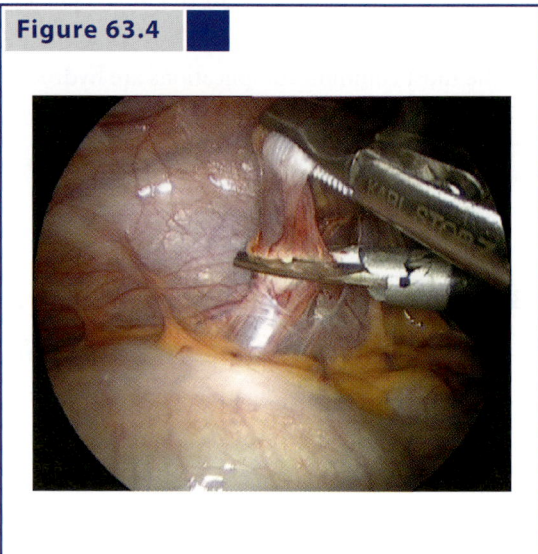

The Ultracision® shears option is used to cauterize the spermatic vessels

Figure 63.5

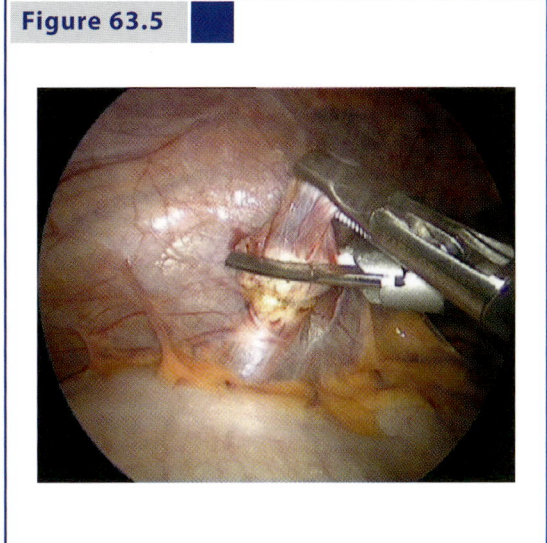

Figure 63.6

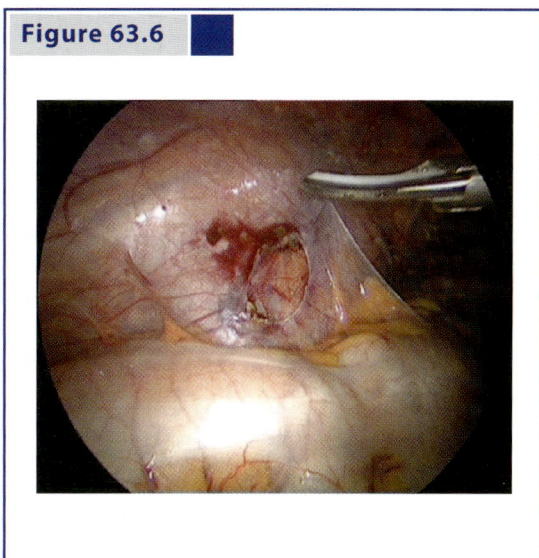

The vessels are divided proximally and distally at the point of cauterization

A section of the vessels between the cauterized sites is removed

Recommended Literature

1. Fretz PC, Sandlow JI (2002) Varicocele: current concepts in pathophysiology, diagnosis, and treatment. Urol Clin North Am 29:921–937
2. Koyle MA, Oottamasathein S, Barqawi A, Rajimwale A, Furness PD 3rd (2004) Laparoscopic Palomo varicocele ligation in children and adolescents: results of 103 cases. J Urol 172:1749–1752
3. Schwentner C, Radmayr C, Lunacek A, Gozzi C, Pinggera GM, Neururer R, Peschel R, Bartsch G, Oswald J (2006) Laparoscopic varicocele ligation in children and adolescents using isosulphan blue: a prospective randomized trial. BJU 98:861–865

Section 6
Miscellaneous Topics

64 Electrosurgical Injuries

Amulya K. Saxena

64.1 Reliance on Electrosurgery

Relatively minimal bleeding, which is a minor obstacle with open procedures, may completely obscure the view in endoscopic surgery and prevent safe dissection. Therefore, in order to perform minimal-access procedures, the surgeon must rely more heavily on the energy source for hemostasis and cutting than in open operations. Several problems are inherent in the use of energy sources during laparoscopy.

64.2 Electrosurgery in Fluids

The conductive properties of blood or saline may be less precise than during an open procedure, where a dry operative field is more readily maintained. Excessive application of energy in a the presence of fluids will distort anatomic planes. Thus, it is important that endoscopic surgeons learn to use energy sources to their fullest potential in order to improve the precision of application and avoid tissue injury.

64.3 Principles of Monopolar Surgery

The effects of monopolar electrosurgery are provided by a rapidly alternating electrical current with a frequency of around 500,000 Hz. These high frequencies generate heat in the tissues to provide a variety of local effects.

Tissue temperatures may vary with current density in the path present between the active surgical electrode and the return pad.

64.4 Generator Settings

1. In most modern generators, the surgeon selects only the wattage; the voltage and amperage vary and are not controlled independently by the surgeon during the application of energy.
2. Voltage increases automatically as tissue is desiccated and leads to an increase in resistance.
3. The surgeon may select varying waveforms from the generator.

64.4.1 "Cut" Waveform

1. At lower voltage the "cut" waveform is continuous and uninterrupted.
2. The "cut" mode causes intense heating and boiling of intracellular contents as a result of the to-and-fro motion of an alternating electrical field.
3. The superficial cells vaporize giving the cutting effect when the electrode is held near the tissue, but not in contact. Hemostasis is poor as less desiccation of deeper tissue occurs.

64.4.2 "Coagulation" Waveform

1. The "coagulation" waveform provides interrupted bursts of high-voltage current.
2. The higher voltage of the "coagulation" waveform enables an electrical charge to penetrate deeper into the tissue or arc for a longer distance to the target tissue.
3. For the same power settings, the "coagulation" mode provides a higher voltage and lower amperage compared to the "cut" mode.

64.5   Fulguration

1. Fulguration is a technique that provides superficial desiccation of tissues by arcing current from the electrode through the air to the adjacent tissue.
2. The most effective fulguration occurs with a high-voltage generator operated in the "coagulation" mode, as higher voltages are capable of generating longer arcing to the tissue.

64.5.1   Effects of Fulguration

1. Superficial tissue effects occur because the electrode has not made contact with the tissue and part of the energy is dissipated as lightning.
2. Fulguration is quite useful, but the high-voltage waveforms used increases the risk of insulation failure and capacitive coupling.
3. Spray fulguration may result in acute elevation of intra-abdominal pressures, hypotension, and air embolism of the instilled gas.

64.6   Contact Desiccation

1. Contact desiccation occurs when the activated electrode in contact with tissue provides hemostasis as successive layers of tissue are desiccated.
2. When the superficial tissue is desiccated, the generator voltage output automatically increases to facilitate deeper tissue effects.
3. Contact desiccation leads to the development of eschar, which may distort anatomic planes.

64.7   Coaptive Coagulation

1. Coaptive coagulation occurs when tissue is compressed within a grasper and current is applied.
2. Desiccation occurs along with the development of a collagen weld of the compressed tissue.
3. This tissue effect can be obtained with either the "cut" or "coagulation" mode. The benefit of the "cut" mode is that a lower voltage is employed.

64.8   Instrument Insulation

1. Conventional insulation is based on the incorporation of layers of nonconductors around the electrode.
2. Defects in insulation allows the delivery of the entire current to tissues outside the view of the surgeon and yet remains imperceptible to visual inspection.
3. Insulation defects occur as a result of mechanical trauma, repeated sterilization, manufacturing flaws, and capacitively coupled meltdown.

64.9   Contributors to Insulation Failure

Routine use of the high-voltage "coagulation" current may actually compromise insulation integrity. The higher the voltage, the greater the risk that the current will break through weak insulation. Using a lower voltage may reduce the wear on the insulation and minimize the chance that the current can escape through hairline cracks.

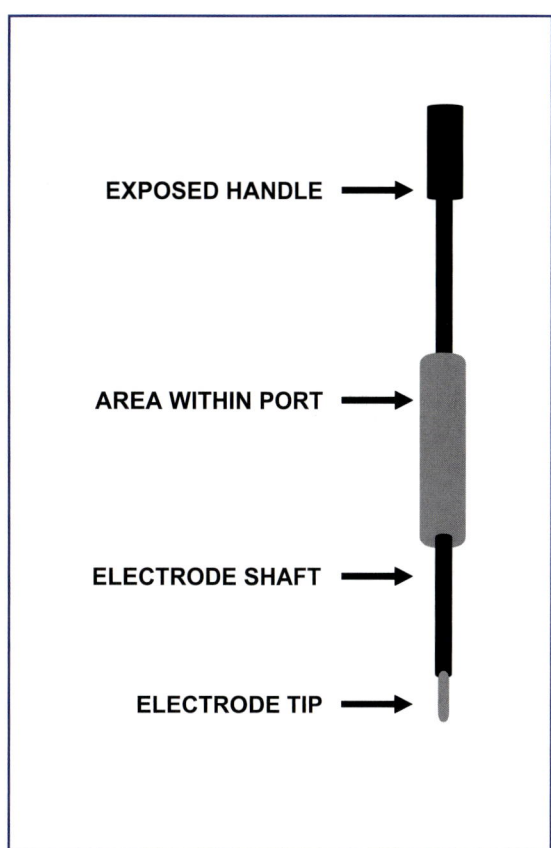

64.10 Areas of Electrode Insulation Failure

The hazards of insulation failure depend on the area of insulation breach. It is important to understand the parts of an electrode in order to have a better overview of the type of injuries that failure of insulation can causes.

An electrode consists of:

1. An exposed handle (in the surgeons' hand).
2. An area within the port.
3. The shaft of the electrode.
4. The electrode tip (desired zone of delivery).

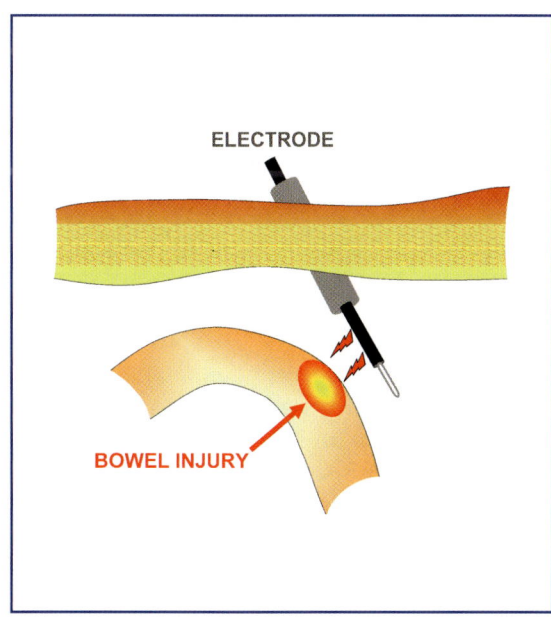

64.10.1 Hazards of Insulation Failure

1. Exposed metal in the handle of the instrument may cause burns to the surgeon's hands.
2. The signs of insulation failure within the port by lower-frequency electrical currents can cause neuromuscular stimulation and jerking of the abdominal wall or diaphragm.
3. Defects in the electrode shaft may cause an injury outside the view of the surgeon.

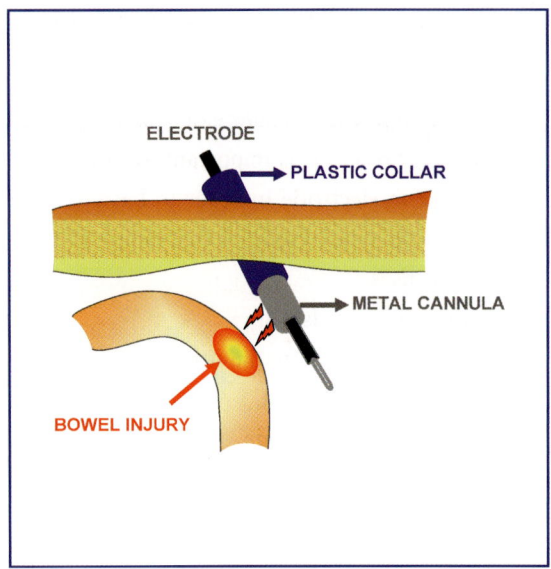

64.11   Capacitive Coupling

1. Capacitive coupling is a mechanism by which electrical current in the electrode induces an unintended current in nearby conductors despite intact insulation.
2. Capacitive coupling is increased by higher voltages.
3. Some degree of capacitive coupling occurs with all monopolar electrosurgical instruments.

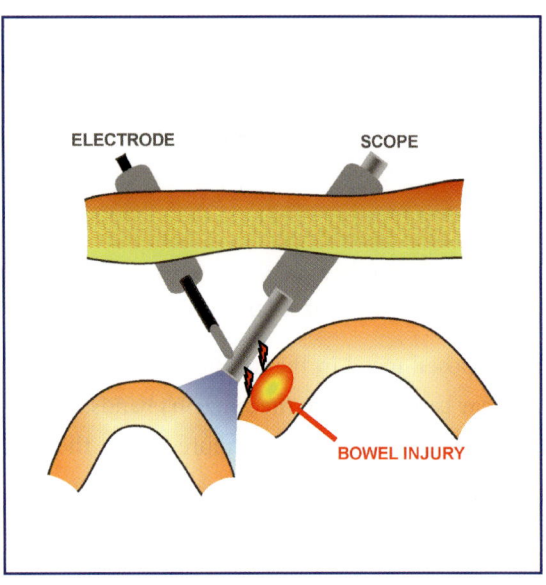

64.12   Direct Coupling

1. Direct coupling is a condition where the activated electrode touches other metal instruments (such as the scope), creating a situation whereby energy can be transferred to tissue outside the laparoscopic field of view.
2. Ports housing conductive instruments should be made of metal to enable dissipation of stray energy over a large area and to reduce the heat production from the stray current.

64.13 Precaution in Injury Prevention

1. The active electrode should not be in close proximity to or touching another metal instrument before the generator is activated.
2. It is important to confirm that the electrode is touching the targeted tissue, and only that tissue, before the generator is activated.
3. When the targeted tissue is coagulated, the impedance increases and the current may arc to adjacent tissue, following the path of least resistance.

64.15 All-Plastic-Port System

When using an all-plastic system, the definition of a capacitor can be eliminated. Instead of two conductors separated by a nonconductor, there is now the conductive electrode, covered by nonconductive insulation, surrounded by the nonconductive port. A capacitor no longer exists and concerns over capacitively coupled current can be eliminated.

64.17 Monopolar Electrosurgery Guidelines

1. All insulations should be inspected for defects.
2. Lower-power settings should be used for both cutting and coagulation to reduce the possibilities of insulation failure, capacitance, and injury.
3. Apply a low-voltage waveform whenever possible.
4. Low-voltage waveforms reduce the amount of capacitively coupled energy that can be produced.
5. Brief activation is better than a prolonged one.
6. Metal-to-metal sparking (direct coupling) should be avoided. The electrode should be activated only when it is touching the target tissue.
7. Hybrid port systems should be avoided.

64.14 All-Metal-Port System

The all-metal-port system is appropriate since all capacitive currents will be safely dispersed through the greater surface area provided by the chest or abdominal wall, thereby reducing current density. The surface area of the metal port will be adequate to safely dissipate any current buildup on the port without significant heat production or tissue damage.

64.16 Hybrid Port (Metal and Plastic)

This system consists of a metal sleeve that is held in place with a plastic anchor. In this system, the coupled current is not able to disperse safely because the port is held in place by a nonconductive plastic anchor. The current that is coupled onto the metal port can only complete the circuit by discharging to tissue that it may encounter within the cavity. This can potentially create a significant injury.

Recommended Literature

1. Jones CM, Pierre K, Nicoud I, Stain S, Melvin W 3rd (2006) Electrosurgery. Curr Surg 63:458–463
2. Meijer DW (2006) Safety of the laparoscopy setup. Minim Invasive Ther Allied Technol 12:125–128
3. Wang K, Advincula AP (2007) "Current thoughts" in electrosurgery. Int J Gynaecol Obstet 97:245–250

65 Complications in Endoscopic Surgery

Thomas Petnehazy and Amulya K. Saxena

65.1 Incidence of Complications

The true incidence of complications in endoscopic surgery is not known. However, awareness of the possible complications at various levels of procedures is important in providing safer endoscopic surgical expertise. Technical difficulties encountered during the learning curve should be recognized and accepted. There is no substitute for practice and training to improve skills and outcome.

65.2 Major Areas of Concern

1. Anesthetic-related complications.
2. Insufflated gases.
3. Access-related complications.
4. Instrumentation.
5. Blood loss during the procedure.
6. Visceral injuries.
7. Port-site complications.
8. Thermal damage.

65.2.1 Predisposition to Anesthetic Problems

Some features of endoscopic surgery predispose to specific anesthetic complications.

1. The use of a steep Trendelenburg position and the distension of the abdomen may both reduce excursion of the diaphragm.
2. Carbon dioxide (CO_2) can be absorbed, particularly during prolonged operations.
3. The vasovagal reflex may produce shock and collapse, especially if the anesthesia is not deep enough.

65.2.2 Mediastinal Emphysema

1. Gas may extend from the pneumoperitoneum into the mediastinum and form mediastinal emphysema.
2. Large emphysema may cause cardiac embarrassment, which will be diagnosed by the anesthetist.
3. In cases of large mediastinal emphysema, the endoscopic procedure must be abandoned and as much gas as possible evacuated.

65.2.3   Extraperitoneal Gas Insufflation

1. Failure to introduce the Veress needle or port into the peritoneal cavity may produce extraperitoneal emphysema.
2. The typical spider-web appearance caused by preperitoneal insufflation will be seen when the telescope reaches the end of the port.
3. The scope should be withdrawn and attempts made to express the gas.

65.2.4   Pneumothorax During Laparoscopy

1. Pneumothorax should be suspected if there is difficulty in ventilating the patient during high port insertion during a laparoscopic procedure.
2. There may be a contralateral mediastinal shift and increased tympanism over the affected area.
3. The procedure should be abandoned and the gas allowed to escape.
4. Occasionally, postoperative mechanical ventilation and insertion of a pleural tube may be necessary.

65.2.5   Pneumo-omentum

1. This occurs when the omentum is penetrated by the Veress needle or port.
2. A raised insufflation pressure should lead the surgeon to suspect an error in the position of the needle or port.
3. The condition does not pose any major problems unless an omental blood vessel is punctured.

65.2.6   Urinary Bladder Injuries

1. Routine catheterization of the bladder should prevent bladder-penetration injuries.
2. The bladder peritoneum should be carefully inspected to ensure that no significant injury has been caused.
3. Simple punctures can be treated conservatively with postoperative bladder drainage.
4. Possible "patent urachus" must be kept in mind when opting for an infraumbilical access.

65.2.7   Gastrointestinal Tract Injuries

1. Certain conditions such as distension of the gastrointestinal tract or adhesions of the bowel to the abdominal wall may predispose to injury.
2. Bilious discharge or fecal soiling indicate gastrointestinal tract injuries and efforts must be made to recognize and repair the problem.
3. During commencement of the procedures, the gastrointestinal tract should be examined carefully for injuries or perforation.

65.2.8   Vascular Injuries

1. The Veress needle has been associated more commonly with vascular injuries.
2. The loose areolar tissue anterior to the aorta can allow accumulation of a considerable amount of blood before frank intra-abdominal bleeding is seen.
3. Dramatic collapse may result from penetration of a major vessel, but the bleeding may not be immediately evident if it is retroperitoneal.

65.2.9   Gas Embolism

1. Intravascular insufflation of gas may lead to gas embolism or even death. This can happen when the Veress needle is used.
2. The patient should be turned on to the left lateral position and, if immediate recovery does not take place, cardiac puncture is the last option that can be performed to release the gas.

65.2.10 CO_2-Associated Complications

1. Gas embolism is possible, but uncommon, because CO_2 is highly soluble and is reabsorbed.
2. Cardiac arrhythmia may occur due to excessive absorption of CO_2.
3. Postoperative pain is common with CO_2 insufflation due to peritoneal irritation, which is a result of conversion of CO_2 to carbonic acid.

65.2.11   Hepatic and Splenic Injuries

1. These injuries may occur when ports are placed just above the level of the diaphragm in video-assisted thoracoscopic procedures.
2. Evaluation of the chest film prior to surgery, with special attention paid to the level of the diaphragm, can help avoid this complication.
3. If hepatic or splenic injury is suspected through thoracoscopy, a concomitant laparoscopy should be performed to evaluate the blood loss and, if possible, the extent of the injury.

65.2.12   Abdominal Wall Vessel Injury

1. Severe bleeding can occur from puncture of the deep inferior epigastric artery.
2. The artery is at risk during the insertion of secondary ports and trocars.
3. Injury may be prevented by transilluminating the abdominal wall before insertion in a thin patient, or by visualizing the artery laparoscopically as it runs lateral to the obliterated umbilical artery.

65.2.12.1   Management of Deep Inferior Epigastric Vessel Injury

1. Diagnosis can be made by the observation of blood dripping or spurting, or the presence of a large hematoma at the site of the secondary port insertion.
2. Options in management include:
   a) passing a Foley catheter down the port side and compressing it against the abdominal wall,
   b) placing a long-bodied needle suture under laparoscopic control, and
   c) occasionally the need to widen the wound and control bleeding.

65.2.13   Stomach Injuries

1. Injuries to the stomach or bowel are always serious.
2. The classical treatment is to perform laparotomy and suture the bowel in two layers.
3. A skilled surgeon may perform the repair by laparoscopic suturing.

65.2.14 Omental and Richter's Herniation

1. If the primary port is withdrawn with its valve closed, a piece of omentum can be drawn by the resulting negative pressure into the umbilical wound.
2. Herniation may also occur some hours after the operation.
3. Herniations do not occur commonly with 5-mm skin incisions.
4. Incisions greater than 7 mm should be sutured in layers to prevent formation of a Richter's hernia.

65.2.15 Intra-abdominal Vascular Injury

1. Injury to minor blood vessels is usually self-limiting or can be controlled by bipolar electro-coagulation.
2. A small leak from a major vein may not be apparent immediately, since the intra-abdominal pressure of the pneumoperitoneum and the decreased venous pressure induced by the Trendelenburg position may temporarily control it.

65.2.16 Thermal Injuries with Electrosurgery

1. Lateral heat spread may occur with monopolar or bipolar current.
2. It is important to ensure that no other organ is in contact with or near an organ to which electricity is being applied.
3. Lateral spread may also be minimized by keeping the forceps blades close together.
4. Build-up of thermal energy may be prevented by intermittent application of energy.

65.2.16.1 Monopolar Coagulation Injuries

1. Thermal injury to organs such as the bowel may also result from leakage of current from the shaft of the instrument.
2. Electrosurgical instruments should be passed through ports and not directly through incisions in the chest or abdominal cavity.
3. Long, insulated active electrodes significantly change the physics surrounding the use of high frequency electrosurgical energy.

65.2.17 Thermal Injury to the Bowel

1. The bowel is the most commonly injured organ with electrosurgical applications.
2. Injury may range from minor blanching of the serosa to frank perforation.
3. If blanching is significant, excision of the damaged tissue and surgical repair should be performed.
4. Failure to recognize the injury may result in delayed ischemic necrosis at the site of the burn.

65.3 Operating-Table-Related Injuries

1. Injury can be caused to the nerves of the leg and to the hip and sacroiliac joints.
2. Compression of the leg veins may predispose to venous thrombosis.
3. The brachial plexus may be injured if the arm is abducted for an extended surgical procedure
4. The hands may be caught and trapped in moving parts of the table.

65.4   Foreign Bodies

Occasionally clips, staples, or parts of instruments such as sapphire laser tips may be inadvertently dropped and lost in the peritoneal cavity. They should be removed if they are easily found, but there have been no reports of long-term complications from such foreign bodies.

65.5   Complications with Tissue Spillage

1. Dropped stones from cholecystectomy, or appendicoliths may incite an inflammatory response and can even lead to abscess formation.
2. Tissue rupture and spillage during removal is also a major problem in endoscopic surgery.
3. Implantation of tumor cells can follow. Port-site metastasis may occur in malignancies.
4. Complications related to tissue spillage can be minimized by the use of specimen retrieval bags.

Recommended Literature

1. Philips PA, Amaral JF (2001) Abdominal access complications in laparoscopic surgery. J Am Coll Surg 192:525–536
2. Philosophe R (2003) Avoiding complications of laparoscopic surgery. Fertil Steril 80:30–39
3. Shirk JG, Johns A, Redwine DB (2006) Complications of laparoscopic surgery: how to avoid them and how to repair them. J Minim Invasive Gynecol 13:352–359

66 Lasers in Endoscopic Surgery

Amulya K. Saxena

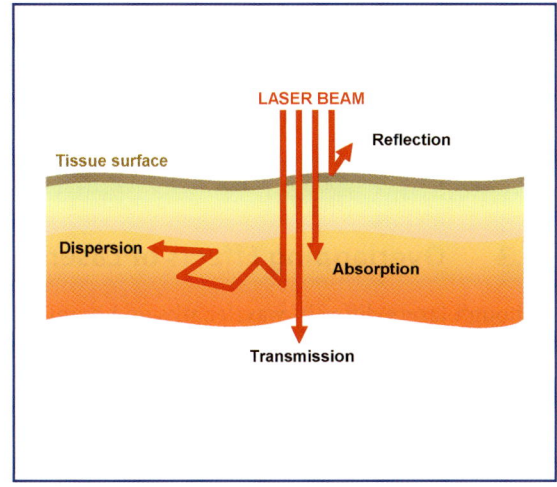

66.1 Schematic Effects of Lasers

Lasers are now being used routinely in the field of endoscopic surgery. The effects of lasers are exhibited on tissues by reflection, absorption, transmission, and dispersion. Understanding of these characteristics is important in the safe use of these tools.

66.2 Laser Wavelengths

Lasers are classified according to their wavelength, which determines their characteristics. The more commonly used lasers in medicine are carbon dioxide (CO_2), neodium-doped:yttrium aluminum garnet (Nd:YAG), argon, and potassium titanyl phosphate (KTP) lasers.

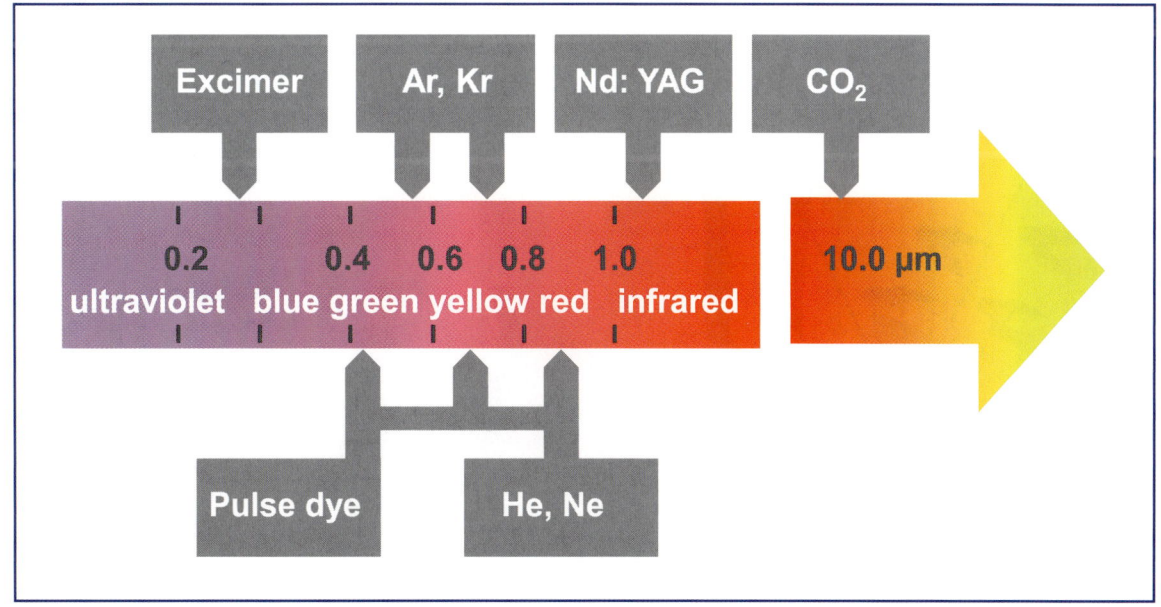

66.2.1 CO$_2$ Lasers

1. The CO$_2$ laser produces an area of injury that is discrete and reproducible with a depth of less than 1 mm and a zone of thermal necrosis less than one-tenth of 1 mm.
2. This laser is highly precise but a poor coagulator.
3. The CO$_2$ laser is used endoscopically to vaporize deposits of endometriosis and adhesions.

66.2.2 Nd:YAG Lasers

1. The Nd:YAG laser produces an effect several millimeters below the tissue surface, providing excellent coagulation but poor precision.
2. This property of the Nd:YAG is potentially dangerous if the underlying tissue heats and explodes.
3. Reduced thermal injury and a more predictable tissue effect has been achieved with the use of sapphire tips or sculpted fibers.

66.2.3 Argon and KTP 532 Lasers

1. Argon and KTP532 lasers have similar tissue effects between those produced by the CO$_2$ and Nd:YAG laser.
2. The Argon laser has less precision but improved coagulating ability.
3. Argon laser has found endoscopic indications in the treatment of polycystic ovarian disease.

66.3 Overlapping Effects of Lasers

Although lasers differ in wavelengths and manifest their effects at specific depths; there is a degree of overlapping in depth penetration.

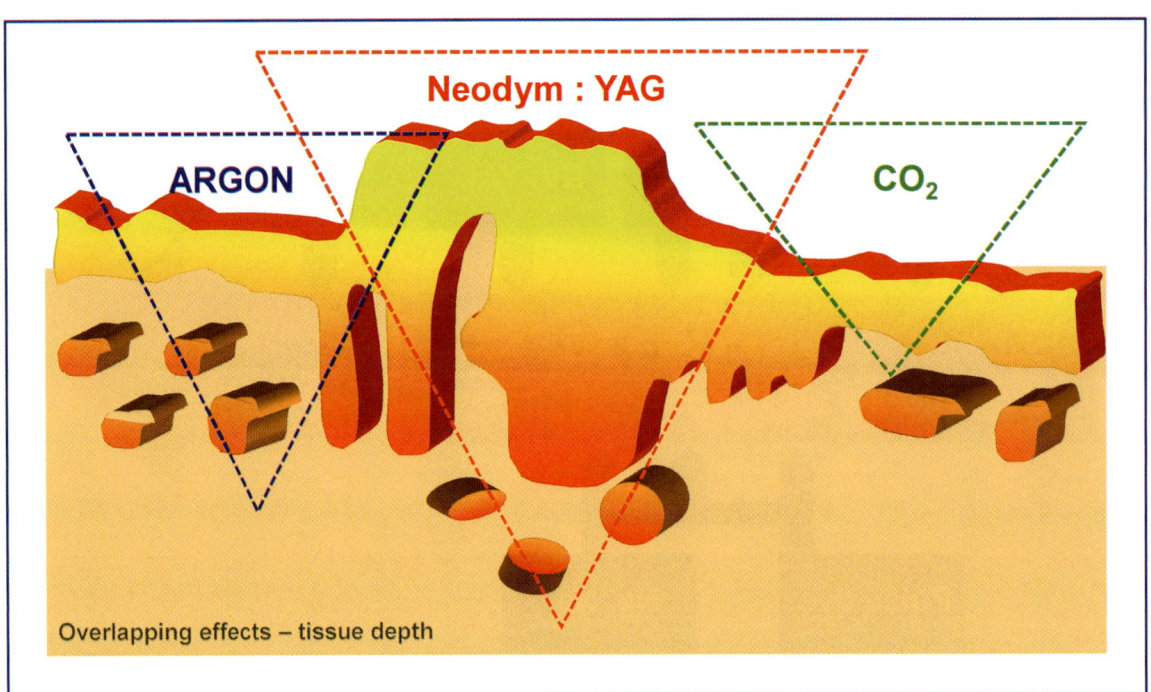

Overlapping effects – tissue depth

66.4 Contact Versus Noncontact Lasers

The CO_2 laser is a noncontact laser and provides the advantage of minimizing tissue trauma due to manipulation. The CO_2 laser can also be used at any distance from the tissue with a fairly constant tissue effect.

Argon, KTP532, and Nd:YAG lasers are contact lasers, whereby the laser beam is focused at the fiber tip. The power density is reduced significantly as the fiber tip moves away from the tissue.

66.5 Comparative Overview of Lasers

Table 66.1

Characteristic	Laser Type		
	CO₂	Argon	Nd:YAG
Wavelength	10,600 nm	514 nm	1064 nm
Absorption	Water	Hemoglobin/melanin	Tissue protein
Penetration	1 mm	2–3 mm	5–7 mm
Coagulation	Low	Medium	High
Cutting	High	Low	Medium

Comparison of lasers with regard to their application, penetration, coagulation, and cutting characteristics

66.6   Injuries Associated with Lasers

66.6.1   Eye Injuries

1. The Nd:YAG, Argon, and KTP lasers can burn the retina, whereas the CO_2 laser can cause corneal burns.
2. The eye is particularly susceptible to retinal burns from the Nd:YAG laser because the light is invisible and does not induce a protective blink response.
3. Tinted eyewear filters the wavelength of the specific laser for which it is designed while allowing as many of the other wavelengths to pass in order to maximize visibility.

66.6.2   Redirection Injuries

1. One mechanism of injury is the redirection of laser energy from reflective surfaces.
2. The unintentional burning of organs in the patient or burning of the surgeon may occur due to reflections off surgical instruments.
3. The surface of most surgical instruments has a convex curve, which usually causes divergence of laser light after reflection
4. Small dents on instrument surfaces could potentially refocus laser energy.

66.6.3   Minimizing Redirection Injuries

In endoscopic surgery, the primary risk of injury by reflection is to the patient's intra-abdominal structures due to the closed nature of surgery. Several methods, such as finely wire-brushed, sand-blasted, or glass-beaded instruments and the use of titanium instead of stainless steel, have helped to reduce the risk of redirection injuries, especially those associated with the CO_2 laser.

66.6.4   Accidental Activation Injuries

Injury can occur from the accidental activation of the laser when it is not in use, especially if another foot pedal is in use for a different instrument such as an electrosurgical instrument. Placing the laser on standby whenever it is not in use will reduce the risk of injury by this mechanism.

66.6.5   Human Error

1. For the CO_2 laser, the He/Ne aiming beam should always be visualized prior to firing the laser. As a blind area exists near the end of the scope, the risk of inadvertent injury to the bowel can be significantly reduced by following this precaution.
2. For contact lasers, the tip should always be visualized, especially immediately after firing the laser, since the tip remains hot and can burn surrounding structures.

66.6.6   Ignition Injuries

1. The liberal use of irrigating solutions to moisten lap packs, gauze bandages, and drapes in the surgical areas reduces the risk of accidental ignition.
2. The use of alcohol and ether solutions should be avoided due to their flammable nature.
3. Anesthesiologists should be informed that flammable anesthetic gases are also to be avoided.

66.6.7   Bowel Injuries

After extensive laser dissection in the cul-de-sac, the bowel should be inspected for perforation injuries. This can be performed by placing a 30-ml Foley catheter into the rectum and clamping the bowel above the site of dissection. The pelvis is then filled with physiologic solution and a 50% solution of Betadine injected through the Foley catheter. Trails of Betadine solution indicate perforation.

66.6.8   Ureteral Injuries

In the case of suspicion of ureteral injury, indigo carmine (5 ml) can be injected intravenously. The appearance of indigo carmine coloring should be present in the Foley catheter and bag within approximately 10 min. As with the detection of bowel injury, underwater trails may be present if injury to the ureter has occurred.

Recommended Literature

1. Gale P, Adeyemi B, Ferrer K, Ong A, Brill AI, Scoccia B (1998) Histologic characteristics of laparoscopic argon beam coagulation. J Am Assoc Gynecol Laparosc 5:19–22

2. Klingler CH, Remzi M, Marberger M, Janetschek G (2006) Haemostasis in laparoscopy. Eur Urol 50:948–956

3. Tulikangas PK, Smith T, Falcone T, Boparai N, Walters MD (2001) Gross and histologic characteristics of laparoscopic injuries with four different energy sources. Fertil Steril 75:806–810

67 Vessel-Sealing Technology

Amulya K. Saxena

67.1 Introduction

LigaSure™ vessel-sealing technology (Valleylab, Boulder, CO, USA) provides a unique combination of pressure and energy to create vessel fusion. It permanently fuses vessels up to and including 7 mm in diameter and tissue bundles without dissection or isolation. The further advantage of this automated system is that it eliminates the guesswork by minimizing seal time and maximizing reliability.

67.2 Technology

1. An optimized combination of pressure and energy creates a seal by melting the collagen and elastin in the vessel walls and reforming it into a permanent, plastic-like seal. It does not rely on a proximal thrombus.
2. The unique energy output results in virtually no sticking or charring.
3. The thermal spread from the point of sealing is minimal and ranges from 1 to 2 mm depending on the type of instrument used.

67.3 Instant Response™ Technology

The patented Instant Response™ technology (Valleylab, Boulder, CO, USA) features an advanced feedback system that recognizes changes in tissue 200 times per second, and adjusts the voltage and current accordingly to maintain the most appropriate power and effectively seal the vessel or tissue bundle. When the instrument determines the seal is complete, a tone sounds and output to the handpiece is automatically discontinued.

The seal can be provided on vessels and tissue bundles without dissection. (Courtesy of Covidien Austria, Brunn am Gebirge, Austria)

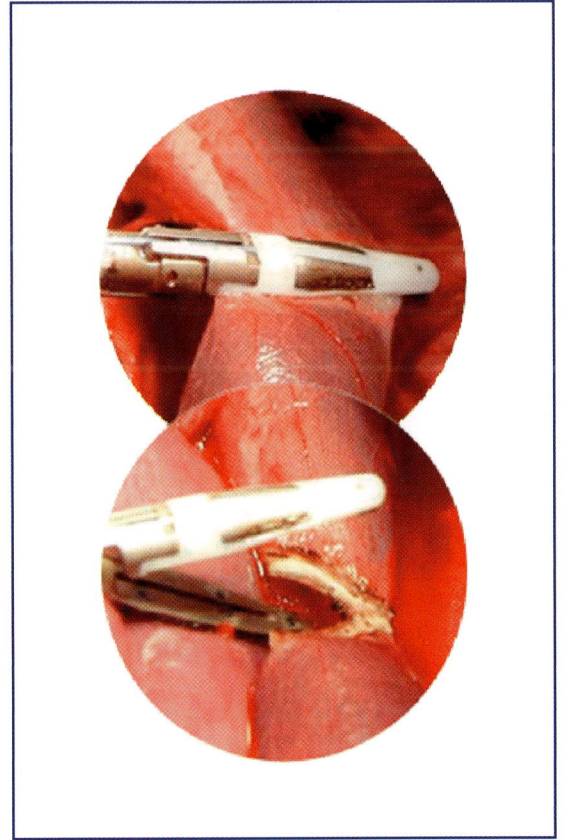

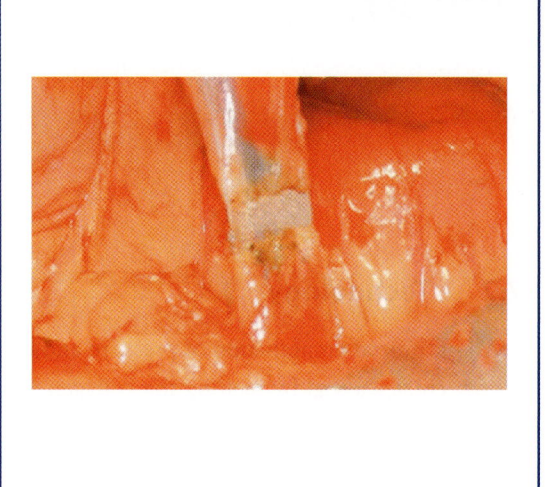

67.4   Characteristics of Vessel Seal

Studies have demonstrated that the seal can withstand pressures three times that of normal systolic blood pressure. (Courtesy of Covidien Austria, Brunn am Gebirge, Austria)

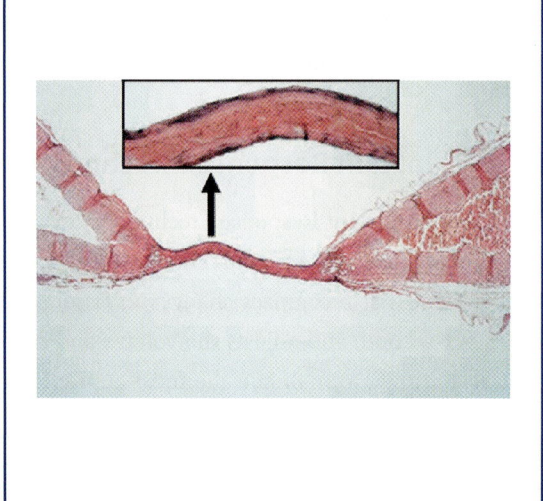

67.5   Histological Evaluation of Seal

This microscopic view of hematoxylin-eosin-stained section shows a sealed renal vessel with notable fusion of the vessel wall lumen. The inset shows a magnified view of the seal demonstrating fusion of the vascular wall. (Courtesy of Covidien Austria, Brunn am Gebirge, Austria)

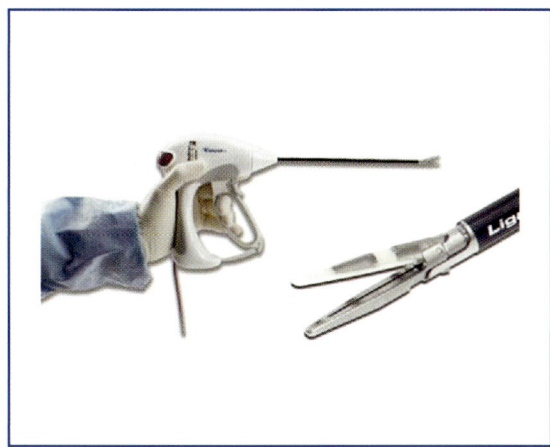

67.6   Instrument Tip

The instrument tips are designed to dissect, seal, and cut. This offers the advantage of fewer instrument exchanges during procedures. (Courtesy of Covidien Austria, Brunn am Gebirge, Austria)

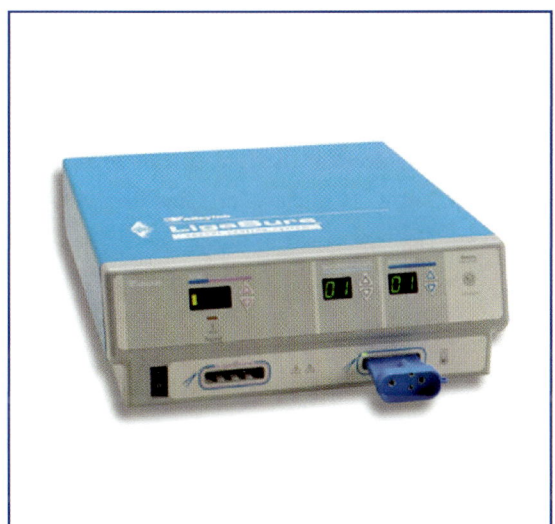

67.7   Generator

The generator produces a high-current, low-voltage output that corresponds to at least four times the current of a standard electrosurgery generator, with one-fifth to one-twentieth the amount of voltage. (Courtesy of Covidien Austria, Brunn am Gebirge, Austria)

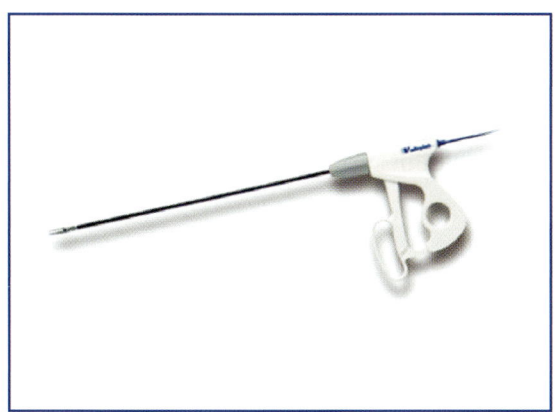

67.7.1   LigaSure™ V Lap

The LigaSure™ V Lap device has a 5-mm diameter with a 32-cm-long shaft. The 15° curved Maryland 18-mm electrode length offers a seal width of 2–4 mm with an average thermal spread of approximately 2 mm. (Courtesy of Covidien Austria, Brunn am Gebirge, Austria)

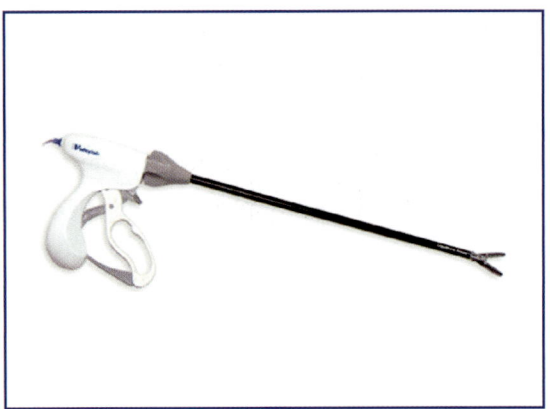

67.7.2   LigaSure™ Atlas Sealer/Divider

The LigaSure™ Atlas sealer/divider device has a 10-mm diameter with a 37-cm-long shaft. The straight, 22-mm long electrode offers a seal width of 6 mm with average thermal spread of approximately 2 mm. (Courtesy of Covidien Austria, Brunn am Gebirge, Austria)

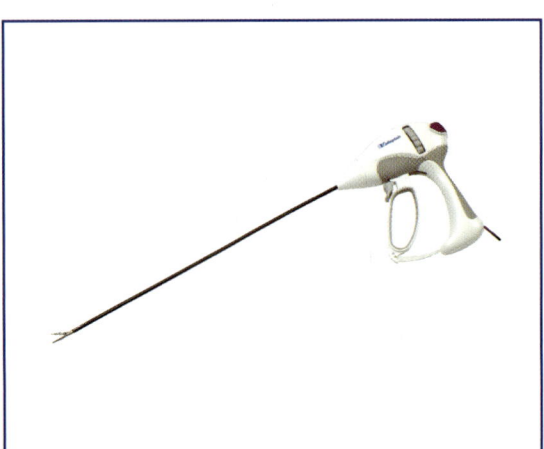

67.7.3   LigaSure™ V Sealer/Divider

The LigaSure™ V sealer/divider device has a 5-mm diameter with a 37-cm-long shaft. The straight, 18-mm-long electrode offers a seal width of 4.62 mm with average thermal spread of approximately 1.5 mm. (Courtesy of Covidien Austria, Brunn am Gebirge, Austria)

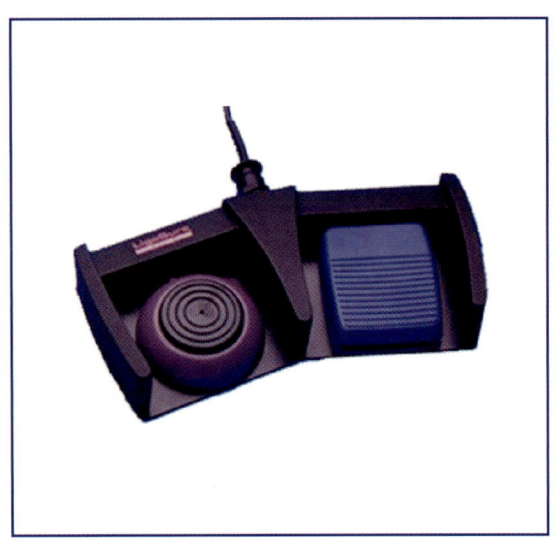

67.8   Foot Pedal Control

The LigaSure™ generator can be operated optionally with a foot pedal control. The LigaSure™ Atlas 20 cm, which was developed for open surgical procedures, is the only instrument that needs to be activated through a foot pedal. (Courtesy of Covidien Austria, Brunn am Gebirge, Austria)

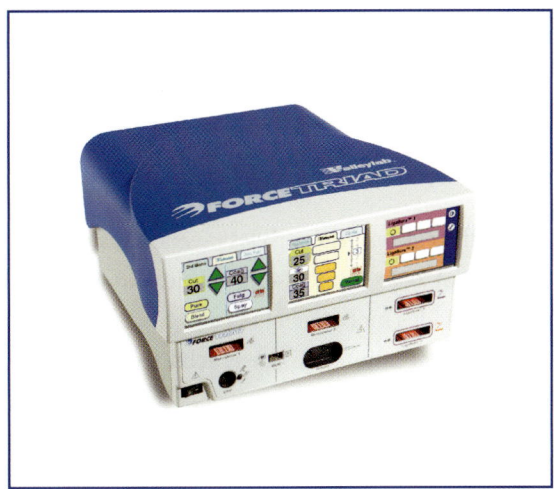

67.9 LigaSure™ Vessel-Sealing Technology Advances

67.9.1 ForceTriad™ Energy Platform

In order to further improve vessel technology, the ForceTriad™ energy (Valleylab, Boulder, CO, USA) platform has been introduced with TissueFect™ sensing technology. (Courtesy of Covidien Austria, Brunn am Gebirge, Austria)

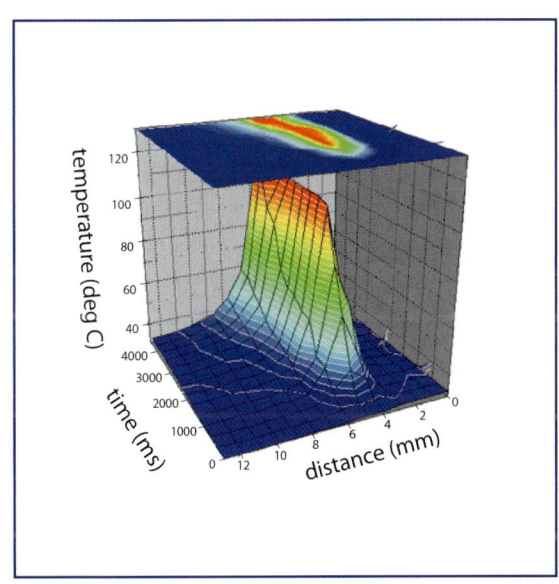

67.9.2 Thermal Spread Profile

Thermal spread can be evaluated using thermography. The histogram profile shown here demonstrates the lateral thermal spread of 2 mm at the point of application. (Courtesy of Covidien Austria, Brunn am Gebirge, Austria)

67.9.3 Advantages of the ForceTriad™

1. The ForceTriad™ energy platform has an improved tissue-sensing, closed-loop control of 3333 decisions per second (vs. 200 decisions per second for the original LigaSure™ generator).
2. The ForceTriad™ energy platform utilizes TissueFect™ sensing technology (Valleylab, Boulder, CO, USA), a control system that was designed to precisely manage energy delivery, creating a range of options for a desired tissue effect.

Acknowledgment

Covidien Austria, Brunn am Gebirge, Austria.

67.9.4 TissueFect™ Sensing Technology

1. TissueFect™ sensing technology actively monitors changes in tissue impedance and provides a real-time adjustment control of the energy output.
2. It offers faster fusion cycles (average fusion cycle time of 2–4 s in most surgical situations).
3. It provides more flexible fusion zones.
4. Less desiccation of tissue is achieved.
5. Consistent controlled tissue effects are possible.

Recommended Literature

1. Hruby GW, Marruffo F, Durak E, Collins S, Pierorazio P, Humphrey P, Mansukhani M, Landman L (2007) Evaluation of surgical energy devices for vessel sealing and peripheral energy spread in a porcine model. J Urol 178:2689–2693
2. Matthews BD, Pratt BL, Backus CL, Kercher KW, Mostafa G, Lentzner A, Lipford EH, Sing RF, Heniford BT (2001) Effectiveness of the ultrasonic coagulating shears, LigaSure vessel sealer, and surgical clip application in biliary surgery: a comparative analysis. Am Surg 67:901–906
3. Romano F, Caprotti R, Franciosi C, De Fina S, Colombo G, Sartori P, Uggeri F (2002) Laparoscopic splenectomy using LigaSure. Preliminary experience. Surg Endosc 16:1608–1611

68 Harmonic Scalpel Technology

Julia Seidel and Amulya K. Saxena

68.1 Introduction

The Ultracision® harmonic scalpel (Johnson & Johnson Medical Products, Ethicon Endosurgery, Cincinnati, OH, USA) is the first ultrasonic surgical device for cutting and coagulation. It provides atraumatic surgical dissection and hemostasis using direct application of ultrasound. With the Ultracision® harmonic scalpel, no electric current is sent through the patient. Hence, all the risks associated with the direct use of electric current are thus avoided.

68.2 Indications

The Ultracision® harmonic scalpel is indicated for soft-tissue incisions when bleeding control and minimal thermal injury are desired. The instrument can be used as an adjunct to or substitute for electrocautery, lasers, and steel scalpels.

68.3 Contraindications

1. Bone incisions.
2. Contraceptive tubal ligation.

68.4 Components

The Ultracision® harmonic scalpel system consists of the following components:
1. Generator.
2. Handpiece with connecting cable.
3. Foot switch.
4. Coagulating shears.
5. Blade system (5 and 10 mm).

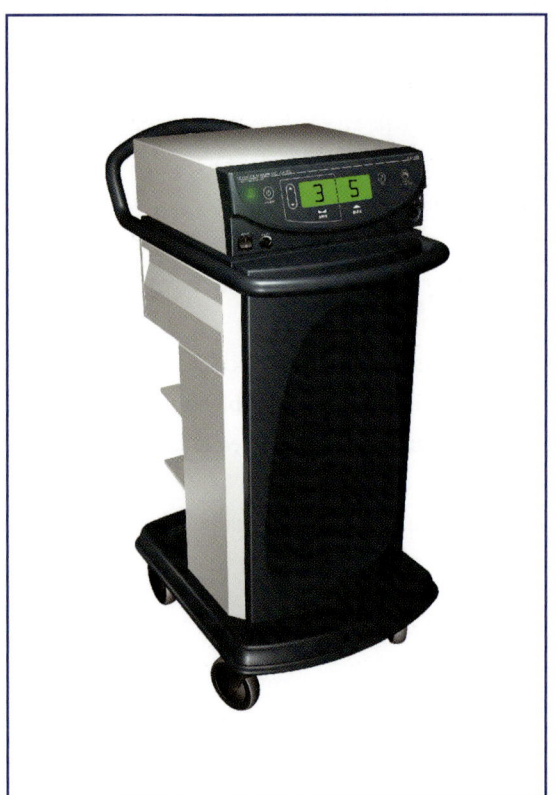

68.4.1 Generator

The Generator is a microprocessor-controlled power supply that drives the acoustic transducer system. (Courtesy of Johnson & Johnson Medical Products, Ethicon Endo-Surgery, Vienna, Austria)

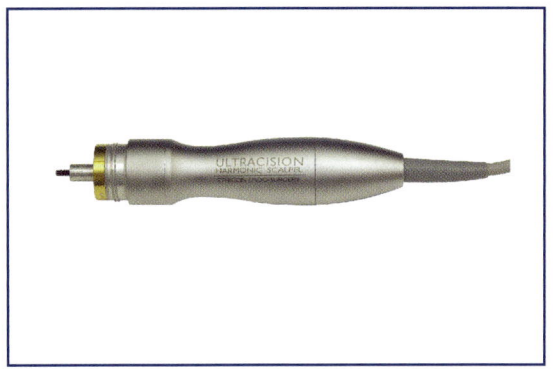

68.4.2 Handpiece

The ergonomic handpiece converts the electrical energy from the generator into mechanical ultrasound vibrations. These vibrations are transmitted to the attached Ultracision® harmonic scalpel device. (Courtesy of Johnson & Johnson Medical Products, Ethicon Endo-Surgery, Vienna, Austria)

68.4.3   Foot switch

The Foot switch is used to activate the output of the generator. It has two pedals: With the left pedal, one of five ultrasound energy levels previously selected on the generator will be activated. The right pedal fixes the level at 5. (Courtesy of Johnson & Johnson Medical Products, Ethicon Endo-Surgery, Vienna, Austria)

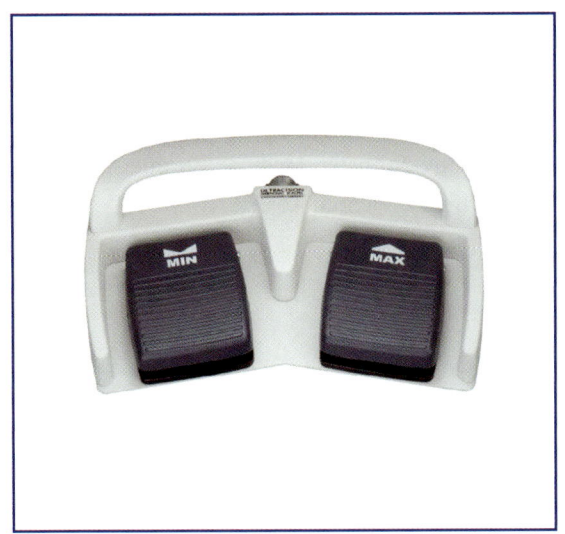

68.4.4   Laparosonic Coagulating Shears

The laparosonic coagulating shears (LCS) is a multi-functional device that has been developed to use the full potential of ultrasound technology. It cuts, coagulates, grasps, and dissects to improve overall procedural efficiency. (Courtesy of Johnson & Johnson Medical Products, Ethicon Endo-Surgery, Vienna, Austria)

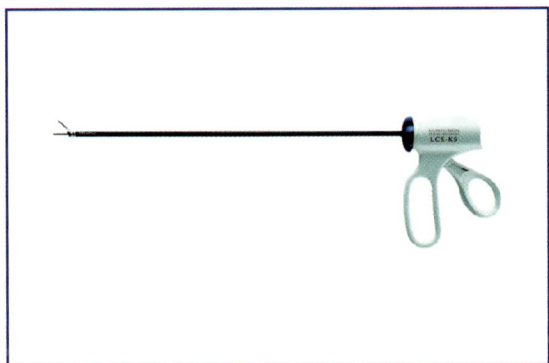

68.4.4.1 Shear Tip Variations

Shear tips may be straight or curved (inset). The straight shear tips are also available in (1) knife-down or (2) blunt variations. (Courtesy of Johnson & Johnson Medical Products, Ethicon Endo-Surgery, Vienna, Austria)

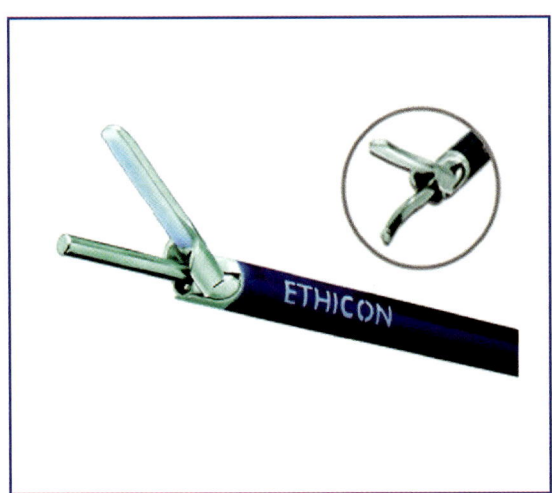

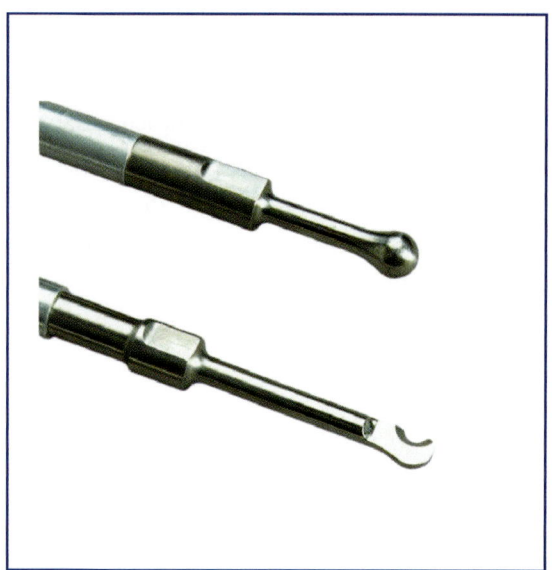

68.4.5   Harmonic Scalpel Blades: 10 mm

There a two types of 10-mm blade: ball coagulator (top) and dissecting hook (bottom). (Courtesy of Johnson & Johnson Medical Products, Ethicon Endo-Surgery, Vienna, Austria)

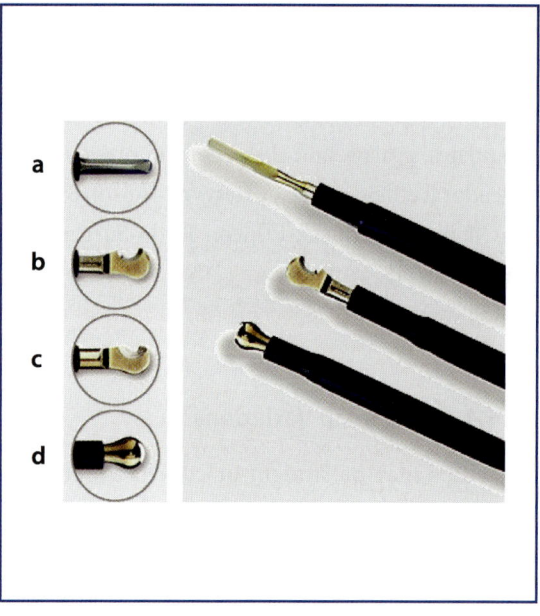

68.4.6   Harmonic Scalpel Blades: 5 mm

There are four types of 5-mm blades: (a) curved blade, (b) sharp hook, (c) dissecting hook, and (d) ball coagulator. (Courtesy of Johnson & Johnson Medical Products, Ethicon Endo-Surgery, Vienna, Austria)

68.5   Comparison of Tissue-Sealing Technologies

Harmonic scalpel technology controls bleeding by captive coagulation at low temperatures ranging from 50 to 100ºC. By contrast, electrosurgery and lasers coagulate by burning (obliterative coagulation) at higher temperatures (150–400ºC). Blood and tissue are desiccated and oxidized (charred), forming eschar that covers and seals the bleeding area. Rebleeding can occur when blades are removed during electrosurgery, as they stick to tissue and disrupt the eschar.

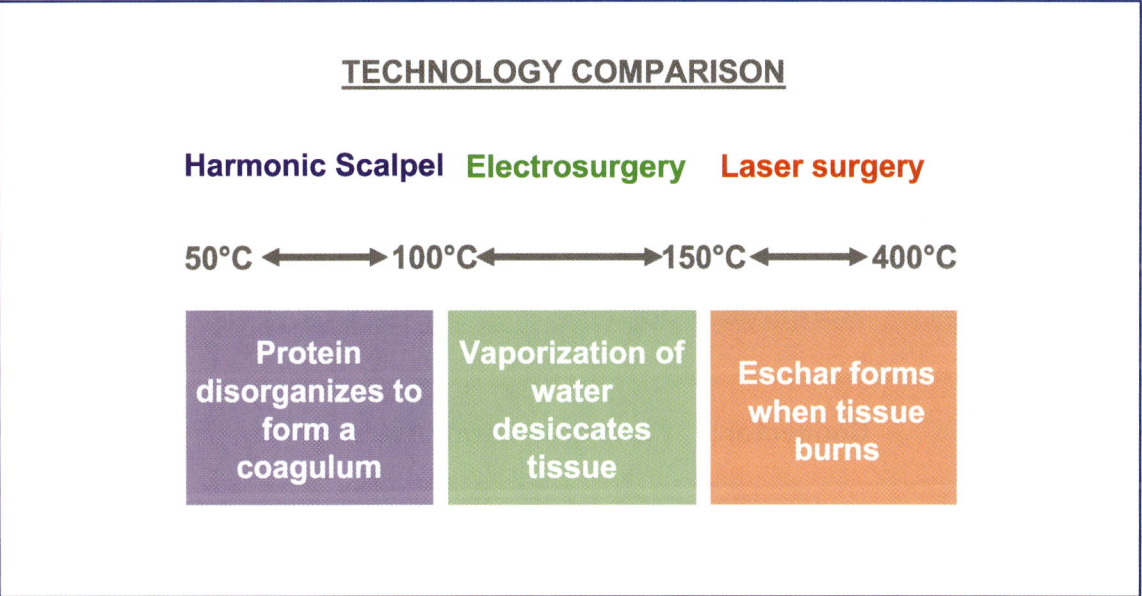

68.6   Transducer Technology

1. The transducer, found in the handpiece, consists of piezoelectric ceramics that expand and contract to convert the electrical energy from the generator into mechanical vibration.
2. The ultrasonic vibration is transmitted from the transducer through an extending rod to the attached blade.
3. The blade extender is supported by silicone rings positioned at nodes to direct the flow of energy in a longitudinal direction and to prevent energy from being dissipated on the sheath.

(Courtesy of Johnson & Johnson Medical Products, Ethicon Endo-Surgery, Vienna, Austria)

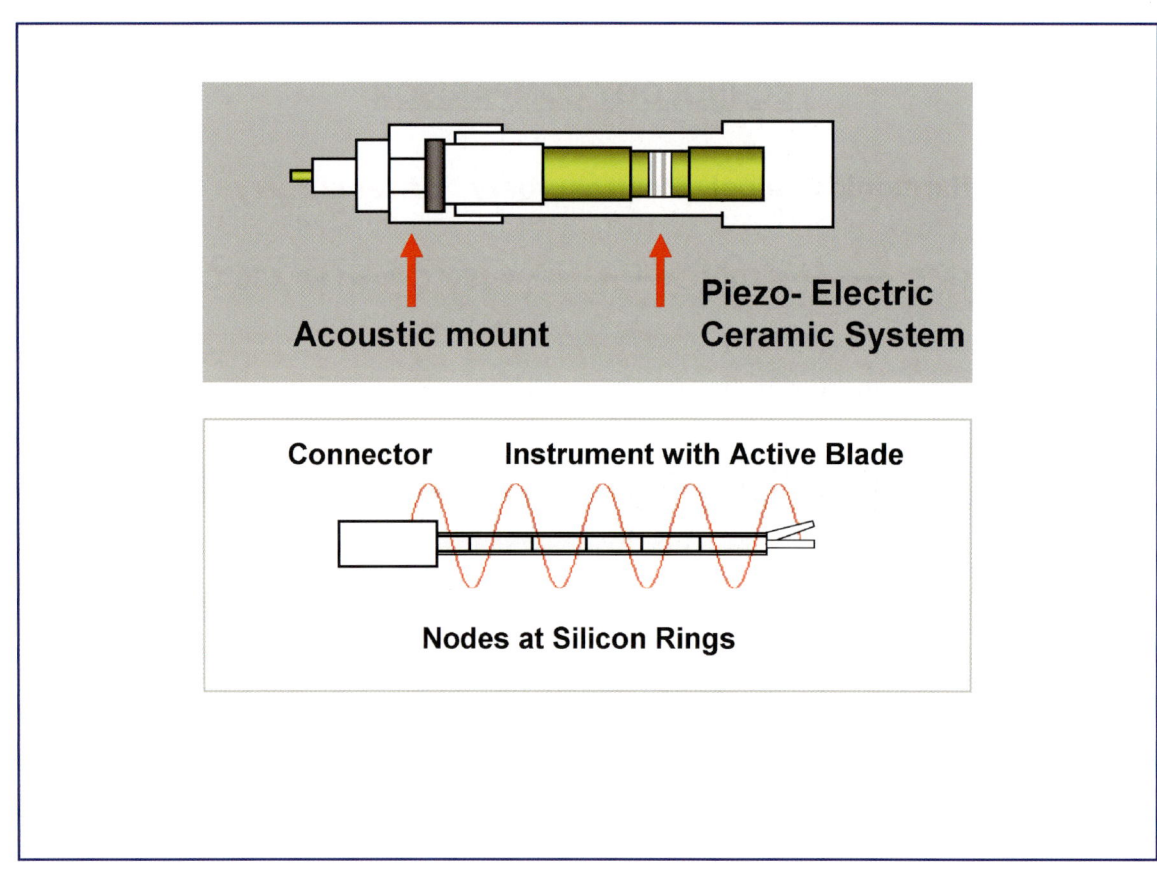

68.7   Power Level and Function

1. The blade or tip of the harmonic scalpel vibrates axially with a constant frequency of 55,500 Hz.
2. The longitudinal extension of the vibration can be varied between 25 and 100 μm in 5 levels by adjusting the power setting of the generator.
3. The maximum longitudinal displacement is 50–100 μm, depending on the type of blade and the set power level.

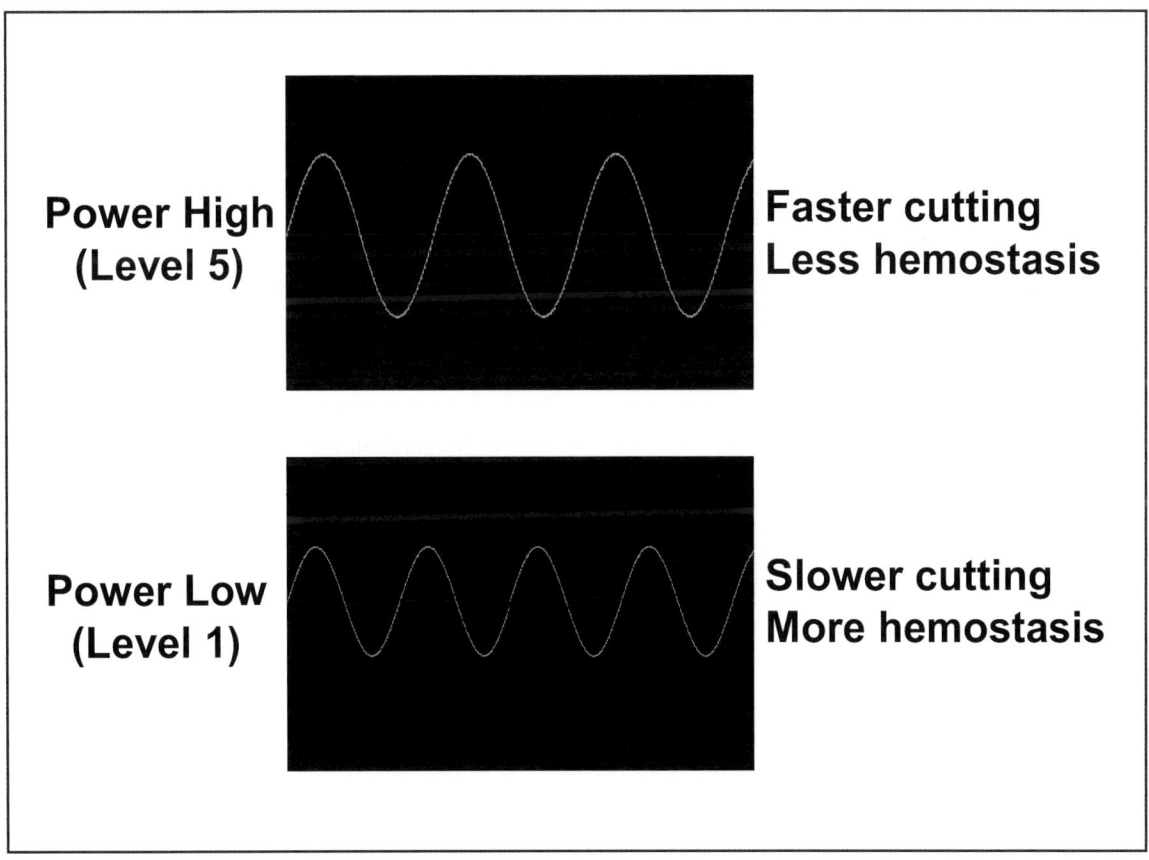

Power High (Level 5) — **Faster cutting Less hemostasis**

Power Low (Level 1) — **Slower cutting More hemostasis**

68.8   Tissue Effects of Harmonic Scalpel

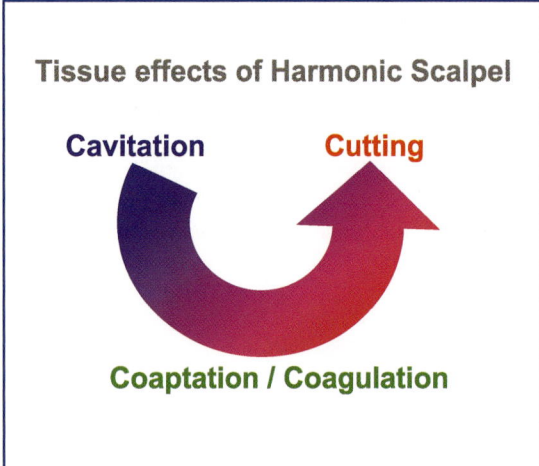

The Ultracision® harmonic scalpel system yields three possible effects: cavitation, coaptation or coagulation, and cutting.

68.8.1   Cavitation

Cavitation is achieved by the formation of vapor bubbles at body temperature due to the rapid volume changes of the tissue and cell fluids, and is induced by the transmitted vibration to the tissues. Cavitation is usually divided into two classes of behavior: inertial and noninertial cavitation. Noninertial cavitation is applied in the harmonic scalpel to achieve the desired tissue effects.

68.8.2   Coaptation and Coagulation

The joint application of pressure and ultrasound to the tissue fragments the protein compounds, leading to the adherence of collagen molecules at low temperatures. Thus, coaptation is achieved at a temperature range of 37–63°C. When the locally applied energy acts for longer periods, the rise in temperature leads to denaturing of protein – coagulation, at a maximum temperature of 150°C.

68.8.3   Cutting

By using tension, pressure, or both, the tissue is rapidly stretched beyond its elastic limit by the high-frequency vibration and is cut smoothly by a sharp blade or instrument tip. The cutting speed and extent of coagulation are easily controlled and can be balanced by varying four factors:

1. Power.
2. Blade sharpness.
3. Tissue tension.
4. Grip force/pressure.

68.8.4   Power Setting and Blade Sharpness

Increasing the power level increases the cutting speed and decreases the coagulation. In contrast, less power decreases the cutting speed and increases coagulation. Cutting speed is also a function of blade sharpness. The shear mode of the LCS cuts faster than the blunt mode; the blunt mode provides more coagulation, assuring coagulation when vascular tissue or vessels are encountered.

68.8.5   Tissue Tension and Grip Pressure

More coagulation can be achieved with slower cutting when tissue tension is reduced. Increased tissue tension leads to faster cutting with less coagulation.

Grip force, or pressure, is another factor controlling the balance between cutting and coagulation. Application of light pressure achieves more coagulation with slower cutting. A firmer grip force achieves less coagulation with faster cutting.

68.9   Injuries with Harmonic Devices

68.9.1   Precautions

A thorough understanding of the principles and techniques involved in ultrasonic procedures is essential to avoid shock and burn hazards to both the patient and medical personnel and damage to the device or other medical instruments.

Electrical connections should be properly checked before any procedure is performed. It should also be ensured that electrical insulation or grounding is not compromised and do not immerse the instruments in liquids.

68.9.2   Handpiece Injuries

1. Handle the handpiece carefully, as damage may shift its resonant frequency.
2. To prevent burn injury, discontinue use if the handpiece temperature makes it uncomfortable to hold.
3. Audible high-pitched tones may indicate blade disconnection and may result in abnormally high sheath temperatures and user or patient injury.

68.9.3   Blade Injuries

1. Do not attempt to bend, sharpen, or otherwise alter the shape of the blade. Doing so may cause blade failure and surgeon or patient injury.
2. During prolonged activation in tissue, the instrument blades may become hot.
3. Blood and tissue build up between the blade and sheath may result in abnormally high temperatures at the distal end of the sheath.

68.9.4   Generator-Related Injuries

1. To prevent overheating during use, ensure that the air vents on the base and back panels of the generator are not blocked.
2. Avoid placing the generator on a soft surface.
3. Place the generator in the "standby" mode before removing or replacing an instrument, hand switching adapter, or handpiece, or when the system is not in use.

Acknowledgment

Johnson & Johnson Medical Products, Ethicon Endosurgery, Vienna, Austria.

Recommended Literature

1. Geis WP, Kim HC, McAfee PC, Kang JG, Brennan EJ Jr (1996) Synergistic benefits of combined technologies in complex, minimally invasive surgical procedures. Clinical experience and educational processes. Surg Endosc10:1025–1028
2. Koch C, Borys M, Fedtke T, Richter U, Pohl B (2002) Determination of the acoustic output of a harmonic scalpel. IEEE Trans Ultrason Ferroelectr Freq Control 49:1522–1529
3. Langer C, Markus P, Liersch T, Fuezesi L, Becker H (2001) UltraCision or high-frequency knife in transanal endoscopic microsurgery (TEM)? Advantages of a new procedure. Surg Endosc15:513–517

69 Instrument and Device Options

Amulya K. Saxena

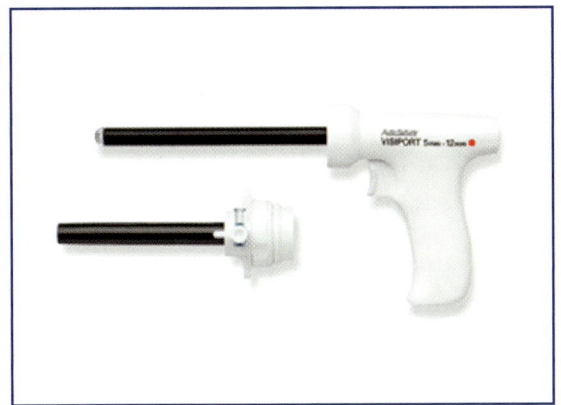

69.1   Optical Port System

AutoSuture™ Visiport™ (Auto Suture, Norwalk, CT, USA) consists of a pistol-grip handle with a trigger and an opening to accommodate a 10-mm laparoscope. When the trigger is pulled, the blade extends approximately 1 mm and immediately retracts, permitting tissue dissection. The 10-mm, 0° laparoscope permits visualization as the obturator passes through the body wall. (Courtesy of Covidien Austria, Brunn am Gebirge, Austria)

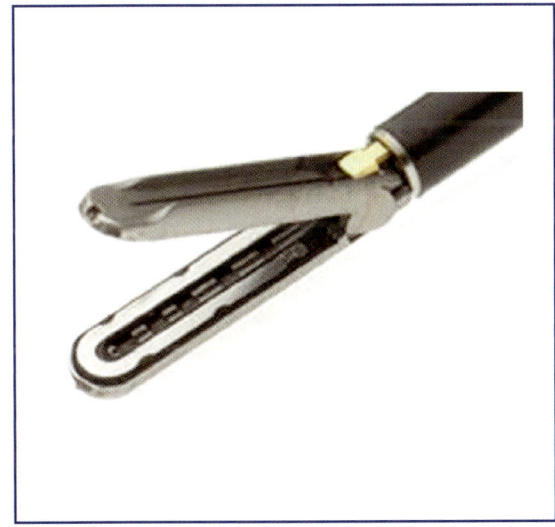

69.2   SurgRx™ Enseal™ Tissue Sealer

EnSeal™ (SurgRx, Redwood City, CA, USA) vessel-sealing nanopolar technology offers a high-compression jaw design to provide secure, rapid vessel sealing with virtually no unwanted thermal effects. It is the first and only system that controls energy deposition at the electrode–tissue interface. The patented polymer temperature control (PTC) electrode can control the energy delivery at the tip.

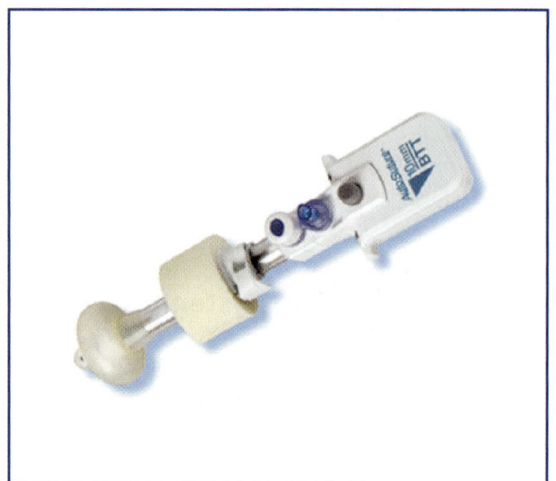

69.3   Locking Port with Balloon

The AutoSuture™ blunt-tip, 10-mm trocar (Auto Suture, Norwalk, CT, USA) has a balloon at the distal end of the sleeve that is complemented by a proximal foam collar assembly to minimize leakage and secure the port to the body wall. (Courtesy of Covidien Austria, Brunn am Gebirge, Austria)

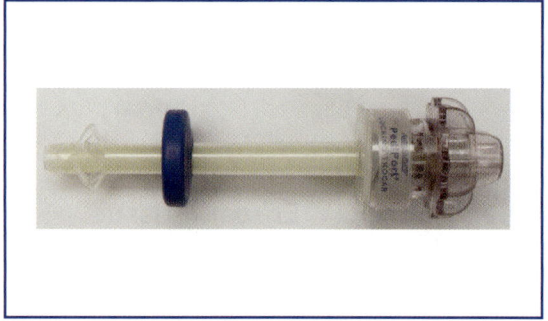

69.4   Pediatric Locking Port

AutoSuture™ Pediport™ Locking Trocar (Auto Suture, Norwalk, CT, USA) is a 5mm disposable port system with a locking mechanism. Once inserted inside the abdominal cavity, the trocar is removed and the head of the port is twisted which in turn opens an umbrella at the tip of the port. From the outside a rubber seal can be pushed to the skin which ensures a bidirectional securing of the port.

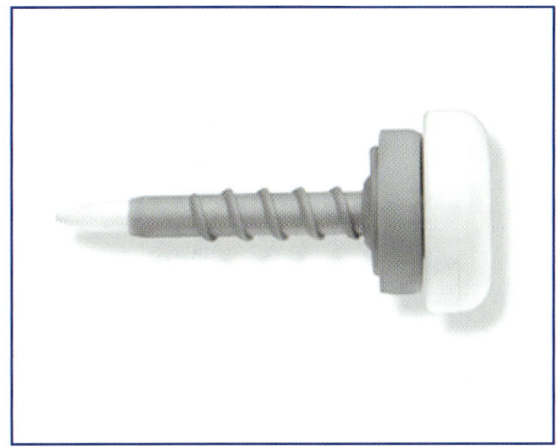

69.5   Thoracic Port System

The Thoracoport™ (Auto Suture, Norwalk, CT, USA) single use trocar (5.5, 10.5, 11.5 and 15 mm) consists of a blunt-tipped obturator and a threaded sleeve with a shroud at its proximal end. Once inserted into the chest cavity, the threaded sleeve is turned clockwise until securely seated in the tissue. The threaded sleeve will grip tissue to reduce slippage during instrument manipulation. (Courtesy of Covidien Austria, Brunn am Gebirge, Austria)

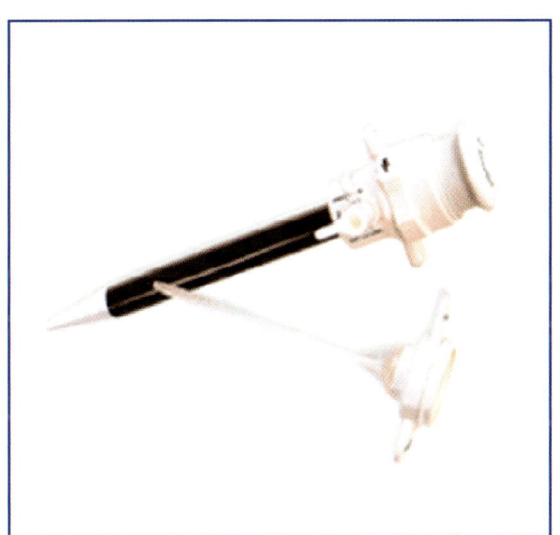

69.6   Step Trocar

The AutoSuture™ VersaStep™ (Auto Suture, Norwalk, CT, USA) port is used to provide dilation access to the cavities. With VersaStep™, the initial needle tract accessed is expanded radially, and tissues are stretched not cut. (Courtesy of Covidien Austria, Brunn am Gebirge, Austria)

69.7   The Veroscope: Veress Needle Insertion Under Endoscopic Control

The Veroscope (Richard Wolf, Knittlingen, Germany) consists of: (a) a 1.9-mm 0° scope, (b) a spring-loaded 3-mm transparent tip, (c) a 3-mm Veress needle, and (d) a 3-mm port sleeve. The system is assembled *a-d* and introduced into the subcutaneous tissue. It is pushed forward under visual aid with slight pressure until the fascia and peritoneum are opened. Once inside, insufflation is started. A 3-mm dilatation sleeve (Veroscout, see next section) is placed and the Veroscope system retracted. Using dilatation trocars, the port tract is dilated and replaced with a larger port. (Courtesy of Richard Wolf, Knittlingen, Germany)

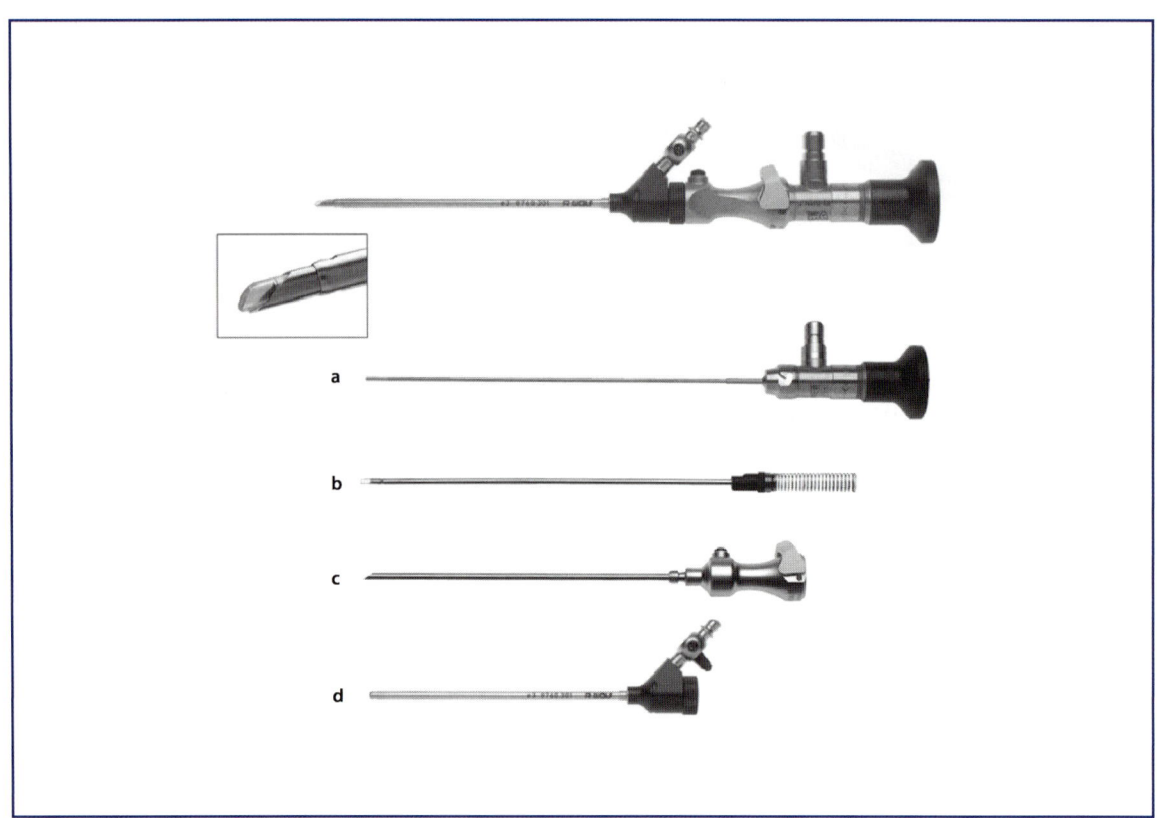

69.8   Veroscout: Incision Dilatation Sleeve

The Veroscout (Richard Wolf, Knittlingen, Germany) is a 3-mm dilatation port sleeve that is placed in the port tract after abdominal access has been established using the Veress needle. Dilatation of the port tract and placement of a larger port is achieved by using a special "nose" dilatation trocar (inset). The trocar is inserted into a port, after which the two are introduced as a set in the Veroscout and guided as far as the abdomen. The Veroscout opens along its length and the trocar and port are inserted without any problem. (Courtesy of Richard Wolf, Knittlingen, Germany)

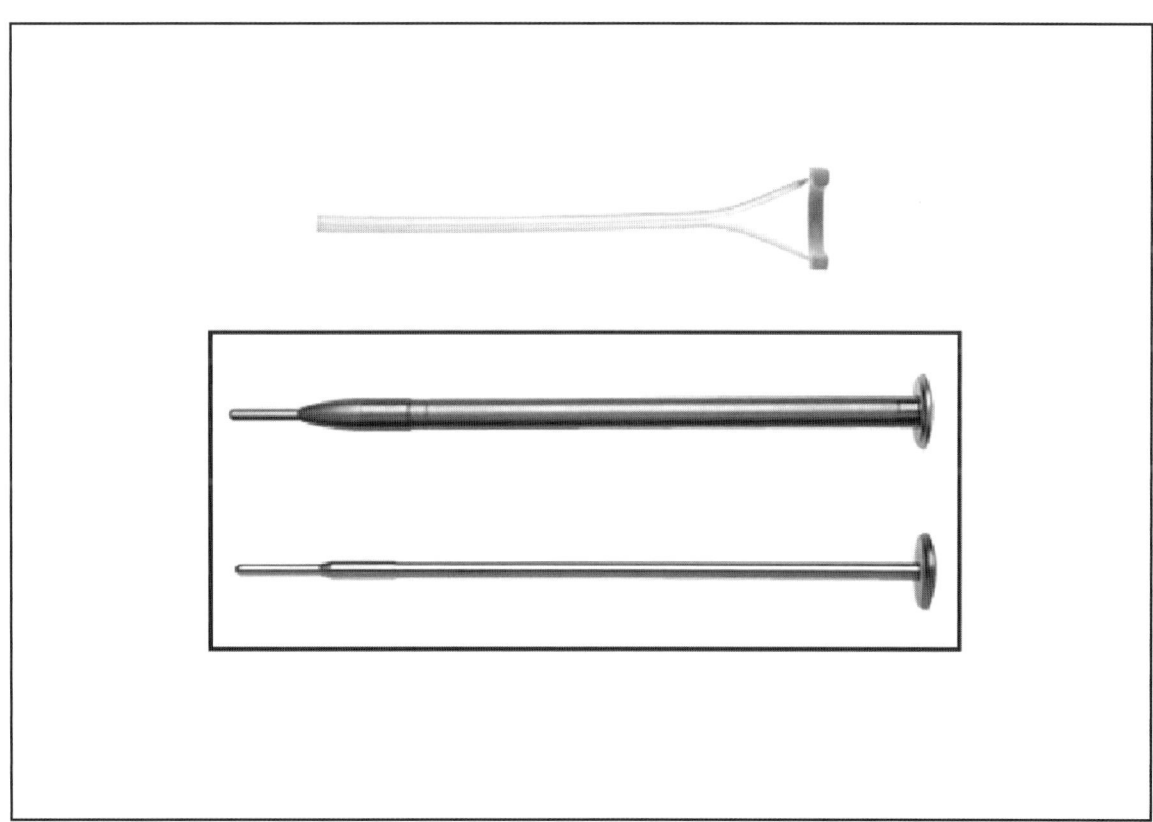

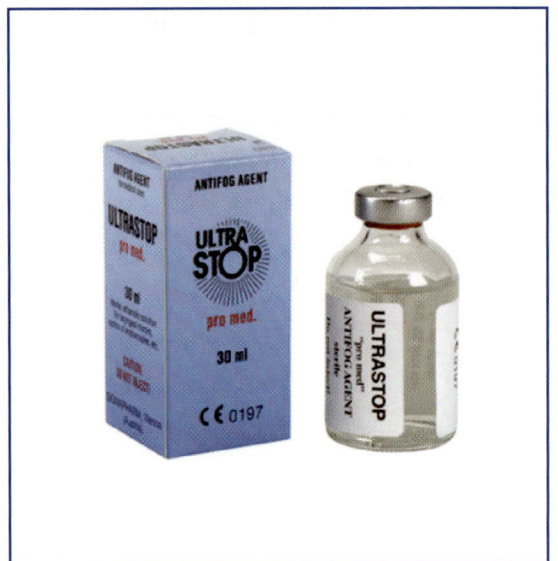

69.9   Antifogging Agents

The active components of antifogging agents, such as Ultrastop (Sigmapharm, Vienna, Austria), form a transparent film on glass surfaces that reduces the surface tension of water to such a degree that the water molecules are unable to form droplets. (Courtesy of Sigmapharm Arzneimittel, Vienna, Austria)

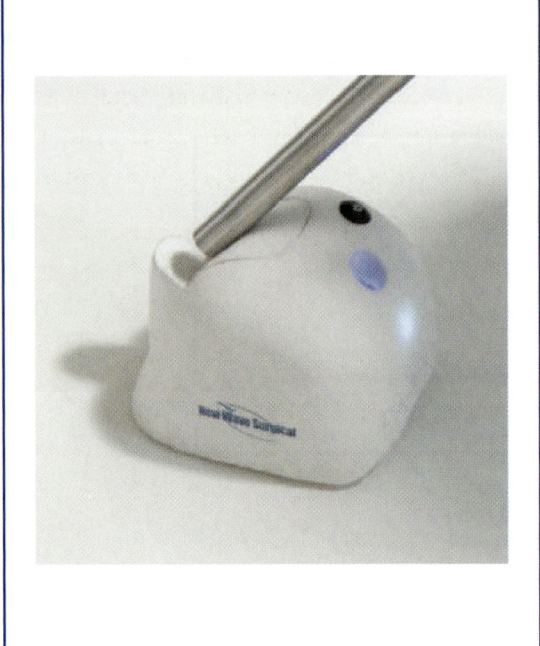

69.10   Defogging Heated Endoscope Lens Protector

Defogging Heated Endoscope Lens Protector (DHELP®; New Wave Surgical, Rego Park, NY, USA) bathes the scope in a warm anti-fog solution until its ready for use. The combination of heat and the antifog-solution eliminates fogging for the entire procedure. (Courtesy of New Wave Surgical, Rego Park, NY, USA)

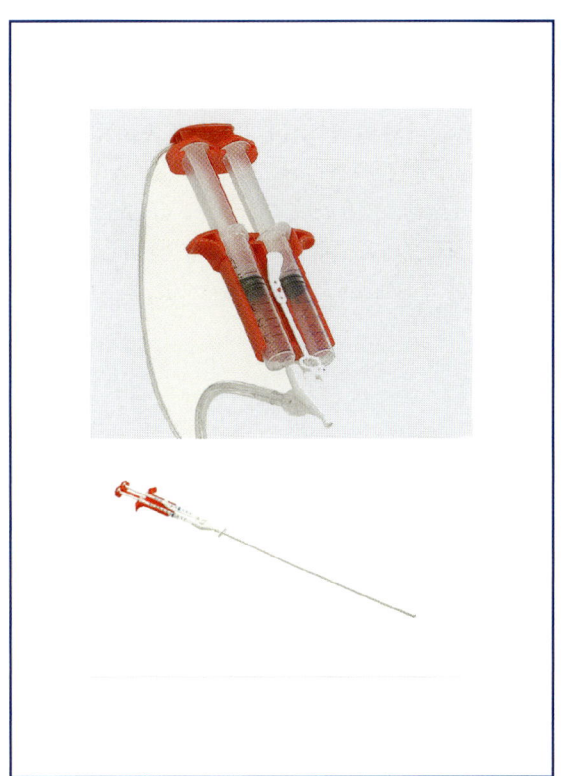

69.11   Fibrin Glue Applicator

The Duplocath™ 35 MIS (Baxter Healthcare, Deerfield, IL, USA) catheter can be passed through a 5mm port for endoscopic application of fibrin glue. The catheter works with the Duplojet™ application device. (Courtesy of Baxter Biosurgery/Bioscience Austria, Vienna, Austria)

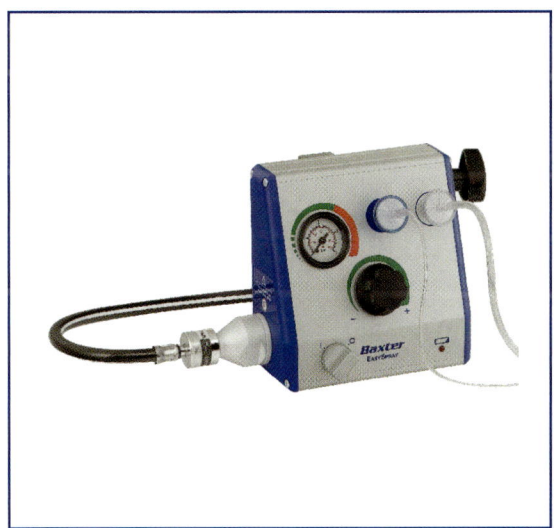

69.12   Fibrin Spray Applicator Device

The Easy Spray™ device (Baxter Healthcare, Deerfield, IL, USA) is a compressed gas controller for spraying fibrin sealant with the appropriate spray set. (Courtesy of Baxter Biosurgery/Bioscience Austria, Vienna, Austria)

Recommended Literature

1. Anidjar M, Desgrandchamps F, Martin L, Cochand-Priollet B, Cissenot O, Teillac P, Le Duc A (1996) Laparoscopic fibrin glue ureteral anastomosis: experimental study in the porcine model. J Endourol 10:51–56
2. Melzer A, Riek S, Roth K, Buess G (1995) Endoscopically controlled trocar and cannula insertion. Endosc Surg Allied Technol 3:63–68
3. Saxena AK, van Tuil C (2007) Advantages of fibrin glue spray in laparoscopic liver biopsies. Surg Laparosc Endosc Percutan Tech17:545–547

70 Suturing Aids in Endoscopic Surgery

Amulya K. Saxena

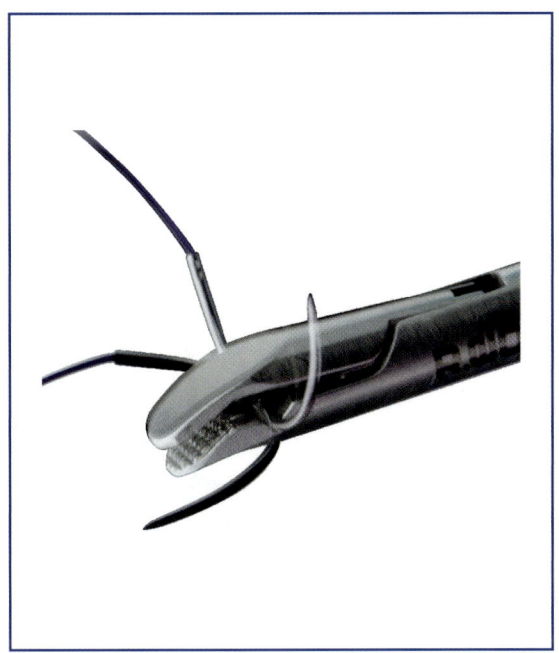

70.1 Self-Righting Needle Holders

Smart needle holders are designed to automatically self-right the needle to the correct position in the holder when the jaws of the needle holder are closed (Sarbu™; Richard Wolf, Knittlingen, Germany). Furthermore, they have a built-in suture cutter to avoid instrument changes once the suture has been tied. (Courtesy of Richard Wolf, Knittlingen, Germany)

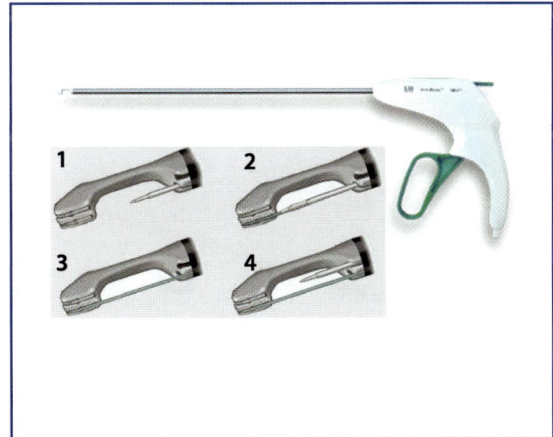

70.2 Sew-Right Sewing Device

The Sew-Right® SR•5 (LSI Solutions, Victor, NY, USA) is a reloadable 5-mm sewing device. To sew: (1) the needle is passed through tissue, (2) after which it automatically captures the suture, (3) and pulls it back through the tissue; (4) The second needle can be selected to take the second bite; after which the two ends are tied.

70.3   Quik-Stitch® Suturing System

The Quik-Stitch® endoscopic suturing system (Pare Surgical, Englewood, CO, USA) is a 5-mm delivery system with a pretied Roeder knot. It consists of a 5-mm reusable, stainless-steel handle, 2.1-mm reusable needle driver, and a patented suture spool with a straight taper point or blunt-tip needle. (Courtesy of Pare Surgical, Englewood, CO, USA)

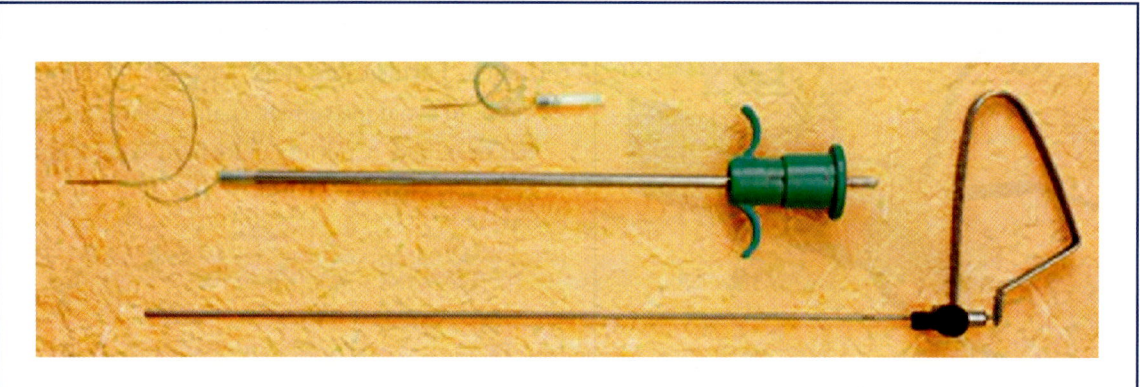

70.4   Clip Knots
for Continuous Sutures

Lapra-Ty-II™ (Ethicon, Somerville, NJ, USA) are absorbable suture clips made of polydiaxanone polymer to secure the ends of suture. A special clip applicator is necessary to secure the clip on the suture ends. (Courtesy of Johnson & Johnson Medical Products, Ethicon, Vienna, Austria)

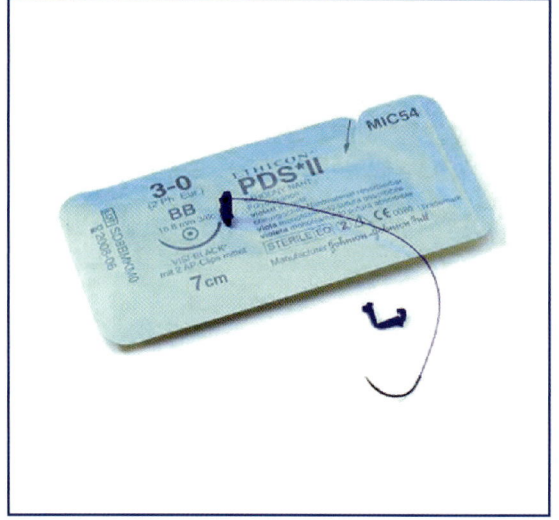

70.5   Busche Port-Site Closure Device

Port sites > 5 mm have to be closed to prevent port-site hernias, especially in adolescent bariatric surgery. The Busche port-site closure device (Richard Wolf, Knittlingen, Germany) comprising of a guide (top) and a grasping forceps (bottom) with a sharp tip (inset) is a useful tool for port-site closure. (Courtesy of Richard Wolf, Knittlingen, Germany)

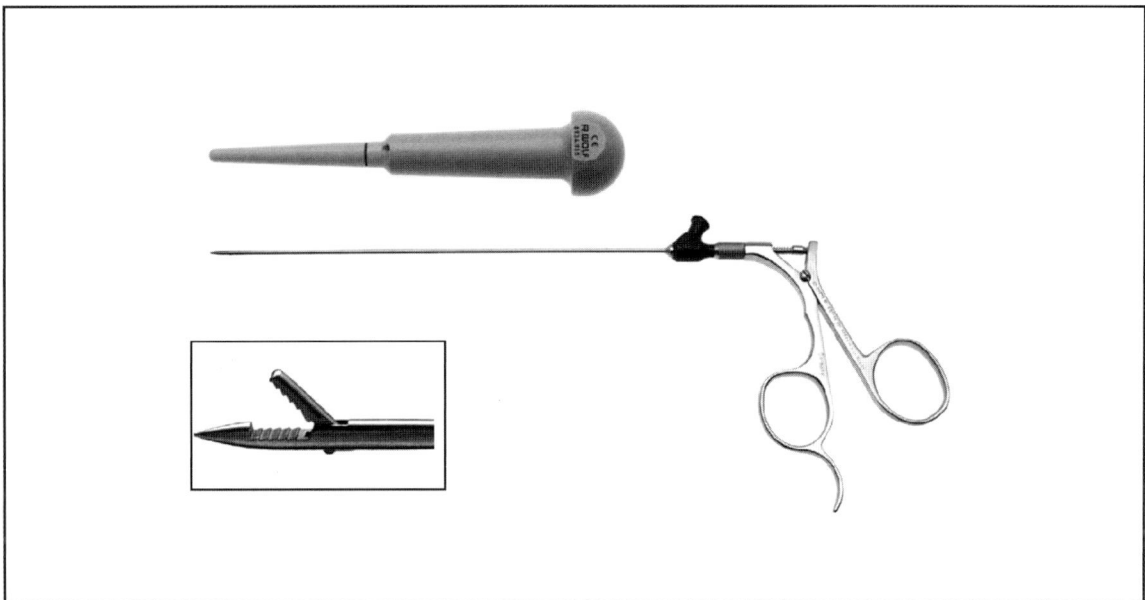

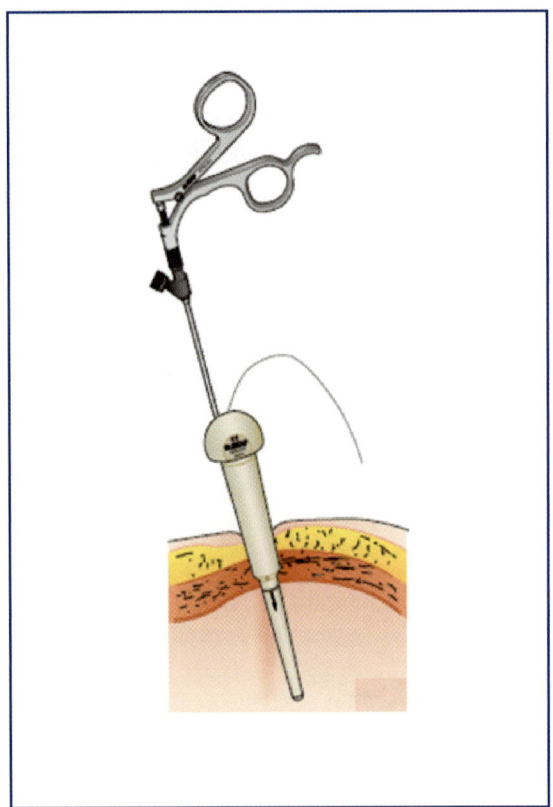

70.5.1   Technique of Port-Site Closure with the Busche Device

Step 1: The guide is first introduced into the port site, after which the grasping forceps with suture is inserted through it. (Courtesy of Richard Wolf, Knittlingen, Germany)

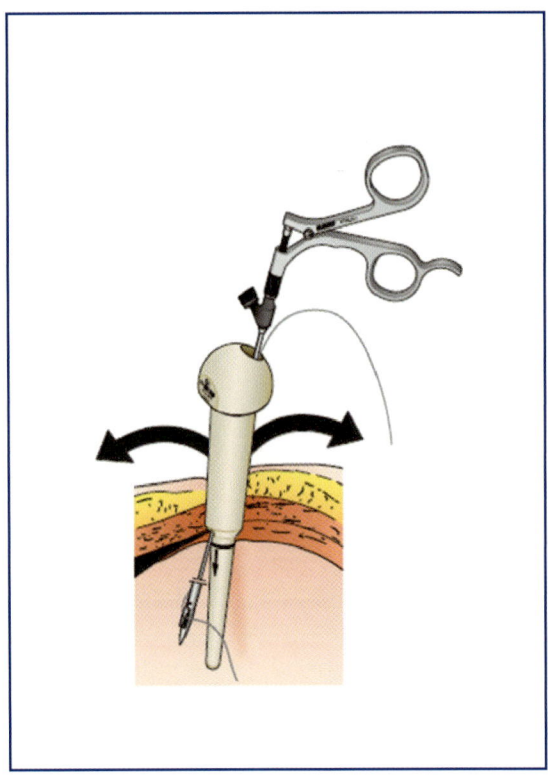

Step 2: The Forceps exit point must not be close to the defect edge to ensure full-thickness closure. The suture is released with ~4 cm length in the abdomen. (Courtesy of Richard Wolf, Knittlingen, Germany)

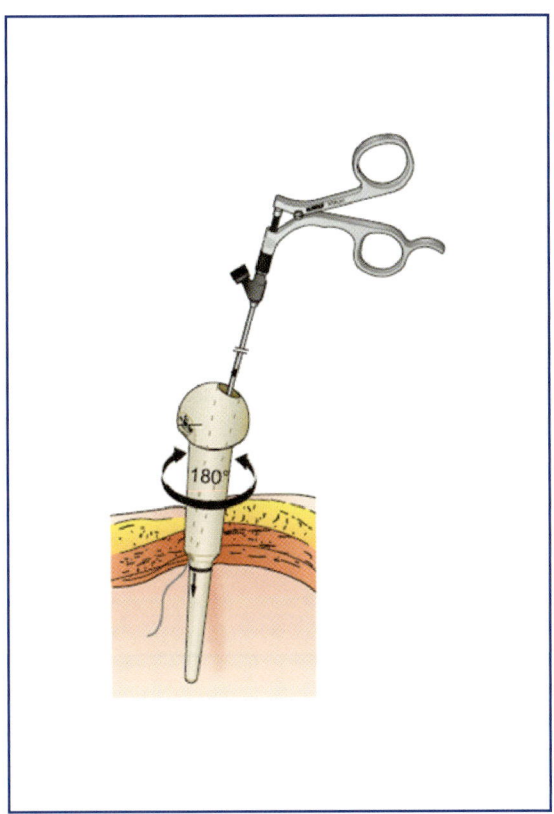

Step 3: The forceps is partially retracted into the guide. With the retracted forceps, the guide is rotated 180° and the forceps reintroduced in the abdomen. (Courtesy of Richard Wolf, Knittlingen, Germany)

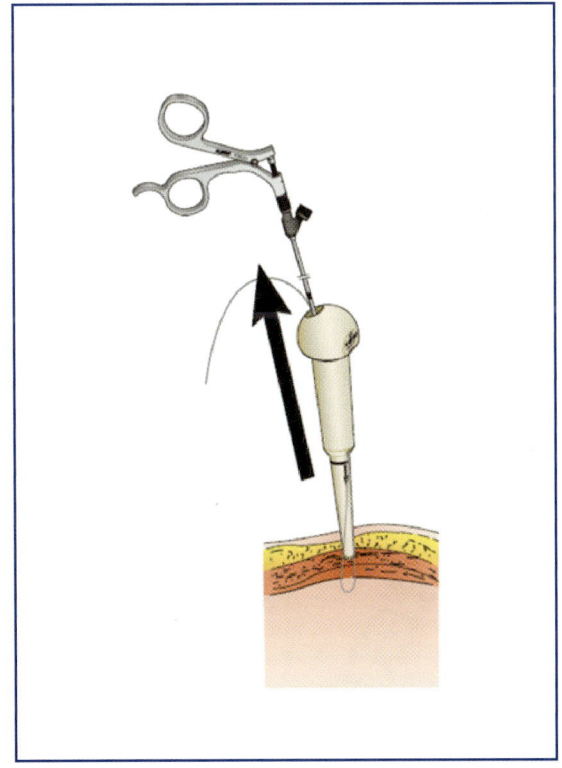

Step 4: The forceps grasps the suture and then is then partially retracted into the guide. The guide and the forceps are removed and the knot tied extracorporeally. (Courtesy of Richard Wolf, Knittlingen, Germany)

70.6   EndoStitch Suturing Device

The Autosuture™ EndoStitch™ (Auto Suture, Norwalk, CT, USA) is a 10-mm, single-use suturing device for intracorporeal knot tying. To create an intracorporeal knot at the end of the suture line, the needle is placed in the left jaw position and passed under the suture line at the end of the incision (a). The needle is toggled to the right jaw to create a loop. With the needle in the right jaw, a loop of suture is placed between the jaws of the EndoStitch™ (b). The needle is then toggled to the left jaw and pulled around the loop by passing under the suture on the right side (c) and tied (d). (Courtesy of Covidien Austria, Brunn am Gebirge, Austria)

Recommended Literature

1. Bermas H, Fenoglio M, Haun W, Moore JT (2004) Laparoscopic suturing and knot tying: a comparison of standard techniques to a mechanical assist device. JSLS 8:187–189
2. Johnson WH, Fecher AM, MacMahon RL, Grant JP, Pryor AD (2006) VersaStep trocar hernia rate in unclosed fascial defects in bariatric patients. Surg Endosc 20:1584–1586
3. Sahin M, Eryilmaz R, Okan I (2006) Closure of fascial defect at trocar sites after laparoscopic surgery. Minim Invasive Ther Allied Technol 15:317–318

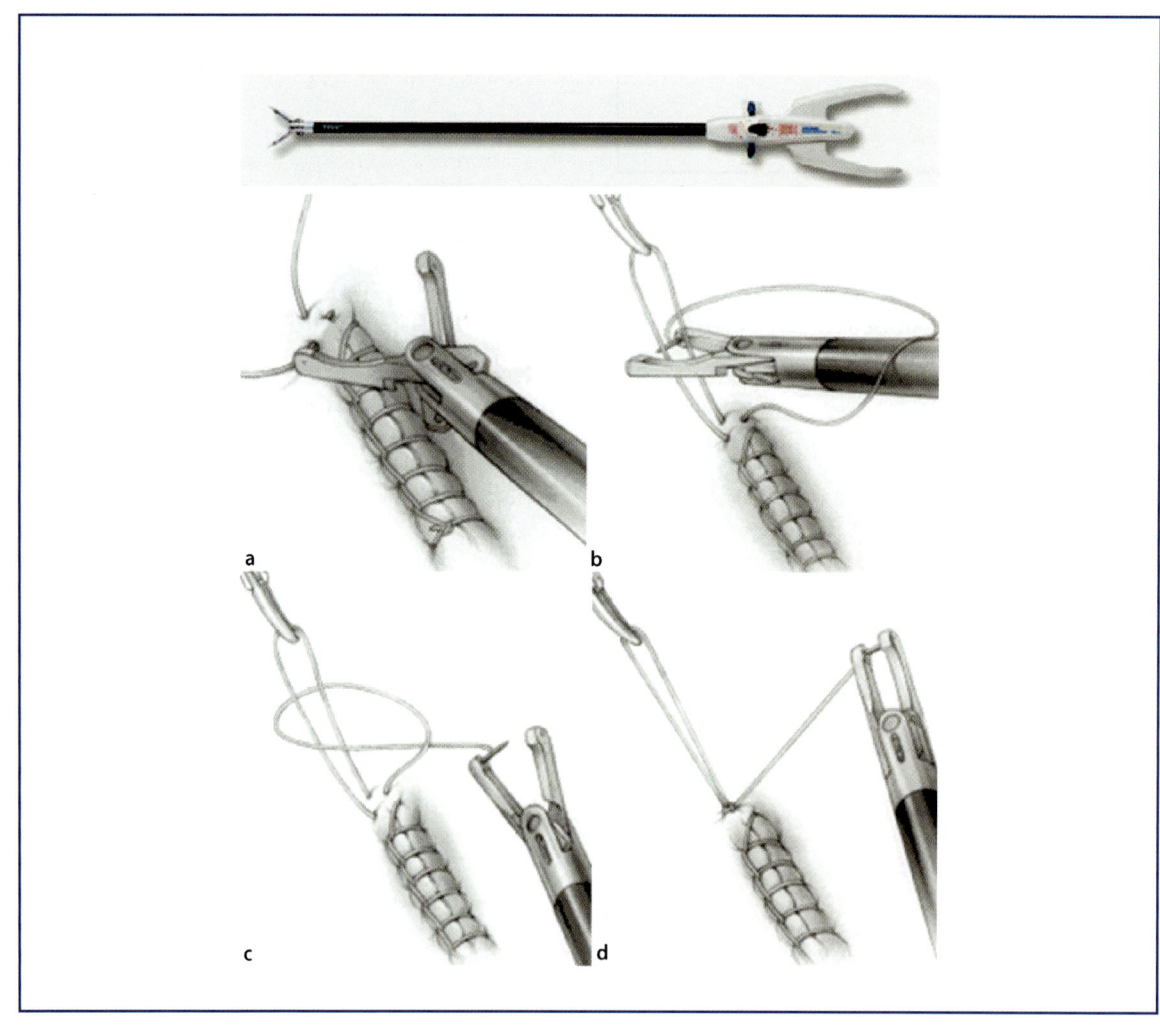

a   b

c   d

71 Slip Knot Techniques

Amulya K. Saxena

71.1 Slip Knots

Surgical knot configuration is determined by the alternating or repetitive direction of rotation of sequential throws of suture to form a knot. Once a knot is configured, it can be conformed into either a flat knot or a slip knot as it is secured.

Slip knots, also known as hitched knots, are formed when one end of suture is rotated around the other end that remains straight. The most common extracorporeally tied slip knots are Roeder, Melzer, and Tayside.

71.2 Extracorporeal Slip Knot Material

Extracorporeal knots are secure if braided materials are used:

1. Dacron (Ethibond™‡, Ti-Cron™† or Ethiflex™‡).
2. Lactomer (Polysorb™†, Dexon™†, Vicryl™‡).
3. Melzer and Tayside knots are resonably secure with polydiaxone.

    († Syneture, Norwalk, CT, USA; ‡ Ethicon, Somerville, NJ, USA)

It is important to note that slip knots must be pushed down. They should never be pulled up on like a lasso. The length of the suture must be at least 75 cm or more.

71.3   Roeder Knot
(Extracorporeal Knot)

Please see Figs. 1–4.

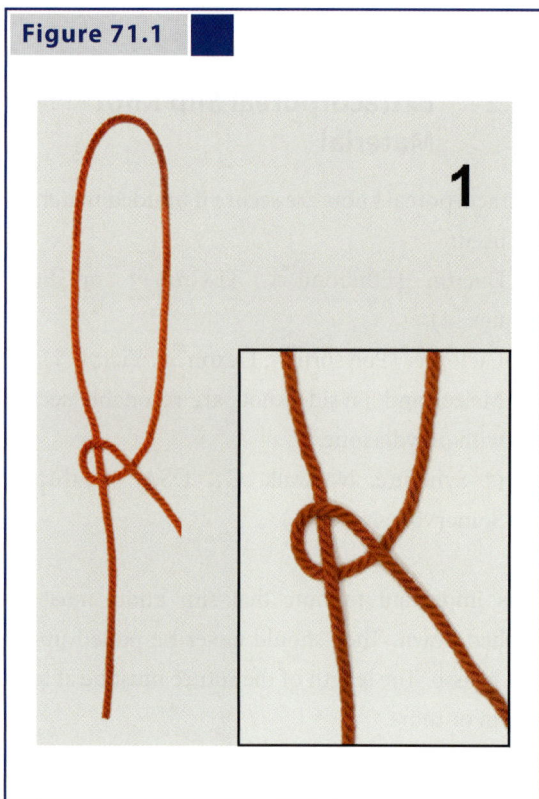

One half knot is taken first

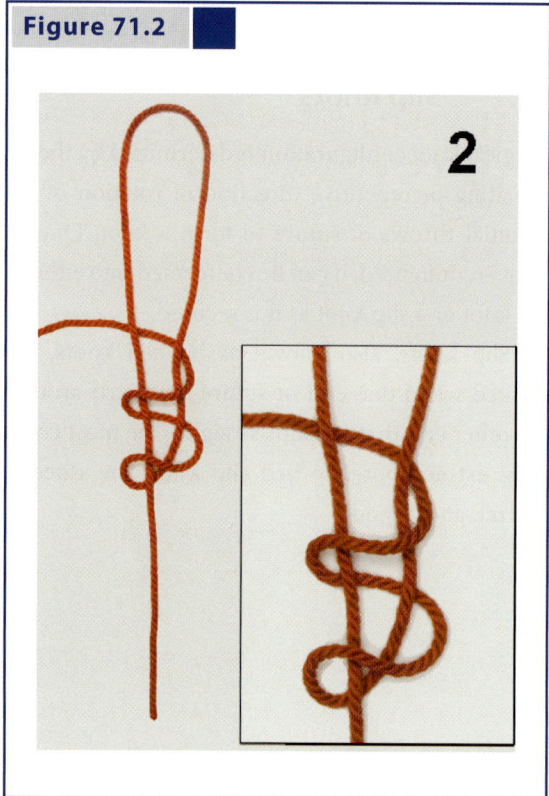

Two rounds over both the limbs

Figure 71.3

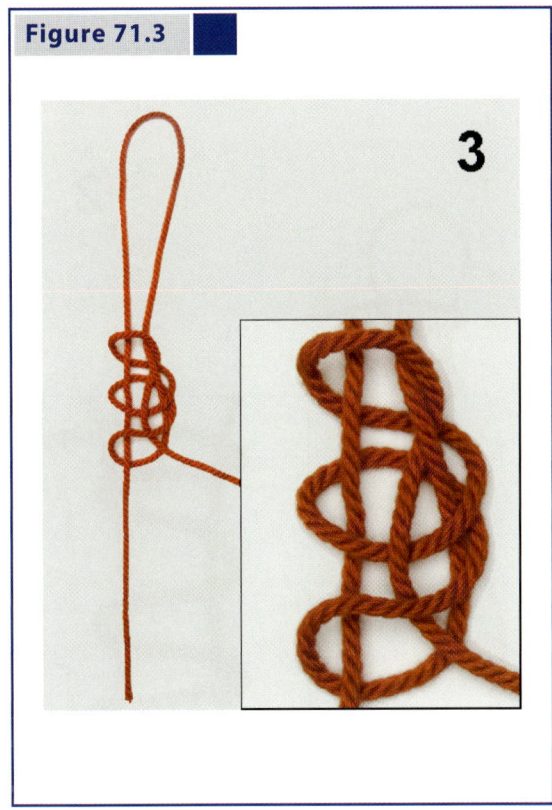

Second half knot on one loop

Figure 71.4

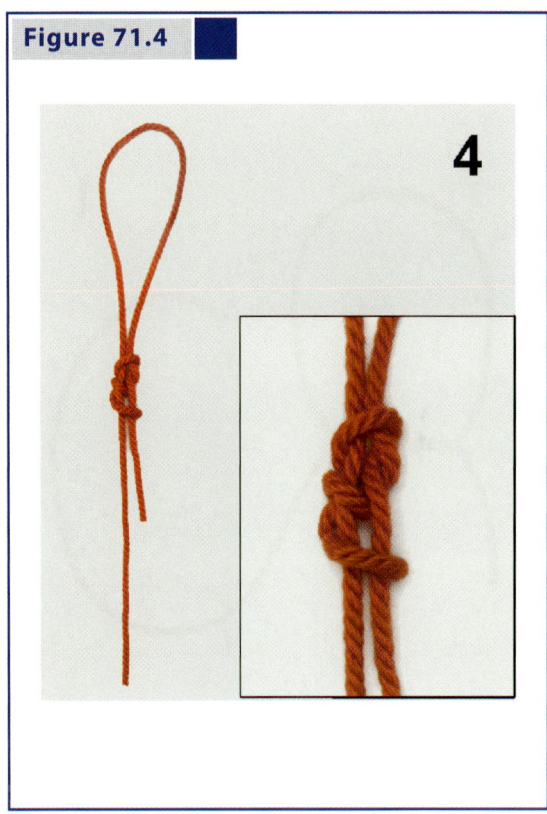

Knot is stacked and pushed

71.4   Metzler Slip Knot (Extracorporeal Knot)

Please see Figs. 5–8.

Figure 71.5

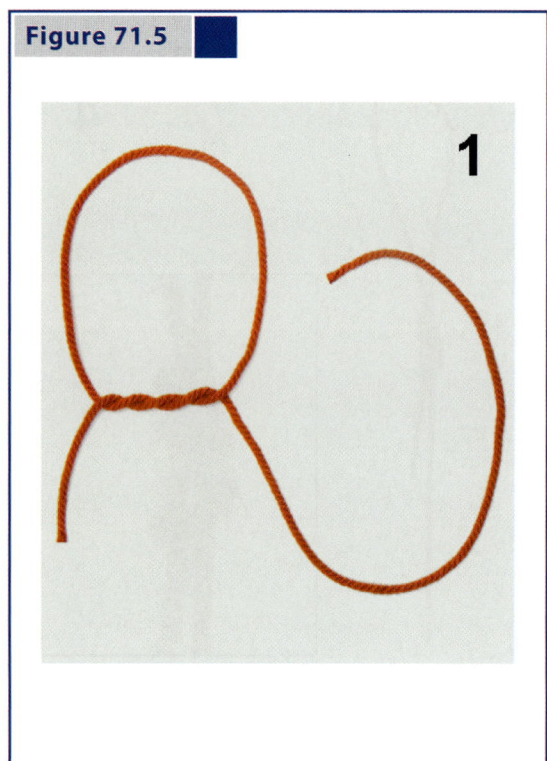

1

Two half knots are taken first

Figure 71.6

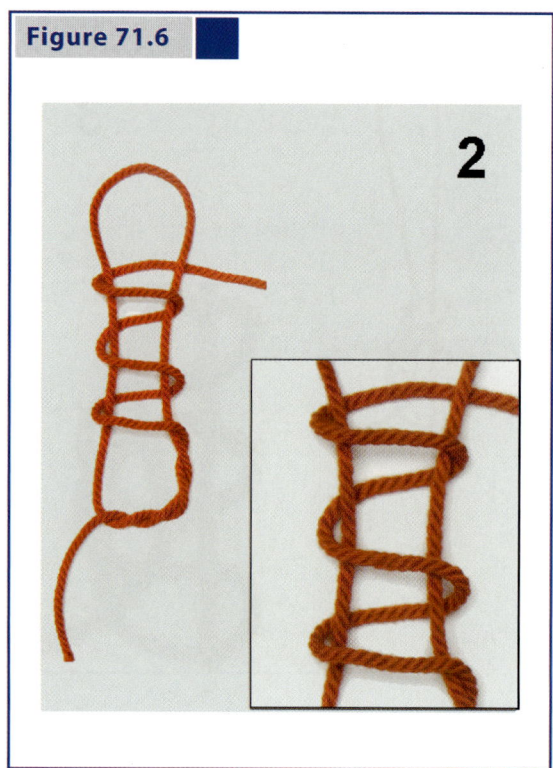

2

Three rounds over both limbs

Figure 71.7

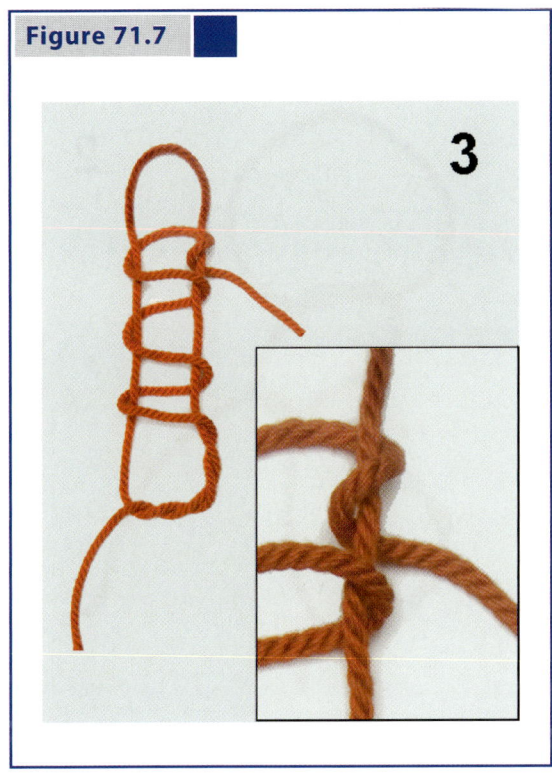

First half hitch on one loop

Figure 71.8

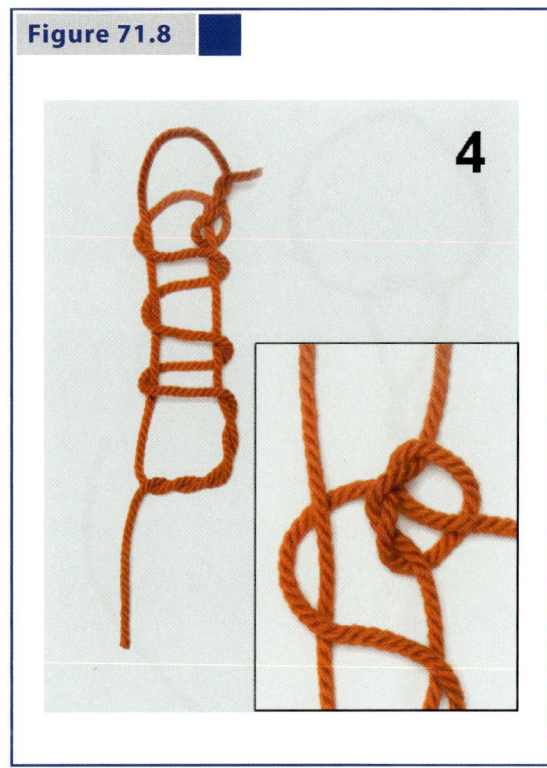

Followed by a second half hitch

71.5   Tayside Knot (Extracorporeal Knot)

Please see Figs. 9–12.

Figure 71.9

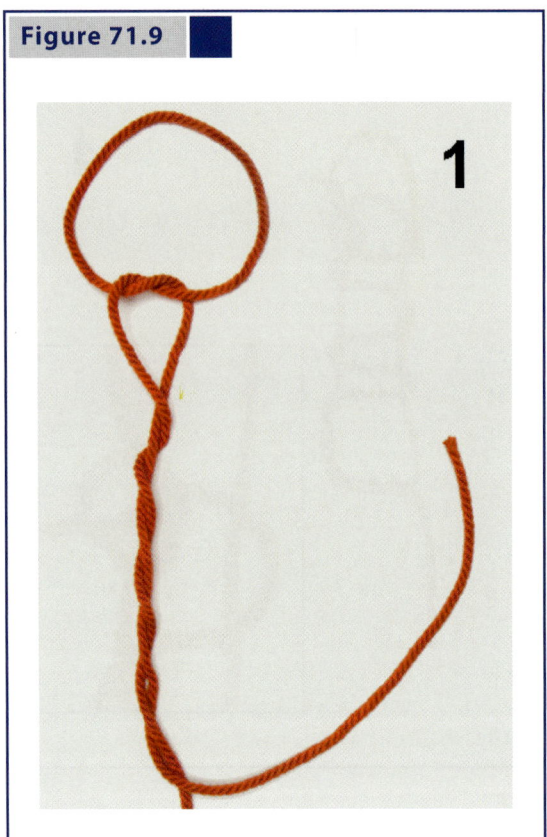

One half knot and four half turns around the longer suture limb

Figure 71.10

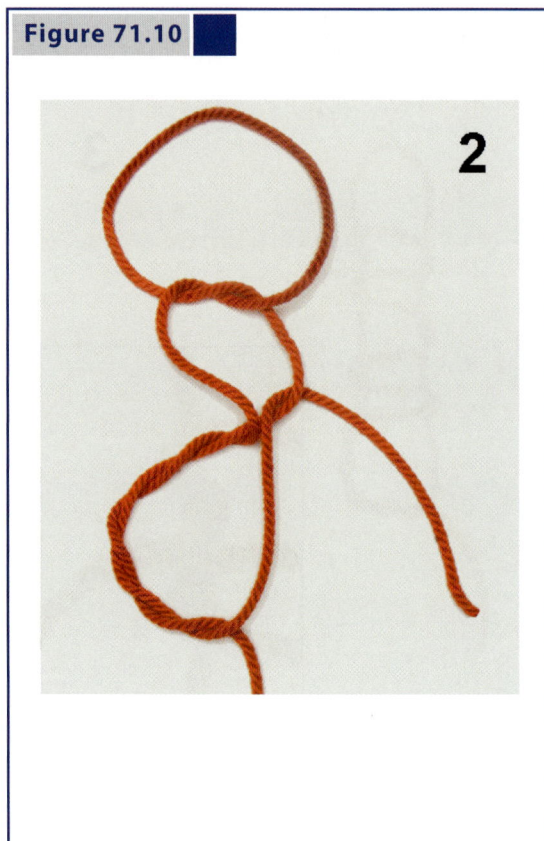

The tail is passed through the second and third loop

Figure 71.11

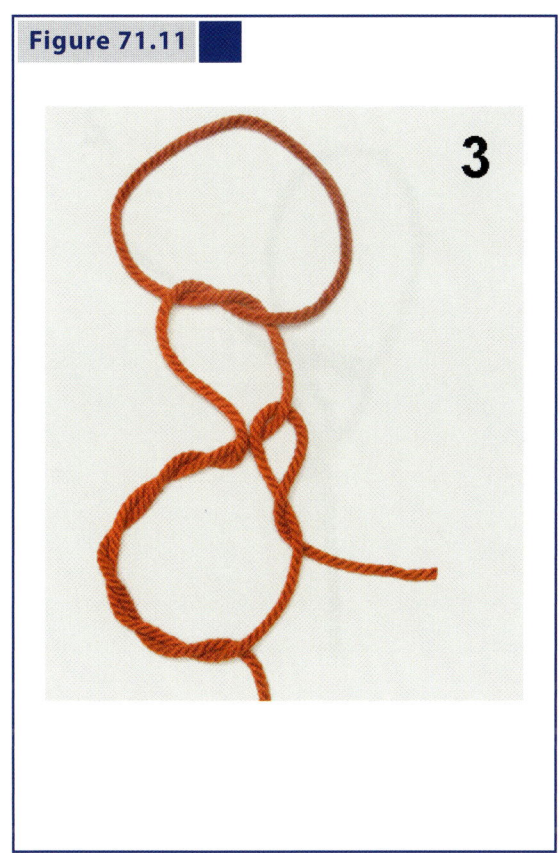

A locking hitch is made

Figure 71.12

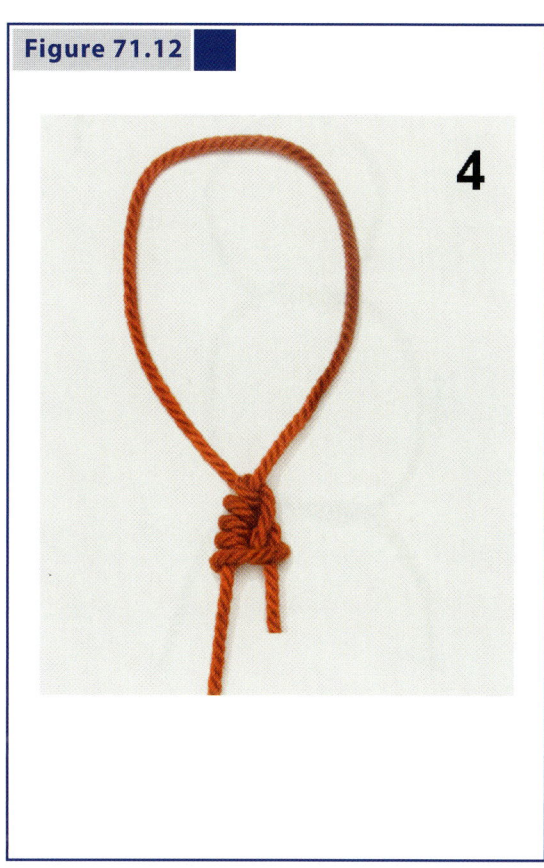

The knot is stacked and the excess tail cut off

71.6 Slipping Square Knot (Intracorporeal Knot)

Please see Figs. 13 and 14.

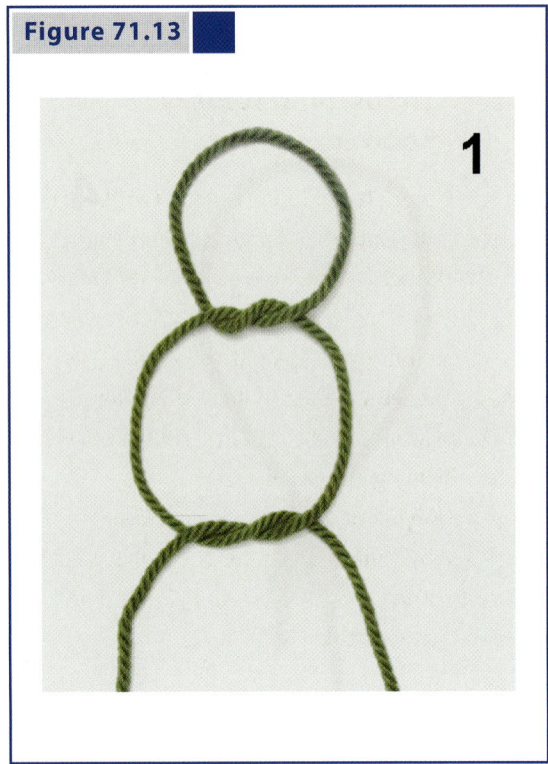

Figure 71.13

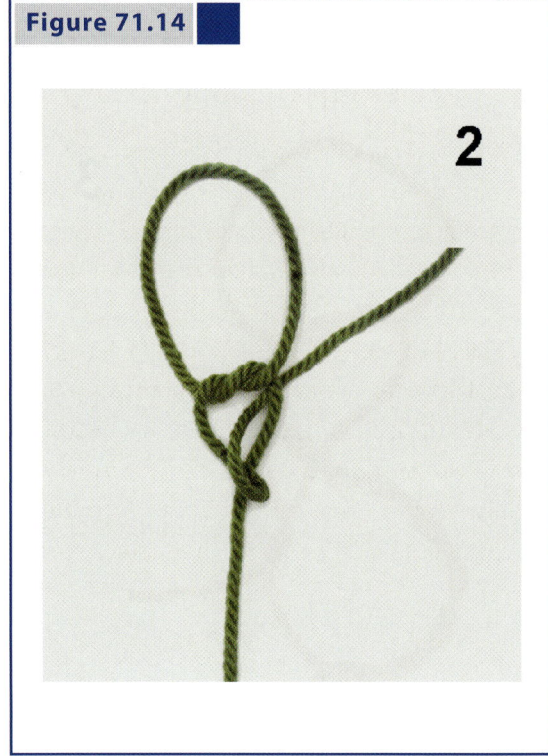

Figure 71.14

The first and second throws are placed, but left loose

The long end is pulled and the tail pushed to slip and snug the knot

Recommended Literature

1. Sharp HT, Dorsey JH, Chovan JD, Holtz PM (1996) A simple modification to add strength to the Roeder knot. J Am Assoc Gynecol Laparosc 3:305–307
2. Shimi SM, Lirici M, van der Velpen G, Cuschieri A (1994) Comparative study of the holding strength of slipknots using absorbable and nonabsorbable ligature materials. Surg Endosc 8:1285–1291
3. Lo IK, Burkhart SS, Chan KC, Athnansiou K (2004) Arthroscopic knots: determining the optimal balance of loop security and knot security. Arthroscopy 20:489–502

72 Developments in Robotic Systems

Amulya K. Saxena

72.1 Milestones in Robotic Surgery

In 1985, the *Puma 560* was the first robot in surgery that was used to place a needle for a brain biopsy using computed tomography guidance. Three years later, in 1988, the *Probot* was developed at Imperial College London and used to perform prostatic surgery. Later in 1992, the *Robodoc* from Integrated Surgical Systems was introduced to mill out precise fittings in the femur for hip replacement. However, robotic systems for endoscopic surgery were developed in 1994 by Computer Motion (*Aesop* and the *Zeus*) and in 1997 by Intuitive Surgical (*da Vinci*).

72.2 Endoscopic Surgery Robotic Systems

In 2003, Computer Motion (Goleta, CA, USA) was merged with Intuitive Surgical (Sunnyvale, CA, USA). Although the *da Vinci* surgical system is currently the only robotic system in endoscopic surgery being offered by Intuitive Surgical, reports with experiences on the robotic systems supplied by Computer Motion – *Aesop*, *Zeus*, and *Hermes* – are constantly being published.

The *Aesop*, *Zeus*, and *Hermes* robotics systems purchased by many medical centers in the late 1990s and early 2000s are still operational and hence deserve to be mentioned.

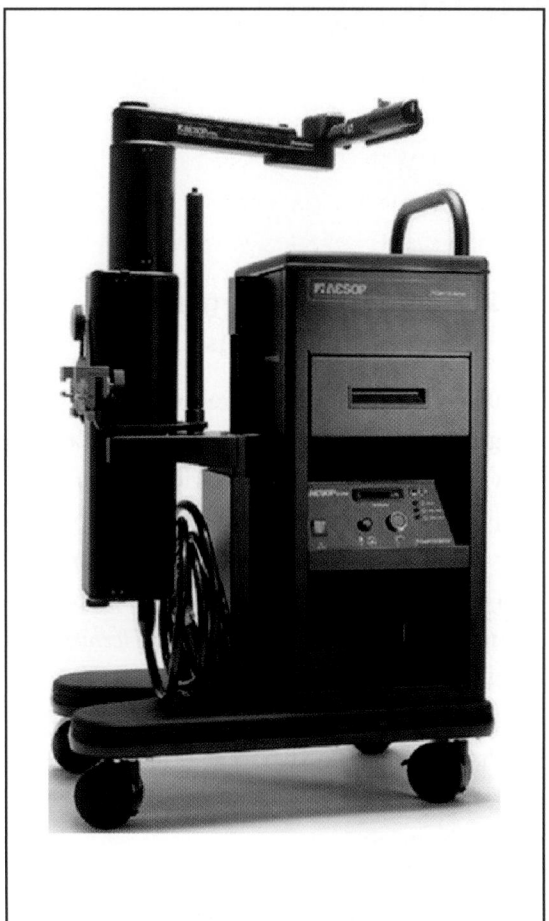

72.3   *Aesop* Robotic System

Aesop (Computer Motion) was a robot system for holding cameras in endoscopic surgery. In 1994, the *Aesop-1000* system became the world's first surgical robot certified by the US Food and Drug Administration. Computer Motion followed with *Aesop-2000* in 1996, with the enhancement of voice control, and in 1998, the *Aesop-3000*, with seven degrees of freedom. The introduction of the *Aesop-3000* provided more flexibility with regard to how surgeons and nurses could position the endoscope. By 1999, over 80,000 surgical procedures had been performed using *Aesop* technology. (Courtesy of Intuitive Surgical, Sunnyvale, CA, USA © 2007)

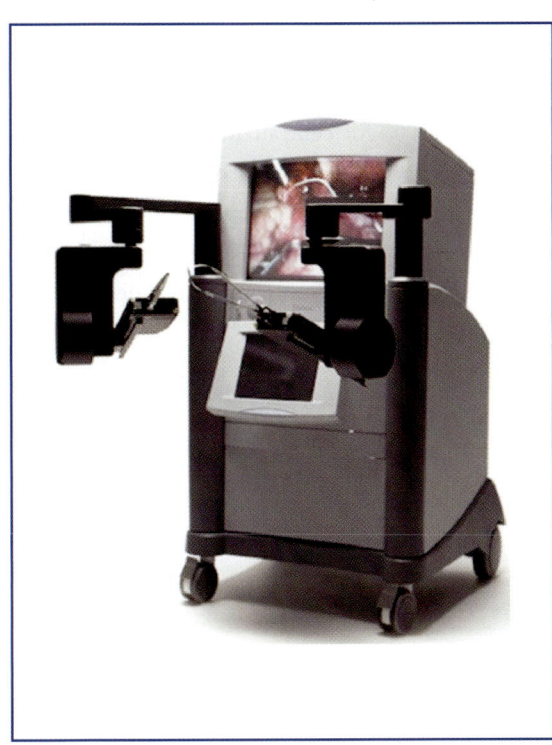

72.4   *Zeus* Robotic System

The *Zeus* robotic system (Computer Motion) made an impact on endoscopic surgery in late 1999 and early 2000. With the *Zeus* system, all of the instruments were robotic. The surgeon could sit comfortably at a master console and control the slave robotic instruments using a pair of master manipulators. Laborde, in Paris, performed the first pediatric cardiac procedure using the *Zeus* robotic system, closure of the patent ductus arteriosus. (Courtesy of Intuitive Surgical, Sunnyvale, CA, USA © 2007)

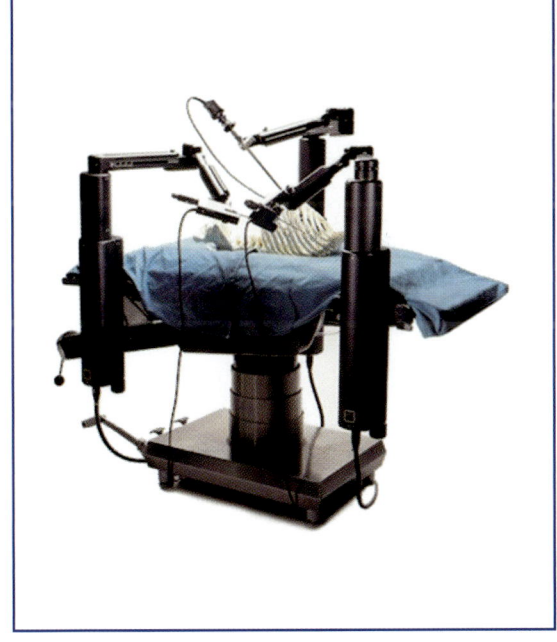

72.4.1   *Zeus* Robot Arms

Set up of the *Zeus* robotic system showing the placement of the robotic arms on the operation table. (Courtesy of Intuitive Surgical, Sunnyvale, CA, USA © 2007)

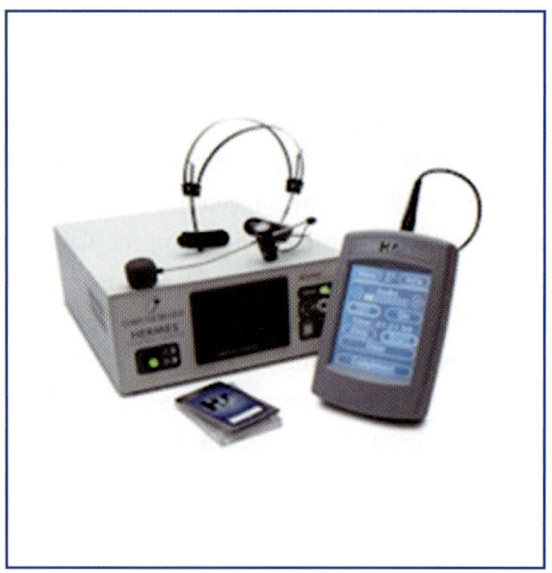

72.5   *Hermes* Platform

The *Hermes* (Computer Motion) platform was developed in 1998 for centralizing the control of devices (using voice command or a handheld pendant) inside or outside the operating room. It offered the concept of an "intelligent operating room." (Courtesy of Intuitive Surgical, Sunnyvale, CA, USA © 2007)

Recommended Literature

1. Klein MD, Langenburg SE, Kabeer M, Lorincz A, Knight CG (2007) Pediatric robotic surgery: lessons from a clinical experience. J Laparoendosc Adv Surg Tech A 17:265–271
2. Nguan C, Kwan K, Al Omar M, Beasley KA, Luke PP (2007) Robotic pyeloplasty: experience with three robotic platforms. Can J Urol 14:3571–3576
3. Panait L, Rafiq L, Mohammed A, Mora F, Merell R (2007) Robotic assistant for laparoscopy. J Laparoendosc Adv Surg Tech A 16:88–93

73 Concept of the Integrated Endoscopic Operation Room

Amulya K. Saxena

73.1 Integrated Operation Room Concept

The aim of integrated operation rooms is to provide the ideal room layout for performing minimally invasive and conventional procedures. Customized to specific fields, these operating rooms have solutions to offer the best possible ergonomics to the surgeon and the team along with direct interactive control of the equipment.

Integrated operation suites provide intuitive control of all functions of the equipments via remote control, touch screen and/or speech control – fast, easy, and safe, directly from the sterile area.

73.2 Advantages

There are many advantages of integrated operation suites:

1. Improved operation room layout.
2. Integration of endoscopic equipment.
3. Direct device control from sterile area.
4. Freedom of device setting.
5. Improved efficiency in device control.
6. Shorter set-up and change-over times.
7. Integration of existing systems.
8. Cost reduction by optimal workflow.
9. Better ergonomics for the team.
10. Concentration of equipment.

73.3   Ergonomics of an Integrated Endoscopic Surgery Room

Integrated endoscopic surgery rooms allow the set up of surgical equipments without overcrowding with mobile carts and cables. The risk of tripping over a thicket of cables is eliminated by one central cable outing for the power supply, carbon dioxide, compressed air, vacuum, and video signals. Suspended flat-screen monitors overcome the problem of positioning endoscopic carts toward the head of the patient (an area occupied by the anesthetist and ventilator) and provide the surgical team with the desired angle and line of vision. (Courtesy of Richard Wolf, Knittlingen, Germany)

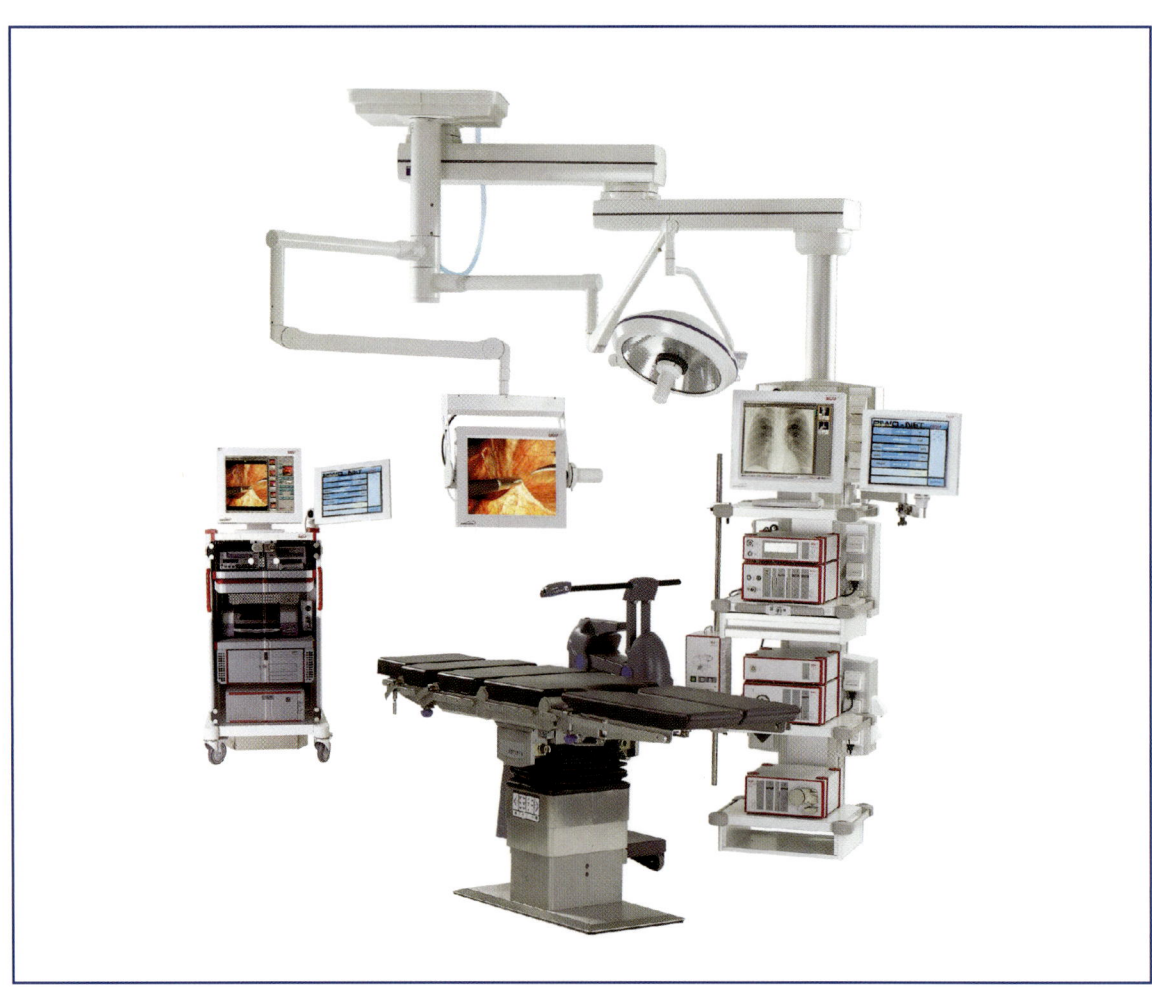

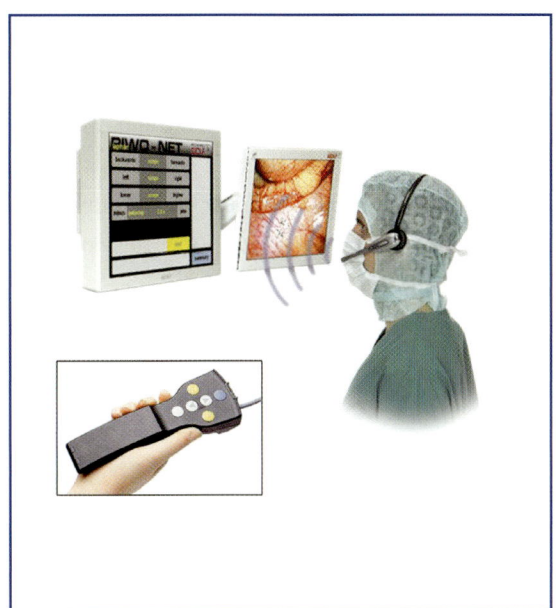

73.4 Voice-/Remote-Control Option

The designations of the device functions on the screen are simply spoken clearly by the operator for voice-controlled operation. Otherwise, the auto-clavable remote (inset) provides direct control from the sterile area. (Courtesy of Richard Wolf, Knittlingen, Germany)

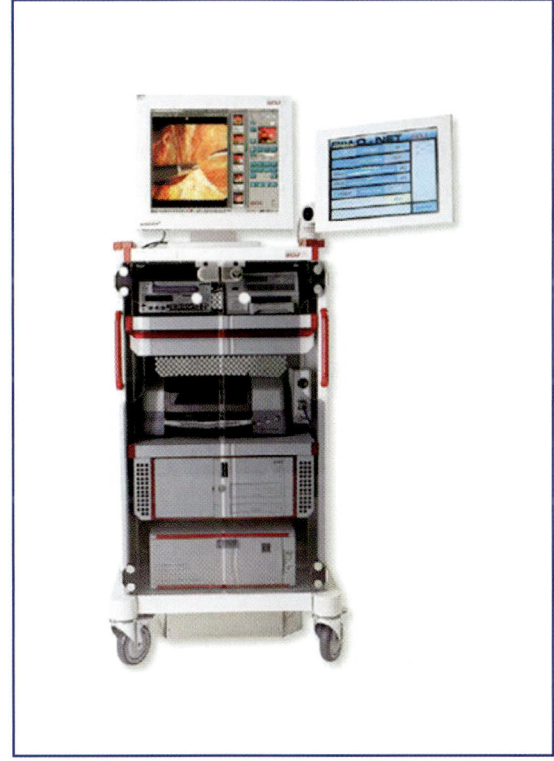

73.5 Nurse Station: Touch-Screen Control

The touch-screen nurse station allows centralized device control for personnel. (Courtesy of Richard Wolf, Knittlingen, Germany)

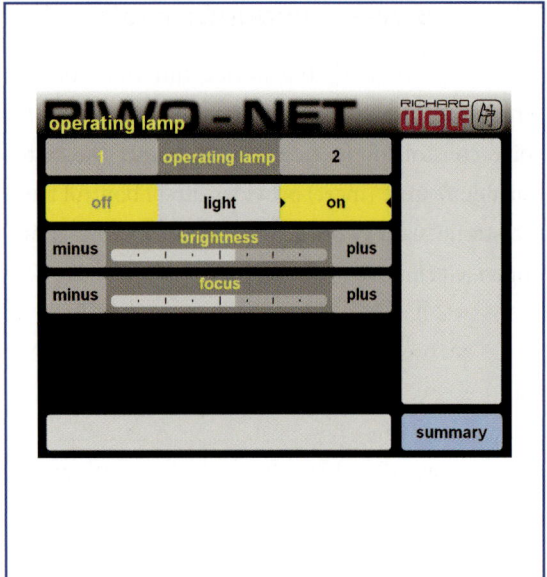

73.6   Centralized Equipment Control

All devices (from the operation table and operation lamp to the endoscopic surgery equipment) to be controlled in the network appear on the monitor as a simple intuitive guided menu. (Courtesy of Richard Wolf, Knittlingen, Germany)

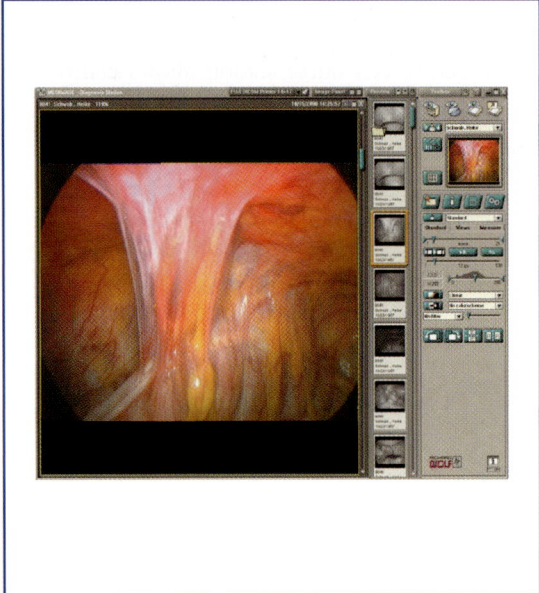

73.7   Image Management System

This feature provides the ability to combine images and reports from all medical disciplines. It allows image acquisition, processing, and archiving to a server or recording device. (Courtesy of Richard Wolf, Knittlingen, Germany)

73.8   Concept of Telemedicine

Telemedicine is an application of clinical medicine whereby medical information is transferred via telephone, the Internet, or other networks for the purpose of consulting, and sometimes remote surgical procedures. It may be as simple as discussing a case over the telephone, or as complex as using satellite technology and video-conferencing equipment to conduct a real-time operative procedure. Telemedicine is based on two concepts: real time (synchronous) and store-and-forward (asynchronous).

73.8.1   Synchronous/Asynchronous Telemedicine

Synchronous telemedicine requires the presence of the communicating groups at the same time and a communications link between them that allows a real-time interaction to take place. Video-conferencing equipment is one of the most common forms of technologies used in synchronous telemedicine.

Asynchronous telemedicine does not require the presence of the communicating groups at the same time. It involves acquiring medical data and then transmitting this data at a convenient time for offline assessment.

73.9   Endoscopic Room Telemedicine

Present capabilities allow transmission and switching of live videos between endoscopic camera, operation room cameras as well as radiological data directly from the operation room. (Courtesy of Richard Wolf, Knittlingen, Germany)

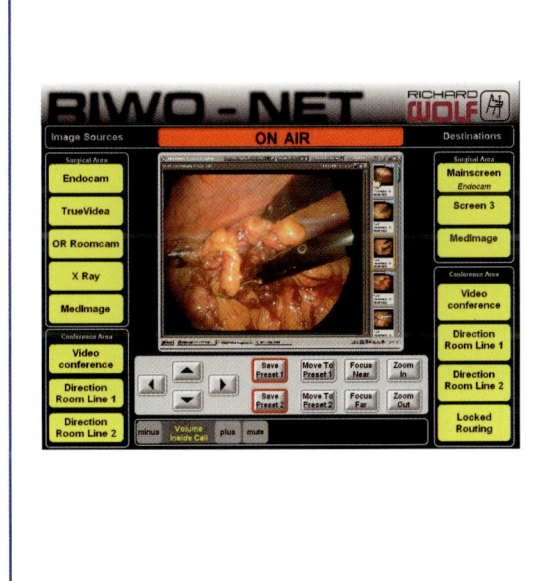

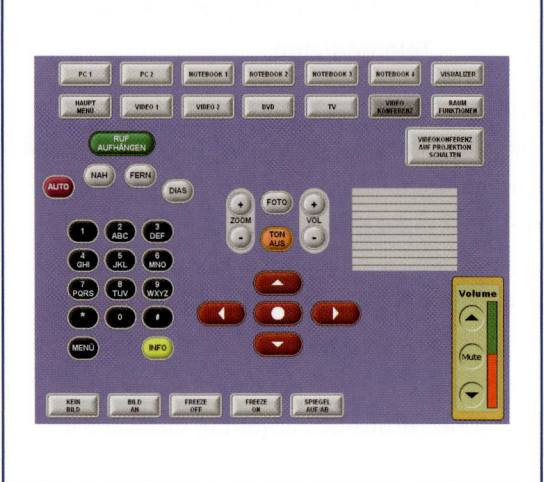

73.10   Video Conferencing

Video conference services offer the establishment of a direct "dial" access link from the operation room. It may either be a direct two-way communication or multipoint exchange. (Courtesy of Richard Wolf, Knittlingen, Germany)

Recommended Literature

1. Gallagher AG, Smith CD (2003) From the operating room of the present to the operating room of the future. Human-factors lessons learned from the minimally invasive surgery revolution. Semin Laparosc Surg 10:127–139
2. Kenyon TA, Urbach DR, Speer JB, Waterman-Hukari B, Foraker GF, Hansen PD, Swanstrom LL (2001) Dedicated minimally invasive surgery suites increase operating room efficiency. Surg Endosc 15:1140–1143
3. Marohn MR, Hanley EJ (2004) Twenty-first century surgery using twenty-first century technology: surgical robotics. Curr Surg 61:466–473

74 Virtual Reality

Amulya K. Saxena

74.1 Why is Virtual Reality Required?

74.1.1 Implant Basic Skills

Virtual reality simulators focus on implanting and complementing basic skills that would be needed by the trainee toward performing a bigger procedure.

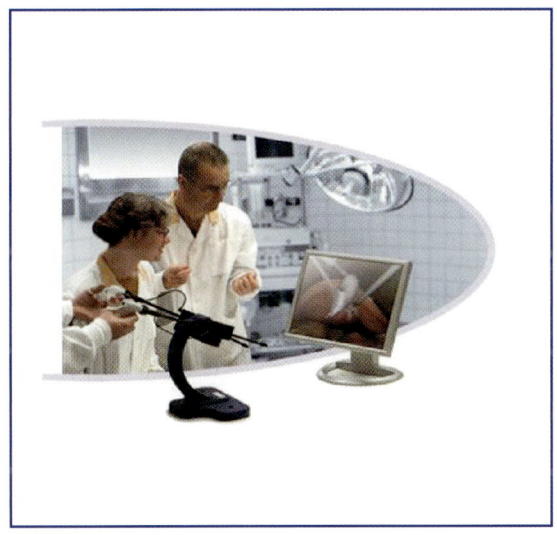

74.1.2 Evaluate Skills

The simulators allow the objective evaluation of surgical skills in practice sessions that can vary in graphic complexity as well as level of difficulty, and can pose challenges to even well-versed surgeons.

Similar to flight simulators, endoscopic virtual reality simulators such as LapSim® (Surgical Science Sweden, Göteborg, Sweden) shown here are employed in the training of operative skills in endoscopic surgery. (Courtesy of Surgical Science Sweden, Göteborg, Sweden)

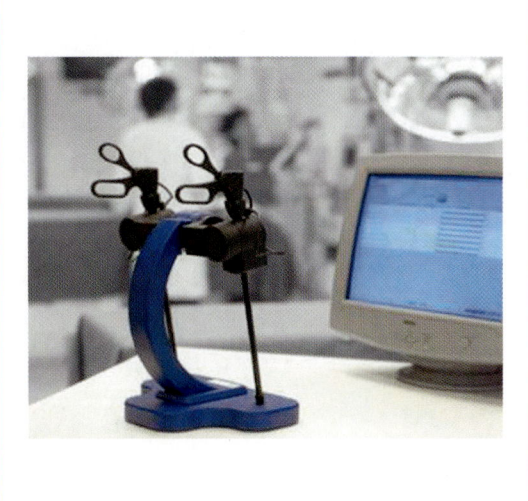

Endoscopic surgery simulators are personal-computer-based systems that assist trainees to repeat procedures and overcome handicaps. LapSim® (Courtesy of Surgical Science Sweden, Göteborg, Sweden).

74.2   Which Skills Can Be Trained?

1. Camera navigation.
2. Instrument navigation.
3. Movement coordination.
4. Object manipulation.
5. Depth estimation.
6. Cutting and dissection action.
7. Suture and knot tying.
8. Precision and speed.

74.2.1 Camera Navigation

Simulators enable trainees to subconsciously realize and accept correct scope positions.

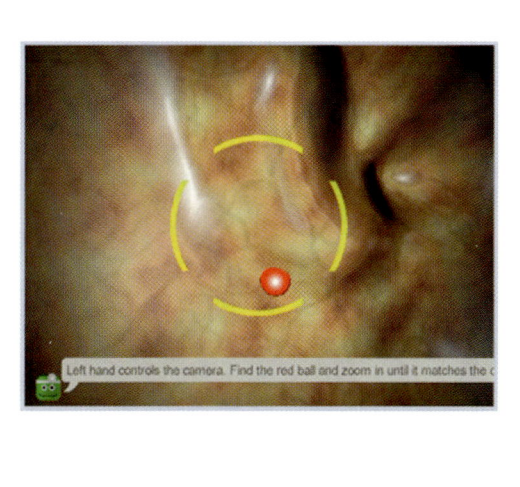

74.2.2 Instrument Navigation

Precision in instrument navigation and synchronization is important in endoscopic surgery procedures.

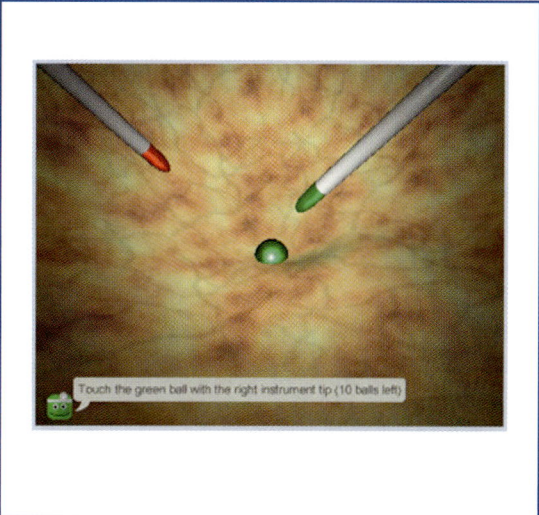

74.2.3 Coordination

This involves three aspects:
1. Hand–eye (virtual coordination).
2. Hand–hand (handling coordination).
3. Image-anticipation (cameraman and surgeon coordination).

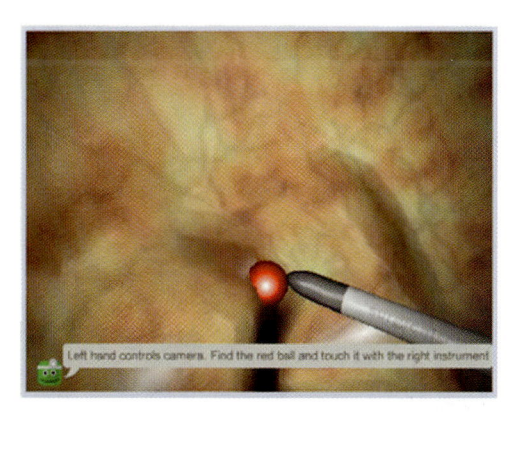

74.2.4 Object Manipulation

Object manipulations helps to differentiate grasping forces from shear forces. It also helps in the estimation of the freedom of movement.

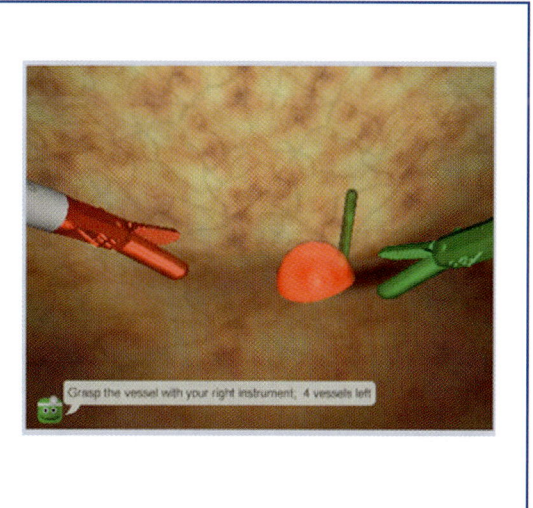

74.2.5   Depth Estimation

Accurate estimation of depth can be learnt. Depth estimation in two dimensions for a three-dimensional manipulation can be improved.

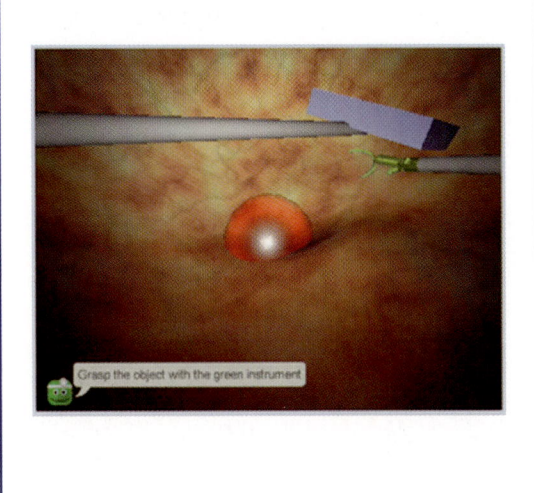

74.2.6   Cutting and Dissection

This requires good coordination since one part of the instrument edge vanishes or is hidden behind the tissue.

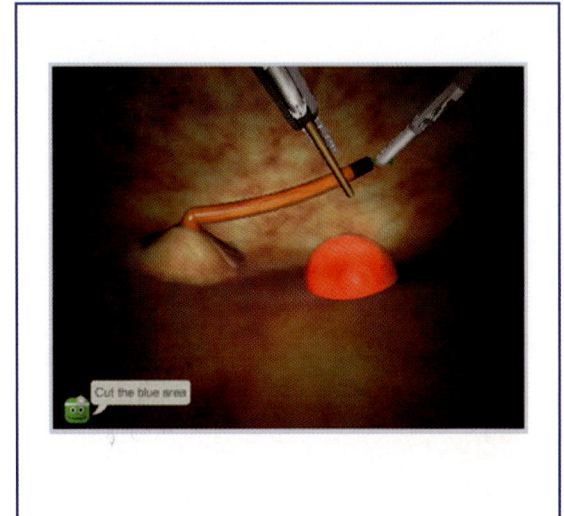

74.2.7   Suture and Knot Tying

There is no substitute but to put in hours of practice on trainers, as it is not advisable to learn suturing on a patient during a surgery.

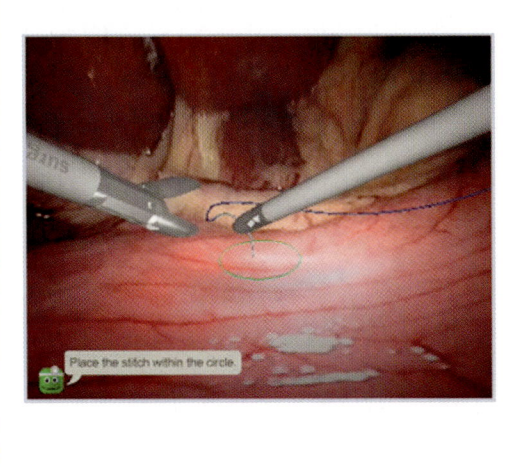

74.2.8   Precision and Speed

These two factors help not only for the speedy completion of the procedure, but also come in extremely handy in trouble shooting, when a rapid response is required during complications.

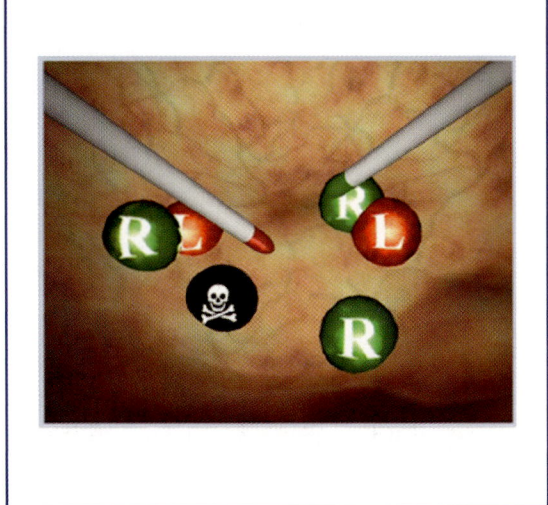

74.3 Procedures that Can Be Simulated on LapSim

74.3.1 Cholecystectomy

This exercise simulates the critical steps during a laparoscopic cholecystectomy procedure. In the first part, the cystic duct and artery are clipped and dissected. In the second part, the gall bladder is separated and removed from the liver.

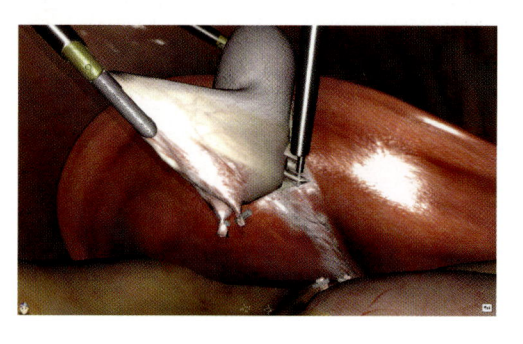

74.3.2 Intestinal Handling

The objective in this training exercise is to measure a predetermined length of the upper intestine using a suction device with markings of one centimeter in width for orientation. The camera is controlled by the computer and the instruments consists of two graspers.

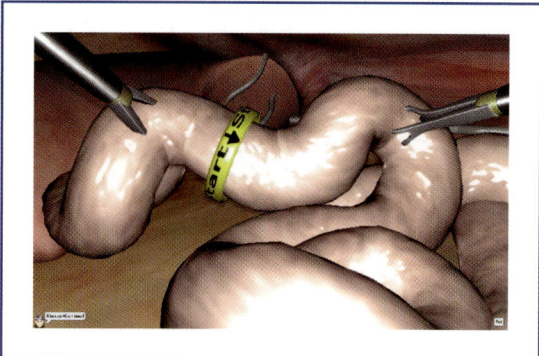

74.3.3 Myoma Suturing

This training task has the highest level of difficulty in the Gynecology package, requiring the trainee to suture and close the uterine wall cavity caused by a myectomy. The procedure is performed using two graspers, needle and thread.

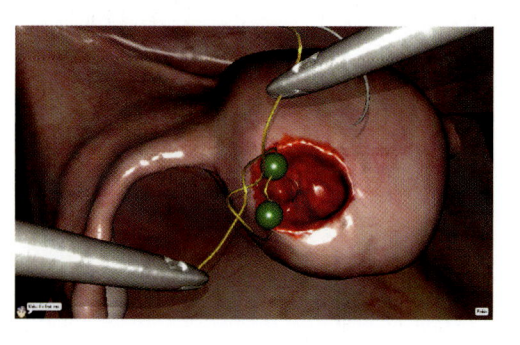

74.3.4 Salpingectomy

This exercise involves rinsing and suction of a bleeding ectopic pregnancy. After control of bleeding, the ectopic pregnancy has to be cut free from the Fallopian tube using bipolar graspers and/or clip applicators and diathermic scissors. The task ends by placing the ectopic pregnancy in the endoscopic basket.

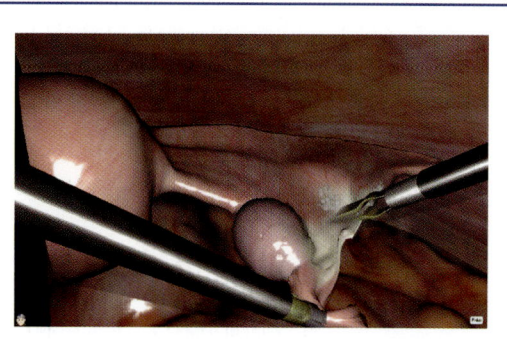

Acknowledgment

Surgical Science Sweden, Göteborg, Sweden.

Recommended Literature

1. Aggarwal R, Grantcharov TP, Eriksen JR, Blirup D, Kristiansen V, Funch-Jensen P, Darzi A (2006) An evidence-based virtual reality training program for novice laparoscopic surgeons. Ann Surg 244:310–314

2. Cosman PH, Hugh HJ, Shearer CJ, Merrett ND, Biankin AV, Cartmill JA (2007) Skills acquired on virtual reality laparoscopic simulators transfer into the operating room in a blinded, randomised, controlled trial. Stud Health Technol Inform 125:76–81

3. van Dongen KW, Tournoij E, van der Zee DC, Schijven MP, Broeders IAMJ (2007) Construct validity of the LapSim: can the LapSim virtual reality simulator distinguish between novices and experts? Surg Endosc 21:1413–1417

Subject Index

C